Anesthesia for Spine Surgery

Anesthesia for Spine Surgery

Ehab Farag, M.D., F.R.C.A.
Staff Anesthesiologist, Departments of General Anesthesia and Outcomes Research, Cleveland Clinic, Ohio, USA

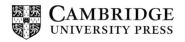
CAMBRIDGE
UNIVERSITY PRESS

CAMBRIDGE UNIVERSITY PRESS
Cambridge, New York, Melbourne, Madrid, Cape Town,
Singapore, São Paulo, Delhi, Mexico City

Cambridge University Press
The Edinburgh Building, Cambridge CB2 8RU, UK

Published in the United States of America by Cambridge University Press, New York

www.cambridge.org
Information on this title: www.cambridge.org/9781107005310

First published 2012

Printed in the United Kingdom at the University Press, Cambridge

A catalogue record for this publication is available from the British Library

Library of Congress Cataloguing in Publication data
Anesthesia for spine surgery / [edited by] Ehab Farag.
    p. ; cm.
  Includes bibliographical references and index.
  ISBN 978-1-107-00531-0 (hbk.)
  I. Farag, Ehab.
  [DNLM: 1. Spine–surgery.   2. Anesthesia–methods.   3. Postoperative Care. WE 725]
  617.4′71–dc23   2012007357

ISBN 978-1-107-00531-0 Hardback

To my wife, my daughters, and my mother for their incessant prayers, help, and support and in memory of my late father

Contents

Contents

Contributors

Alaa A. Abd-Elsayed
Resident Physician, Department of Anesthesiology, University of Cincinnati, Cincinnati, OH, USA

Basem Abdelmalak
Staff Anesthesiologist and Director, Anesthesia for Bronchoscopic Surgery, Anesthesiology Institute, Cleveland Clinic, Cleveland, OH, USA

Kalil G. Abdullah
Cleveland Clinic Lerner College of Medicine, Cleveland Clinic, Cleveland, OH, USA

Maged Argalious
Medical Director, PACU and Same Day Surgery; Assistant Professor, Cleveland Clinic Lerner College of Medicine, Case Western Reserve University, Cleveland, OH, USA

Rafi Avitsian
Section Head, Neurosurgical Anesthesiology; Program Director, Neuroanesthesia Fellowship; Assistant Professor of Anesthesiology, Cleveland Clinic Lerner College of Medicine Anesthesiology and Neurological Institutes, Cleveland Clinic, Cleveland, OH, USA

Maria Bauer
Clinical Research Fellow, Department of Outcomes Research, Institute of Anesthesiology, Cleveland Clinic, Cleveland, OH, USA

Edward C. Benzel
Chairman, Department of Neurosurgery, Neurological Institute, Cleveland Clinic, Cleveland, OH, USA

Dani S. Bidros
Cerebrovascular Center, Department of Neurosurgery, Cleveland Clinic, Cleveland, OH, USA

William Bingaman
Vice-Chairman, Neurological Institute, Department of Neurosurgery, Cleveland Clinic, Cleveland, OH, USA

Jay B. Brodsky
Professor, Department of Anesthesia, Stanford University School of Medicine, Stanford, CA, USA

David Brown
Chairman, Anesthesiology Institute, Cleveland Clinic, Cleveland, OH, USA

Patrick M. Callahan
Assistant Professor of Anesthesiology, University of Pittsburgh School of Medicine, Department of Anesthesiology, Children's Hospital of Pittsburgh, Pittsburgh, PA, USA

Juan P. Cata
Instructor, Department of Anesthesiology and perioperative Medicine, Division of Anesthesiology and Critical Care, The University of Texas MD Anderson Cancer Center, Houston, TX, USA

Chakorn Chansakul
Clinical Neurophysiology Fellow, Epilepsy Center, Cleveland Clinic Neurological Institute, Cleveland, OH, USA

Jianguo Cheng
Program Director of Pain Medicine Fellowship, Departments of Pain Management and Neurosciences, Cleveland Clinic, Cleveland, OH, USA

Jeffrey G. Clark
Cleveland Clinic Lerner College of Medicine, Cleveland Clinic, Cleveland, OH, USA

ix

Peter J. Davis
Professor of Anesthesiology and Pediatrics,
University of Pittsburgh School of Medicine,
Anesthesiologist-in-Chief, Department of
Anesthesiology, Children's Hospital of Pittsburgh,
Pittsburgh, PA, USA

Stacie Deiner
Assistant Professor of Anesthesiology, Neurosurgery,
Geriatrics, and Palliative Care, Mount Sinai School of
Medicine, New York, NY, USA

Xiao Di
Section of Pediatric and Congenital Neurosurgery,
Department of Neurosurgery, Cleveland Clinic,
Cleveland, OH, USA

Karen B. Domino
Professor, Department of Anesthesiology and
Pain Medicine, University of Washington, Seattle,
WA, USA

D. John Doyle
Staff Anesthesiologist, Cleveland Clinic, Cleveland,
OH, USA

Zeyd Ebrahim
Vice-Chair for Operating Affairs, Department of
General Anesthesiology, Cleveland Clinic, Cleveland,
OH, USA

Ehab Farag
Staff Anesthesiologist, Departments of General
Anesthesia and Outcomes Research, Cleveland
Clinic, OH, USA

Gordon Finlayson
Clinical Instructor, Department of Anesthesiology,
Pharmacology, and Therapeutics, Division of Critical
Care Medicine, University of British Columbia,
Vancouver, BC, Canada

Elizabeth A. M. Frost
Professor of Anesthesia, Mount Sinai Medical Center,
New York, NY, USA

Matthew Grosso
Center for Spine Health, Cleveland Clinic, Cleveland,
OH, USA

David P. Gurd
Staff Physician, Department of Orthopedic Surgery,
Cleveland Clinic, Cleveland, OH, USA

Rodolfo Hakim
Section of Pediatric and Congenital Neurosurgery,
Department of Neurosurgery, Cleveland Clinic,
Cleveland, OH, USA

Robert Helfand
Staff Anesthesiologist, Anesthesiology Institute,
Cleveland Clinic, Cleveland, OH, USA

Iain H. Kalfas
Surgeon, Center for Spine Health, Cleveland Clinic,
Cleveland, OH, USA

Rami Karroum
Associate Staff Member, Department of Pediatric
Anesthesiology, Cleveland Clinic, Cleveland,
OH, USA

Michael Kelly
Department of Neurosurgery, Center for Spine
Health, Cleveland Clinic, Cleveland, OH, USA

Stephen J. Kimatian
Chair, Pediatric Anesthesiology, Children's Hospital,
Cleveland Clinic Foundation, Cleveland, OH, USA

Christian Koopman
Neuroradiology Fellow, Cleveland Clinic, Cleveland,
OH, USA

Ajit A. Krishnaney
Associate Staff Physician, Center for Spine Health;
Associate Staff Physician, Neurological Surgery;
Associate Staff Physician, Cerebrovascular Center,
Cleveland Clinic, Cleveland, OH, USA

Andrea Kurz
Department of Outcomes Research, Institute of
Anesthesiology, Cleveland Clinic, Cleveland, OH,
USA

Lorri A. Lee
Assistant Professor, Department of Anesthesiology
and Pain Medicine, University of Washington,
Seattle, WA, USA

Brian P. Lemkuil
Assistant Clinical Professor, Department of Anesthesia,
University of California San Diego, CA, USA

James K. C. Liu
Resident, Department of Neurosurgery, Cleveland
Clinic, Cleveland, OH, USA

Sara P. Lozano
Staff, Pediatric Anesthesiology, Cleveland Clinic, Cleveland, OH, USA

Daniel Lubelski
Cleveland Clinic Lerner College of Medicine, Cleveland Clinic, Cleveland, OH, USA

Mark Luciano
Head, Pediatric and Congenital Neurosurgery, Pediatric Neurosciences, Cleveland Clinic, Cleveland, OH, USA

Ramez Malaty
Neuroradiology Fellow, Cleveland Clinic, Cleveland, OH, USA

Mariel R. Manlapaz
Associate Staff, Department of General Anesthesiology, Cleveland Clinic, Cleveland, OH, USA

Edward M. Manno
Cerebrovascular Center, Department of Neurosurgery, Cleveland Clinic, Cleveland, OH, USA

Virgilio Matheus
Resident, Department of Neurosurgery, Cleveland Clinic, Cleveland, OH, USA

Robert F. McLain
Professor of Surgery and Director, Spine Surgery Fellowship Program, Cleveland Clinic Center for Spine Health, Cleveland, OH, USA

Nagy Mekhail
Professor of Anesthesiology, Cleveland Clinic Lerner College of Medicine of Case Western Reserve University and Cleveland Clinic Spine Center, Cleveland, OH, USA

Doksu Moon
Staff Neuroradiologist, Cleveland Clinic, Cleveland, OH, USA

Loran Soliman Mounir
Staff Member, Departments of General Anesthesia and Pediatric Anesthesia, Cleveland Clinic, Cleveland, OH, USA

Raghu Mudumbai
Associate Professor, Department of Opthalmology, University of Washington, Seattle, WA, USA

Thomas E. Mroz
Director, Spine Surgery Fellowship Program, Neurological Institute, Center for Spine Health, Departments of Orthopedic and Neurological Surgery, Cleveland Clinic, Cleveland, OH, USA

Dileep R. Nair
Section Head, Epilepsy Center, Cleveland Clinic Neurological Institute, Cleveland, OH, USA

Julie Niezgoda
Staff, Pediatric Anesthesiology, Cleveland Clinic, Cleveland, OH, USA

R. Douglas Orr
Staff Physician, Center for Spine Health and Department of Orthopedic Surgery, Cleveland Clinic Foundation, Cleveland, OH, USA

Piyush M. Patel
Professor of Anesthesiology, Department of Anesthesia, University of California, San Diego; Staff Anesthesiologist, Veterans Affairs Medical Center, San Diego, CA, USA

Jason E. Pope
Napa Pain Institute, Napa, CA, USA

Manuel Saavedra
Division of Plastic Surgery and Neurosurgery Section, Department of Surgery, University of Puerto Rico, Medical Sciences Campus, San Juan, Puerto Rico

Kenneth J. Saliba
Surgeon, Department of Pediatric Anesthesiology, Children's Hospital, Cleveland Clinic Foundation, Cleveland, OH, USA

Richard Schlenk
Neurosurgery Residency Program Director, Center for Spine Health, Cleveland Clinic, Cleveland, OH, USA

John Seif
Associate Staff, Department of Pediatric Anesthesiology, Cleveland Clinic, Cleveland, OH, USA

John H. Shin
Department of Neurosurgery, Center for Spine Health, Neurological Institute, Cleveland Clinic, Cleveland, OH, USA

Jeffrey Silverstein

Professor of Anesthesiology, Neurosurgery, Geriatrics, and Palliative Care, Mount Sinai School of Medicine, New York, NY, USA

Dmitri Souzdalnitski

Clinical Fellow of Pain Medicine, Department of Pain Management, Cleveland Clinic, Cleveland, OH, USA

Michael Steinmetz

Center for Spine Health, Cleveland Clinic, Cleveland, OH, USA

Tunga Suresh

Assistant Professor of Anesthesiology, University of Pittsburgh School of MedicineDepartment of Anesthesiology, Children's Hospital of Pittsburgh, Pittsburgh, PA, USA

John E. Tetzlaff

Professor of Anesthesiology, Cleveland Clinic Lerner College of Medicine of Case Western Reserve University; Staff Anesthesiologist, Department of General Anesthesia, Cleveland Clinic, Cleveland, OH, USA

Sherif Zaky

Staff Anesthesiologist, Department of Anesthesiology, Cleveland Clinic, Cleveland, OH, USA

Foreword by Dr. Edward Benzel

Ehab Farag has assembled an incredible group of authors for this "first of a kind" book, *Anesthesia for Spine Surgery*. This book is the first comprehensive text devoted to the anesthetic management of the spine surgery patient. It addresses both the adult and pediatric domains. It is comprehensive in scope and detailed in content.

Anesthesia for Spine Surgery addresses all aspects of the subject at hand. It begins with a group of dissertations on the variety of surgical procedures and the complications that can ensue. Chapters on imaging and surgical technique-specific nuances follow. These are followed by a variety of chapters that address specific spine anesthesia techniques and complications. The book closes with a number of discussions regarding pediatrics-related issues.

How good is this book? It is a "must read." Why is it a "must read"?

First, it is a "first of its kind." Hence, there is no competition. I am virtually certain that others will follow. They always do when pioneers open and develop a field.

Second, it "covers the field." This cannot be underestimated as an attribute. *Anesthesia for Spine Surgery* is both deep and broad in content. It truly "covers the field" in many regards. It is thorough. It is comprehensive. It is organized both to facilitate a reading from cover to cover and to function as a reference.

Third, it is "a great read." This book feels good in my hands and I feel at home while reading it. It is, in fact, difficult to put down. This is, in part, related to its unique position in the spine surgery and anesthesia domain. It is also related to its wonderful presentation.

This book covers everything, and I do mean everything, from visual complications to spinal cord injury. No stones are left unturned. It is a complete, comprehensive, and user-friendly text. It will soon become a great addition to the libraries of all spine surgeons, neurosurgeons, and orthopedic surgeons, and of all neuro-anesthesiologists, anesthesiologists, and related professionals. It is, indeed, a classic in the making.

Foreword by Dr. David Brown

It is a real pleasure to be asked to contribute a foreword to *Anesthesia for Spine Surgery* by Dr. Ehab Farag and colleagues. This useful text covers the entire spectrum of surgical and anesthetic procedures required to be at the forefront of clinical care for our patients requiring spine care. Ehab has assembled an outstanding list of contributors; all true experts in their area of clinical coverage. Many are colleagues at the Cleveland Clinic and others are recognized national experts.

Spinal surgery has developed over the last 20 years into a specialized field in which increasingly complex and lengthy surgical procedures are being carried out; these clearly demand an anesthetic approach that is equally intricate. The willingness of surgeons and anesthesiologists to share their approaches to complex and straightforward spinal surgical patients allows readers of this book to apply the most current approaches to minimizing morbidity and optimizing safety in their patients. The contributors to this book are made up of individuals with whom I would be fully comfortable in having them providing care for myself or members of my family at any time. They truly are experts.

I congratulate all involved in creating this important work and hope that it really adds value to your care of this important group of patients.

Preface

Spine surgery has evolved in the last two decades into a multidisciplinary specialty including surgery, pain management, neuromonitoring, and neuroradiology. This book is the first comprehensive textbook for anesthesia for spine surgery in both adults and pediatric patients. I believe that in order for the anesthesiologist to provide adequate perioperative care, the anesthesiologist should be armed with the proper knowledge of the different facets of the specialty for which he or she administers the anesthetic. This book serves that belief, for it covers the techniques of surgical procedures described to the anesthesiologist in a simple approach by world-renowned surgeons. The other aspects of the spine surgery specialty (pain management for acute and chronic pain after spine surgery, intraoperative neuromonitoring, and neuroimaging) are fully covered by well-versed experts in those fields.

This book is a very useful resource for anesthesiologists involved in anesthesia for spine surgery, spine surgeons, neurologists, and other health care providers caring for spine surgery patients. Included are chapters for perioperative anesthetic management in adult and pediatric patients, which cover the preoperative evaluation, airway management, lung isolation, fluid management, and postoperative care both in the postanesthesia care unit and in intensive care. The book has chapters that cover in full detail the intraoperative anesthetic management from cervical to lumbosacral regions. The anesthetic and surgical complications during spine surgery are discussed in full detail as well.

I would like to express my gratitude to my colleagues for their hard work and dedication in accomplishing this book. I would also like to acknowledge the help and support of my editorial assistants at Cleveland Clinic and the Cambridge University Press team.

Ehab Farag, M.D., F.R.C.A.

Chapter

1

Preoperative assessment of the adult patient

Elizabeth A. M. Frost

Key points

- Tests should be ordered only as indicated.
- History and physical examination should precede laboratory studies.
- Variability of spinal anatomy and physiology dictate that cases involving spine surgery should be considered on an individual basis.
- General "cardiac clearance" is rarely useful.
- Many diseases and comorbidities involve the spine and must be considered separately.

Introduction

Procedures on the spine vary in complexity from simple discectomy to multi level reconstruction and fusion with instrumentation. Moreover, the level of surgery from the cervical area to the coccyx further impacts planning for anesthetic management. Procedures may be planned for months or occur emergently as part of multiple trauma. Thus many factors determine appropriate preoperative anesthetic assessment.

General guidelines

In 2002 the American Society of Anesthesiologists developed a practice advisory to assist in decision making regarding appropriate preanesthetic assessment and care.[1] The advisory is the synthesis of opinions from experts, open forums, public sources, and literature review. It is to be applied to all anesthesiologists and those who provide care under the direction of an anesthesiologist including residents, certified registered nurse anesthetists (CRNA) or students. It applies to all age groups and all types of anesthesia and deep sedation for both surgical and nonsurgical situations. The advisory does not address emergency situations.

Preanesthetic evaluation is the process of clinical assessment preceding the delivery of anesthesia. It is the responsibility of the anesthesiologist or CRNA practicing alone. The process must consider information from multiple sources including, among others, the patient, surgical and medical records, nurse evaluations, and laboratory tests and other tests. As appropriate, consultations may be sought and preoperative tests ordered as indicated. In some departments of anesthesia, informed consent is obtained separately from surgical consent; in others consent is signed as part of general hospital consent. In either case, the preanesthetic record must note that the anesthetic options, risks and benefits of anesthesia have been explained to the patient, and he/she has agreed and accepted the plan.

Obtaining a history and physically examining the patient should precede the ordering or performance of preanesthesia tests. Such a process includes evaluation of pertinent medical records, patient interview, assessment of the risk/benefit for different anesthetic techniques and a plan for postoperative pain management, which is especially important for the patient scheduled to undergo complex lower spine surgery. The timing of the evaluation depends on the degree of surgical invasiveness, where highly invasive procedures should be done prior to the day of surgery (multilevel laminectomies with instrumentation) and medium or low risk surgery (minimally invasive single-level laminectomy) may be done on the day before or day of surgery. Analysis of the Practice Advisory of the ASA provides a good indication of minimal standard of care in the United States. Airway assessment and documentation was considered essential by 100% of consultants and 100% of ASA members. Pulmonary and cardiovascular examination was cited by 81–88% of respondents as required. In addition, the health care system should provide appropriate assessment of the severity of the patient's medical condition and the invasiveness of surgery. In other words, the diagnosis and planned surgery should be identified prior to operation.

Routine testing implies tests that are performed without clinical indication and include such items as hemoglobin, urinalysis, chest radiograph (CXR), electrocardiogram, coagulation profile and basic metabolic panel. The reasons for ordering these tests as a "shotgun" approach are varied and include such arguments as:

1. The approach represents good screening (although for what, is not specified).
2. It may save an annual physical examination (although mammography, colonoscopy, and prostatic screening are usually recommended in annual physical examinations, these results do not impact anesthetic management).
3. Preoperative testing is medicolegally sound (but tests may cause more harm than good, may produce false positives or may not be reviewed, thus resulting in even more adverse situations).
4. Testing is required (most hospital do not have mandated tests written into the policies and procedures).
5. Multiple testing provides income for hospitals and laboratories (true).

A study done 20 years ago showed that routine testing cost >$60 billion annually and >60% of tests were not indicated. Approximately 0.2% revealed pertinent abnormalities, that is, a finding that might change the anesthetic or surgical plan.[2] There has been little change in many areas.

Site of surgery

Pathology, usually resulting in pain may occur throughout the cervical spine due to trauma, degenerative changes, tumors, lytic lesions, and compression. Levels for surgery may be upper cervical (C1–2), middle and lower cervical, thoracic, lumbar and, more rarely, sacral/coccygeal. The approaches at each level are shown in Tables 1.1–1.3. Anterior upper cervical approaches are used to relieve compression at the cervicomedullary junction and stabilize odontoid fractures. They may also be indicated in resection of tumors such as clival chordomas. Posterior approaches are used to correct atlantoaxial or occipitalatlanto instability, odontoid and spinal fractures, and cervical instability.

Supine approach to the middle lower cervical spine is indicated in the removal of osteophytes or herniated discs. Fusion and/or instrumentation allow the disc space height to be maintained. The posterior approach

Table 1.1 Upper cervical approaches

Anterior	Posterior
Transoral	Craniocervical fusion/fixation
Transpalatal	Atlantoaxial fusion
Transmandibular	C1–C2 wiring/plating
Anterior retropharyngeal	C1–C2 transarticular screw fixation

Table 1.2 Middle and lower cervical approaches

Supine	Prone
Anterior cervical discectomy	Laminectomy, foraminotomy, laminotomy
Cloward procedure, includes insertion of autologous or bank bone or methylmethacrylate	Wiring: interspinous, sublaminar
	Plating, pedicle screws

Table 1.3 Other levels and approaches

Anterior cervicothoracic
Anterior thoracic: thorascopic techniques
Posterior thoracic
Anterior lumbar/lumbosacral
Posterior lumbar
Combined anterior posterior
Minimally invasive and microdiscectomies

is used in cases of cervical radiculopathy due to degenerative disease and in cases of cervical canal stenosis or removal of intraspinal masses such as ependymomas. Multiple levels may be involved.

Lumbar fusion is performed to relieve pain due to intervertebral movement. Segmental instability, spondylolisthesis, and iatrogenic instability are other indications. Pedicle screw stabilization involves creation of a rigid three-column spinal fixation. Posterolateral fusions include laminectomy, discectomy, and grafted bone to decorticated bone. Posterior lumbar interbody fusion includes bilateral laminectomies with removal of the inferior and part of the superior facets, discectomies, autologous or banked bone placement or cages to the disc spaces. Combined anterior posterior approaches are indicated for correction of multilevel collapse, unstable three-column injury, severe kyphosis, scoliosis, or infective or neoplastic conditions. Surgery involves complete circumferential decompression, rigid short segment fixation, and maximal correction of deformities.

It is clear that preanesthetic assessment varies depending on the approach required, the pathology involved, the invasiveness of the procedure, and the presence of other comorbidities, which may be part of the spinal disease. Assessment also varies depending on whether the surgery is elective or emergent

Cervical and elective surgery

Upper levels

High cervical cord tumors such as chordomas or ependymomas may be resected through the mouth – an approach rarely used today. Many of these patients are young and relatively healthy and require little preoperative testing. However, psychological preparation includes the awareness that a tracheostomy is usually placed prior to surgery. The approach requires bisection of the tongue and mandible allowing direct access to the back of the mouth. Surgery necessitates the cooperation of several specialties and is generally very long, lasting 24 hours or more. Decannulation of the trachea can usually be accomplished within 72 hours as swelling subsides in the upper airway. Blood loss is minimal.

Indicated tests: Complete radiographic series to determine the extent of the pathology.

Trisomy 21 is one of the most common chromosomal abnormalities in humans, occurring in 1:6–800 live births in the United States. The anomaly affects many organ systems with implications that require close preanesthetic assessment (Table 1.4). As life expectancy of these patients has improved, the number of adult patients with Down's syndrome presenting for surgery is increasing. Muscle hypotonia and ligamentous laxity with atlantoaxial instability occur frequently and patients may present for stabilization with plating, wiring, or some other means of fusion of C1–2.

Approximately 15% of patients with Down's syndrome have atlantoaxial instability and the majority of them are asymptomatic.[3] However, they are predisposed to subluxation and cervical cord compression especially during endoscopy and intubation. Specific history and physical examination are important to seek out such symptoms as gait abnormalities, clumsiness and increased fatigue when walking. Other findings include abnormal neck motion (very mobile), upper and lower motor neuron signs such as spasticity, hyperreflexia, extensor plantar reflexes, loss of bowel or bladder control, and neck posturing (torticollis).[4] The Sharp and Purser test may also be applied. With the patient in a sitting position, and the neck flexed, backward pressure is applied against the forehead while the spinous process of the axis is palpated. A gliding motion may be felt as subluxation is reduced. The test is positive in about 50% of patients with atlantoaxial instability. Posterior stabilization is recommended for patients with subluxation prior to any other elective surgery. Intubation should be performed with head stabilization including two-point pin fixation.

Approximately 40% of Down's syndrome patients have some form of congenital heart disease, the most prevalent of which is endocardial cushion defect. Other anomalies include ventricular and atrial septal defects. All three of these lesions may result in pulmonary hypertension. Adults appear to have a higher incidence of aortic insufficiency and mitral valve prolapse. Those with previously repaired congenital heart disease may have conduction defects, usually left anterior hemiblock and right bundle branch block. Cardiology consultation may be indicated.

There is a general predisposition towards hypoxia. Respiratory tract infections secondary to airway anomalies, immunologic deficiencies and institutional living are contributing factors. Hypotonia and sleep apnea with both mechanical and central nervous

Table 1.4 Trisomy 21. Perianesthetic considerations

Anatomic	Short stature, obesity, small mouth, large tongue, high arched palate, small mandible and maxilla, short neck
Musculoskeletal	Hypotonia, lax joints, unstable atlantoaxial joint, temporomandibular joint disease
Cardiac	Congenital defects, aortic insufficiency, mitral valve prolapse
Respiratory	Frequent infections, pulmonary hypertension, sleep apnea, atelectasis, airway obstruction
Immune system	Altered response, infections, hepatitis B, lymphocytic leukemia increased incidence
Neurologic	Mental retardation, seizures, early onset presenile dementia, perioperative agitation
Gastrointestinal system	Gastroesophageal reflux
Hematologic	Polycythemia
Endocrine	Thyroid anomalies, especially in adults; decreased central and peripheral sympathetic activity

system factors add to hypoventilation and hypoxia. Preoperative assessment should include blood gas analyses, pulmonary function testing, and training in basic respiratory therapeutic maneuvers.

Patients of all ages with Down's syndrome tend to have lower blood pressures than normal and mentally handicapped controls, perhaps related to a decrease in central and peripheral sympathetic activity. Resting and stress levels of dopamine beta-hydroxylase, which converts dopamine to norepinephrine, are decreased. Excretion of epinephrine is decreased, which may be due to decreased adrenal production even though plasma epinephrine levels are normal.

Indicated tests: Chest radiography to exclude aspiration or atelectasis, complete blood count to assess polycythemia and leukocytosis indicating infection, room air oxygen saturation, electrocardiogram to assess conduction defects, thyroid function tests, neck radiography, blood glucose to exclude diabetes.

Syringomyelia is the development of a fluid-filled cyst (syrinx) within the spinal cord (Fig. 1.1). Over time, the cyst may enlarge, damaging the spinal cord and causing pain, weakness, and stiffness, among other symptoms. If left untreated, symptoms may worsen and require surgery. There are several possible causes. The majority of syringomyelia cases are associated with Arnold–Chiari malformation, a condition in which brain tissue protrudes into the spinal canal. The malformation consists of a downward displacement of the cerebellar tonsils through the foramen magnum, sometimes causing noncommunicating hydrocephalus as a result of obstruction of cerebrospinal fluid (CSF) outflow. The cerebrospinal fluid outflow is caused by phase differences in outflow and influx of blood in the vasculature of the brain. Any obstruction can cause headaches, fatigue, muscle weakness in the head and face, difficulty swallowing, dizziness, nausea, impaired coordination, and, in severe cases, paralysis. While the Chiari malformation may be present at birth, symptoms are often delayed until the 2nd–4th decade. Often symptoms may appear to be triggered by a fall or minor trauma. Other causes of syringomyelia include spinal cord tumors, spinal cord injuries such as tethered cord syndrome, and meningitis. Early signs and symptoms of syringomyelia may affect the back of the neck, shoulders, arms, and hands and include:

- Muscle weakness and wasting (atrophy)
- Loss of reflexes
- Loss of sensitivity to pain and temperature

Later signs and symptoms of syringomyelia are:

- Stiffness in the back, shoulders, arms, and legs
- Pain in the neck, arms, and back
- Bowel and bladder function problems
- Muscle weakness and spasms in the legs
- Facial pain or numbness
- On neck flexion, a tingling sensation rapidly spreading down the trunk and into the legs (Lhermitte's sign)

Syringomyelia can become a progressive disorder and lead to complications such as scoliosis, Horner's syndrome, and chronic pain. In other cases, there may be no associated symptoms and no intervention is necessary. Typically, surgery for syringomyelia, usually in the upper cervical spine with a posterior and prone approach (especially for Chiari malformations) includes one or more of the following:

- Treatment of a Chiari malformation. A suboccipital craniectomy is performed and a dural graft may be added around C1–2 to enlarge the opening of the foramen magnum and restore the flow of cerebrospinal fluid.

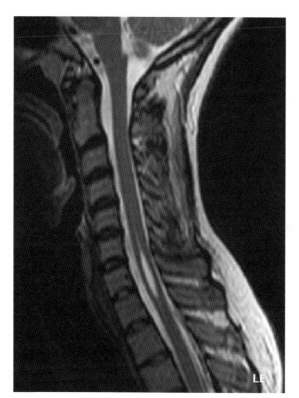

Figure 1.1 Syringomyelia. The thin gray curved line indicates extravasated cerebrospinal fluid.

- Draining of the syrinx. A shunt may be inserted from the syrinx to the abdomen or chest (syringoperitoneal or syringopleural shunt). Less commonly, the syrinx can be drained at surgery.
- Removal of the obstruction. If there is blockage within the cord such as might be caused by adhesions or a tumor, surgical removal of the obstruction may restore the normal flow and allow fluid to drain from the syrinx.
- Correction of an abnormality. If a spinal abnormality is hindering the normal flow of cerebrospinal fluid, surgery to correct it – such as releasing a tethered spinal cord – may be corrective.

Preanesthetic assessment centers on history and physical examination. Duration and amount of symptoms as well as drug ingestion including narcotics and antidepressants should be documented. All nonsteroidal analgesics should be discontinued 1–2 weeks before surgery if possible. Frequently the diagnosis of syringomyelia is delayed and the patient may have received multiple consultations and many therapies. Neurologic examination should include a review of any preexisting deficits. Muscle and nerve assessments and electromyelography may be indicated to gauge the extent of paresthesias or numbness. Range of motion of the neck may indicate a sharp increase in symptoms during flexion. Nausea, vomiting, and difficulty swallowing should be assessed and prophylactic therapy given as indicated.

Indicated tests: MRI of the syrinx, CXR if a shunt is to placed in the thorax, complete blood count, and coagulation profile if the patient has received analgesic medications.

Middle and lower levels; elective surgery

Anterior cervical discectomy is commonly performed in the treatment of nerve root or spinal cord compression. By decompressing the spinal cord and nerve roots of the cervical spine the corresponding vertebrae can be stabilized and pain and paresthesias relieved. This procedure is used when other nonsurgical treatments have failed.

The nucleus pulposus of the herniated disc bulges out through the annulus and presses on the nerve root next to it (Fig. 1.2). This nerve root becomes inflamed and causes pain. The problem can also be caused by degenerative disc disease (spondylosis). The disc consists of about 80% water and with age dries out and shrinks, causing small tears in the annulus and inflammation of the nerve root. At surgery, the disc is completely removed as well as any arthritic bone spurs. To prevent the vertebrae from collapsing and to increase stability, the open space is filled with bone graft, taken from the pelvis or cadaveric bone or methylmethacrylate. Occasionally a titanium plate is screwed on the vertebrae to increase stability during fusion, especially when there is more than one disc involved.

Recently, endoscopic anterior cervical discectomy under epidurogram guidance has been described.[5] Contrast dye through a cervical discectomy is used to generate an epidurogram. Using fluoroscopy, endoscopic instruments are advanced to the epidural space and both soft and hard discs can be removed.

As with other surgery on the spine, ingestion of all nonsteroidal anti-inflammatory medicines (Advil,

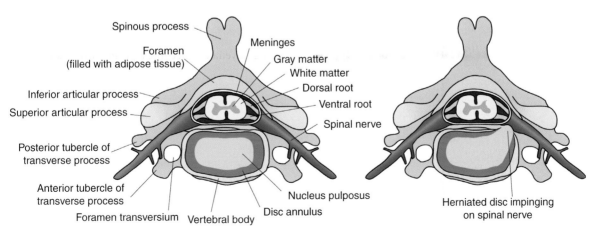

Figure 1.2 Vertebra and disc: normal (left) and herniated situation (right) (from http://en.wikipedia.org/wiki/Anterior_cervical_disectomy and fusion).

Motrin, Nuprin, Aleve, etc.) and anticoagulants (Coumadin, clopidogrel, aspirin) should be stopped 1 to 2 weeks before surgery. In some instances, as for example recent placement of a drug eluding stent, discontinuing of clopidogrel may be ill advised. The cardiologist and surgeon should be consulted and the preferred therapy determined. Ingestion of herbs that can interfere with coagulation should also be stopped. For example, garlic decreases platelet aggregation, ginger inhibits thromboxane synthetase, gingko inhibits platelet activating factor, ginseng interacts with all the anticoagulants to increase their effectiveness, and feverfew inhibits serotonin release from platelets. Additionally, the patient should be advised to stop smoking (pipes and cigarettes), inhaling snuff, and chewing tobacco at least 1 week before and 2 weeks after surgery (although complete cessation is preferable) as these activities can cause bleeding problems. Also, nicotine interferes with bone metabolism through induced calcitonin resistance and decreased osteoblastic formation. Patients who smoked had failed fusions in up to 40% of cases, compared with only 8% among nonsmokers.[6] Smoking also retards wound healing and increases the risk of infection.[7]

Because risk of damage to the recurrent laryngeal nerve is a complication of this surgery, its function should be ascertained preoperatively. Many patients with spinal disc disease are smokers and may have other causes of hoarseness. The recurrent laryngeal nerve is a branch of the vagus nerve that supplies motor function and sensation to the larynx. It is referred to as "recurrent" because the branches of the nerve innervate the laryngeal muscles in the neck through a rather circuitous route: it descends into the thorax before rising up between the trachea and esophagus to reach the neck. The left laryngeal nerve branches from the vagus nerve to loop under the arch of the aorta, posterior to the ligamentum arteriosum before ascending. The right branch loops around the right subclavian artery. Both nerves give off several cardiac filaments to the deep part of the cardiac plexus. As they ascend in the neck, branches – more numerous on the left than on the right side – are given off to the mucous membrane and muscular coat of the esophagus; branches also supply the mucous membrane and muscular fibers of the trachea, and some pharyngeal filaments go to the superior pharyngeal constrictor muscle. The nerve splits into anterior and posterior rami before supplying muscles in larynx and supplies all laryngeal muscles except for the cricothyroid, which is innervated by the external branch of the superior laryngeal nerve. The recurrent laryngeal nerve enters the pharynx, along with the inferior laryngeal artery, below the inferior constrictor muscle to innervate the intrinsic muscles of the larynx responsible for controlling the movements of the vocal folds.

Unilateral damage may cause hoarseness. Although the right recurrent laryngeal nerve is more susceptible to damage due to its relatively medial location, surgery is generally performed on the right side more for convenience of the right-handed surgeon. Indeed, the total rate of persisting recurrent laryngeal nerve damage using a right-sided approach approximates 13%, a number that can be reduced to 6.5% with a left-sided incision.[8] The complication can be further reduced by controlling endotracheal tube (ETT) cuff pressure to <20 mmHg.[9] Noting that cuff pressures are often much higher than realized and may increase intraoperatively, proper control by manometer reduced ETT related postprocedural respiratory complications, even in procedures of short duration. Problems such as cough and sore throat were significantly reduced.[10] However, the significance of reducing and controlling cuff pressure in reducing the incidence of vocal cord immobility has been questioned by one study.[11] Laryngeal damage may also relate to excessive pressures of the retractors on the esophagus. The patient should be advised preoperatively that while a short period of soreness in the throat is not unusual, should it be accompanied by hoarseness or last longer than 2–3 days then further consultation should be sought.

A preoperative plan for pain control should be in place. To this end it is important to know whether autologous bone grafting is intended. Acute postoperative pain and nerve injuries after anterior iliac crest bone graft can lead to neuropathic chronic pain. A small study evaluated the efficacy of preoperative placement of transversus abdominis plane (TAP) block under ultrasound-guided technology.[12] The authors considered TAP to be an appropriate technique for postoperative analgesia after bone harvest as about 80% of patients had no pain at 18 months. Whatever the approach, a plan for pain relief must be detailed as the discomfort experience from the hip is significantly greater than that felt in the neck. Other techniques include local infiltration, patient-controlled analgesia, and opioid or nonsteroidal injections.

Blood loss during this procedure is minimal, although there are rare instances of delayed bleeding from vessel damage and retropharygeal hematomas.

Indicated tests: Coagulation profile to ensure no adverse effects of medications or herbs; cervical radiologic studies to assess the extent of the disease; type and screen to check for antibodies; complete blood count to ensure adequate hemoglobin levels for optimal wound healing.

Thoracic levels: elective surgery

Scoliosis (from Greek: skoliōsis, "crooked") is an abnormal lateral curvature of the spine. It is a complex three-dimensional deformity that is typically classified as either congenital (caused by vertebral anomalies present at birth), idiopathic (cause unknown, subclassified as infantile, juvenile, adolescent, or adult according to when onset occurred), or neuromuscular (having developed as a secondary symptom of another condition, such as spina bifida, cerebral palsy, spinal muscular atrophy, or physical trauma). The condition affects approximately 20 million people in the United States.[13] Although surgery is more often performed in children in whom growth retardation is a significant problem as the disease progresses, a significant number of adults also undergo the operation. Scoliosis may be associated with other conditions such as Ehlers–Danlos syndrome (hyperflexibility, "floppy baby" syndrome, and other variants including a high incidence of mitral valve prolapse), Charcot–Marie–Tooth, Prader–Willi syndrome, kyphosis, cerebral palsy, spinal muscular atrophy, muscular dystrophy, familial dysautonomia, CHARGE syndrome (coloboma, heart abnormalities, atresia of the nasal choanae, growth retardation, genital and urinary anomalies, ear deformities, and deafness), Friedreich's ataxia, proteus syndrome, spina bifida, Marfan's syndrome, neurofibromatosis, connective tissue disorders, congenital diaphragmatic hernia, hemihypertrophy, and craniospinal axis disorders (e.g., syringomyelia, Arnold–Chiari malformation).

Depending on the existence of comorbidities that may be present in >50% of patients, preanesthetic assessment may be complex.[14] Of most importance is the assessment of ventilatory function, which may be considerably compromised if the curvature exceeds 40°. Several comorbidities such as Duchenne muscular dystrophy and spinal muscular atrophy are often associated with poor pulmonary function tests and the simultaneous development of scoliosis will further aggravate the situation. However, at least one study showed that despite preoperative forced vital capacity of <30% and further slight decreases postoperatively, there were no major pulmonary complications

postoperatively and functional ability improved markedly.[15] Nevertheless, lung function should be assessed preoperatively to allow a program of respiratory therapy to be instituted.

Cardiac assessment is also critical as many of these patients may have other problems that affect cardiac function such as Marfan's syndrome. Also, severe curvatures affect heart rhythm by altering the position of the heart within the chest. Echocardiographic and stress tests as far as the patient can manage are indicated. It is doubtful whether the patient can be made into any better condition based on results of these tests except that pulmonary infection or aspiration might be identified and corrected.

As with iliac crest grafting, pain control becomes a major problem postoperatively. Thoracic epidural–general analgesia has been shown to be effective.[14]

Typically the surgery, performed in a prone position and with instrumentation, involves many levels and lasts some 6–8 h. Blood loss may be considerable. Occasionally patients predonate which may make them relatively anemic preoperatively. As a complementary surgical procedure a thoracoplasty (or costoplasty) may be performed to reduce the rib hump that affects most scoliosis patients with a thoracic curve. Thoracoplasty may also be performed to obtain bone grafts from the ribs instead of the pelvis, regardless of whether a rib hump is present. Thoracoplasty can be performed as part of a spinal fusion or as a separate surgery and involves the resection of typically four to six segments of adjacent ribs that protrude. Each segment is 2.5–5 cm long, (the ribs grow back, straight). The most common complication of thoracoplasty is increased pain in the rib area during recovery. Another complication is temporarily reduced pulmonary function (10–15% is typical) following surgery. This impairment can last anywhere from a few months to 2 years. Hemothorax and pneumothorax may also occur. Because thoracoplasty may lengthen the duration of surgery, patients may also lose more blood or develop complications from the prolonged anesthesia.

Indicated tests: Type and crossmatch blood, which will almost certainly be required; coagulation profile if the patient has been receiving analgesics; complete blood count, especially if predonation has taken place; CXR to rule out infection, pulmonary function tests as a baseline of ventilatory function; cardiology consult for other (often rare) comorbidities; assessment of Cobb and pelvic angles.

Tumors may metastasize to the thoracic spine. Other pathologies that arise in the thoracic area and require surgery include infection such as tuberculosis, and hemangiomas. Pott's disease (named after Percivall Pott, 1714–1788, a London surgeon) is a presentation of extrapulmonary tuberculosis that affects the intervertebral joints. It is most commonly localized in the thoracic portion of the spine. Pott's disease results from hematogenous spread of tuberculosis from other sites, often pulmonary. The infection then spreads from two adjacent vertebrae into the adjoining intervertebral disc space. If only one vertebra is affected, the disc is normal, but if two are involved the disc, which is avascular, cannot receive nutrients and collapses to be broken down by caseation, leading to vertebral narrowing and eventually to vertebral collapse and spinal damage. A soft tissue mass may form.

Spinal metastasis is common in patients with cancer. The spine is the third most common site for cancer cells to metastasize, following the lung and the liver. Approximately 60–70% of patients with systemic cancer develop spinal metastasis of which only 10% are symptomatic and 94–98% have epidural and/or vertebral involvement.[16]

Spread from primary tumors is mainly by the arterial route. Retrograde spread through the Batson plexus during Valsalva maneuver is postulated. Direct invasion through the intervertebral foramina also can occur. Besides mass effect, an epidural mass can cause cord distortion, resulting in demyelination or axonal destruction. Vascular compromise produces venous congestion and vasogenic edema of the spinal cord, resulting in venous infarction and hemorrhage.

About 70% of symptomatic lesions are found in the thoracic region of the spine, particularly at the level of T4–T7. Of the remainder, 20% are found in the lumbar region and 10% are found in the cervical spine. More than 50% of patients with spinal metastasis have several levels of involvement. About 10–38% of patients have involvement of several noncontiguous segments. Intramural and intramedullary metastases are not as common as those of the vertebral body and the epidural space. Isolated epidural involvement accounts for less than 10% of cases; it is particularly common in lymphoma and renal cell carcinoma. Most of the lesions are localized at the anterior portion of the vertebral body (60%). Rarely is there disease in both posterior and anterior parts of the spine.

Primary sources for spinal metastatic disease are as follows:

- Lung 31%
- Breast 24%
- GI tract 9%
- Prostate 8%
- Lymphoma 6%
- Melanoma 4%
- Unknown 2%
- Kidney 1%
- Others, including multiple myeloma, 13%

Preanesthetic assessment depends on the cause. Often surgery for the primary tumor has been undertaken, but if vertebral collapse and pain have become the prominent feature then attempts may be undertaken to stabilize the thoracic spine. The approach is usually prone and may be prolonged with considerable blood loss. Many patients have already undergone chemotherapy or radiation therapy and may be debilitated.

Indicated tests: Identification of primary tumor; complete blood count and metabolic panel for cancer patients; CXR to rule out infection or metastasis; cardiac evaluation for patient with general debility.

Vertebroplasty is a minimally invasive procedure performed in the thoracic area in which a filler material (traditionally polymethylmethacrylate, PMMA) is injected percutaneously into a vertebral body for treatment of vertebral fractures associated with osteoporosis, malignant conditions, hemangiomas, and acute trauma.[17]

Osteoporosis, or porous bone, is a disease characterized by low bone mass and structural deterioration of bone tissue. The resulting bone fragility increases fractures of all bones, especially the hip, spine, and wrist, (especially the spine). These fragility fractures cause both acute and chronic pain and are a major source of morbidity and mortality. One in every two women and one in four men over 50 years of age will have an osteoporosis-related fracture in their lifetime. The demographics of this population are predominantly whites and females of Asian descent, many with the comorbidities of the geriatric group. Other risk factors include poor nutritional status, a history of a primary relative with bone fragility, inactive lifestyle, early menopause, smoking, steroid use, and alcohol use. Diagnosis depends on a bone mineral density test and a dual-energy X-ray absorptiometry (DEXA) test.

In vertebroplasty, the PMMA is injected directly into the bone, whereas in kyphoplasty it is injected after establishment of a cavity by inflation of a balloon tamp.

As the ability of the procedure to dramatically decrease pain has been repeatedly demonstrated, it has been applied to many more and sicker patients. It is used as a palliative treatment for osteoporotic and malignant vertebral lesions, which weaken vertebrae and cause chronic pain.

Preanesthetic assessment is critical in these patients as many of them have significant comorbidities. Some of the considerations include:

1. Cardiac disease
2. Pulmonary compromise
3. Urinary tract infection
4. Multiple medications and interactions, including herbal therapies
5. Metastatic disease
6. Poor nutritional status
7. Narcotic dependency
8. Limited mobility
9. Communication difficulties

As age increases so do cardiovascular and pulmonary comorbidities. The decrease in pulmonary function associated with osteoporotic vertebral fracture may be clinically significant in a patient with already reduced pulmonary and cardiovascular reserve. Previously pulmonary function in the osteoporotic patient was described as normal, perhaps because height at age 25 years and not current height was used in pulmonary function test calculations.[18] On adjusting for this change, a statistically significant decrease in vital capacity and FEV_1 suggesting restrictive lung pattern may be identified. Also, the mortality rate from pulmonary disease (not lung cancer) is increased with osteoporotic vertebral fractures. Significant improvement in pulmonary function has been shown after vertebroplasty and kyphoplasty, improvement that might increase for up to 3 months.[19] Metastatic lesions may cause vertebral fractures. The primary source may or may not have been identified. In addition to the effects upon the pulmonary system, vertebral fractures also affect the gastrointestinal system. Loss of vertebral height decreases abdominal space and compromises gastrointestinal function. Prophylactic antacid therapy is indicated. Long-term opioid use causes constipation and decreases nutrient absorption. Insomnia and depressive effects of chronic pain adversely affect psychological well-being and many patients are also maintained with antidepressants, especially such herbal preparations as St. John's Wort.

Indicated tests: Cardiac evaluation in an elderly debilitated patient; assessment of volume status; complete blood count to exclude anemia; basic metabolic panel to exclude renal and hepatic disease; CXR to exclude pneumonia and aspiration; assessment of multiple medications for drug interactions especially narcotic patches; urine analysis to exclude urinary tract infection; availability of an interpreter as many patients are of Asian descent

Lumbar level: elective surgery

Many surgical procedures are performed on the lumbar spine ranging from a simple minimally invasive and endoscopic discectomy to multilevel reconstructive procedure with complex instrumentation. Similarly, anesthetic management varies from little more than local anesthesia with some sedation to general anesthesia. Recently there has been resurgence in the use of regional anesthesia, especially for single-level discectomies. Advantages for this approach are decreased blood loss, better pain management (especially if epidural clonidine is added to the technique), less nausea and vomiting, and a decreased incidence of deep venous thrombosis.[20] Endoscopy may be used posteriorly for discectomy and anteriorly for instrumentation.

Spinal stenosis is the single most common diagnosis leading to any type of spine surgery, and laminectomy is a basic part of the surgical treatment. The lamina of the vertebra, which itself is not damaged, is removed to widen the spinal canal and create more space for the spinal nerves and thecal sac. Surgical treatment that includes laminectomy is the most effective remedy for severe spinal stenosis; however, most cases of spinal stenosis are not severe and respond to bed rest, nonsteroidal anti-inflammatory agents, and steroids. Should symptoms include numbness, loss of function, and neurogenic claudication, laminectomy is generally indicated. If the spinal column is unstable then fusion with instrumentation is required.

Spondylolisthesis describes the anterior displacement of a vertebra or the vertebral column in relation to the vertebrae below (Fig. 1.3). This pathology occurs most commonly in the lumbar spine. A hangman's fracture is a specific type of spondylolisthesis where the C1 vertebra is displaced anteriorly relative to the C2 vertebra due to fractures of the C2 vertebra's pedicles.

Patients presenting for major spinal surgery are more likely to be male with truncal obesity and frequently have multisystem disease. Some of the more typical findings are shown in Table 1.5.

Table 1.5 The patient for major spine surgery often has many comorbidities

Findings and symptoms	Anesthetic implications
Hypertension	Well controlled? Medications? Effects of general anesthesia?
Smoking	Respiratory function? Wound healing? Postoperative care?
Obesity	Obstructive sleep apnea? Airway difficulties? Pulmonary hypertension?
Diabetes mellitus	Perioperative glucose control?
Multiple pain managements	Drug interactions?
Renal disease	Diuretic therapy? Coronary artery disease?
Hematologic anomalies	Anemia? polycythemia?

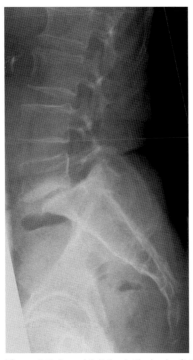

Figure 1.3 Spondylolisthesis. The body of L5 can be seen slipped over the sacrum.

Spinal fusion and instrumentation is major surgery that is generally planned for many months. Thus patients have often undergone extensive evaluation before they are even seen in a preanesthetic assessment clinic. However, in consultations key questions should be identified to ensure that all of the perioperative caregivers are considered when providing a response.[21]

Several studies suggest that such an approach is not always taken. A multiple-choice survey regarding the purposes and utility of cardiology consultations was sent to randomly selected New York metropolitan area anesthesiologists, surgeons, and cardiologists.[22] There was disagreement on the importance and purposes of a cardiology consultation on topics such as intraoperative monitoring, "clearing the patient for surgery," and advising as to the safest type of anesthesia and avoidance of hypoxia and hypotension. This advice was regarded as important by most cardiologists and surgeons but as unimportant by anesthesiologists. Also, the charts of 55 consecutive patients aged more than 50 years who received preoperative cardiology consultations were examined to determine the stated purpose of the consultation, recommendations made, and concordance by surgeons and anesthesiologists with the recommendations. Of the cardiology consultations, 40% contained no recommendations other than "proceed with case," "cleared for surgery," or "continue current medications." A review of 146 medical consultations suggested that the majority of such consultations give little advice that impacted either perioperative management or outcome of surgery.[23] In only 5 consultations (3.4%) did the consultant identify a new finding; 62 consultations (42.5%) contained no recommendations. Therefore, careful history taking and physical evaluation by the anesthesiologist is essential as not only can situations change over a few weeks but factors that are critical in anesthetic management may appear of less significance to the cardiologist.

The history should seek to identify cardiac conditions that have been shown to impact perioperative morbidity and mortality such as unstable coronary syndromes, prior angina, recent or past myocardial infarction, decompensated heart failure, significant dysrhythmias, and severe valvular disease.[21] A prior history of placement of a pacemaker or implantable cardioverter defibrillator (ICD) or a history of orthostatic intolerance is important. Modifiable risk factors for coronary heart disease (CHD) should be recorded, along with evidence of associated diseases, such as peripheral vascular disease, cerebrovascular disease, diabetes mellitus, renal impairment, and chronic pulmonary disease. In patients with established cardiac disease, any recent change in symptoms must be ascertained. Accurate recordings of current medications used, including herbal and other nutritional supplements, and dosages are essential. Alcohol and tobacco use and ingestion of over-the-counter and illicit drugs

Table 1.6 METS chart for energy cost of activities

Level	Self-care	Housework	Recreation	Work
METS 1–3	Bathe, dress, comb hair, put on shoes	Wash dishes, dust, set table	Walk 2 mph, read, TV, play piano	Type, desk, occasional lifting up to 10 lbs
METS 3–4	Shower, climb stairs, wash hair, driving	Laundry, weeding, vacuuming, make bed	Walk 3 mph, bowl, golf with cart, fish from boat	Light repair work, painting small jobs, occasionally lift to 20 lbs
METS 4–5	Sexual intercourse	Digging, wax floors, move furniture, wash car	Walk 3.5 mph, golf and carry clubs, doubles tennis, bicycling	Mix cement, occasionally lift to 50 lbs, painting exteriors
METS 5–7	Hanging clothes	Split wood, climb ladder, put up storm windows	Walk 4–5 mph, singles tennis, softball, cross-country skiing	Heavy farming, occasionally lift 50–100 lbs, heavy industry
METS >8		Saw hardwood by hand, push and pull hard, move furniture	Jogging 5 mph, football, downhill skiing, cross-country running	Heavy construction, frequent lifting and carrying (>50 lbs)

should be documented. The history should also seek to determine the functional capacity (Table 1.6).

Assessment of a patient's capacity to perform a spectrum of common daily tasks correlates well with maximum oxygen uptake by treadmill testing.[24] A patient classified as high risk owing to age or known CAD but who is asymptomatic and runs for 30 minutes daily may need no further evaluation. In contrast, a sedentary patient, such as one immobilized by severe back pain, without a history of cardiovascular disease but with clinical factors that suggest increased perioperative risk, may benefit from a more extensive preoperative evaluation.

Physical examination should include a review of general appearance. Cyanosis, pallor, dyspnea during conversation or with minimal activity, Cheyne–Stokes respiration, poor nutritional status, obesity, skeletal deformities, tremor, and anxiety are indicators of underlying disease and/or coronary artery disease. A long-standing history of hypertension and hyperlipidemia is common, usually treated with several medications including diuretics, angiotensin-converting enzyme (ACE) inhibitors, calcium channel and beta blockers, and a statin. In assessing blood pressure, several values should be taken from both arms. An elevated blood pressure may indicate "white coat" syndrome or failure to adhere to the prescribed regimen. Some patients (and other health care workers) believe that an order "nothing to eat or drink" excludes all medications. If the blood pressure is indeed recorded within a normal range, it is important to remember that, as in a diabetic patient in whom one measurement is normoglycemic, the disease is still present. In other words, even though a mean blood pressure of 60–70 mmHg may be well tolerated by a young man with normal vasculature, such a level may well be too low for someone who may have a baseline mean pressure of 110 (140/90)

with medication. Also, the long-term ingestion of antihypertensive agents, especially ACE inhibitors, may cause a decrease in blood pressure intraoperatively, necessitating early administration of vasopressors. Other signs that should be sought include carotid pulse contour and bruits, jugular venous pressure and pulsations, auscultation of the lungs, precordial palpation and auscultation, abdominal palpation, and examination of the extremities for edema and vascular integrity. The finding of weak or absent arterial pulses confirms the diagnosis of underlying cardiovascular disease.

Although rales and chest radiographic evidence of pulmonary congestion correlate well with elevated pulmonary venous pressure in acute heart failure, in patients with chronic failure these findings may be absent and an elevated jugular venous pressure or a positive hepatojugular reflux are more reliable signs. Peripheral edema is not a reliable indicator of chronic failure unless the jugular venous pressure is elevated or the hepatojugular test is positive. During cardiac auscultation, a third heart sound at the apical area suggests a failing left ventricle, but its absence is not a reliable indicator of good ventricular function. Presence of a cardiac murmur may or may not be significant. For example, aortic stenosis poses a higher risk for noncardiac surgery.[25] Even if aortic regurgitation and mitral regurgitation are minimal, they predispose the patient to infective endocarditis should bacteremia occur.

The basic clinical evaluation obtained by history, physical examination, and review of the ECG usually provides sufficient data to estimate cardiac risk. The resting 12-lead ECG has been examined perioperatively to evaluate its prognostic value. Lee *et al.* studied 4135 patients aged 50 years or older undergoing major noncardiac surgery (more than-2 day stay).[26] The presence of a pathological Q wave on the preoperative ECG was associated with an increased risk of major cardiac complications, defined as an infarction, pulmonary edema, ventricular fibrillation, primary cardiac arrest, or complete heart block. Pathological Q waves were found in 17% of the patient population. Based on these findings, the authors derived a "simple index" for the prediction of cardiac risk for stable patients undergoing nonurgent major noncardiac surgery. Independent risk factors included:

1. Ischemic heart disease (history of myocardial infarction, positive treadmill test, use of nitroglycerin, chest pain, or ECG with abnormal Q waves)
2. Congestive heart failure (history of failure, pulmonary edema, paroxysmal nocturnal dyspnea, peripheral edema, bilateral rales, S3, radiography with pulmonary vascular diease
3. Cerebral vascular disease (transient ischemic attack or stroke)
4. High-risk surgery (major vascular or orthopedic surgery)
5. Need for insulin treatment for diabetes mellitus
6. Preoperative creatinine greater than 2 mg/dl.

Increasing numbers of risk factors correlate with increased risk, yet the risk was lower than described in many of the original indices. Improvements in outcome may reflect selection bias in surgery, advances in surgical technique, anesthesia, and perioperative management of coronary artery disease. The Revised Cardiac Risk Index has become one of the most widely used risk indices.[26]

In contrast to these findings, Liu and colleagues studied the predictive value of a preoperative 12-lead ECG in 513 patients aged 70 years or older undergoing elective or urgent noncardiac surgery.[27] In this cohort, 75% of the patients had a baseline ECG abnormality, and 3.7% of the patients died. Electrocardiographic abnormalities were not predictive of outcome. The optimal time interval between obtaining a 12-lead ECG and elective surgery is unknown, but general consensus suggests that an ECG within 30 days of surgery is adequate for those with stable disease.

Cardiac conditions indicating the need for further evaluation prior to noncardiac surgery are summarized in Table 1.7.

Two main techniques are used in preoperative evaluation of patients who cannot exercise:

1. Increasing myocardial oxygen demand (by pacing or intravenous dobutamine)

Table 1.7 Cardiac conditions that require further evaluation

Unstable coronary syndrome	Decompensated cardiac failure
Severe angina	Worsening or new onset failure
Recent myocardial infarction	Symptomatic dysrhythmias
High-grade AV block	Severe valvular disease
Mobitz II AV block	

2. Inducing a hyperemic response by pharmacological vasodilators such as intravenous dipyridamole or adenosine.

The most common examples presently in use are dobutamine stress echocardiography and intravenous dipyridamole/adenosine myocardial perfusion. Results of these studies have shown that reversible perfusion defects, which reflect jeopardized viable myocardium, carry the greatest risk of perioperative cardiac death or magnetic imaging with both thallium-201 and technetium-99m.

Dobutamine stress echocardiography (DSE) is the method of choice for pharmacological stress testing with ultrasound imaging. Incremental infusion of supratherapeutic doses of dobutamine increase myocardial contractility and heart rate, thus inducing left ventricular ischemic regional wall-motion abnormalities within the distribution of stenotic vessels. The dobutamine infusion may be supplemented with intravenous atropine to optimize chronotropic response to stress. Intravenous contrast imaging for left ventricular opacification may enhance the image and improve diagnostic interpretation

Several reports have documented the accuracy of DSE to identify patients with significant angiographic coronary disease and indicate that DSE can be performed safely with acceptable patient tolerance. Positive test results range from 5% to 50%. The predictive value of a positive test is 0% to 33% for events such as myocardial infarction or death. Negative predictive value range from 93% to 100%.[21] The presence of a new wall-motion abnormality appears to be a powerful determinant of an increased risk for adverse perioperative events after multivariable adjustment for different clinical and echocardiographic variables.[28] The value of DES in prediction of perioperative events is further enhanced by integration with other risk factors such as angina or diabetes. An ischemic response at 60% or more of maximal predicted heart rate was associated with only a 4% event rate if no clinical risk factors were present versus a 22% event rate in patients with more than 2 risk factors.[29] These findings have been shown to be predictors of long-term and short-term outcomes.[30] Beattie *et al.* conducted a meta-analysis (68 studies) comparing stress myocardial perfusion imaging versus stress echocardiography in 10,049 patients at risk for MI before elective noncardiac surgery and concluded that both myocardial perfusion imaging and stress echocardiography detected a moderate-to-large defect in 14% of patients that was predictive of myocardial infarction and/or death.[31] Mondillo *et al.* compared the predictive value and determined that the predictors were the severity and extent of ischemia (dipyridamole, $p < 0.01$; dobutamine, $p < 0.005$).[32] Only reversible perfusion defects at scintigraphy were significantly related to perioperative events. The strongest predictor of cardiac events was the presence of more than three reversible defects ($p < 0.05$). A meta-analysis of 58 studies indicated that perioperative cardiac risk appears to be directly proportional to the amount of myocardium at risk as reflected in the extent of reversible defects found on imaging.[33] Because of the overall low positive predictive value of stress nuclear imaging, it is best used selectively in patients with a high clinical risk of perioperative cardiac events.

Current recommendations regarding continuing drug therapies are:

1. If the patient is medicated with statins and or beta-blockers these medications should be continued.
2. Beta-blocking therapy should not be started de novo.
3. Some clinicians advise discontinuing ACE inhibitors on the day before surgery.
4. Patients with a bare metal stent should not have surgery for a month, and patients with a drug-eluting stent should continue clopidogrel for a year and perhaps even longer.[34]

Smoking

The presence of either obstructive or restrictive pulmonary disease places the patient at increased risk of developing perioperative respiratory complications, compounded by placement in the prone position for several hours during surgery. Hypoxemia, hypercapnia, acidosis, and increased work of breathing can all lead to further deterioration of an already compromised cardiopulmonary system. If significant pulmonary disease is suspected, documentation of response to bronchodilators and/or evaluation for the presence

Table 1.8 Estimated times for return of lung function after stopping smoking

Elimination of nicotine	12 h
Elimination of carboxyhemoglobin	1–3 days
Return of ciliary function	6–7 days
Decrease of sputum production	6–8 weeks
Normalization of immune system	>8 weeks

of carbon dioxide retention through arterial blood gas analysis may be justified. If there is evidence of infection, appropriate antibiotic therapy is critical. Steroids and bronchodilators may be indicated, although the risk of producing dysrhythmias or myocardial ischemia by beta-agonists and hyperglycemia must be considered. Complete abstinence from tobacco intake for several weeks prior to surgery would be ideal to allow regeneration of lung function but is rarely possible. Times required for regeneration of various functions are approximated in Table 1.8.

A carboxyhemoglobin level of 15% can reduce the availability of oxygen by up to 25% and while this level may not be significant in asymptomatic patients, it may present a considerable risk for patients with coronary artery disease in whom a favorable myocardial balance is critical. These patients should be advised to refrain from smoking for at least 24 h prior to surgery. While pulmonary function tests are not usually helpful in predicting postoperative pulmonary events or the need for mechanical ventilation, a low preoperative oxygen room air saturation, or low partial pressure of arterial oxygen may identify patients at higher risk. Other important factors in determining postoperative pulmonary complications include the site and duration of the surgical procedure and the amount of blood lost. Preoperative pulmonary therapy might be useful, if only to acquaint the patient with the several tools that may be used in the postoperative period to maintain oxygenation. Clinical studies suggest that smoking is a risk factor in the progression of kidney disease, especially diabetic nephropathy. Nicotine promotes mesangial cell proliferation and fibronectin production, and smoking may promote the progression of diabetic nephropathy by increasing the expression of profibrotic cytokines such as transforming growth factor and the extracellular matrix proteins fibronectin and collagen IV.[35] Thus, evaluation of kidney function and glycemic status, especially in diabetic patients, is important in the smoker and limitation of the use or doses of drugs dependent on the kidney for excretion is indicated.

Examination of the airway is a prerequisite of all anesthetic encounters. Nicotine is a significant risk factor for the development and progression of periodontal disease.[36] The drug probably acts by decreasing gingival blood flow, increasing cytokine production, and adversely affecting the immune system to cause loosening of teeth and actual tooth loss. Chewing tobacco also causes tooth decay due to the high sugar content. Oral cancers and leukoplakia may interfere with intubation or oral airway placement due to bleeding or ulceration. Additional exposure to ethanol appears to enhance adverse changes in the buccal mucosa in vitro in more than an additive effect.[37] Noting that surgery might present a teachable moment, several studies have been undertaken to assess the benefit of referring patients preoperatively to telephone quitlines.[38,39] While many of these reports are on small groups, there is benefit in advising patients on the adverse effects of tobacco and referring them for further help, especially by facilitating referral of smokers for counseling and follow-up. Indeed, the preanesthetic assessment interview has been deemed the "teachable moment." Smoking has been identified as a major factor in failure to fuse and continued pain after lumbar surgery.[40–41]

Obesity

The obese patient presents many perioperative problems ranging from the initial assurance of a satisfactory airway, to position difficulties, to a high incidence of obstructive sleep apnea and pulmonary hypertension. During the preanesthetic assessment, the airway must be carefully assessed for ease of intubation. Neck circumference >40 cm (17 inches) and heavy jowls, often combined with small mouth opening and a large tongue may compromise the situation. Appropriate plans should be made, including informing the patient of a possible awake intubation technique. As spinal disease is rarely confined to only the lumbar area, assessment of a range of motion of the neck must also be documented as must notation be made of the patient's ability to lie flat.

Obstructive sleep apnea syndrome. The American Society of Anesthesiologists has introduced guidelines for anesthetic management of an increasing population of patients who snore and are obese but who have not been formally diagnosed as suffering from sleep apnea, a syndrome that can have serious complications perioperatively.[42] Knowledge of these potential problems is required for all anesthesiologists. A recent retrospective, case control study of patients having joint replacement surgery at the Mayo Clinic found that 24% of OSAS patients vs. 9% of controls had serious postoperative complications (dysrhythmias, myocardial ischemia, re-intubations, and unplanned intensive care unit admissions) – with most occurring within 72 h of surgery, and resulting in increased hospital length of stay.[43] Evidence-based risk-screening tools that facilitate preoperative risk stratification of the undiagnosed OSAS patient, thereby allowing appropriate perioperative care, may help reduce the above-mentioned complications. Once the potential for OSAS has been identified, the patient may have a formal polysomnographic sleep study, which defines the patient's apnea/hypopnea index (AHI), categorizes the severity of OSAS as mild, moderate, or severe, and makes recommendations for appropriate continuous positive airway pressure CPAP or nasal CPAP (nCPAP). The use of nCPAP for several weeks preoperatively has been found to be highly effective at preserving airway patency during sleep and anesthesia as well as diminishing reflex responses to hypoxia and hypercapnia. This effect may result from upper airway stabilization, a residual effect of nCPAP that begins to occur within as little as 4 h of continuous use of nCPAP. Chronic nCPAP preoperatively has been found to abolish mean, systolic, and diastolic blood pressure fluctuations in OSAS patients.[43] As a result, the risk of cardiac ST segment depression and recurrent atrial fibrillation is reduced. It is recommended that nCPAP and oral appliances be continued during the postoperative period. It is also important to note that patients who have had corrective surgery for OSAS, such as uvulopalatopharyngoplasty, may still harbor the disease despite lessening or absence of current symptoms.[43]

The undiagnosed OSAS patient proves to be a greater diagnostic dilemma during the preoperative screening clinic examination because these patients seldom have sleep studies, which makes accurate risk stratification (low, moderate, or severe) to guide intra- and postoperative management difficult. A presumed diagnosis of OSAS can be inferred from a history of abnormal breathing during sleep (e.g., loud snoring and witnessed apnea by a bed partner), frequent arousals from sleep to wakefulness (e.g., periodic extremity twitching, vocalization, turning, and snorting), severe daytime sleepiness, a BMI of $\geq 35 \, kg/m^2$, increased neck circumference (≥ 40 cm [17 inches] for males, ≥ 38.5 cm [16 inches] for females), and the presence of coexisting morbidities (e.g., essential systemic hypertension, pulmonary hypertension, cardiomegaly).

The ASA task force on OSAS (May 2006) recommended a risk scoring system.[42] The risk score was achieved through expert opinion, literature review, and consensus – but it remains to be validated. The ASA Risk Score considers the following with points being assigned for each of three categories (a, b, c) and then totaled (d):

(a) Severity of sleep apnea: Based on a sleep study (i.e., AHI) or clinical indicators if a sleep study is not available (i.e., presumptive diagnosis). Points: 0 = none; 1 = mild OSA; 2 = moderate OSA; 3 = severe OSA.

   One point may be subtracted if a patient has been on CPAP or bilevel positive airway pressure (BiPAP) prior to surgery and will be using this consistently during the postoperative period. One point should be added if a patient with mild or moderate OSA has a resting P_aCO_2 exceeding 50 mmHg.

(b) Invasiveness of the surgical procedure and anesthesia: Based on type of surgery/anesthesia. Points: 0 = superficial surgery under local or peripheral nerve block, anesthesia without sedation; 1 = superficial surgery with moderate sedation or general anesthesia or peripheral surgery with spinal or epidural anesthesia (with no more than moderate sedation); 2 = peripheral surgery with general anesthesia or airway surgery with moderate sedation; 3 = major surgery under general anesthesia or airway surgery under general anesthesia.

(c) Requirement for postoperative opioids: Points: 0 = none; 1 = low-dose oral opioids; 3 = high-dose oral opioids or parenteral or neuraxial opioids.

(d) Estimation of perioperative risk: Based on the overall score (0–6) derived from the points assigned to (a) added to the greater of the points assigned to (b) or (c).

Patients with overall score of ≥ 4 may be at increased perioperative risk from OSA. Patients with a score of ≥ 5 may be at significantly increased perioperative risk from OSA.

Recently, a study was conducted to evaluate a new abbreviated version of the ASA questionnaire – the STOP Questionnaire.[44] Four questions are asked related to Snoring, Tiredness during the day, Observed apnea, and high blood Pressure. After screening 2467 patients, the authors concluded that this screening tool was reliable and easy to use. Combined with body mass index, age, neck size, and sex it had a high sensitivity, especially in patients with moderate to severe OSAS

In summary, clinical suspicion of OSAS may be the only preoperative tool available to the anesthesiologist as formal and widely used; preoperative validated questionnaires have not been established.

Pulmonary hypertension

Symptoms of pulmonary hypertension may develop very gradually and include shortness of breath, fatigue, nonproductive cough, angina pectoris, fainting or syncope, peripheral edema, and rarely hemoptysis, all of which may be confused by immobility due to back pain, obesity, and myocardial ischemia. Pulmonary venous hypertension typically presents with shortness of breath while lying flat or sleeping (orthopnea or paroxysmal nocturnal dyspnea), while pulmonary arterial hypertension (PAH) usually does not.

A history of exposure to drugs such as cocaine, methamphetamine, alcohol leading to cirrhosis, and tobacco leading to emphysema is significant. Typical signs of pulmonary hypertension, include a widely split S_2 or second heart sound, a loud P_2 or pulmonic valve closure sound (part of the second heart sound), sternal heave, possible S_3 or third heart sound, jugular venous distension, pedal edema, ascites, hepatojugular reflux, and clubbing. Tricuspid insufficiency is consistent with the presence of pulmonary hypertension.

Procedures to confirm the presence of pulmonary hypertension and exclude other possible diagnoses include pulmonary function tests; blood tests to exclude HIV, autoimmune diseases, and liver disease; electrocardiography (ECG); arterial blood gas analyses; CXR (followed by high-resolution CT scanning if interstitial lung disease is suspected); and ventilation-perfusion or V/Q scanning to exclude chronic thromboembolic pulmonary hypertension. Biopsy of the lung is usually not indicated unless the pulmonary hypertension is thought to be due to an underlying interstitial lung disease. Lung biopsies are fraught with risks of bleeding due to the high intrapulmonary blood pressure. Brain natriuretic peptide level is also used to follow the progress of patients with pulmonary hypertension.

Diagnosis of PAH requires the presence of pulmonary hypertension with two other conditions. Pulmonary artery occlusion pressure (PAOP or PCWP) must be less than 15 mmHg (2000 Pa) and pulmonary vascular resistance (PVR) must be greater than 3 Wood units (240 dyn s cm^{-5} or 2.4 mN s cm^{-5}).

Although pulmonary arterial pressure can be estimated on the basis of echocardiography, pressure measurements with a pulmonary artery provide the most definite assessment. PAOP and PVR cannot be measured directly with echocardiography. Therefore diagnosis of PAH requires right-sided cardiac catheterization. Cardiac output is more important in measuring disease severity than pulmonary arterial pressure. Normal pulmonary arterial pressure in a person living at sea level has a mean value of 12–16 mmHg (1600–2100 Pa). Pulmonary hypertension is present when mean pulmonary artery pressure exceeds 25 mmHg (3300 Pa) at rest or 30 mmHg (4000 Pa) with exercise. Mean pulmonary artery pressure (mPAP) should not be confused with systolic pulmonary artery pressure (sPAP), which is often recorded on echocardiogram reports. A systolic pressure of 40 mmHg typically implies a mean pressure of more than 25 mmHg. Roughly, $mPAP = 0.61 \cdot sPAP + 2$.

Diabetes mellitus

Type 2 or insulin-resistant diabetes is a common finding in patients presenting for major back surgery and its presence heightens the suspicion for cardiac disease; Lee *et al.* identified insulin therapy as a significant risk factor for cardiac morbidity.[26] Older patients with diabetes mellitus are more likely to develop cardiac failure postoperatively than those without diabetes mellitus even after adjustment for treatment with ACE inhibitors.[45] Perioperative management of blood glucose levels may be difficult as stress and steroid administration will cause hyperglycemia. However, many studies have shown that wound healing is impaired and neurologic damage increased when excess sugar is metabolized.[46–47]

Patients need careful treatment with adjusted doses or infusions of short-acting insulin based on frequent blood sugar determinations.

Drug interactions

Commonly patients presenting for major back surgery have been in severe and chronic pain for years. They have attended many clinics and have undergone multiple therapies. They may have resorted to over-the-counter medications and herbal remedies. Frequently they receive multiple narcotic patches and may have become relatively resistant to the effects of opioids (in fact, they are addicts). Antidepressants including monoamine oxidase inhibitors and selective serotonin reuptake inhibitors are often among their drug armamentarium. Identification and documentation of ingested substances is essential for safe selection of agents intra- and postoperatively. Patients should be advised to discontinue the use of herbal preparations such as ginseng, garlic, gingko, and ginger, all of which may interfere with coagulation. Most patients presenting for laminectomy have received steroids either as a 7-day pack to decrease swelling or as part of pain management (epidural steroid injections). While perioperative supplementation of steroids is no longer advocated, ingestion of this class of drugs should be noted to perhaps explain hyperglycemia or cardiovascular instability intraoperatively.

Renal impairment

Renal dysfunction is associated with cardiac disease, diabetes, and an increased risk of cardiovascular events. Preexisting renal disease (preoperative serum creatinine levels >2 mg/dl or greater or reduced glomerular filtration rate) has been identified as a risk factor for postoperative renal dysfunction and increased long-term morbidity and mortality compared with patients without renal disease.[21,48] Coronary artery bypass patients who are more than 70 years old with preoperative creatinine levels greater than 2.6 mg/dl are at much greater risk for chronic dialysis postoperatively than those with creatinine levels below 2.6 mg/dl. One large study has confirmed that a preoperative creatinine level greater than 2 mg/dl is a significant, independent risk factor for cardiac complications after major noncardiac surgery.[21]

Creatinine clearance, which incorporates serum creatinine, age, and weight to provide a more accurate assessment of renal function than serum creatinine alone has been used to predict postoperative complications.[49] After major surgery, mortality increased when both serum creatinine increased and creatinine clearance decreased, with creatinine clearance providing a more accurate assessment

Hematologic disorders

Patients are often advised to predonate their blood prior to major back surgery. As a result they may come to the hospital relatively anemic. Smokers generally have a higher hematocrit and thus these patients while presenting with values of 36% or even higher may normally have values of >50%. Notation should be made of available autologous blood with a plan to replace it promptly. Anemia imposes a stress on the cardiovascular system and was also identified in the American Society of Anesthesiologists Postoperative Visual Loss Registry as a risk factor.[50]

Hematocrit <28% is associated with an increased incidence of perioperative ischemia and postoperative complications. In the VA National Surgical Quality Improvement Program database, mild degrees of pre-operative anemia or polycythemia were associated with an increased risk of 30-day postoperative mortality and cardiac events in older, mostly male veterans undergoing major noncardiac surgery.[51] The adjusted risk of 30-day postoperative mortality and cardiac morbidity begins to rise when hematocrit levels decrease to less than 39% or exceed 51%.

Polycythemia, thrombocytosis, and other conditions that increase viscosity and hypercoagulability may increase the risk of thromboembolism or hemorrhage. Appropriate steps to reduce these risks should be considered and tailored to the individual patient's particular circumstances.

Consent issues

Several issues require special acknowledgement during the preanesthetic assessment. The patient should be aware that there will most probably be a need for blood transfusion. Awake fiberoptic intubation may be indicated and the patient may require continued ventilatory support postoperatively. In practice guidelines, The American Society of Anesthesiologists have recommended the placement of an arterial cannula but not of a central venous catheter or pulmonary artery catheter, given the limited amount of useful information obtained from these two monitors in determining therapy.[50] Anesthesiologists are also advised to tell patients that there is a low but real risk of postoperative blindness. The American College of Surgeons has been silent on this issue to date. Postoperative visual loss is probably not a single entity with a single cause. Rather multiple factors have been associated including long surgery in the prone position, blood loss, relative hypotension, diabetes, excessive fluid administration, comorbidities including hypertension, and obesity, among others.

Indicated tests: Type and crossmatch blood for intraoperative use; complete blood count to establish baseline; coagulation profile to ensure reversal of effects of all anticoagulant medications; room air saturation to assess pulmonary function; appropriate cardiac evaluation depending on the patient's status; CXR to ensure there are no infective processes that require preoperative treatment; basal metabolic panel to obtain electrolyte and sugar levels; creatinine clearance for renal function; brain natriuretic peptide as further assessment of cardiac function; carotid and deep venous Doppler scan to assess other vascular disease.

Emergency spine surgery

Emergency spine surgery is generally related to cervical injuries. However, among individuals suffering general traumatic injury, the cervical spine is involved in 4.3% of cases, the thoracolumbar spine in 6.3% of cases, and the spinal cord in 1.3% of cases.[52] In adults, the most susceptible areas of injury include C5–C7 and the thoracolumbar junction, T12–L1, areas of the vertebral column with the greatest mobility. While patients may present for release of epidural hematomas after neuraxial anesthesia (very rarely) or after vertebroplasty or other retroperitoneal surgeries, these procedures are often not diagnosed or undertaken for several hours.

The incidence of cervical spine injury (CSI) associated with blunt trauma is about 0.9–3%.[53] Types of trauma cases include motor vehicle accidents (50–75%), falls (6–10%), and recreational injuries (5–15%).[52–54] About 20% of patients have more than one cervical spine fracture. Approximately 20–75% of cervical spine fractures are considered unstable and 30–70% are associated with neurologic injuries. Prognosis for recovery from complete cervical cord lesions is poor and emphasis must be placed on preventing extension of neurologic injury once trauma has occurred. Factors include: level of consciousness, need for respiratory assistance, level of the lesion, and severity of neurologic injury, among others. The primary causes of CSI-related deaths are cardiac and respiratory complications.[52–54] Perhaps the most convincing case of the importance of early care of CSI is that of actor Christopher Reeves. A sports-related cervical CSI, Reeves' injury brought to national attention the plight of the patient suffering from trauma-related respiratory, cardiovascular, and sustained systemic damage. Thanks in no small part to his acute trauma care, Reeves was able to regain some peripheral nervous function before his untimely death in October 2004 due to cardiovascular complications.

Acute injury

Thirty-nine percent of fractures occur at C6 and C7, with the vertebral body being the most common anatomical site of fracture and 24% of injuries occurring at C2.[53] Instability occurs when vertebral displacement jeopardizes the spinal cord or nerve roots. To maintain stability, one element of the injured column must be preserved. The anterior column contributes more to the stability of the spine in extension. The posterior column adds more during flexion. In hyperextension injuries, the anterior elements tend to be disrupted, whereas in hyperflexion injuries the posterior elements are disrupted. Both columns may be disrupted with extreme flexion or extension or if either compressive or rotational forces are added.[52] Primary mechanical injury is caused by compression, penetration, laceration, shear and/or distraction forces, resulting in immediate neural damage due to avulsion and devitalization of tissues. Spinal cord blood flow is severely reduced within the first 30–60 minutes of injury due to hypertensive vasogenic edema as a result of initial catecholamine release. Loss of autoregulation leads to ischemia and tissue hypoxia. Global perfusion compromise from systemic hypotension and tissue hypoxemia from hypoventilation associated with head injury exacerbate existing perfusion deficits.[53]

Fracture and dislocation cause cord compression and ischemia. Cord injury may also occur from laceration, contusion, or concussion by bony fragments.[52] Mechanisms responsible for secondary cord injury including vascular compromise lead to reduced blood flow, loss of autoregulation, vasospasm, thrombosis, and hemorrhage. Electrolyte shifts, permeability changes, loss of cellular membrane integrity, edema, and loss of energy metabolism all contribute to progressive injury. Biochemical changes including neurotransmitter accumulation, arachidonic acid release, free radical production, prostaglandin production, and lipid peroxidation cause axonal disruption and cell death.[52,54] Glutamate release from damaged cells of the CNS is responsible for the excitotoxic component of secondary injury. Increased protease activity, loss of mitochondrial function, and increased oxidative stress as a result of overactivation of glutamate receptors begin a cascade of events resulting in selective cell death and demyelination around the site of injury leading to an increase in lesion size and scar development.[52]

Clinical features

Although victims of multiple trauma including head injury usually present to the Emergency Room with a neck collar in place, traumatic injury to the cervical spine alone only occurs in about 20%. Systemic injuries cause hypotension and hypoxia and necessitate urgent airway management to preserve cerebral function. Intubation and ventilation should be achieved as expeditiously as possible. Patients with cord injury and systemic injury typically show reduced neurologic recovery and increased mortality. However, it is uncertain whether this poorer outcome is due to more severe primary injury or the progression of secondary injury.[54]

Spinal shock occurs rapidly after a complete lesion of the spinal cord as sympathetic tone is interrupted below the level of the injury. Symptoms include hypotension, bradycardia, decreased peripheral resistance, loss of bowel/bladder function, loss of sensation and deep tendon reflexes (DTRs), and total paralyses below the level of the lesion with flail limbs.[55] Respiratory insufficiency and pulmonary dysfunction are common in injuries to the cervical spinal cord. Marked reductions in expected vital capacity, inspiratory capacity, and relative hypoxemia occur in severely injured patients exacerbating cord ischemia.[53] A few key landmarks of spinal trauma aid in localization:

1. C3,4,5 innervate the diaphragm; apnea indicates injury above this level.
2. Diaphragmatic breathing alone suggest injury at C5–T1.
3. Presence of the biceps reflex with absence of triceps function suggests integrity of C6 and loss of C7 function.
4. Injury above T5 may see the conversion of flaccid paralysis to spastic paralysis, positive Babinski sign, return of deep tendon reflexes, smaller vesical capacity with accompanying frequency of micturition, and the mass reflex which may occur 2–3 weeks after injury.

Diagnosis/treatment

Although there is considerable variation in imaging of the patient at risk for cervical spine injury, most centers rely on multiple plain radiographs (at least three views) of the cervical spine supplemented by CT scan of areas that are difficult to visualize or suspicious for injury. Obtundation, coexisting distracting (i.e., painful) injuries, head injuries, and intoxication make it impossible to clinically assess many patients without imaging. If there is evidence of neurologic deficit suggesting cervical injury despite normal radiographs and CT imaging, MRI may be useful.[53]

The goals of treatment of injuries to the spinal cord are to protect the cord from secondary damage, maintain alignment of bony structures, and to stabilize the spinal column to allow for rehabilitation. Considerable controversy has existed over the timing of surgical intervention, but current practice is to operate within 24 h of injury.[56] Surgical indications include: decompression with or without fusion in a patient with neurologic deterioration, reduction and stabilization when conservative management has failed, and surgical intervention for other life-threatening conditions.[55]

Methylprednisolone was advocated some years ago as treatment for primary and secondary injury in acute spinal cord injury.[57] However, current opinion has moved away from this therapy.[58] A recent survey reported that 76% of spine surgeons do not use methylprednisolone for acute spinal cord injury, a reversal from the practice 5 years previously. In fact, one-third of physicians report they administer methylprednisolone only out of fear of litigation.[59] Practice guidelines and the role of methylprednisolone in the treatment of acute spinal cord injury had been based on the National Acute Spinal Cord Injuries Studies (NASCIS I, II, and III). However, evidence-based medicine now suggests that although methylprednisolone results in neurologic improvement in certain types of acute spinal cord injury, its role in prevention of secondary spinal cord injury remains unclear.[60] Furthermore, in light of the proven harmful side effects of high-dose steroids including an increased incidence of wound infection, pulmonary embolism, hyperglycemia, and gastrointestinal hemorrhage, further study would define benefits and limitations of steroid use in acute spinal cord injury.[61] Yet a recent study once more indicated improvement in spinal cord function when methylprednisolone was combined with mouse nerve growth factor.[62]

A number of treatments that may require anesthetic involvement on a semi-emergent basis have bridged the "translational gap" and currently either are in the midst of human CSI trials or are about to begin such clinical evaluation. These include minocycline, Cethrin, anti-Nogo antibodies, systemic hypothermia, Riluzole, magnesium chloride in polyethylene glycol, intraperitoneal octreotide, modulation of growth factors, intrathecal administration of magnesium sulfate, and human embryonic stem cell-derived oligodendrocyte progenitors.[63–65]

In all cases airway, breathing, and circulation must be assessed and addressed even if surgery is not immediately planned or to facilitate placement of a patient in traction as a temporizing treatment. Resuscitation and stabilization followed by prevention of secondary damage to the spinal cord by spinal immobilization and airway management are priorities. Cervical spine injury should be suspected in all mechanisms of injury involving blunt trauma.

Continuous reassessment of the patient with suspected cervical spine injury that is fully awake, talking, and maintaining their own airway is warranted as the status may deteriorate suddenly. Several categories of trauma patients require a definitive secured airway immediately including those with apnea, a Glasgow coma scale <9 or sustained seizure activity, unstable mid-face trauma, airway injuries, large flail chest segment(s) or respiratory failure, high aspiration risk, or inability to maintain an airway or oxygenation. For both complete and incomplete lesions of the spinal cord, manipulation can aggravate the injury and cause ascending deterioration. Therefore, the goal is to establish endotracheal intubation without causing further damage to the spinal cord.[54] Perhaps the most important factor in determining the best technique for intubation is the urgency of the situation. The anesthesiologist must evaluate and assess the risk of further cord injury taking into consideration head and neck movement, the degree of cooperation from the patient, anatomy of and trauma to the airway, and his or her expertise with airway techniques (fiberoptic intubation, Glidescope®, Eschmann or Shikani stylets, etc). A cricothyrotomy kit should be available. Collars whether soft or rigid do not effectively eliminate movement of the neck during intubation. Manual in-line stabilization is more effective in immobilizing the neck during intubation, but may cause excessive distraction in C1–C2 fractures.[52] If possible a neurologic assessment after intubation may assure that there has been no change in neurologic status. However, no data suggest that better neurologic outcomes are achieved by this means. In fact, failed awake intubation has been identified as a cause of morbidity and mortality according to the latest analysis of difficult airways claims by the American Society of Anesthesiologists' Closed Claims Project (www.asaclosedclaims.org,).[1]

Direct laryngoscopy after induction of anesthesia is considered an acceptable option encouraged in emergent and urgent situations.[52] The American Society of Anesthesiologists algorithm should be followed (www.asahq.org). Use of axial in-line stabilization reduces cervical movement by 60% and is preferred to leaving a hard collar in place. However, direct laryngoscopy may cause greater spinal movement than indirect techniques such as fiberoptic intubation. Atlantooccipital extension is necessary to bring the vocal cords into the line of sight of the mouth. Therefore, patients with unstable C1–C2 injuries might be at more risk with direct laryngoscopy. While not ruled out for C-spine injury, an awake and alert patient without neck pain has minimal risk of such injury. In an intoxicated, comatose patient, the risk of C-spine injury must be assumed until a complete diagnostic work-up can prove otherwise. A patient able to shrug the shoulders and outwardly rotate the arms is deemed to have intact C5 innervation. If no other injuries present, acute ventilatory support may not be needed. Hypotension when seen with bradycardia and hypothermia would suggest a high injury, whereas hypotension could also be a sequelae of any of the following conditions: myocardial injury, pneumothorax, or occult bleeding.[55] In the case of a high injury, serial analyses of forced vital capacity (FVC) and negative inspiratory force is helpful in determining respiratory functioning. During the comprehensive evaluation, opioids and benzodiazepines should be avoided because of possible depressed ventilation; however, atropine may be necessary to treat bradycardia.

As noted, not all cases come to surgery urgently and some may be delayed for days or longer. However, in all cases successful surgical management can only be addressed after a comprehensive preoperative evaluation. Airway, breathing, and circulation must be first assessed and addressed as noted above. Both anterior and posterior surgical approaches may be used. Cervical discectomy and fusion are often indicated in the repair of trauma to the vertebral body. The immediate management of every penetrating spinal cord injury is the main indication for neurosurgical intervention using laminectomy. Objectives for laminectomy are to relieve spinal cord or spinal root pressure made by comminuted bone fragments, blood clots, or foreign bodies. Especially in cervical cord injury, decompression of the one or two roots above the transecting lesion and the subsequent restoration of function could mean the difference between quadriplegia and paraplegia.

Patients with transection above T6 may present later in the course of their injury for stabilizing procedures. Autonomic hyperreflexia (AH) may be present, characterized by hypertension, bradycardia, and vasodilation. It is characterized by hypertension associated with throbbing headaches, profuse sweating, nasal stuffiness, and flushing of the skin above the level of the lesion. Bradycardia, apprehension, and anxiety, sometimes accompanied by cognitive impairment are common. AH is believed to be triggered by afferent stimuli which originate below the level of the spinal cord lesion. The stimulus is mediated through the central and peripheral (somatic and autonomic) nervous systems. As the name implies, the autonomic nervous system is responsible for the signs and symptoms of AH. Normally there is a balance between sympathetic and parasympathetic systems lost in spinal cord injury above T6. It is believed that afferent stimuli trigger and maintain an increase in blood pressure via a sympathetically mediated vasoconstriction in muscle, skin, and splanchnic vascular beds. Ascending information reaches the major splanchnic sympathetic outflow (T5–T6) and stimulates a sympathetic response. The sympathetic response causes vasoconstriction below the level of the injury, resulting in hypertension. This hypertension stimulates the baroreceptors in the carotid sinuses and aortic arch. The parasympathetic system is unable to counteract these effects through the injured spinal cord. However, instead, through the brainstem it attempts to maintain homeostasis by stimulation of the vagus nerve causing bradycardia and vasodilation above the level of the spinal injury. The parasympathetic impulses are unable to descend past the lesion, and therefore no changes occur below the level of injury.

Thus should a noxious stimulus inhibit local vasoconstriction, the body responds with autonomic hyperreflexia and causes a generalized vasoconstriction. This response can be severe enough to require vasoactive drugs as treatment. Additionally, autonomic hyperreflexia will not occur during spinal shock. If a history of spasticity is present, or if elicitation of sustained motor responses upon reflex testing occurs without history of spasticity, then the patient is considered at risk for autonomic hyperreflexia. Using either general or spinal anesthesia, as opposed to epidural or axillary analgesia, or sedation, can prevent the reflex. Autonomic dysreflexia presents as headache, sweating, severe hypertension, and bradycardia. While it has been recognized that sufficient general anesthesia is effective at controlling spasms and autonomic dysreflexia, the adverse effects of hypotension and respiratory dysfunction necessitate caution. If a patient with a low-level complete CSI presents without a history of autonomic dysreflexia or troublesome spasms, anesthesia may not be necessary.

It should be noted that the cardiovascular response to intubation might change over time, especially in paraplegics where the pressor response may become exaggerated but is abolished in quadriplegics.[66]

Systems assessment

Respiratory system

The diaphragm is innervated by C3–C5 and contributes about 65% of ventilation; therefore a spinal cord injury above C4 causes respiratory failure. In acute cases of spinal cord injury, there is a high risk of pulmonary edema.[52] The edema may be caused by fluid overload and further exacerbated by efforts of resuscitation. Aspiration often occurs. Coexisting chest injury may be present. As the patient cannot generate an effective cough to clear secretions, atelectasis and pneumonia develop rapidly following acute injury

Treatment with diuretics, antibiotics, bronchoscopy, or positive end-expiratory pressure is indicated.[55]

Chronic CSI patients commonly suffer from decreased respiratory function due to muscle weakness. Consequently, many of these patients depend on mechanical ventilation and are vulnerable to ventilation-associated pneumonia, involving bacterial stasis in uncleared pulmonary secretions. A major complication of chronic CSI is hypoxemia secondary to decreased functional residual capacity, where the administration of supplemental O_2 is necessary. Chronic CSI patients are also at an increased risk for aspiration due to an impaired airway.[52]

Cardiovascular system

If the spinal cord injury is sufficiently high, sympathetic innervation is interrupted, leaving parasympathetic input unopposed and leading to an increased vascular space and pooling of blood in compliant vessels as alpha-receptor-mediated vasoconstriction from sympathetic input is virtually absent, resulting in hypothermia, hypotension, and bradycardia. Hypothermia is exacerbated in the patient unable to vasoconstrict in response to cold. Bradycardia results due to unopposed M2 muscarinic receptor action in cardiac myocytes, unopposed by sympathetic input to beta-1 receptors, which normally increase heart rate. These changes can lead to complications such as circulatory instability and hypotension. Atropine is the drug of choice to block bradycardia.

Lack of adequate perfusion to the spinal cord secondary to hypotension can cause more insult to an already injured area.[55] Adequate cardiac output should be maintained at an arterial blood pressure >85 mmHg to prevent additional injury to the spinal cord. Administering fluids and vasopressors will offset the pooling of the blood that is caused by vasodilation. However, care must be taken not to fluid overload. An inotropic agent such as dopamine or dobutamine may be the drug of choice but care should be taken in the use of potent alpha agonists such as phenylephrine, as substantial increases in cardiac afterload may impair cardiac output and precipitate left ventricular

failure.[52] Invasive monitoring is often required while transesophageal echocardiography can monitor the changes in chamber size of the heart when adding fluid. But controversy remains: while many prefer a pulmonary artery catheter, others weigh the benefits of fluid administration – and consequent raising of pulmonary wedge pressure – over inotropic vasoconstrictor agents, mindful that fluids can precipitate the risk of pulmonary edema and extravascular lung water.[52]

Musculoskeletal system

Musculoskeletal complications involve peripheral cholinergic responses and osteopenia. Acetylcholine receptors are upregulated, and patients can suffer from spasticity. Succinylcholine is contraindicated due to the risk of hyperkalemia. Moreover, the bone density of these patients is in a compromised state and leaves the patient vulnerable to osteoporosis, hypercalcemia, heterotropic ossification, and muscle calcification.[55] Decubitus ulcers and infection are common

Genitourinary system

Patients may suffer long-term problems with bladder function, leaving them vulnerable to ascending and recurring urinary tract infections. Bladder obstruction and infections can lead to further complications such as pyelonephritis, sepsis, and amyloidosis, which can ultimately lead to renal insufficiency and failure. Management of urinary tract infections and sepsis is complicated by an immunocompromised state.[55] Using less invasive procedures can reduce the risk of nosocomial infection.

Gastrointestinal system

Gastrointestinal complications occur in up to 11% of patients after CSI consisting of ileus, gastric distension, peptic ulcer disease, hemorrhage, acalculous cholangitis, and pancreatitis.[52] A high index of suspicion must be maintained for occult acute abdomen, as the usual signs of fever, tachycardia, and pain may not develop. The risk for aspiration is increased. A nasogastric tube can prevent regurgitation by decompression.[55]

Hematologic management

Patients are at risk for anemia, deep vein thrombosis (40–100%), or pulmonary embolism (0.5–4.6%).[52] Anticoagulants are indicated to prevent thrombus formation.[55]

Indicated tests: Depending on acuteness of the injury: vital signs to assess level; oxygen saturation to gauge ventilatory ability; complete blood count to assess infection or occult or actual bleeding; urinalysis to determine infection; basic metabolic panel to evaluate electrolyte status; creatinine clearance to assess kidney function; liver profile to assess hepatic and nutritional status; CXR to determine any additional injuries, type and crossmatch blood if the patient is a trauma victim; coagulation profile if head injury; cardiogram if head or neck injury.

Conclusion

Patients with spinal cord pathology presenting for surgery may have many and varied problems that encompass all body systems. Preanesthetic assessment may therefore be extremely complex and must be readily prepared to adapt quickly.

References

1. American Society of Anesthesiologists Task Force on Preanesthesia Evaluation. Practice Advisory for Preanesthesia Evaluation *Anesthesiology* 2002; **96**: 485–96.

2. Roizen M. Preoperative patient evaluation. *Can J Anaesth* 1989; **36** Suppl 1: S13–19.

3. Pueschel SM, Scola FH. Atlantoaxial instability in individuals with Down Syndrome. Epidemiologic, radiographic and clinical studies *Pediatrics* 1987; **80**(4): 555–60.

4. Moore RA, McNicholas KW, Warran SP. Atlantoaxial subluxation with symptomatic cord compression in a child with Down's syndrome. *Anesth Analg* 1987; **66**(1): 89–90.

5. Liu KX, Massoud B. Endoscopic anterior crevical discectomy under epidurogram guidance. *Surg Technol Int* 2010 Oct; **XX**: 373–8.

6. Jenkins LT, Jones AL, Harms JJ. Prognostic factors in lumbar spinal fusion. *Contemp Orthop* 10994; **29**(3): 173–80.

7. Hilibrand AS. Impact of smoking on the outcome of anterior cervical arthrodesis with interbody or strut-grafting. *J Bone Joint Surg Am* 2001; **83-A**: 668–73.

8. Jung A, Schramm J. How to reduce recurrent laryngeal nerve palsy in anterior cervical spine surgery: a prospective observational study. *Neurosurgery* 2010; **67**(1): 10–15.

9. Apfelbaum RI, Kriskovich MD, Haller JR. On the incidence, cause, and prevention of recurrent laryngeal nervepalsies during anterior cervical spine surgery. *Spine (Phila Pa 1976)* 2000; **25**(22): 2906–12.

10. Liu J, Zhang X, Ging W, *et al.* Correlations between controlled endotracheal tube cuff pressure and postprocedural complications: a multicenter study. *Anesth Analg* 2010; **111**(5): 1133–7.

11. Audu P, Artz G, Scheid S, *et al.* Recurrent laryngeal nerve palsy after anterior cervical spine surgery: the impact of endotracheal tube cuff deflation, reinflation and pressure adjustment. *Anesthesiology* 2006; **15**(5): 898–901.

12. Chiono J, Bernard N, Bringuier S, *et al.* The ultrasound-guided transversus abdominis plane block for anterior iliac bone graft postoperative pain relief: a prospective descriptive study. *Reg Anesth Pain Med* 2010; **35**(6): 520–4.

13. Good C. The genetic basis of adolescent idiopathic scoliosis. *J Spinal Res Found* 2009; **4**(1): 13–15.

14. Sundarathiti P, Pasutharnchat K, Jommaroeng P. Thoracic epidural-general analgesia in scoliosis surgery. *J Clin Anesth* 2010; **22**(6): 410–14.

15. Modi HN, Suh SW, Hong JY, *et al.* Surgical correction of paralytic neuromuscular scoliosis with poor pulmonary functions. *J Spinal Disord Tech* 2011; **24**(5): 325–33.

16. Tse V. Spinal metastasis and metastatic disease to the spine and related structures. emedicine from web MD: http://emedicine.medscape.com/article/1157987-overview (accessed November 30, 2010).

17. Peh WC, Munk PL, Rashid F, *et al.* Percutaneous vertebral augmentation: vertebroplasty, kyphoplasty and skyphoplasty. *Radiol Clin North Am* 2008; **46**(3): 611–35, vii.

18. Schlaich C, Minne HW, Wagner G, *et al.* Reduced pulmonary function in patients with spinal osteoporotic fractures. *Osteoporos Int.* 1998; (8): 261–7.

19. Dong R, Chen L, Gu Y, *et al.* Improvement in respiratory function after vertebroplasty and kyphoplasty. *Int Orthop* 2009; **339**(6): 1689–94.

20. Jellish WS, Thalji Z, Srevenson K, *et al.* A prospective randomized study comparing short and intermediate-term perioperative outcome variables after spinal or general anesthesia for lumbar disc and laminectomy surgery. *Anesth Analg* 1996; **83**: 559–64.

21. ACC/AHA Guidelines on Perioperative Cardiovascular Evaluation and care for noncardiac surgery. *J Am Coll Cardiol* 2007; **50**(17): 159–222.

22. Katz RI, Barnhart JM, Ho G, Hersch D, Dayan SS, Keehn L. A survey on the intended purposes and perceived utility of preoperative cardiology consultations. *Anesth Analg.* 1998; **87**: 830–6.

23. Katz RI, Cimino L, Vitkun SA. Preoperative medical consultations: impact on perioperative management and surgical outcome. *Can J Anaesth.* 2005; **52**: 697–702.

24. Fletcher GF, Balady G, Froelicher VF, *et al.* Exercise standards: statement for healthcare professionals from the American Heart Association. *Circulation* 1992; **86**: 340–4.

25. Goldman L, Caldera DL, Nussbaum SR, *et al.* Multifactorial index of cardiac risk in noncardiac surgical procedures. *N Engl J Med* 1977; **297**: 845–50.

26. Lee TH, Marcantonio ER, Mangione CM, *et al.* Derivation and prospective validation of a simple index for prediction of cardiac risk of major noncardiac surgery. *Circulation* 1999; **100**: 1043–9.

27. Liu LL, Dzankic S, Leung JM. Preoperative electrocardiogram abnormalities do not predict postoperative cardiac complications in geriatric surgical patients. *J Am Geriatr Soc* 2002; **50**: 1186–91.

28. Poldermans D, Arnese M, Fioretti PM, *et al.* Improved cardiac risk stratification in major vascular surgery with dobutamine-atropine stress echocardiography. *J Am Coll Cardiol* 1995; **26**: 648–53.

29. Das MK, Pellikka PA, Mahoney DW, *et al.* Assessment of cardiac risk before nonvascular surgery: dobutamine stress echocardiography in 530 patients. *J Am Coll Cardiol* 2000; **35**: 1647–53.

30. Bigatel DA, Franklin DP, Elmore JR, Nassef LA, Youkey JR. Dobutamine stress echocardiography prior to aortic surgery: long-term cardiac outcome. *Ann Vasc Surg* 1999; **13**: 17–22.

31. Beattie WS, Abdelnaem E, Wijeysundera DN, Buckley DN. A meta-analytic comparison of preoperative stress echocardiography and nuclear scintigraphy imaging. *Anesth Analg* 2006; **102**: 8–16.

32. Mondillo S, Ballo P, Agricola E, *et al.* Noninvasive tests for risk stratification in major vascular surgery. *VASA* 2002; **31**: 195–201.

33. Klocke FJ, Baird MG, Lorell BH, *et al.* ACC/AHA/ASNC guidelines for the clinical use of cardiac radionuclide imaging–executive summary: a report of the American College of Cardiology/American Heart Association Task Force on Practice Guidelines (ACC/AHA/ASNC Committee to Revise the 1995 Guidelines for the Clinical Use of Cardiac Radionuclide Imaging). *J Am Coll Cardiol* 2003; **42**: 1318–33.

34. ACC/AHA Focused Update on Perioperative Beta Blockade incorporated into the ACC/AHA 2007 Guidelines in Perioperative Cardiovascular Evaluation: www.americanheart.org/presenter.jhtml?identifier=3004542 (accessed December 1, 2010).

35. Obert DM, Hua P, Pilkerton ME, *et al.* Environmental tobacco smoke furthers progression of diabetic nephropathy. *Am J Med Sci* 2011; **341**(2): 126–30.

36. Malhotra R, Kapoor A, Grover V, *et al.* Nicotine and periodontal tissues. *J Indian Soc Periodontol* 2010; **14**(1): 72–9.

37. Bor-Caymaz C, Bor S, Tobey NA, *et al.* Effects of ethanol and extract of cigarette smoke on rabbit buccal mucosa. *J Oral Pathol Med* 2011; **40**(1): 27–32.

38. Shi Y, Warner DO. Surgery as a teachable moment for smoking cessation. *Anesthesiology* 2010; **112**(1): 102–7.

39. Warner DO, Klesges RC, Dale LC, *et al.* Telephone quitlines to help surgical patients quit smoking and provider attitudes. *Am J Prev Med* 2008; **35**: S486–93.

40. Lee JC, Kim MS, Shin BJ. An analysis of the prognostic factors affecting the clinical outcomes of conventional lumbar open discectomy: clinical and radiological prognostic factors. *Asian Spine J* 2010; **4**(1): 23–31.

41. Harrer SW, Carlson WO. Spinal health and smoking. *S D Med* 2009; **62**(8): 309, 311–13.

42. Gross JB, Bachenberg KL, Benumof JL, *et al.*; American Society of Anesthesiologists Task Force on Perioperative Management. Practice guidelines for the perioperative management of patients with obstructive sleep apnea: A report by the by the American Society of Anesthesiologists Task Force on Perioperative Management of patients with obstructive sleep apnea. *Anesthesiology* 2006; **104**: 1081–93. Available online at: http://www.asahq.org/publicationsAndServices/sleepapnea103105.pdf.

43. Kaw R, Michota A, Jaffer A, *et al.* Unrecognized sleep apnea in the surgical patient: implications for the perioperative setting. *Chest* 2006; **129**(1): 198–205.

44. Chung F, Yeqneswaran B, Liao P, *et al.* STOP questionnaire: a tool to screen patients for obstructive sleep apnea. *Anesthesiology* 2008; **108**(5): 812–21.

45. Charlson ME, MacKenzie CR, Gold JP, Ales KL, Topkins M, Shires GT. Risk for postoperative congestive heart failure. *Surg Gynecol Obstet* 1991; **172**: 95–104.

46. Bilotta F, Rosa G. Glucose management in the neurosurgical patient: are we yet any closer? *Curr Opin Anaesthesiol* 2010; **23**(5): 539–43.

47. Rizvi AA, Chillag SA, Chillag KJ. Perioperative management of diabetes and hyperglycemia in patients undergoing orthopaedic surgery. *J Am Acad Orthop Surg* 2010; **18**(7): 426–35.

48. Brosius FC III, Hostetter TH, Kelepouris E, *et al.* Detection of chronic kidney disease in patients with or at increased risk of cardiovascular disease: a science advisory from the American Heart Association Kidney and Cardiovascular Disease Council; the Councils on High Blood Pressure Research, Cardiovascular Disease in the Young, and Epidemiology and Prevention; and the Quality of Care and Outcomes Research Interdisciplinary Working Group: developed in collaboration with the National Kidney Foundation. *Circulation* 2006; **114**: 1083–7.

49. Kertai MD, Boersma E, Bax JJ, *et al.* Comparison between serum creatinine and creatinine clearance for the prediction of postoperative mortality in patients undergoing major vascular surgery. *Clin Nephrol* 2003; **59**: 17–23.

50. Lee LA, Roth S, Posner KL, *et al.* The American Society of Anesthesiologists Postoperative Visual Loss Registry:

analysis of 93 spine surgery cases with postoperative visual loss. *Anesthesiology* 2006; **105**(4): 652–9.

51. Wu WC, Schifftner TL, Henderson WG, *et al.* Preoperative hematocrit levels and postoperative outcomes in older patients undergoing noncardiac surgery. *JAMA* 2007; **297**: 2481–8.

52. Stier, G.R., Schell, R.M., Cole, D.J. Neurosurgical diseases and trauma of the spine and spinal cord: anesthetic considerations. In: Cottrell JE, Young WL, eds. *Cottrell and Young's Neuroanesthesia*. 5th ed. Mosby: St. Louis; 2010: 355–79.

53. Crosby, Edward T. Airway management in adults after cervical spine trauma. *Anesthesiology* 2006; **104**: 1293–318.

54. Pimental L, Diegelmann L. Evaluation and management of acute cervical spine trauma. *Emerg Med Clin North Am* 2010; **28**(4): 719–38.

55. Hadley MN, Walters BC. Guidelines for the management of acute cervical spine and spinal cord injuries. *Clin Neurosurg* 2003; **50**: 239–48.

56. Fehlings MG, Wilson JR. Timing of surgical intervention in spinal trauma: what does the evidence indicate? *Spine (Phila Pa 1976)* 2010; **35**(21): 159–60.

57. Belegu V, Oudega M, Gary D, McDonald JW. Restoring function after spinal cord injury: promoting spontaneous regeneration with stem cells and activity based therapies. *Neurosurg Clin North Am* 2007; **18**(1): 143–68.

58. Sugimoto IY, Tomioka M, Kai N, *et al.* Does high dose methylprednisolone sodium succinate really improve neurological status in patients with acute cervical cord injury?: a prospective study about neurological recovery and early complications. *Spine (Phila Pa 1976)* 2009; **34**(20); 121–4.

59. Hurlbert RJ, Hamilton MG. Methylprednisolone for acute spinal cord injury: 5-year practice reversal. *Can J Neurol Sci* 2008; **35**(1): 41–5.

60. Rozet, I. Methylprednisolone in acute spinal cord injury: is there any other ethical choice? *J Neurosurg Anesthesiol* 2008; **20**(2): 137–9.

61. Miller, S M. Methylprednisolone in acute spinal cord injury: a tarnished standard. *J Neurosurg Anesthesiol* 2008; **20**(2): 140–2.

62. Zeng Y, Xiong M, Yu H, *et al.* Clinical effect of methylprednisolone sodium succinate and mouse nerve growth factor for injection in treating acute spinal cord injury and cauda equina injury. *Zhongguo Xiu Chong Jian Wai Ke Za Zhi* 2010; **24**(10): 1208–11.

63. Kwon BK, Sekhon LH, Fehlings MG. Emerging repair, regeneration, and translational research advances for spinal cord injury. *Spine (Phila Pa 1976)*. 2010; **35**(21 Suppl): S263–70.

64. Jellish WS, Zhang X, Langen KE, *et al.* Intrathecal magnesium sulfate administration at the time of experimental ischemia improves neurological functioning by reducing acute and delayed loss of motor neurons in the spinal cord. *Anesthesiology* 2008; **108**(1): 78–86.

65. Erol FS, Kaplan M, Tiftikci M, *et al.* Comparison of the effects of octreotide and melatonin in preventing nerve injury in rats with experimental spinal cord injury. *J Clin Neurosci* 2008; **15**(7): 784–90.

66. Yoo, K Y, Jeong CW, Kim SJ, *et al.* Altered cardiovascular response to tracheal intubation in patients with complete spinal cord injuries. *Br J Anaesth* 2010; **105**(6): 753–9.

Chapter

2

Fluid management

Maria Bauer, Andrea Kurz, and Ehab Farag

Key points

- Cardiac index decreases in prone position due to reduced venous return and left ventricle compliance.
- Crystalloid should be used for maintenance and colloid for replacement of blood loss.
- Albumin seems to be the suitable colloid during spine surgery.
- Glycocalyx is better maintained by avoiding hyper- and hypovolemia.
- Goal-directed fluid therapy is the ideal way to guide fluid management during spine surgery especially in prone position.

Introduction

Fluid management during spine surgery is very important and difficult at the same time. Most spine surgeries are performed in prone position. Prone position induces a decrease in cardiac index and cardiac output. Maintaining stable hemodynamics with proper tissue perfusion requires adequate fluid management without fluid overloading. The best way to ensure normovolemia in prone position is by utilizing goal-directed fluid therapy for fluid management during spine surgery in prone position. This chapter will cover the pathophysiological changes during prone position, the physiology and the importance of the endothelial glycocalyx, the different types of fluid, and the most recent advances in goal-directed fluid therapy.

Pathophysiology of prone position

Prone position decreases cardiac index and venous return. Wadsworth et al.[1] measured cardiac index (CI) in unanesthetized volunteers. CI was reduced mostly in the knee-chest position by 20% and decreased by 3% on the Jackson table (the Jackson table allows free abdominal excursion in the prone position, which enhances the venous return). Using transesophageal echocardiography (TEE), Toyota and Amaki[2] demonstrated a decrease in left ventricular volume and compliance in prone position for lumbar laminectomy. These changes can be explained by inferior vena caval compression and decreased left ventricular compliance due to increased intrathoracic pressure in the prone position. These results have been confirmed using a thermodilution pulmonary artery catheter. Cardiac output decreased from 17% to 24% using this technique.[3] It should be mentioned that vena cava pressures vary between 0 – 40 mmH$_2$O in prone position with the abdomen hanging free and >300 mm H$_2$O with abdominal compression in prone position.[4] Consequently the increase in venous pressure not only will increase bleeding during spine surgery but also can impair spinal cord perfusion.

On the other hand, the prone position has a more favorable effect on the respiratory system than the supine position. The prone position enhances ventilation–perfusion matching by recruiting dorsal airways, resulting in an increase in lung units and consequently an increased functional residual capacity (FRC) with near normal ventilation–perfusion matching and reduction in shunt volume. Furthermore, prone position has a beneficial effect of positive end-expiratory pressure (PEEP) without the risks of barotrauma or interference with cardiac functions. It should be noted that respiratory benefits in prone position depend on maintaining a freely moving abdomen during surgery.[5,6]

Endothelial glycocalyx

Since the first description of blood circulation by William Harvey (1578–1657), it has been recognized that an intact barrier is an essential prerequisite for a healthy circulatory system and proper fluid distribution

Anesthesia for Spine Surgery, ed. Ehab Farag. Published by CAMBRIDGE UNIVERSITY PRESS. © Cambridge University Press 2012.

between the intravascular and extravascular compartments. In 1940, Danielli described the existence of a thin layer of proteinaceous material on the endothelial surface, which could be associated with the regulation of vascular filtration. Today this layer is called the endothelial glycocalyx (EG). The structure consists of membrane-bound proteoglycans and glycoproteins building up a network in which plasma or endothelial proteins are retained.[7] The main constituents of the glycocalyx are syndecan, heparan sulfate, and hyaluronan.[8] EG plus bound fluids and plasma proteins form the endothelial surface layer (ESL) with a thickness of about 1 μm. The noncirculating part of the plasma fixed within the ESL is approximately 700–1000 ml in humans.

According to the Starling principle published in 1896, high vascular colloid osmotic pressure (COP) in contrast to low extravascular COP is essential for vascular barrier function. However, it was recently indicated that extravascular COP is almost equal to intravascular COP.[8] According to the Starling principle, high extravascular COP should lead to fluid shifts from the vessel into the interstitial space, resulting in tissue edema. Also, the filtration rate across the vascular barrier is independent of COP in the interstitial space. The presence of an intact EG is an integral factor in order to maintain an intact vascular barrier, proper filtration rate, and avoidance of tissue edema despite high COP in the extravascular space. EG retains plasma proteins and generates the endothelial surface layer with its own high oncotic pressure. In a small gap below the EG, the concentration of proteins is lower than in the interstitial space, allowing small net fluid filtration into the interstitial space[9] (Fig 2.1). The EG structure makes the arteriolar and capillary domains relatively impermeable.

However, venules represent the suitable site for filtration through their gaps and pores. Because colloids are able to escape through venular pores, there are low oncotic pressure differences in addition to low hydrostatic differences. The result is a low net filtration in the venular sections.[10] The latter property is in accordance

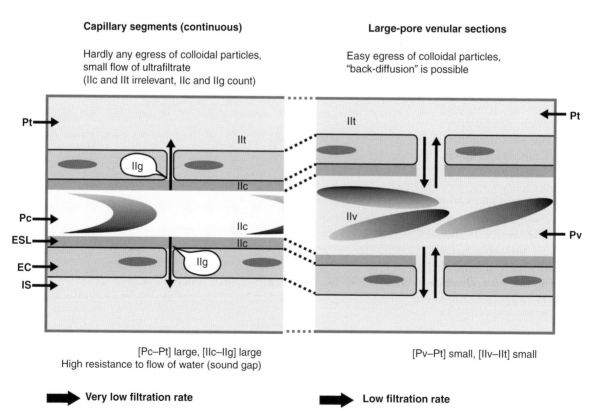

Capillary segments (continuous)

Hardly any egress of colloidal particles, small flow of ultrafiltrate
(IIc and IIt irrelevant, IIc and IIg count)

Large-pore venular sections

Easy egress of colloidal particles, "back-diffusion" is possible

[Pc–Pt] large, [IIc–IIg] large
High resistance to flow of water (sound gap)

[Pv–Pt] small, [IIv–IIt] small

Very low filtration rate

Low filtration rate

Figure 2.1 Low-filtration concept of lymph production. Pt, Pc, and Pv, hydrostatic pressure in tissue, capillary, and venule, respectively; Πt, Πc, Πv, Πe, and Πg, colloid osmotic pressure in tissue, capillary, venule, endothelial surface layer, and beyond the endothelial glycocalyx, respectively; ESL = endothelial surface layer (glycocalyx + bound colloid), EC, endothelial cell, IS, interstitial space. (Reprinted with permission from Jacob M, *et al.*, The endothelial glycocalyx affords compatibility of Starling's principle and high cardiac interstitial albumin levels. *Cardiovascular Research* 2007;73:575–586.)

with the newly appreciated fact that there is no net reabsorption of fluid in the venular segments of the microcirculation.[10]

In summary, a small fluid and protein shift out of the blood vessels occurs at all times, but it is disposed of in a timely manner from the interstitial space via the lymphatic system under normal physiological conditions.[11]

The important functions of glycocalyx

Endothelial glycocalyx plays a very important role in maintaining the proper functions of immune and coagulation systems. Altered functions of EG lead to an increase in the coagulation and the inflammatory response during the perioperative period. Release of tumor necrosis factor (TNF-α) or oxidized lipoproteins mediates disruption of ESL.[12] Furthermore, it has been reported that perioperative ischemia/reperfusion injury induces shedding of the EG depending on the duration of ischemia.[13] Normally, the small vascular adhesion molecules are within the EG. Degradation of the EG exposes adhesion molecules for immunocompetent cells, which enhances leukocyte and platelet adhesion. After shedding of the EG, circulating glycocalyx components like heparan sulfates have a direct chemotactic effect on leukocytes and increase their presence at the site of inflammation. Consequently, the destruction of EG can trigger the inflammatory cascade. Thus, maintaining the integrity of EG might represent a promising therapy for inflammation and ischemic/reperfusion injury.[8] EG has an important mechanosensory role by translating intravascular shear stress into biochemical activation of endothelial cells to release nitric oxide (NO). EG is a crucial component for binding and regulating enzymes involved in the coagulation cascade. In addition, the most important inhibitor of thrombin, factor Xa (antithrombin III), is firmly attached to the endothelium. It is therefore not surprising that hyperglycemia-induced loss of EG is accompanied by activation of coagulation and vascular dysfunction in diabetics[14] (Fig. 2.2).

Perioperative fluid management and glycocalyx

Perioperative fluid management is one of the key factors in maintaining the integrity of EG. It is well known that iatrogenic acute hypervolemia can lead to release of atrial natriuretic peptide (ANP). ANP induces shedding of EG components, mainly syndecan-1, thereby increasing shifts of fluid and macromolecules into the interstitial space. Thus the ability of ANP to increase capillary permeability to water, solutes, and macromolecules might be at least partially explained by its capacity to disturb the EG structure.[15] Recent studies have shown that the classical "third space" does not exist.[16] The average insensible perspiration is only about 0.5 ml/kg/h via skin and airways in the awake adult. During abdominal surgery, insensible fluid losses increase to only 1 ml/kg/h.[17] Avoiding hypovolemia and hypervolemia, which includes a careful indication for perioperative fluid management, is an important element to maintain a healthy EG and therefore to limit perioperative fluid and protein shifts into the interstitial space.

The type of fluid used for perioperative fluid management is also very crucial to maintain a competent vascular barrier and reduce the degree of tissue edema. Isotonic crystalloids are usually used to replace insensible perspiration and urinary output. Colloids, by contrast are indicated to replace plasma deficits due to acute blood loss or protein-rich fluid shifts toward the interstitial space.[17] Albumin seems to be the ideal colloid to maintain the integrity of the vascular barrier. This intrinsic effect of albumin is most likely based on its electrostatic binding properties. The charges exposed by the molecules forming the EG are mainly negative (heparan, dermatan, and chondroitin sulfates, etc.), whereas albumin carries not only negative charges (carboxylate groups) but also positive charges (arginine, lysine) at physiologic pH. The presence of positive charges in albumin will enable it to attach to the EG and provide intact ESL. Jacob et al.[18] have shown in an isolated perfused heart model that providing albumin to the endothelium, before and after ischemia, maintains vascular integrity during reperfusion and alleviates development of tissue edema. It should be mentioned that fluid accumulation may be adequately tolerated by young, vigorous patients. However, in elderly or frail patients it may be seriously jeopardized because of impairment of oxygen delivery to the lungs, myocardium, and brain. It is quite interesting to note in the same study the authors confirmed that hydroxyethyl starch (HES 130/0.4) infusion was proved superior to isotonic saline only in the very late stage of reperfusion.

Intravenous fluids commonly used in spine surgery

Fluid replacement remains a mainstay of perioperative care, especially when altered hemodynamics or large

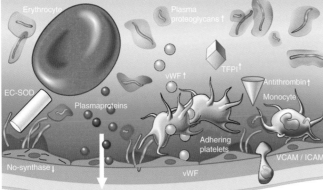

A   *Glycocalyx under physiological condition*

Erythrocyte   Plasma proteoglycan

EC-SOD

Plasmaproteins

Platelet

Monocyte

Glycocalyx

Endothelium

Subendothelial
space

NO-synthase   vWF   TFPI   Antithrombin   VCAM / ICAM

Endothelial function	Permeability	Coagulation	Inflammation
Shear induces NO-sythesis, superoxide dismutation	"Sieving" barrier	Inhibition of platelet adherence, coagulation regulatory factors	Prevention of leukocyte adhesion

B   *Perturbed glycocalyx*

Erythrocyte   Plasma proteoglycans ↑

vWF ↑   TFPI↑

Antithrombin↑

EC-SOD

Plasmaproteins

Monocyte

Adhering platelets

VCAM / ICAM

Perturbed
glycocalyx
Endothelium

Subendothelial
space

No-synthase ↓   vWF

NO availability ↓, oxidative stress ↑	Leakage of macromolecules ↑	Platelet adherence↑, thrombin generation ↑	Leukocyte adhesion↑, and diapedesis

Figure 2.2 (a) Physiological role of the glycocalyx. Endothelial glycocalyx regulates nitric oxide synthase activity, harbors superoxide dismutase, and serves as a physical barrier for macromolecules, including plasma proteins and lipoproteins. In addition, the glycocalyx attenuates platelet as well as leukocyte adhesion. (b) Consequence of glycocalyx perturbation. Glycocalyx perturbation results in a pro-atherogenic state, characterized by endothelial dysfunction, increased vascular permeability, as well as the activation of coagulation and cellular adhesion/migration. AT, antithrombin; EC-SOD, extracellular superoxide dismutase; ICAM, intercellular cell adhesion molecule; NO, nitric oxide; TFPI, tissue factor pathway inhibitor; VCAM, vascular cell adhesion molecule; vWF, von Willebrand factor. (Reprinted with permission from Nieuwdorp M, *et al.*, The endothelial glycocalyx: a potential barrier between health and vascular disease. *Current Opinion in Lipidology* 2005;16:507–511.)

fluid shifts are anticipated. Adequate hemodynamic management in patients undergoing major surgery is paramount; however, much controversy exists about the composition and amount of fluids replaced perioperatively. The debate is of long standing; available data do not provide conclusive evidence to establish universally accepted guidelines from any consensus group or professional society. Focus has been shifting from fluid types, cost, and availability, and standard/liberal/restrictive regimens to individualized (goal-directed) fluid management strategies; the latter, especially with colloid administration, appearing to potentially decrease perioperative morbidity and mortality by improving microcirculatory flow and tissue oxygenation.[19] Complex spine surgery in the prone position, especially if characterized by substantial blood loss

and fluid requirements, necessitates careful selection of intraoperative fluids, and an approach for volume substitution that is adapted to the patient's needs.

Of the possible causes, trauma and surgery bring about the most severe blood loss in the greatest frequency in the medical setting. Spinal procedures carry a high risk of significant surgical bleeding. The degree of blood loss in spine surgery is highly variable and depends on the presence of predisposing factors. Moller and colleagues reported an average intraoperative blood loss of 861 ml (range 100–3100 ml) and 1517 ml (range 360–7000 ml) in patients undergoing noninstrumented and instrumented spinal fusion, respectively.[20] Advanced age, preexisting coagulation abnormalities and other comorbidities, prolonged surgery, increased intra-abdominal pressure – due to the valveless communication between the inferior vena cava and the vertebral veins,[21] posterior spinal procedures, reconstruction of structural abnormalities of neuromuscular etiology, fusions involving multiple levels, tumor resections, and revision surgeries have been associated with greater surgical blood loss. Bleeding can be considerable even in routine cases. Neither the potentially devastating sequelae of organ hypoperfusion in prone spine surgery, nor the adverse outcomes associated with perioperative blood transfusion should be underestimated. Restoration and maintenance of optimal tissue perfusion is therefore imperative, and, ideally, is tailored to the patient's individual fluid requirements during surgery.

Intraoperative fluid management, for conceptual convenience, can be divided into two separate components: administration of maintenance fluids to meet basic, predictable volume requirements – i.e., fluid losses from the extracellular space due to insensible perspiration and urine production, and administration of resuscitation fluids to respond to volume deficits that exceed maintenance administration – i.e., mainly blood loss occurring during trauma or surgery, accounting for the intravascular deficit. Resuscitation fluids, based on their constituents, fall into the categories of crystalloids and colloids.

The choice of resuscitation fluid type largely depends on the type of volume lost, concurrent electrolyte imbalances, and the distribution of the given fluid within the body; and it may have an impact on the postoperative outcome.[22] *Crystalloids* are safe, non-pyrogenic, nonallergenic solutions that contain differing concentrations of inorganic and/or water-soluble organic (dextrose) particles dissolved in water, with or without bicarbonate or its precursor. Those containing nonorganic particles are used intraoperatively to provide maintenance hydration and electrolytes. The kinetics of crystalloids is determined by sodium diffusion; these solutions therefore primarily distribute in the extracellular space. Their use for aggressive fluid resuscitation elicits a delayed hemodynamic response, and may carry an increased risk of fluid overload, dilutional hypoalbuminemia, and subsequent pulmonary and tissue edema.[23,24] Crystalloids contain a sufficient amount of free water to cause reduction in plasma osmolarity, and may therefore cause or worsen edematous states and compromise oxygen delivery and organ function. *Protein and nonprotein colloids* are solutions of large-molecule substances homogeneously dispersed in an isotonic or hypertonic vehicle that do not freely cross the vascular endothelium. Iso-oncotic colloids are commonly used plasma substituents – usually in combination with crystalloids – in cases when the risk of acute blood loss is high, or large amounts of protein-rich fluid shifts are present or anticipated. Their attributed potential to produce or restore oncotic pressure designates their main area of indication: rapid restitution and maintenance of intravascular volume, hemodynamic stabilization, and improvement of microcirculation.[25] Compared with crystalloids, their use is costly and has been associated with several adverse effects. Serious adverse effects of plasma-derived albumin are rare, but despite its preparation method and the lack of case reports of transmission of viral infections following albumin administration, the potential risk of transmitting infections cannot be fully eliminated.[26–28] An association has been found between synthetic colloids (such as starches, dextrans, or gelatins) and hypersensitivity reactions,[29] coagulation disorders,[30] and kidney dysfunction.[31] However, these adverse effects may potentially be provoked by the infusion of any type of colloidal solution. Although its advantages over crystalloids remains questioned by prospective randomized trials and meta-analyses,[32–34] colloid administration has been found to carry a lesser risk of hypoalbuminemia and pulmonary edema.[23] Colloids remain in the intravascular space for longer, are more effective plasma expanders, and in the presence of an intact endothelium, are known to restore intravascular volume with a prompt and prolonged hemodynamic response and – due to their, albeit minimal, ability to pass through the intercellular pores of the endothelial cells – a decreased risk of tissue deposition. In the presence of a suspected or evident disruption of the blood–brain barrier, although highly controversial, colloids should be avoided or used with caution.[35,36] Although numerous types are available, the most commonly used colloids are human albumin and hydroxyethyl starch solutions.

Crystalloids

Normal saline

Normal (physiological, 0.9%) saline is an unbalanced isotonic solution of the major extracellular cation and anion, with no effect on plasma osmolarity. Saline is indicated to replenish anticipated or ongoing sodium-containing fluid losses. Normal saline distributes in the extracellular space: about 25% of the administered volume tends to remain intravascularly, about 75% distributes extravascularly. Its volume-expanding potential is low; for every unit of blood volume lost, a 4-fold replacement of normal saline is required. As an easily available, inexpensive, isotonic solution, it is a preferred fluid in the perioperative care of the neurosurgical patient; however, its composition is nonphysiological in the following ways: as an unbalanced solution, it contains a concentration of chlorine higher than physiological. Evidence supports that massive infusion of normal saline or normal saline-based fluids alone may predictably induce hyperchloremic, non-anion-gap metabolic acidosis, with observed reductions in plasma pH of as much as 0.3 units.[37,38] Normal saline is devoid of bicarbonate or a bicarbonate precursor to buffer acid–base abnormalities, and lacks other electrolytes and organic particles present in the plasma, potentially worsening any preexisting abnormalities.

The phenomenon of developing metabolic acidosis upon the infusion of large amounts of crystalloids was first discussed in a randomized trial in 1994 by McFarlane and Lee,[39] whose findings have been confirmed in subsequent studies.[37,40] The phenomenon has traditionally been explained by the concept of dilutional acidosis: dilutional acidosis occurs when excessive amounts of resuscitation solutions devoid of buffer reduce the concentration of plasma bicarbonate.[40,41] The traditional explanation for the mechanism of acid–base derangements was challenged in 1978 by Peter A. Stewart, who introduced the term "strong ion difference."[42] Stewart's nontraditional approach is based on three physicochemical principles: first, the law of electroneutrality (i.e., in a solution, all positively and all negatively charged ions must be equal), second, the principle of mass conservation (i.e., the mass of a closed system will remain constant over time), and third, the equilibrium constraints on dissociation reactions. According to his approach, any changes in the H^+ and HCO_3^- concentration resulting in acid–base derangements are secondary to alterations of (1) pCO_2, (2) nonvolatile weak acid concentration (acids partially ionized at physiological pH, such as albumin and inorganic phosphate), and (3) strong ion concentration (ions that remain dissociated, thus nearly completely ionized within the ranges of physiological pH, such as Na^+, K^+, Ca^{2+}, Mg^{2+}, Cl^-, lactate, sulfate, and ketone bodies). In the plasma, however, adding up all the strong ions does not result in zero. This accounts for the concept of strong ion difference (SID). Stewart originally described this equation as

$$SID = (Na^+ + K^+) - (Cl^- \text{ lactate}) = 40\text{–}44 \text{ mEq/l}$$

To account for further ions, the above equation has been modified:[43]

$$SID \text{ (apparent)} = (Na^+ + K^+ + Mg^{2+} + Ca^{2+}) - (Cl^- \text{ lactate}) \qquad (2.1)$$

Strong ion difference is therefore a function of both the charge and the concentration of electrolytes, and its driving force is considered to be an independent mechanism imposed on the acid–base regulation. The electrochemical driving forces generated by the strong ion difference will ultimately cause alterations of the H^+ concentration. SID, as well as weak acids and pCO_2, will determine the final H^+ ion concentration: any decrease in SID will result in acidosis, any increase in SID will result in alkalosis (resulting from an increase or a decrease, respectively, in $[H^+]$ to maintain electrochemical neutrality). The acid–base disorder after administration of unbalanced solutions can thus be explained by acidosis resulting from a decrease in the strong ion difference.[42]

Since the severe pathophysiological implications of this transient hyperchloremic metabolic acidosis are not convincingly supported by currently available evidence, translation of its development into clinical significance should be done with appropriate caution. It should be remembered that the presence of hyperchloremic metabolic acidosis may potentially aggravate any preexisting acidosis of different etiology. Acidosis, regardless of the underlying mechanism, may impair end organ perfusion and performance, blunts inotropic responsiveness to catecholamines, causes coagulopathy, and, with concomitant hypothermia, increases morbidity and mortality.[38,44,45] Hyperchloremia, as suggested by animal studies, has the potential to selectively induce renal vasoconstriction by modulation of renin release and increased sensitivity of the afferent arteriole to angiotensin II; and it may further decrease renal blood flow and glomerular filtration rate, and prolong time to first urination, compared with balanced fluids.[46–48] Recognition of the phenomenon and the avoidance of further increase in the Cl^- load are therefore expected. Additional effects of excessive saline administration include increased bleeding, coagulation derangements, and transfusion requirement, when compared to balanced fluids.[37,49] One possible explanation may lie with the lack of calcium – an important cofactor of the coagulation cascade – in the physiological saline. Another possible mechanism may be the reduced levels of von Willebrand factor antigen and impaired platelet function.[50]

Lactated Ringer's

Lactated Ringer is an inexpensive, widely available physiological solution that equilibrates freely across the intravascular and extravascular fluid compartments, and restores extracellular fluid deficit associated with blood loss. Its constituents and their concentrations match those of the plasma, accounting for less fluid shifts. Although lactated Ringer's has a lesser volume-expanding effect than normal saline, a significant advantage of lactated Ringer's over saline is that due to its lactate (bicarbonate precursor) content it does not bring about hyperchloremic acidosis as does normal saline,[51] even in large volumes: bicarbonate is generated by both oxidation (70%) and gluconeogenesis (30%), both biochemical processes taking place predominantly in the liver. Both mechanisms result in OH^- production, which, when combined with CO_2, generates bicarbonate over a period of 1–2 h.[52] A healthy volunteer study noted a decreased time to first urine output in the group infused with lactated Ringer's with little electrolyte imbalance, and significantly less abdominal discomfort, as compared with the normal saline group.[53] For fluid maintenance, however, with regard to its potential to improve tissue perfusion, lactated Ringer's has not been proven to have advantages over normal saline: when compared with 0.9% NaCl, no difference in urine output, serum creatinine change, blood loss and transfusion requirements, or coagulation markers was observed.[40,54,55] Administration of larger volumes of lactated Ringer's required for adequate volume resuscitation carries the risk of fluid overload, especially in patients with poor cardiac reserve, as well as decreased colloid osmotic pressure, iatrogenic metabolic alkalosis, and dilutional coagulation disorders. Furthermore, consideration should be given to the use of alternative crystalloids in certain patient populations. Patients with severely impaired liver function are at risk of developing metabolic alkalosis resulting from the impaired hepatic metabolism of the lactate. Metformin, however, was found to have no effect on the rate of lactate turnover and oxidation, or gluconeogenesis from lactate.[56]

Colloids

Albumin

Albumin, a natural plasma protein with a molecular weight of 69 000 kDa, accounts for the greatest proportion of plasma colloid osmotic pressure. For preparations commonly used in clinical practice, albumin is isolated from pooled human plasma, and has been considered to be the "gold standard" solution for fluid resuscitation in the critically ill patient population.[57] Of note, the findings of the landmark Saline versus Albumin Fluid Evaluation (SAFE) study, evaluating the effect of albumin versus normal saline administration for fluid resuscitation on overall 28-day mortality in critically ill patients, demonstrated clinical equivalency between albumin and saline.[36] Preparations are available in the form of hypo-oncotic (4%), iso-oncotic (5%) and hyperoncotic (20%, 25%) solutions. As a natural plasma derivative, albumin can be administered in large amounts;[27] however, its potential to induce anaphylaxis exceeds that of starches.[58,59] Albumin, possibly due to its ability to prolong the antiplatelet activity of nitric oxide (NO), has mild antithrombotic and anticoagulant effects.[60]. This natural colloid, contrasting with artificial preparations, exhibits anti-inflammatory properties by (1) suppressing the neutrophil oxidative burst and spreading,[61,62] and (2) the reduction of inflammatory cytokine release.[63] Albumin administration favorably affects the endothelial barrier function, possibly in a concentration-dependent manner and by modulating molecular charge. Also, it reduces subendothelial and interstitial permeability by binding to these layers.[64,65] Studies evaluating the renal effects of albumin versus hydroxyethyl starch have found no difference in urine output and serum levels of retention markers;[66,67] however, decreased urine output was observed in patients receiving albumin, as opposed to those who received lactated Ringer's, in the early postoperative course of abdominal aortic surgery.[34] The glomerular filtration rate has been found to decrease with both hyperoncotic albumin and 10% hydroxyethyl starch administration; acute tubular necrosis may also occur due to the accumulation of small molecules in the renal tubuli.[68] Albumin has the capacity to reduce necrotic tissue volume in the ischemic brain, and to improve cortical perfusion, as demonstrated in animal models.[69,70] Furthermore, in a recent meta-analysis, the use of albumin-containing solutions in septic patients was associated with lower mortality than were other fluid resuscitation regimens.[71]

Hydroxyethyl starch

Hydroxyethyl starch (HES) is a hydrolyzed and hydroxyethylated derivative of the natural corn starch amylopectin, dissolved in normal saline or other balanced solvents, and has been developed to serve as an alternative colloid to albumin. HES solutions have been

31

shown to have favorable effects on microcirculation.[19] They decrease plasma viscosity,[72] reduce inflammatory response by decreasing TNFα, IL-1β, ICAM-1, and myeloperoxidase activity along with nuclear factor-κB activation, decrease pulmonary capillary leakage,[73,74] and improve postoperative outcome.[75] Although HES solutions are not indicated to treat or reverse hypoalbuminemic states, their potential to restore colloid osmotic pressure in the intravascular space is comparable to that of albumin.[76,77] Hydroxyethyl starches are characterized by their molecular weight, degree of molar substitution (referring to the average number of hydroxyethyl residues per glucose subunit) and the C_2/C_6 ratio (referring to the site of hydroxyethylation on the glucose constituent). The traditional classification of these solutions is based on the above-mentioned physicochemical properties of HES. The range comprises the high- (≥ 400 kDa), medium- (200–400 kDa), and low-molecular weight (<200 kDa) solutions; highly substituted (hetastarch, 0.6–0.75), intermediately substituted (pentastarch, 0.5), or low-substituted (tetrastarch, 0.4) solutions, and solutions with a high (>8) or low (<8) C_2/C_6 ratio.[25,78] Generally, the higher the molecular weight, the molar substitution, and the C_2/C_6 ratio, the slower is the degradation of the HES solution. Slowly degradable, high molecular weight, old generation starches (for example, HES 200/0.5) entail the risk of severe kidney dysfunction,[31] as well as delayed, dose-dependent, HES-induced pruritus due to tissue deposition, predominantly in macrophages.[77] Although the etiology of acute tubular necrosis is multifactorial, volume resuscitation with HES 200/0.62 increased the risk of renal failure, and caused a 2.6-fold increase in the risk of acute kidney failure in severely septic patients.[79] Besides their adverse effect on renal function, the overall side effect profile of hydroxyethyl starches appears less advantageous, compared with albumin. Adverse effects of slowly degradable HES administration include coagulation abnormalities, bleeding, and allergic reactions. HES 200/0.5 has been shown to decrease the level of circulating von Willebrand factor and coagulation factor VIII in healthy volunteers, even when the administered amounts remained below the recommended cumulative daily dose,[80] as well as to inhibit platelet aggregation.[81,82] These side effects, however, are much less pronounced with the administration of low-molecular weight, low-molar substitution hydroxyethyl starch solutions (HES 130/0.4).[25,28,83–86] Until the results of ongoing randomized controlled trials using HES 130/0.4 are known, albumin should be considered the preferred colloid for fluid management during spine surgery.

Goal-directed fluid therapy

Maintenance of perioperative normovolemia, adequate tissue perfusion, and tissue oxygenation is paramount in the care of the surgical patient. However, the amount and type of resuscitation fluids remains controversial. The fluid of choice largely depends on the type and amount of fluid lost, but evidence suggests that focusing on individualized volume replacement strategies may have a greater impact on postoperative outcome improvement than fluid types.

Perioperative volume replacement has traditionally been guided by static circulatory parameters. Static hemodynamic parameters, such as blood pressure, heart rate, or central venous pressure, however, have not been found to be reliable predictors of mild hypovolemia.[87] Suboptimal intraoperative volume status (volume overload, as well as hypovolemia) has been associated with adverse postoperative outcomes. Optimization of intravascular volume by optimizing flow-related dynamic variables, such as cardiac preload, has been hypothesized to improve microcirculation and tissue oxygenation, and therefore to improve clinical outcomes. Minimally invasive esophageal Doppler-guided fluid bolusing has the potential to assess fluid responsiveness in the anesthetized patient, as well as to optimize the amount of fluid administered intraoperatively, to reduce postoperative complications. Clinical studies demonstrated that Doppler-guided fluid replacement decreased length of hospital stay and reduced unfavorable outcomes in patients undergoing major abdominal, orthopedic, cardiac, and vascular surgery, especially in elderly patients.[88] Intraoperative fluid optimization, a fluid replacement strategy adapted to the patient's individual needs, may therefore be the strategy of choice to improve patient outcomes and, as such, may be more important than the choice of fluid type. The following subsection will discuss the principles and techniques for different methods for goal-directed fluid therapy.

Static variables of preload and fluid responsiveness

Cardiac filling pressures

Numerous studies have shown that cardiac filling pressures such as central venous pressure (CVP) and pulmonary artery occlusion pressure (PAOP) are not suitable to accurately reflect the preload. A recent

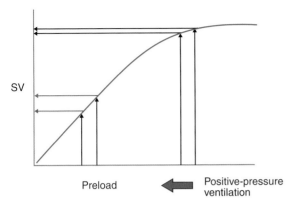

Figure 2.3 The cyclic changes in RV and LV stroke volume are greater when the ventricles operate on the steep rather than the flat portion of the Frank–Starling curve. (Reprinted with permission from Marik PE, Techniques for assessment of intravascular volume in critically ill patients. Journal of Intensive Care Medicine 2009;24:329–337.)

systemic review by Marik *et al.*[89] demonstrated a very poor relationship between CVP and blood volume, as well as the inability of CVP/change of CVP to predict the hemodynamic response to a fluid challenge. The authors recommend that CVP should not be used to make clinical decisions regarding fluid management. The cardiac filling pressures measured by either CVP and/or PAOP failed to be a reliable predictor of fluid responsiveness. First, the response of stroke volume to enhanced preload depends on cardiac function. The fluid bolus will enhance the stroke volume if it is given in the steep part of the Frank–Starling curve of normal heart function, while it will have no effect or even be harmful if it has been given in flat part of the Frank–Starling curve or the failing heart (Fig. 2.3). Second, the filling pressures are highly dependent on left ventricular compliance, which is frequently altered in critically ill patients. The relationship between cardiac filling pressures and end-diastolic volumes is curvilinear and varies between individuals. Consequently, there are no absolute filling pressure values that would produce specific end-diastolic volumes; all depend on ventricular compliance. During spine surgery in prone position, there is an increase in intrathoracic pressure, which is accompanied by an increase in pericardial pressure and consequently by an increase in filling pressures, making them an unsuitable tool to guide the fluid management in prone position. In conclusion, static cardiac filling pressures are not appropriate to assess intravascular volume status or to predict the fluid responsiveness in spine surgery, especially in prone position.[90,91]

Pulmonary artery occlusion pressure

Recent studies have demonstrated that PAOP is a poor predictor of preload and volume responsiveness.[92] The use of POAP with a rapid thermistor and electrocardiogram (ECG) electrode allows recognition along the rewarming phase of the thermodilution curve of a series of plateaus, which are due to pulsatile ejections of blood from the right ventricle (RV). The temperature drop between two successive beats allows computation of the RV ejection fraction (RVEF). Knowledge of RVEF allows the calculation of the right ventricular end-systolic and end-diastolic volumes from the stroke volume.[93]

The left ventricular end–diastolic area (LVEDA) has been measured by transesophageal echocardiography (TEE) in patients undergoing mechanical ventilation. However, the LVEDA has the same limitations as those reported for invasive cardiac filling pressures. Subcostal transthoracic echocardiography (TTE) has been used to measure the diameter of the inferior vena cava (IVC) as it enters the right atrium. A collapsed IVC is assumed to be indicative of volume depletion while a distended IVC is reflective of high right atrial pressure. However, measurement of IVC diameter is an indirect indicator of the CVP and is associated with all the limitations of CVP measurement.[93] It has been clearly stated by Vincent and Weil.[94] that estimates of intravascular volume based on any given level of filling pressure do not reliably predict a patient's response to fluid administration.

Global end-diastolic volume obtained by transpulmonary thermodilution

The measurement of global end-diastolic volume (GEDV) is considered a volumetric static variable of preload using the mathematical analysis of the transpulmonary indicator dilution curve. Transpulmonary indicator dilution curves are used in all commercial available monitors. Temperature in the PiCCO system and lithium in the LidCO system are the most popular ones. The technique for measurement of GEDV requires injection of cold solutions via the central venous catheter in the PiCCO system or lithium via the peripheral venous catheter in the LidCO system, followed by calculation of mean transit time (MTt) of the thermal indicator (detection of the downstream changes in temperature), which is usually measured at a central artery (femoral, axillary, brachial) in the PiCCO system or a peripheral artery in the LidCO system. The product of cardiac output (CO) and MTt is the volume of distribution of the thermal indicator, which is considered the intrathoracic thermal volume

(ITTV), which theoretically represents the sum of intrathoracic blood volume (ITBV) and extravascular lung water (EVLW). The product of CO and the exponential down-slope time of the thermodilution curve (DStT) is the pulmonary thermal volume (PTV), which is composed of pulmonary blood volume and EVLW.

$$ITTV = CO \times MTt \quad\quad (2.2)$$

$$PTV = CO \times DStT \quad\quad (2.3)$$

$$PTV = \text{Pulmonary blood volume} + EVLW \quad (2.4)$$

$$GEDV = ITTV - PTV \quad\quad (2.5)$$

Global end-diastolic volume is the difference between ITTV and PTV and is supposed to be the sum of the right and left heart end-diastolic volumes.

Sakka et al.[95] demonstrated that the ITBV index was closely correlated with the stroke volume index (SVI, $r = 0.66$), whereas neither CVP nor PAOP showed significant correlation ($r = 0.10$ and 0.06, respectively). Changes in SVI were also more likely to be mirrored by changes in ITBV in this study. GEDV was used as a useful indicator of preload and potentially as a variable to predict fluid responsiveness with acceptable sensitivity and specificity.[96] It should be mentioned that GEDV is a static indicator of preload and may prove less useful than dynamic measures of preload responsiveness such as systolic and pulse pressure variation. However, the use of dynamic measures for preload responsiveness is limited to mechanically controlled patients. GEDV is a particularly useful tool in spontaneously breathing patients and thus puts GEDV in a unique position for guidance of fluid administration[96,97] (Fig. 2.4).

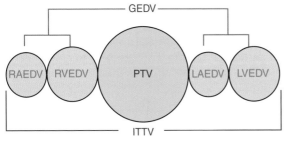

Figure 2.4 Schematic diagram of the relevant intrathoracic fluid compartments and their derivation. RAEDV, right atrial end-diastolic volume; RVEDV, right ventricular end-diastolic volume; PTV, pulmonary thermal volume. LAEDV, left atrial end-diastolic volume; LVEDV, left ventricular end-diastolic volume; GEDV, global end-diastolic volume; ITTV, intrathoracic thermal volume. (Reprinted with permission from Renner J, et al. Monitoring fluid therapy. Best Practice & Research. Clinical Anaesthesiology 2009;23:159–171.)

FloTrac/Vigileo

The FloTrac/Vigileo system can be used to continuously measure CO from a peripheral arterial catheter. The system measures the pulsatility of the arterial waveform by calculating the standard deviation of the arterial pressure wave over a 20-second period. This is multiplied by a constant quantifying arterial compliance and vascular resistance based on patient demographic data (age, sex, height, and weight). The system is based on the principle that if pressure is measured directly and the resistance is known, flow (CO) can then be calculated. The system constantly fine-tunes itself on the basis of the character of the arterial waveform and autocalibrates every minute.[98] The disadvantage of the system is that it uses autocalibration based on experimental data and is not calibrated for every patient.

Dynamic variables of fluid responsiveness

Positive pressure ventilation induces cyclic changes in the loading conditions of the left and right ventricles. Mechanical ventilation decreases preload and increases afterload of the right ventricle (RV) and consequently decreases left ventricle (LV) preload in response to a reduction in venous return. Observing and analyzing the resulting effects on stroke volume (SV), or its surrogates such as pulse pressure (PP) or systolic pressure (SP), is known as functional hemodynamic monitoring.

Systolic and pulse pressure variation

Mechanical ventilation induces cyclic changes in systolic and pulse pressures, referred to as systolic pressure variation (SPV) and pulse pressure variation (PPV). These parameters are surrogates for stroke volume (SV) variation (SVV). During the positive pressure breath of mechanical ventilation, LV preload is enhanced by squeezing of blood from the pulmonary capillaries and veins into the left side of the heart. Simultaneously, there is a decrease in LV afterload.[99] At the same time, inspiration raises intrathoracic pressure, causing a reduction in right ventricular preload and an increase in afterload. Over the course of a few heartbeats (because of the long blood pulmonary transit time), the consequent reduction in right ventricular SV impacts on LV filling as the RV and LV are in series. The LV preload reduction may induce a decrease in LV stoke volume, which is at its minimum during the expiratory period of mechanical ventilation.[93] The variation across the respiratory cycle is normal and is essentially the opposite physiology of pulsus paradoxus; this reduction is

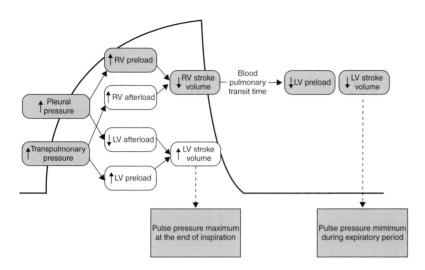

Figure 2.5 The effect of respiratory changes on the magnitude of biventricular preload dependence.

exaggerated during hypovolemic states due to collapsibility of the venae cavae and therefore reduces the RV preload. Also, the transmission of pressure through the RV in low-volume states reduces right heart filling. The cyclic changes in RV and LV stroke volume are greater when the ventricles operate on the steep rather than the flat portion of the Frank–Starling curve. Therefore, the magnitude of the respiratory changes in LV stroke volume is an indicator of biventricular preload dependence[100] (Fig. 2.5).

The arterial systolic pressure variation is defined as the difference between maximal and minimal systolic arterial pressure during one mechanical breath. Its Δdown component is calculated as Δdown = (apneic − minimum systolic blood pressure). SVV and its Δdown component have been shown to be sensitive indicators of hypovolemia. The increase in systolic pressure above baseline (baseline is measured at apnea) is defined as Δup, and the decrease in systolic pressure below baseline is known as the Δdown component. SPV is the sum of Δup and Δdown. SPV is influenced by transmitted changes in pleural pressure, meaning that increasing inspiratory pressures may falsely accentuate SPV. PPV is not influenced in the same way, as inspiratory pressure changes are transmitted to both systolic and diastolic components of the arterial waveform, and pulse pressure remains unchanged. Consequently, PVV will reflect changes in cardiac output more accurately, and may be a better index of preload responsiveness. (Figs. 2.6 and 2.7)

Stroke volume variation and pulse contour analysis

SPV and PPV are helpful to differentiate between hypovolemia and vasodilatation as the cause of hypotension. Pizov et al.[101] induced hypotension in ventilated animals either by hypovolemia or sodium nitroprusside infusion. PAOP and CVP were similarly reduced in both groups, whereas SPV and Δdown were significantly increased only in the hemorrhagic group, distinguishing between preload and vasodilatation as the cause of hypotension. Identifying the cause of hypotension as either drug induced or hypovolemia is crucial to correctly treating hemodynamic changes in anesthetized patients.

Stroke volume can be calculated continuously by the PiCCO system by measuring the systolic portion of the aortic pressure waveform and dividing the area under the curve by the aortic impedance, which is determined initially by transpulmonary thermodilution.[96] SVV measured by PiCCO has been shown to correlate well with SPV and to predict fluid responsiveness, being superior in this regard to CVP and PAOP.[97] In neurosurgical patients, Berkenstadt et al.[102] found that a SVV of 9.5% or more predicted a SV increase of more than 5% in response to standard fluid challenge, with a sensitivity of 79% and a specificity of 93%. It is interesting to note that SVV was able to predict fluid response equally well in patients with reduced left ventricular function (ejection fraction ≤35%) and those with normal cardiac function, as demonstrated by Reuter et al.[103] (Fig. 2.8 and Table 2.1)

Limitations of heart–lung interaction as a predictor of fluid responsiveness

The first limitation of using SVV, SPV, and PPV is its restriction to mechanically ventilated patients with no spontaneous breathing activity. The second limitation is its tidal volume dependence. Since respiratory

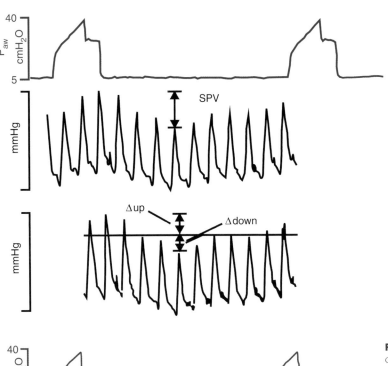

Figure 2.6 Respiratory cycle-induced changes in arterial systolic pressure. The reference line indicates apnea and allows for measurement of the Δup and Δdown components of systolic pressure variation. P_{aw}, positive airway pressure; SPV, systolic pressure variation. (Reprinted with permission from Renner J, *et al.*, Monitoring fluid therapy. *Best Practice & Research. Clinical Anaesthesiology* 2009;23:159–171.)

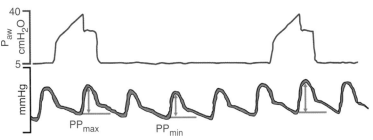

Figure 2.7 Respiratory cycle-induced changes in pulse pressure (PP). Pulse pressure variation is calculated between the maximal (PP_{max}) and minimal (PP_{min}) values of pulse pressure. P_{aw}, positive airway pressure. (Reprinted with permission from Renner J, *et al.*, Monitoring fluid therapy. *Best Practice & Research Clinical Anaesthesiology* 2009;23:159–171.)

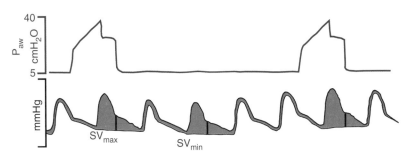

Figure 2.8 Respiratory cycle-induced changes in stroke volume variation is calculated between the maximal (SV_{max}) and minimal (SV_{min}) values of stroke volume. P_{aw}, positive airway pressure. (Reprinted with permission from Renner J, *et al.*, Monitoring fluid therapy. *Best Practice & Research. Clinical Anaesthesiology* 2009;23:159–171.)

changes in preload are induced in pleural pressure, lower tidal volumes reduce the magnitude of SVV or PPV. Therefore, using tidal volume ≥8 ml/kg is currently recommended while SVV or PPV are being monitored. The Respiratory Systolic Variation Test (RSVT) is suggested as a solution to this problem. RSVT is conducted by delivering three consecutive mechanical breaths of 10, 20, and 30 cmH₂O causing a progressive swing in the arterial trace. The minimum systolic blood pressure

during each breath is measured from the arterial pressure waveform, and the slope of the line of best fit of these three points is calculated. The steeper the gradient, the emptier the circulation and better response to fluid challenge. Combined RSTV with PPV was found to be the most sensitive and specific predictor of a response to a fluid challenge as assessed by TEE. The third limitation of PPV or SVV is that it cannot be used in patients with arrhythmias.

Table 2.1 Dynamic variables of fluid responsiveness

Variable	Description	Calculation	Monitoring
Delta down (Δdown)	Difference between systolic arterial pressure (SAP) in apnea and at end-expiration (minimal value during one mechanical ventilatory cycle)	$SAP_{apnoea} - SAP_{exp}$	Invasive arterial pressure recordings and appropriate monitor
Delta up (Δup)	Difference between maximal SAP value during mechanical ventilatory cycle and apneic SAP	$SAP_{insp} - SAP_{apnoea}$	Invasive arterial pressure recordings and appropriate monitor
Systolic pressure variation (SPV)	Systolic arterial pressure variation during one mechanical ventilatory cycle: sum of Δup + Δup	$SAP_{insp} - SAP_{exp}$	Invasive arterial pressure recordings and appropriate monitor
Pulse pressure variation (PPV)	Pulse pressure (PP) variation calculated from the mean values of four minimum and maximum SVs averaged during the previous 30 s	$\dfrac{PP_{max} - PP_{min}}{\frac{1}{2}\left(PP_{max} - PP_{min}\right)} \times 100$	Invasive arterial pressure recordings and appropriate monitor (PiCCO*, LIDCO*)
Stroke volume variation (SW)	Stroke volume (SV) variation calculated from the mean values of 4 minimum and maximum 4 SVs averaged during the previous 30 s	$\dfrac{SV_{max} - SV_{min}}{\frac{1}{2}\left(SV_{max} - SV_{min}\right)} \times 100$	PiCCO*, LIDCO*
Variation in pulse oxymetric plethysmographic waveform (ΔPOP)	Pleth variability index (PVI) calculates the respiratory variations in the plethysmography waveform amplitude	$\dfrac{PI_{max} - PI_{min}}{PI_{max}}$	PVI, Masimo* Radical-7™
Peak aortic flow velocity variation (ΔV_{peak})	Peak aortic blood flow velocity variation (ΔV_{peak}) during one mechanical ventilatory cycle	$\dfrac{Vpk_{max} - Vpk_{min}}{\frac{1}{2}\left(Vpk_{max} - Vpk_{min}\right)} \times 100$	Echocardiography

* PiCCO, Pulse Contour Cardiac Output monitoring system.

Dynamic changes in aortic flow velocity/stroke volume assessed by esophageal Doppler

Esophageal Doppler permits rapid, minimally invasive, and continuous estimation of cardiac output. Cardiac output measurements by esophageal Doppler compare acceptably with the direct Fick method, and are even more reliable than the thermodilution method.[104]

The esophageal Doppler technique measures blood flow velocity in the descending aorta by means of a Doppler transducer (4 MHz continuous wave or 5 MHz pulsed wave, depending on manufacturer) placed at the tip of a flexible probe. The probe is introduced into the esophagus of the mechanically ventilated patient and then rotated so that the transducer faces the aorta, and a characteristic aortic velocity signal is obtained. The cardiac output is calculated based on the diameter of the aorta (measured or estimated) and the measured flow velocity of blood in the aorta. The duration of the aortic velocity corrected for heart rate is called flow time corrected (FTc) and is considered a static indicator of cardiac preload.[93] The esophageal Doppler allows the optimization of SV based on the FTc, and the change in

SV following a fluid challenge[105] demonstrated that use of an esophageal Doppler probe in multiple-trauma patients was associated with a decrease in blood lactate levels, a lower incidence of infectious complications, and a reduced duration of intensive care and hospitals stays. A meta-analysis by Walsh *et al.*[88] demonstrated that intraoperative goal-directed fluid therapy (GDT) using an esophageal Doppler probe significantly reduces postoperative complication rates and length of hospital stay.

Suitable and practical techniques for goal-directed fluid therapy during spine surgery

Fluid management during spine surgery in the prone position represents a challenge due to decreased RV preload induced by increased intrathoracic pressure, and consequently SV. The use of GDT is considered the preferred method to maintain proper intravascular filling without fluid overload. Fluid overload during spine surgery is a major problem resulting in increased facial edema, delayed postoperative extubation, and even in increased length of hospital stay.

During spine surgery, GDT can be easily conducted using either SVV or PPV. SVV can be measured by pulse contour analysis using the FloTrac/Vigileo system. Fluid boluses of 200 ml over 2 minutes are usually given to the patient when SVV increases by more than 14% (sensitivity = 94%, specificity = 80%).[106] The other technique for SVV is measuring dynamic changes of descending aortic blood flow and SV by esophageal Doppler probe. Doppler is used to guide the fluid boluses to maintain FTc >0.35 s and/or to keep giving fluid boluses as long as SV still increases by more than 10%. In the PPV technique fluid boluses are usually given if PPV is >15% (sensitivity = 100%, specificity = 80%).[106] In our practice, we prefer to use esophageal Doppler probe or PPV to guide fluid management during spine surgery, especially in the prone position. It should be remembered that tidal volume should be 8–10 ml/kg during the measurement period. If the blood pressure remains lower than the required target even after fluid supplementation, we administer vasopressors or inotropes to reach target blood pressure.

Conclusion

Fluid management during spine surgery in the prone position is a very difficult but important task to ensure patient safety and successful outcome. Fluid management should be informed by a goal-directed approach. The basal fluid maintenance should not exceed 1 ml/kg/h using crystalloid solution. This can be supplemented by crystalloids or colloids according to hemodynamic goals. Colloids are indicated to replace plasma deficits due to blood loss or as boluses to maintain normovolemia using a goal-directed approach.

References

1. Wadsworth R, Anderton JM, Vohra A. The effect of four different surgical prone positions on cardiovascular parameters in healthy volunteers. *Anaesthesia* 1996; **51**: 819–22.

2. Toyota S, Amaki Y. Hemodynamic evaluation of the prone position by transesophageal echocardiography. *J Clin Anesth* 1998; **10**: 32–5.

3. Kim KA, Wang MY. Anesthetic considerations in the treatment of cervical myelopathy. *Spine J* 2006; **6**: 207S–11S.

4. Pearce DJ. The role of posture in laminectomy. *Proc R Soc Med* 1957; **50**: 109–12.

5. Nyren S, Mure M, Jacobsson H, Larsson SA, Lindahl SG. Pulmonary perfusion is more uniform in the prone than in the supine position: scintigraphy in healthy humans. *J Appl Physiol* 1999; **86**: 1135–41.

6. Tobin A, Kelly W. Prone ventilation – it's time. *Anaesth Intensive Care* 1999; **27**: 194–201.

7. Nieuwdorp M, Meuwese MC, Vink H, Hoekstra JB, Kastelein JJ, Stroes ES. The endothelial glycocalyx: a potential barrier between health and vascular disease. *Curr Opin Lipidol* 2005; **16**: 507–11.

8. Paptistella M, Chappell D, Hoffmann-Kiefer K, Kammerer T, Conzen P, Rehm M. The role of the glycocalyx in transvascular fluid shifts. *Transfus Altern Transfus Med* 2010; **11**: 92–101.

9. Hu X, Weinbaum S. A new view of Starling's hypothesis at the microstructural level. *Microvasc Res* 1999; **58**: 281–304.

10. Jacob M, Bruegger D, Rehm M, *et al.* The endothelial glycocalyx affords compatibility of Starling's principle and high cardiac interstitial albumin levels. *Cardiovasc Res* 2007; **73**: 575–86.

11. Fleck A, Raines G, Hawker F, *et al.* Increased vascular permeability: a major cause of hypoalbuminaemia in disease and injury. *Lancet* 1985; **1**: 781–4.

12. Vink H, Constantinescu AA, Spaan JA. Oxidized lipoproteins degrade the endothelial surface layer: implications for platelet-endothelial cell adhesion. *Circulation* 2000; **101**: 1500–2.

13. Rehm M, Bruegger D, Christ F, *et al.* Shedding of the endothelial glycocalyx in patients undergoing major vascular surgery with global and regional ischemia. *Circulation* 2007; **116**: 1896–906.

14. Nieuwdorp M, van Haeften TW, Gouverneur MC, *et al.* Loss of endothelial glycocalyx during acute hyperglycemia coincides with endothelial dysfunction and coagulation activation in vivo. *Diabetes* 2006; **55**: 480–6.

15. Bruegger D, Jacob M, Rehm M, *et al.* Atrial natriuretic peptide induces shedding of endothelial glycocalyx in coronary vascular bed of guinea pig hearts. *Am J Physiol Heart Circ Physiol* 2005; **289**: H1993–9.

16. Jacob M, Chappell D, Rehm M. The 'third space' – fact or fiction? *Best Pract Res Clin Anaesthesiol* 2009; **23**: 145–57.

17. Chappell D, Jacob M, Hofmann-Kiefer K, Conzen P, Rehm M. A rational approach to perioperative fluid management. *Anesthesiology* 2008; **109**: 723–40.

18. Jacob M, Bruegger D, Rehm M, Welsch U, Conzen P, Becker BF. Contrasting effects of colloid and crystalloid resuscitation fluids on cardiac vascular permeability. *Anesthesiology* 2006; **104**: 1223–31.

19. Kimberger O, Arnberger M, Brandt S, *et al.* Goal-directed colloid administration improves the microcirculation of healthy and perianastomotic colon. *Anesthesiology* 2009; **110**: 496–504.

20. Moller H, Hedlund R. Instrumented and noninstrumented posterolateral fusion in adult

spondylolisthesis – a prospective randomized study: part 2. *Spine (Phila Pa 1976)* 2000; **25**: 1716–21.

21. Batson OV. The function of the vertebral veins and their role in the spread of metastases. *Ann Surg* 1940; **112**: 138–49.

22. Rose B, Post T, eds. *Clinical Physiology of Acid–Base and Electrolyte Disorders*. 5th ed. New York: McGraw-Hill; 2001.

23. Rackow EC, Falk JL, Fein IA, *et al.* Fluid resuscitation in circulatory shock: a comparison of the cardiorespiratory effects of albumin, hetastarch, and saline solutions in patients with hypovolemic and septic shock. *Crit Care Med* 1983; **11**: 839–50.

24. McIlroy DR, Kharasch ED. Acute intravascular volume expansion with rapidly administered crystalloid or colloid in the setting of moderate hypovolemia. *Anesth Analg* 2003; **96**: 1572–7, table of contents.

25. Kozek-Langenecker SA. Effects of hydroxyethyl starch solutions on hemostasis. *Anesthesiology* 2005; **103**: 654–60.

26. von Hoegen I, Waller C. Safety of human albumin based on spontaneously reported serious adverse events. *Crit Care Med* 2001; **29**: 994–6.

27. Kozek-Langenecker SA. Influence of fluid therapy on the haemostatic system of intensive care patients. *Best Pract Res Clin Anaesthesiol* 2009; **23**: 225–36.

28. Barron ME, Wilkes MM, Navickis RJ. A systematic review of the comparative safety of colloids. *Arch Surg* 2004; **139**: 552–63.

29. Kannan S, Milligan KR. Moderately severe anaphylactoid reaction to pentastarch (200/0.5) in a patient with acute severe asthma. *Intensive Care Med* 1999; **25**: 220–2.

30. Herwaldt LA, Swartzendruber SK, Edmond MB, *et al.* The epidemiology of hemorrhage related to cardiothoracic operations. *Infect Control Hosp Epidemiol* 1998; **19**: 9–16.

31. Cittanova ML, Leblanc I, Legendre C, Mouquet C, Riou B, Coriat P. Effect of hydroxyethylstarch in brain-dead kidney donors on renal function in kidney-transplant recipients. *Lancet* 1996; **348**: 1620–2.

32. Choi PT, Yip G, Quinonez LG, Cook DJ. Crystalloids vs. colloids in fluid resuscitation: a systematic review. *Crit Care Med* 1999; **27**: 200–10.

33. Alderson P, Schierhout G, Roberts I, Bunn F. Colloids versus crystalloids for fluid resuscitation in critically ill patients. *Cochrane Database Syst Rev* 2000: CD000567.

34. Virgilio RW, Rice CL, Smith DE, *et al.* Crystalloid vs. colloid resuscitation: is one better? A randomized clinical study. *Surgery* 1979; **85**: 129–39.

35. Jungner M, Grande PO, Mattiasson G, Bentzer P. Effects on brain edema of crystalloid and albumin fluid resuscitation after brain trauma and hemorrhage in the rat. *Anesthesiology* 2010; **112**: 1194–203.

36. Finfer S, Bellomo R, Boyce N, French J, Myburgh J, Norton R. A comparison of albumin and saline for fluid resuscitation in the intensive care unit. *N Engl J Med* 2004; **350**: 2247–56.

37. Waters JH, Gottlieb A, Schoenwald P, Popovich MJ, Sprung J, Nelson DR. Normal saline versus lactated Ringer's solution for intraoperative fluid management in patients undergoing abdominal aortic aneurysm repair: an outcome study. *Anesth Analg* 2001; **93**: 817–22.

38. Ho AM, Karmakar MK, Contardi LH, Ng SS, Hewson JR. Excessive use of normal saline in managing traumatized patients in shock: a preventable contributor to acidosis. *J Trauma* 2001; **51**: 173–7.

39. McFarlane C, Lee A. A comparison of Plasmalyte 148 and 0.9% saline for intra-operative fluid replacement. *Anaesthesia* 1994; **49**: 779–81.

40. Scheingraber S, Rehm M, Sehmisch C, Finsterer U. Rapid saline infusion produces hyperchloremic acidosis in patients undergoing gynecologic surgery. *Anesthesiology* 1999; **90**: 1265–70.

41. Mathes DD, Morell RC, Rohr MS. Dilutional acidosis: is it a real clinical entity? *Anesthesiology* 1997; **86**: 501–3.

42. Stewart PA. Independent and dependent variables of acid-base control. *Respir Physiol* 1978; **33**: 9–26.

43. Figge J, Rossing TH, Fencl V. The role of serum proteins in acid-base equilibria. *J Lab Clin Med* 1991; **117**: 453–67.

44. Burch JM, Ortiz VB, Richardson RJ, Martin RR, Mattox KL, Jordan GL, Jr. Abbreviated laparotomy and planned reoperation for critically injured patients. *Ann Surg* 1992; **215**: 476–83; discussion 483–4.

45. Yudkin J, Cohen RD, Slack B. The haemodynamic effects of metabolic acidosis in the rat. *Clin Sci Mol Med* 1976; **50**: 177–84.

46. Wilcox CS. Regulation of renal blood flow by plasma chloride. *J Clin Invest* 1983; **71**: 726–35.

47. Wilkes NJ, Woolf R, Mutch M, *et al.* The effects of balanced versus saline-based hetastarch and crystalloid solutions on acid-base and electrolyte status and gastric mucosal perfusion in elderly surgical patients. *Anesth Analg* 2001; **93**: 811–16.

48. Thompson RC. 'Physiological' 0.9% saline in the fluid resuscitation of trauma. *J R Army Med Corps* 2005; **151**: 146–51.

49. Martin G, Bennett-Guerrero E, Wakeling H, *et al.* A prospective, randomized comparison of

thromboelastographic coagulation profile in patients receiving lactated Ringer's solution, 6% hetastarch in a balanced-saline vehicle, or 6% hetastarch in saline during major surgery. *J Cardiothorac Vasc Anesth* 2002; **16**: 441–6.

50. Schramko A, Suojaranta-Ylinen R, Kuitunen A, Raivio P, Kukkonen S, Niemi T. Hydroxyethylstarch and gelatin solutions impair blood coagulation after cardiac surgery: a prospective randomized trial. *Br J Anaesth* 2010; **104**: 691–7.

51. Phillips CR, Vinecore K, Hagg DS, *et al.* Resuscitation of haemorrhagic shock with normal saline vs. lactated Ringer's: effects on oxygenation, extravascular lung water and haemodynamics. *Crit Care* 2009; **13**: R30.

52. White SA, Goldhill DR. Is Hartmann's the solution? *Anaesthesia* 1997; **52**: 422–7.

53. Williams EL, Hildebrand KL, McCormick SA, Bedel MJ. The effect of intravenous lactated Ringer's solution versus 0.9% sodium chloride solution on serum osmolality in human volunteers. *Anesth Analg* 1999; **88**: 999–1003.

54. O'Malley CM, Frumento RJ, Hardy MA, *et al.* A randomized, double-blind comparison of lactated Ringer's solution and 0.9% NaCl during renal transplantation. *Anesth Analg* 2005; **100**: 1518–24, table of contents.

55. Boldt J, Haisch G, Suttner S, Kumle B, Schellhase F. Are lactated Ringer's solution and normal saline solution equal with regard to coagulation? *Anesth Analg* 2002; **94**: 378–84, table of contents.

56. Cusi K, Consoli A, DeFronzo RA. Metabolic effects of metformin on glucose and lactate metabolism in noninsulin-dependent diabetes mellitus. *J Clin Endocrinol Metab* 1996; **81**: 4059–67.

57. Miletin MS, Stewart TE, Norton PG. Influences on physicians' choices of intravenous colloids. *Intensive Care Med* 2002; **28**: 917–24.

58. Laxenaire MC, Charpentier C, Feldman L. Anaphylactoid reactions to colloid plasma substitutes: incidence, risk factors, mechanisms. A French multicenter prospective study. *Ann Fr Anesth Reanim* 1994; **13**: 301–10.

59. Dieterich HJ, Kraft D, Sirtl C, *et al.* Hydroxyethyl starch antibodies in humans: incidence and clinical relevance. *Anesth Analg* 1998; **86**: 1123–6.

60. Simon DI, Stamler JS, Jaraki O, *et al.* Antiplatelet properties of protein *S*-nitrosothiols derived from nitric oxide and endothelium-derived relaxing factor. *Arterioscler Thromb* 1993; **13**: 791–9.

61. Nathan C, Xie QW, Halbwachs-Mecarelli L, Jin WW. Albumin inhibits neutrophil spreading and hydrogen peroxide release by blocking the shedding of CD43 (sialophorin, leukosialin). *J Cell Biol* 1993; **122**: 243–56.

62. Rhee P, Wang D, Ruff P, *et al.* Human neutrophil activation and increased adhesion by various resuscitation fluids. *Crit Care Med* 2000; **28**: 74–8.

63. Horstick G, Lauterbach M, Kempf T, *et al.* Early albumin infusion improves global and local hemodynamics and reduces inflammatory response in hemorrhagic shock. *Crit Care Med* 2002; **30**: 851–5.

64. Qiao R, Siflinger-Birnboim A, Lum H, Tiruppathi C, Malik AB. Albumin and Ricinus communis agglutinin decrease endothelial permeability via interactions with matrix. *Am J Physiol* 1993; **265**: C439–46.

65. Haraldsson B, Rippe B. Serum factors other than albumin are needed for the maintenance of normal capillary permselectivity in rat hindlimb muscle. *Acta Physiol Scand* 1985; **123**: 427–36.

66. Vogt NH, Bothner U, Lerch G, Lindner KH, Georgieff M. Large-dose administration of 6% hydroxyethyl starch 200/0.5 total hip arthroplasty: plasma homeostasis, hemostasis, and renal function compared to use of 5% human albumin. *Anesth Analg* 1996; **83**: 262–8.

67. Vogt N, Bothner U, Brinkmann A, de Petriconi R, Georgieff M. Peri-operative tolerance to large-dose 6% HES 200/0.5 in major urological procedures compared with 5% human albumin. *Anaesthesia* 1999; **54**: 121–7.

68. Rozich JD, Paul RV. Acute renal failure precipitated by elevated colloid osmotic pressure. *Am J Med* 1989; **87**: 359–60.

69. Belayev L, Busto R, Zhao W, Clemens JA, Ginsberg MD. Effect of delayed albumin hemodilution on infarction volume and brain edema after transient middle cerebral artery occlusion in rats. *J Neurosurg* 1997; **87**: 595–601.

70. Belayev L, Liu Y, Zhao W, Busto R, Ginsberg MD. Human albumin therapy of acute ischemic stroke: marked neuroprotective efficacy at moderate doses and with a broad therapeutic window. *Stroke* 2001; **32**: 553–60.

71. Delaney AP, Dan A, McCaffrey J, Finfer S. The role of albumin as a resuscitation fluid for patients with sepsis: a systematic review and meta-analysis. *Crit Care Med* 2011; **39**: 386–91.

72. Boldt J, Zickmann B, Rapin J, Hammermann H, Dapper F, Hempelmann G. Influence of volume replacement with different HES-solutions on microcirculatory blood flow in cardiac surgery. *Acta Anaesthesiol Scand* 1994; **38**: 432–8.

73. Rittoo D, Gosling P, Simms MH, Smith SR, Vohra RK. The effects of hydroxyethyl starch compared with gelofusine on activated endothelium and the systemic inflammatory response following aortic aneurysm repair. *Eur J Vasc Endovasc Surg* 2005; **30**: 520–4.

74. Feng X, Yan W, Wang Z, *et al.* Hydroxyethyl starch, but not modified fluid gelatin, affects inflammatory

response in a rat model of polymicrobial sepsis with capillary leakage. *Anesth Analg* 2007; **104**: 624–30.

75. Brandstrup B, Tonnesen H, Beier-Holgersen R, *et al.* Effects of intravenous fluid restriction on postoperative complications: comparison of two perioperative fluid regimens: a randomized assessor-blinded multicenter trial. *Ann Surg* 2003; **238**: 641–8.

76. Treib J, Baron JF, Grauer MT, Strauss RG. An international view of hydroxyethyl starches. *Intensive Care Med* 1999; **25**: 258–68.

77. Bork K. Pruritus precipitated by hydroxyethyl starch: a review. *Br J Dermatol* 2005; **152**: 3–12.

78. Niemi TT, Miyashita R, Yamakage M. Colloid solutions: a clinical update. *J Anesth* 2010; **24**: 913–25.

79. Schortgen F, Lacherade JC, Bruneel F, *et al.* Effects of hydroxyethylstarch and gelatin on renal function in severe sepsis: a multicentre randomised study. *Lancet* 2001; **357**: 911–16.

80. de Jonge E, Levi M, Buller HR, Berends F, Kesecioglu J. Decreased circulating levels of von Willebrand factor after intravenous administration of a rapidly degradable hydroxyethyl starch (HES 200/0.5/6) in healthy human subjects. *Intensive Care Med* 2001; **27**: 1825–9.

81. Omar MN, Shouk TA, Khaleq MA. Activity of blood coagulation and fibrinolysis during and after hydroxyethyl starch (HES) colloidal volume replacement. *Clin Biochem* 1999; **32**: 269–74.

82. Franz A, Braunlich P, Gamsjager T, Felfernig M, Gustorff B, Kozek-Langenecker SA. The effects of hydroxyethyl starches of varying molecular weights on platelet function. *Anesth Analg* 2001; **92**: 1402–7.

83. Westphal M, James MF, Kozek-Langenecker S, Stocker R, Guidet B, Van Aken H. Hydroxyethyl starches: different products – different effects. *Anesthesiology* 2009; **111**: 187–202.

84. Wilkes MM, Navickis RJ, Sibbald WJ. Albumin versus hydroxyethyl starch in cardiopulmonary bypass surgery: a meta-analysis of postoperative bleeding. *Ann Thorac Surg* 2001; **72**: 527–33; discussion 534.

85. Porter SS, Goldberg RJ. Intraoperative allergic reactions to hydroxyethyl starch: a report of two cases. *Can Anaesth Soc J* 1986; **33**: 394–8.

86. Huttner I, Boldt J, Haisch G, Suttner S, Kumle B, Schulz H. Influence of different colloids on molecular markers of haemostasis and platelet function in patients undergoing major abdominal surgery. *Br J Anaesth* 2000; **85**: 417–23.

87. Shippy CR, Appel PL, Shoemaker WC. Reliability of clinical monitoring to assess blood volume in critically ill patients. *Crit Care Med* 1984; **12**: 107–12.

88. Walsh SR, Tang T, Bass S, Gaunt ME. Doppler-guided intra-operative fluid management during major abdominal surgery: systematic review and meta-analysis. *Int J Clin Pract* 2008; **62**: 466–70.

89. Marik PE, Baram M, Vahid B. Does central venous pressure predict fluid responsiveness? A systematic review of the literature and the tale of seven mares. *Chest* 2008; **134**: 172–8.

90. Hollenberg SM, Ahrens TS, Annane D, *et al.* Practice parameters for hemodynamic support of sepsis in adult patients: 2004 update. *Crit Care Med* 2004; **32**: 1928–48.

91. Pinsky MR. Clinical significance of pulmonary artery occlusion pressure. *Intensive Care Med* 2003; **29**: 175–8.

92. Michard F, Teboul JL. Predicting fluid responsiveness in ICU patients: a critical analysis of the evidence. *Chest* 2002; **121**: 2000–8.

93. Marik PE. Techniques for assessment of intravascular volume in critically ill patients. *J Intensive Care Med* 2009; **24**: 329–37.

94. Vincent JL, Weil MH. Fluid challenge revisited. *Crit Care Med* 2006; **34**: 1333–7.

95. Sakka SG, Bredle DL, Reinhart K, Meier-Hellmann A. Comparison between intrathoracic blood volume and cardiac filling pressures in the early phase of hemodynamic instability of patients with sepsis or septic shock. *J Crit Care* 1999; **14**: 78–83.

96. Renner J, Scholz J, Bein B. Monitoring fluid therapy. *Best Pract Res Clin Anaesthesiol* 2009; **23**: 159–71.

97. Benington S, Ferris P, Nirmalan M. Emerging trends in minimally invasive haemodynamic monitoring and optimization of fluid therapy. *Eur J Anaesthesiol* 2009; **26**: 893–905.

98. Manecke GR, Jr., Auger WR. Cardiac output determination from the arterial pressure wave: clinical testing of a novel algorithm that does not require calibration. *J Cardiothorac Vasc Anesth* 2007; **21**: 3–7.

99. Pinsky MR. Cardiovascular issues in respiratory care. *Chest* 2005; **128**: 592S-7S.

100. Michard F, Teboul JL. Using heart-lung interactions to assess fluid responsiveness during mechanical ventilation. *Crit Care* 2000; **4**: 282–9.

101. Pizov R, Ya'ari Y, Perel A. Systolic pressure variation is greater during hemorrhage than during sodium nitroprusside-induced hypotension in ventilated dogs. *Anesth Analg* 1988; **67**: 170–4.

102. Berkenstadt H, Margalit N, Hadani M, *et al.* Stroke volume variation as a predictor of fluid responsiveness in patients undergoing brain surgery. *Anesth Analg* 2001; **92**: 984–9.

103. Reuter DA, Kirchner A, Felbinger TW, *et al.* Usefulness of left ventricular stroke volume variation to assess fluid responsiveness in patients with reduced cardiac function. *Crit Care Med* 2003; **31**: 1399–404.

104. Espersen K, Jensen EW, Rosenborg D, *et al.* Comparison of cardiac output measurement techniques: thermodilution, Doppler, CO_2-rebreathing and the direct Fick method. *Acta Anaesthesiol Scand* 1995; **39**: 245–51.

105. Chytra I, Pradl R, Bosman R, Pelnar P, Kasal E, Zidkova A. Esophageal Doppler-guided fluid management decreases blood lactate levels in multiple-trauma patients: a randomized controlled trial. *Crit Care* 2007; **11**: R24.

106. Biais M, Bernard O, Ha JC, Degryse C, Sztark F. Abilities of pulse pressure variations and stroke volume variations to predict fluid responsiveness in prone position during scoliosis surgery. *Br J Anaesth* 2010; **104**: 407–13.

Chapter

3

Blood conservation

Robert Helfand

Key points

- All blood conservation techniques work better with higher preoperative hemoglobin concentrations.
- ESA should be used with caution in spine surgery due to increased risk of DVT.
- Antifibrinolytic therapy is an underutilized technique.
- Cell savers are key elements of blood conservation programs.
- Blood conservation requires multidisciplinary involvement.

Blood management during spine surgery remains a challenge. Perioperative blood administration is expensive, and exposes the recipient to a number of risks. A number of methods are available to decrease the need to administer blood during the perioperative period (Table 3.1). We will discuss the current techniques and controversies with the goal of lessening the patient's exposure to blood transfusions.

The spectrum of blood component-related complications has changed significantly in the last few years. Enhanced technology has allowed for better screening of donated blood units with a dramatic decrease in many infectious complications. Estimates of viral transmission in the blood donor system range from 1:205 000 for hepatitis B to 1:2 135 000 for HIV.[1] Extremely sensitive nucleotide screening systems have led to remarkable gains in the safety of administration of allogeneic blood units.

We now recognize that there are other transfusion risks that are far greater problems than the previously feared viral infections. The West Nile Virus demonstrated that new, emerging threats remain ongoing problems. Bacterial contaminations, particularly with platelet products, have now attracted new attention and

Table 3.1 Methods of blood conservation in spine surgery

Preoperative optimization of hemoglobin levels
Preoperative autodonation
Antifibrinolytic therapy
Acute normovolemic hemodilution
Intraoperative cell salvage
Point of care testing of coagulation

new efforts at mitigation. Immunologic complications have now taken a more key role in the complication profile of transfusions. Transfusion-associated acute lung injury (TRALI) is now recognized as a major complication of transfusions. Increased duration of blood storage has been suggested as a source of poor outcomes in cardiac surgery.[2] Even autologous blood can suffer from clerical errors or infectious complications (see Table 3.2). The only way to eliminate transfusion-related complications is to lessen a patient's exposure to transfusions.

The remarkable safety of blood administration has come at a considerable cost. Each additional screening test drives up the cost of each unit of blood products. Restrictions on who can donate limit our pool of candidates. In an era of sicker patients facing more complex surgery, we now face an increasingly limited, expensive, risk-laden resource.

One of the most common questions is "what does blood cost?". Unfortunately, the answer is not straightforward. Shander *et al.* looked at this question at an American and several European sites.[3] Cost estimates ranged from $522 to $1183 dollars per unit of blood. Costs for additional blood products are also considerable and difficult to estimate. A successful blood conservation program would have to show a decrease in transfusions, better patient outcomes, and overall lower costs. Given the complexity of measuring each cost, blood conservation becomes part of the increasingly complex health care accounting and must prove its success.

Anesthesia for Spine Surgery, ed. Ehab Farag. Published by Cambridge University Press. © Cambridge University Press 2012.

Table 3.2 Potential transfusion risks by type[a]

Type	Potential transfusion risk
Infectious	Viral: hepatitis A, B, C, E, G; HIV, HTLV-I, HTLV-II, cytomegalovirus, Epstein–Barr virus, parvovirus B19
	Bacterial
	Variant Creutzfeldt–Jakob disease[b]
	Parasitic: malaria, babesiosis, Chagas' disease
	Risk of viral contamination with viruses not yet screened for
Noninfectious	Hemolytic transfusion reactions
	Transfusion errors leading to blood type incompatibility reactions
	Febrile nonhemolytic transfusion reactions
	Anaphylaxis and urticarial allergic reactions
	Posttransfusion purpura
	Risks of old blood vs. fresh blood (e.g., microcirculatory occlusion, lack of effect)
	Transfusion-related acute lung injury
	Circulatory overload
	Iron overload
	Air embolism
	Fat embolism (intraoperative administration of salvaged blood)
	Hypotensive reactions (with ACE inhibitors negatively charged leukoreduction filters)
	Metabolic disturbances: citrate toxicity, hypocalcemia, hyperkalemia, acidosis, and hyperammonemia
	Hypothermia
Immunologic	Multiple organ dysfunction syndrome or multiple organ failure attributed to cytokine release
	Postoperative infection
	Transfusion-associated sepsis
	Increased risk of cancer recurrence
	Downregulation of macrophage and T-cell function
	Alloimmunization: HLA, especially in patients undergoing chronic transfusion
	Transfusion-associated graft versus host disease in immunocompromised and nonimmunocompromised hosts

HIV = human immunodeficiency virus; HTLV = human T cell lymphoma virus; ACE = angiotensin-converting enzyme; HLA = human leukocyte antigen.

[a] This table presents a broad sampling of potential risks from transfusion of blood products; neither is it all-inclusive nor is it intended to imply that causality has been proved. Because of limitations in the number of references that can be cited, those associated with this information are available on request to the corresponding author.

[b] Classic Creutzfeldt–Jakob disease is probably not transmissible through blood products.

Reprinted with permission from reference 16: Shander A and Goodnough LT, Update on transfusion medicine. *Pharmacotherapy* 2007;27(9 Pt2):57S–68S.)

Predicting which patients are appropriate for aggressive blood conservation measures is also crucial for successful blood management. Just as transfusion has its costs and limitations, not every patient should receive the same level of conservation techniques. Current evidence supports several factors that predict the need for transfusion in adult spine surgery: advanced age, preoperative anemia, osteotomy, and fusion. These have been confirmed by Lenoir *et al.* with their predictive model of transfusion in spine surgery.[4] It is these patients and procedures that will be the best targets for blood-conserving interventions.

Preoperative measures

All blood conservation methods work better with patients who have higher hemoglobin concentrations. However, the estimates of anemic patients presenting for major surgery range from 5% to 75.8%. In patients presenting for total hip, knee, or hip fracture surgery anemia rates ranged from 24% to 44%.[5] Lower preoperative hemoglobin correlates with increased transfusion requirements. While there are a great range of patients presenting for spine surgery, undoubtedly a sizable number will be anemic. Correction of preoperative anemia is the first step in blood management.

Figure 3.1 shows a targeted anemia work-up for preoperative patients. This focused evaluation should be done as soon as it is identified that a patient for a major blood loss surgery is anemic. Most preoperative anemia is a combination of nutritional deficiencies and ongoing chronic inflammation. Therefore it is unlikely that a single treatment will consistently treat the majority of patients.

In the absence of a specifically identified reason for the anemia, the common treatment approaches involve supplementation with iron and administration of erythropoietic stimulating agents (ESAs). Iron supplementation is needed frequently even with seemingly normal iron stores. Chronic inflammatory conditions limit the body's ability to mobilize iron from storage sites. This functional iron deficiency can be overcome by pharmacologic iron administration. Figure 3.2 shows a targeted preoperative anemia treatment protocol.

Oral iron is poorly tolerated in most patients. Therefore, while it seems simple to administer PO iron, the limited absorption from the GI tract as well as the common occurrence of significant side effects limits the effectiveness of this treatment. Intravenous iron supplementation is much more effective, but requires considerable additional resources to administer safely. Currently there are five parenteral iron compounds available. Iron dextran is available in both high- and low-molecular weight compounds. The high-molecular weight version has a poor safety record with a high risk of anaphylaxis. The advantage of this preparation is the ability to administer a large dose of iron in one sitting. The other preparations, low-molecular weight iron dextran, iron sucrose, ferric gluconate, and ferumoxytol have at least a 10-fold lower risk of serious allergic reactions. These preparations are generally well tolerated but require multiple dosings due to the more rapid iron release and lower dose that can be administered in one sitting.[6]

ESAs are commonly used to prepare anemic orthopedic patients for major surgery. More recently it has been appreciated that these agents increase the perioperative risk of deep venous thrombosis (DVT). The FDA published an advisory warning against the use of these drugs in surgical patients who cannot receive pharmacologic DVT prophylaxis.[7] Most spine patients are not candidates for pharmacologic DVT prophylaxis due to the risk of postoperative epidural hematoma formation. Therefore, the use of ESA for the preparation of anemic spine patients needs to be viewed with extreme caution.

The safest overall preoperative preparatory regimen for spine surgery is intravenous iron supplementation.

If hemoglobin is less than 10 gm/dl, then obtain a standard anemia work-up

Iron and TIBC, T_{sat}
Ferritin
Reticulocyte count
Vitamin B_{12}, if borderline low–normal then MMA
Folic acid, if borderline low–normal then RBC folate+/– homocysteine
RBC smear

Figure 3.1 Preoperative anemia evaluation.

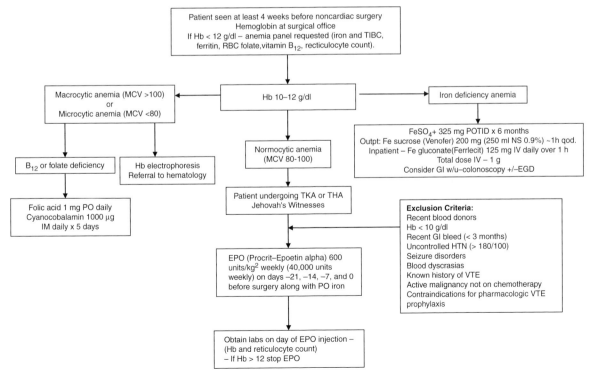

Figure 3.2 Targeted preoperative anemia treatment protocol.

In 7–14 days, irons stores can be replenished such that effective erythropoiesis can correct preoperative anemia. Since most spine procedures are elective in nature, many patients are candidates for this treatment.

Antifibrinolytic treatments

ε-Aminocaproic acid (Eaca) and tranexamic acid (TXA) are two lysine analogs that are inexpensive and safe agents to decrease perioperative blood loss in spine surgery. Aprotinin is no longer available after reports of excessive renal failure in cardiac surgery[8] and will not be further discussed. Antifibrinolytic agents act to mitigate the increased fibrinolysis frequently seen during surgery. Both agents prevent the conversion of plasminogen to plasmin and also directly inhibit plasmin's ability to degrade fibrinogen.

Both drugs are administered intravenously as a continuous infusion during surgery due to their rapid renal excretion. TXA is 6–10 times more potent than Eaca and is administered in a correspondingly lower dose. Typical protocols are:[9]

Eaca loading dose 100–150 mg/kg, infusion 10–15 mg/kg/h.

TXA loading dose 10 mg/kg, infusion 1 mg/kg/h.

Antifibrinolytic treatment has been studied in both pediatric and adult spine surgery.[10] Both have demonstrated efficacy in decreasing intraoperative, postoperative, and transfusion requirements in complex spine surgery. Excessive thrombosis has not been a major finding in most trials to date. Therefore the use of lysine analogs represents a safe, low-cost, easy means of lowering perioperative blood loss and transfusion in spine surgery.

Recombinant activated factor VII

The off-label use of recombinant activated factor VII to control bleeding in a wide variety of settings (trauma, intracranial hemorrhage, surgery, bleeding in the setting of anticoagulant therapy) is quite common. This drug can activate the coagulation system directly, bypassing many of the early steps in the clotting cascade. Anecdotal use and small series describe successful control of bleeding when other usual methods have failed. However, its use in spine surgery is largely unexplored. Only one phase IIa study has been published on safety in spine surgery.[11] This trial reported nonsignificant differences in blood loss and transfusion volume. A recent analysis of the off-label uses of this agent highlights the small but significant increased risk of arterial thrombosis in those receiving the drug.[12] Therefore there is no current indication for this drug unless all reasonable means of controlling hemorrhage have been exhausted, and then this is at the risk of potentially devastating arterial thrombotic events.

Preoperative autodonation

Preoperative autodonation (PAD) enjoyed great interest in the late 1980s and early 1990s. Currently, it is a technique that has a much more limited benefit. While the emotional appeal of storing blood for the patient's own use is considerable, many problems exist. First, without supplemental agents, patients will not replace the donated red cells adequately. The result is that the patient will likely become anemic and therefore would be more likely to need transfusions. Transfusing back their donated red cells will expose the patient to a risk of clerical error. Stored red cells, whether autologous or not, do not transport oxygen normally. PAD is not free, and can be inconvenient for the patient. The platelets and plasma are discarded and usually about half the units are discarded. As the safety of allogeneic blood has increased, the utility of PAD has decreased considerably.

Acute normovolemic hemodilution

Acute normovolemic hemodilution (ANH) is in principle a very simple and elegant approach to red cell conservation as well as sequestration of platelets and plasma. Before surgery, blood is drained into blood bags containing a citrate anticoagulant while asanguinous fluid is administered to maintain circulating intravascular volume. As a result, during surgery the patient will lose blood during surgery that contains fewer red cells. When the bleeding has stopped, the stored whole blood is re-administered. This whole blood contains red cells, platelets, and plasma. Since the blood is otherwise not processed and is stored in the operating room in immediate proximity to the patient, issues of clerical error and storage problems are eliminated. Cost is minimal, although the collection of the blood needs good vascular access and some time. The key questions are how low to take the hemoglobin and how much blood can be saved. The more aggressively you withdraw blood, the more likely you are to be successful, but at the risk of exposing a patient to lower red cell levels than they may be able to tolerate.[13]

As with other blood-conservation strategies, ANH only works well if the patient has a normal starting hemoglobin. Withdrawal of anemic blood results in storage of relatively fewer red cells and leaves the patient with a low hemoglobin level. This will result in the need to transfuse the stored blood relatively soon, largely negating any benefit of the effort to store the blood. Since blood loss in spine surgery is rarely in sudden, large volumes, ANH can be an effective technique to minimize the spine surgery patient's exposure to allogeneic blood.

Intraoperative red cell salvage

The mainstay of most blood conservation programs in the use of intraoperative cell salvage, commonly referred to as cell savers. A cell saver is a system consisting of a means to collect shed intraoperative blood, store it until enough has been collected to process, and then concentrate and wash the salvaged material so that a clean, safe product can be returned to the patient.

Initially the shed blood is removed with special surgical suction devices. The vacuum tubing has a channel to immediately mix the shed blood with an anticoagulant, generally either heparin or citrate. The vacuum level must be regulated to lessen the physical trauma and resultant hemolysis. This frequently results in objections from the surgical team about the effectiveness of the suction systems. Suctioning is also best done in a manner that removes the liquid from pools with less entrainment of air, also to lessen the resultant red cell trauma. The recovered blood is filtered upon entry to the storage canister to remove large contaminants. The shed blood is stored in the reservoirs until sufficient material is available to process in the centrifuge. The storage time should be monitored subject to reasonable times set forth by blood banking policies.

The centrifuge bowls are specifically designed to allow the heaviest elements, the red cells to collect in the bottom of the bowl. Shed blood is pumped into the spinning bowl until a sufficient volume of packed red cells forms and is usually detected by a photo eye on the device. Once the bowl is full, saline is pumped through the red cell pack to wash out residual debris and proteins so that the resultant product contains concentrated red cells suspended in saline. See Fig. 3.3.

Typically for spine surgery, a small or medium-sized bowl is chosen so that the blood can be processed at reasonable time intervals. Fill and wash protocols are chosen that typically fill the bowl slowly so that less material is lost due to too rapid filling, and slow washing with large volumes of wash saline is chosen to remove as much bone debris and fat as reasonable.

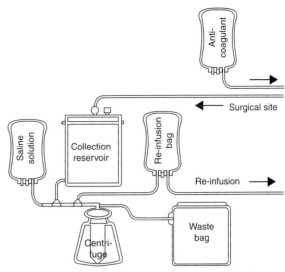

Figure 3.3 Schematic of a cell saver system. From Noblood.org

The efficiency of cell salvage is limited, especially during spine surgery. If surgical sponges are used to dry the field, these should be soaked in saline and the blood-contaminated saline suctioned into the cell saver reservoir. Also the suctioning should be done to minimize air entrapment. Despite the most meticulous efforts at cell salvage, typically only 60–70% of the lost blood can be returned. Operations with large amounts of blood loss will ultimately need allogeneic red cells to prevent anemia, even with meticulous cell salvage.

Cell savers should not be used when material that should not be administered systemically is given in the wound. Cell savers should not be used when the wound is irrigated with antibiotics that are not supposed to be systemically administered. During these times, discard suction should be used. Also, cells savers should not be used when topical hemostatic agents have been used. If these materials are administered systemically through the cells saver, disseminated intravascular coagulation can result.

Cell salvage in controversial in several areas, the most commonly sited being cancer surgeries and bacterial infections.[14] Cell salvage in cancer surgery exposes the patient to the possibility of returning viable cancer cells to the circulation from the re-administration of salvaged blood. There is little proof that these transfused cancer cells will inevitably produce hematogenous spread of the cancer. Furthermore, there is some suggestion that transfusion of allogeneic blood may worsen the prognosis in cancer patients. Therefore some centers have decided that it is reasonable to administered salvaged intraoperative blood from

47

cancer surgeries, particularly if techniques are used to decrease the burden of cancer cells. The two techniques are the use of leukodepletion filters to remove a burden of the cancer cells or irradiation of the salvaged blood prior to re-infusion.

Similar arguments can be made for the use of cell savers in operations with bacterial contamination. The physical process of aggressive cell washing as well as the use of leukodepletion filters may allow for the re-infusing of all but the most contaminated of shed blood. Most of these patients are receiving systemic antibiotics that can also lessen the chance of disseminating the infectious elements. Since allogeneic blood can be immunosuppressive in its own right, lessening the patient's exposure by using cell savers, even in controversial areas, may improve the patient's outcome.

A final use of the cell saver is to acutely fractionate the patient's blood into its elements in the OR. Some cell savers have protocols that allow for the collection of red cells, plasma, and platelets. Depending on the anticipated need in the surgery, for example the need for platelets and plasma, the patient's blood can either be collected and centrifuged or directly drawn into the centrifuge and the desired elements separated. This process is more complicated than ANH, but allows the team to collect the elements most needed for the specific surgery.

Postoperative cell salvage

Some surgeons leave drains in place after certain surgeries. It is very tempting to re-administer this wound drainage as a means of supplementing the patient's red cells. Unfortunately, there are several issues with administration of wound drainage. This material has a hematocrit typically less than 15%. Therefore, a large volume of wound drainage will need to be administered before any significant amount of blood is given back to the patient. Direct so-called "flip and drip" type systems administer this fluid to the patient without any processing.[15] The wound drainage contains a large number of inflammatory mediators that should not be administered systemically in an ideal world. There are commercial systems that can collect and wash this material prior to administration. Whether it is cost effective given the low yields needs to be considered.

Point of care testing

The management of intraoperative coagulation disorders during spine surgery can have a large impact on control of bleeding and the quantity of blood products utilized. Frequently empirical methods are employed with unclear end points. Laboratory testing such as PT/INR, PTT, fibrinogen, and platelet counts can be helpful but frequently involves considerable delay. Quantitative measurement of intraoperative coagulation can provide a better guide as to the type of coagulation disorder and the required treatment. Techniques of viscoelastic monitoring of coagulation can be done in the operating room and provide more defined diagnosis of the clotting disorder.

There are two main technologies for measuring intraoperative clotting: the Sonoclot® (Sienco, Inc.) and the Thromboelastogram TEG® (Haemoscope Corp.) or a similar technique called ROTEM® (Rotem, Inc.). Both techniques follow the in vitro rheologic changes in blood during the coagulation process. Characteristic changes can be seen that can diagnose clotting factor depletion, hypofibrinogenemia, thrombocytopenia, fibrinolysis, and anticoagulant administration. Specific therapy can be administered based on the characteristic findings.

These methods are all moderately complex point of care testing systems. This requires an infrastructure of qualified personnel, and comprehensive quality control systems for test validation. Most clinical literature exists in the cardiac surgery arena.[17] There is comparatively little literature to support the use of these techniques in spine surgery.[18] Viscoelastic measurement of coagulation is a potentially useful but is currently a poorly validated point of care testing method for spine surgery.

Quality management

Blood banks adhere to strict procedures to ensure the best outcomes from transfusions. Many of the blood conservation techniques in spine surgery interface closely with the blood banking system. Therefore, quality assurance mechanisms frequently derived from blood bank techniques should be used to monitor blood conservation methods. Suggestions include monitoring the quality of cell saver products and watching for complications from other techniques. Transfusions have significant risks and, likewise, haphazard use of blood conservation may be harmful to patients.

Summary

Spine surgery patients frequently need transfusions. Effective blood conservation starts by making sure that most patients are not anemic when they start surgery. The risk of DVT with preoperative administration of ESA needs to be considered. ANH can be used for patients who can tolerate the acute volume shifts and the forced anemia that is incumbent for appropriate use. Antifibrinolytic agents can be used safely for many patients. Intraoperative cell salvage is a cornerstone for most blood conservation programs.

References

1. Centers for Disease Control and Prevention (CDC). HIV transmission through transfusion – Missouri and Colorado, 2008. *MMWR Morb Mortal Wkly Rep* 2010 Oct 22; **59**(41): 1335–9.

2. Koch CG, Li L, Sessler DI, *et al.* Duration of red-cell storage and complications after cardiac surgery. *N Engl J Med* 2008 Mar 20; **358**(12): 1229–39.

3. Shander A, Hofmann A, Ozawa S, *et al.* Activity-based costs of blood transfusions in surgical patients at four hospitals. *Transfusion* 2010 Apr; **50**(4): 753–65.

4. Lenoir B, Merckx P, Paugam-Burtz C, *et al.* Individual probability of allogeneic erythrocyte transfusion in elective spine surgery: the predictive model of transfusion in spine surgery. *Anesthesiology* 2009 May; **110**(5): 1050–60.

5. Spahn DR. Anemia and patient blood management in hip and knee surgery: a systematic review of the literature. *Anesthesiology.* 2010 Aug; **113**(2): 482–95.

6. Auerbach M, Goodnough LT, Picard D, Maniatis A. The role of intravenous iron in anemia management and transfusion avoidance. *Transfusion* 2008 May; **48**(5): 988–1000.

7. Shander A, Spence RK, Auerbach M. Can intravenous iron therapy meet the unmet needs created by the new restrictions on erythropoietic stimulating agents? *Transfusion* 2010 Mar; **50**(3): 719–32.

8. Mangano DT, Tudor IC, Dietzel C; Multicenter Study of Perioperative Ischemia Research Group; Ischemia

Research and Education Foundation. The risk associated with aprotinin in cardiac surgery. *N Engl J Med* 2006 Jan 26; **354**(4): 353–65.

9. Eubanks JD. Antifibrinolytics in major orthopaedic surgery. *J Am Acad Orthop Surg* 2010 Mar; **18**(3): 132–8.

10. Henry DA, Carless PA, Moxey AJ, *et al.* Anti-fibrinolytic use for minimising perioperative allogeneic blood transfusion. *Cochrane Database Syst Rev* 2007 Oct 17; (4): CD001886.

11. Sachs B, Delacy D, Green J, *et al.* Recombinant activated factor VII in spinal surgery: a multicenter, randomized, double-blind, placebo-controlled, dose-escalation trial. *Spine (Phila Pa 1976)* 2007 Oct 1; **32**(21): 2285–93.

12. Levi M, Levy JH, Andersen HF, Truloff D. Safety of recombinant activated factor VII in randomized clinical trials. *N Engl J Med* 2010 Nov 4; **363**(19): 1791–800.

13. Shander A, Perelman S. The long and winding road of acute normovolemic hemodilution. *Transfusion* 2006 Jul; **46**(7): 1075–9.

14. Waters JH. Indications and contraindications of cell salvage. *Transfusion* 2004 Dec; **44**(12 Suppl): 40S-4S.

15. Hansen E, Hansen M. Reasons against the retransfusion of unwashed wound blood. *Transfusion* 2004 Dec; **44**(12 Suppl): 45S–53S.

16. Shander A, Goodnough, LT. Update on transfusion medicine. *Pharmacotherapy* 2007 Sep; **27**(9 Pt 2): 57S–68S.

17. Shore-Lesserson L, Manspeizer HE, DePerio M, *et al.* Thromboelastography-guided transfusion algorithm reduces transfusions in complex cardiac surgery. *Anesth Analg* 1999; **88**: 312–19.

18. Horlocker TT, Nuttall GA, Dekutoski MB, Bryant SC. The accuracy of coagulation tests during spinal fusion and instrumentation. *Anesth Analg.* 2001 Jul; **93**(1): 33–8.

Airway management in spine surgery

Basem Abdelmalak and D. John Doyle

Key points

- Flexible fiberoptic bronchoscope is the device of choice for many clinicians for unstable neck or difficult airway management in spine surgery, because this technique is associated with minimal movement of the cervical spine in comparison with other methods.
- While many clinicians fear untoward consequences from cervical spine movement during intubation in the setting of an unstable neck, these movements are typically small, and the clinical implications of such a degree of cervical spine movement are not well established.
- When anesthesiologists in the United States and Canada were surveyed regarding their preference in airway management of patients with cervical spine disease, *awake* flexible fiberoptic intubation was the first choice.
- Caution should be exercised with the use of succinylcholine in patients with trauma to the spine, especially those with neurologic symptoms from spinal cord injury.
- Edema and hematoma formation may sometimes make extubation risky following cervical spine surgery.
- Every effort should be made to prevent inadvertent extubation during spine surgery, especially in the prone position. Inserting a supraglottic airway can be a quick temporizing measure in these situations.

Introduction

This chapter deals with clinical airway management in the context of spine surgery. However, although the focus is on spine surgery, many of the principles discussed here also apply to clinical airway management in general, regardless of the surgical procedure. In particular, the American Society of Anesthesiologists Difficult Airway Algorithm, briefly outlined in this chapter and shown in Fig. 4.1 should be an important starting point for all aspects of clinical airway management.

To a large extent, the airway management technique employed for anesthesia for spine surgery will depend on clinical circumstances as well as on the airway management skills of the anesthesiologist. Three options are employed: (1) general endotracheal anesthesia; (2) general anesthesia using a supraglottic airway device such as a laryngeal mask airway; and (3) neuraxial anesthesia, for instance, spinal anesthesia. The first option is undoubtedly the most preferred.

Tracheal intubation in patients undergoing spine surgery

Most patients undergoing spine surgery have their airway managed via tracheal intubation, especially if they are undergoing surgery in the prone position. Under ordinary circumstances, tracheal intubation is straightforward; therefore, ordinary laryngoscopic techniques work well. However, patients are occasionally encountered who are potentially difficult to intubate, and these patients are usually managed using video laryngoscopy or flexible fiberoptic intubation. Three key decisions must be made in such cases. The first concerns whether intubation should be carried out awake or following the induction of general anesthesia (Fig. 4.1). The second concerns the tools to employ if difficulty is encountered with ventilation or with intubation (Table 4.1). Finally, there is the question of how to manage a patient with an unstable cervical spine – a vital issue that will be discussed later in the chapter.

The trachea of a patient in the supine position is often intubated with an ordinary polyvinylchloride

Anesthesia for Spine Surgery, ed. Ehab Farag. Published by Cambridge University Press. © Cambridge University Press 2012.

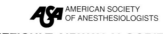

AMERICAN SOCIETY OF ANESTHESIOLOGISTS

DIFFICULT AIRWAY ALGORITHM

1. Assess the likelihood and clinical impact of basic management problems:
   - A. Difficult Ventilation
   - B. Difficult Intubation
   - C. Difficulty with Patient Cooperation or Consent
   - D. Difficult Tracheostomy

2. Actively pursue opportunities to deliver supplemental oxygen throughout the process of difficult airway management

3. Consider the relative merits and feasibility of basic management choices:

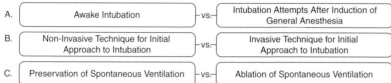

A. Awake Intubation —vs.— Intubation Attempts After Induction of General Anesthesia

B. Non-Invasive Technique for Initial Approach to Intubation —vs.— Invasive Technique for Initial Approach to Intubation

C. Preservation of Spontaneous Ventilation —vs.— Ablation of Spontaneous Ventilation

4. Develop primary and alternative strategies:

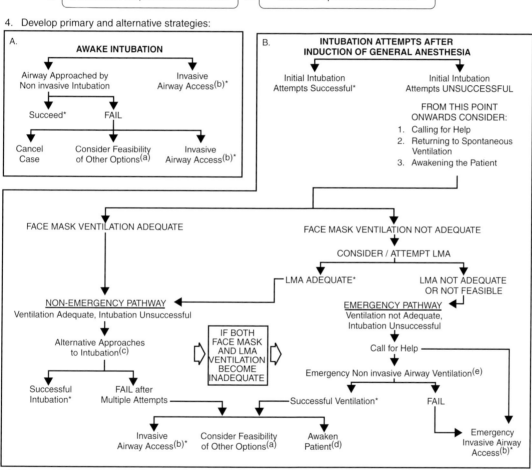

* Confirm ventilation, tracheal intubation, or LMA placement with exhaled CO_2

a. Other options include (but are not limited to): surgery utilizing face mask or LMA anesthesia, local anesthesia infiltration or regional nerve blockade. Pursuit of these options usually implies that mask ventilation will not be problematic. Therefore, these options may be of limited value if this step in the algorithm has been reached via the Emergency Pathway.

b. Invasive airway access includes surgical or percutaneous tracheostomy or cricothyrotomy.

c. Alternative non-invasive approaches to difficult intubation include (but are not limited to): use of different laryngoscope blades, LMA as an intubation conduit (with or without fiberoptic guidance), fiberoptic intubation, intubating stylet or tube changer, light wand, retrograde intubation, and blind oral or nasal intubation.

d. Consider re-preparation of the patient for awake intubation or canceling surgery.

e. Options for emergency non-invasive airway ventilation include (but are not limited to): rigid bronchoscope, esophageal-tracheal combitube ventilation, or transtracheal jet ventilation.

Figure 4.1 Synopsis of the 2003 ASA difficult airway algorithm. It is expected that future editions of the algorithm will place special emphasis on the use of video laryngoscopy for situations in which direct laryngoscopy produces an unsatisfactory view of the glottic structures.

Table 4.1 Techniques for difficult airway management
This table, from the 2003 ASA difficult airway algorithm, lists some commonly cited techniques. Since the time of publication, the use of video laryngoscopy (e.g., GlideScope, McGrath video laryngoscope, Storz video laryngoscope, Pentax AWS) has become commonplace and therefore belongs to the left-hand column. Naturally, the tools used in any particular situation will depend on the specific circumstances.

Techniques for difficult intubation	Techniques for difficult ventilation
Alternative laryngoscope blades	Esophageal tracheal Combitube®
Awake intubation	Intratracheal jet stylet
Blind intubation (oral or nasal)	Invasive airway access
Fiberoptic intubation	Laryngeal mask airway (LMA)
Intubating stylet or tube changer	Oral and nasopharyngeal airways
Intubation via LMA	Rigid ventilating bronchoscope
Invasive airway access	Transtracheal jet ventilation
Light wand	Two-person mask ventilation
Retrograde intubation	

(PVC) endotracheal tube. Three precautions are required here: the tube should be firmly secured with tape or other means; the tube tip should not be too close to the carina (or worse, positioned endobronchially); and the tube should be situated so that kinking is unlikely to occur with head movement. Many anesthesiologists employ wire-reinforced endotracheal tubes for spine cases, especially for patients in the prone position. The principal advantage of such tubes is that they are unlikely to kink. Finally, it is important that cuff pressures in the endotracheal tube be maintained under 25 cmH$_2$O to avoid damage to the tracheal mucosa.

Role of the ASA Difficult Airway Algorithm

The American Society of Anesthesiologists (ASA) has issued guidelines for management of the difficult airway. The guidelines began with an algorithm originally published in 1993,[1] followed by a revision in 2003.[2] These guidelines, as well as similar guidelines from other organizations,[3,4] offer considerable advice to the clinician facing potentially difficult airway challenges. The advice emphasizes, for example: (1) the importance of performing an airway evaluation prior to inducing anesthesia; (2) the importance of providing oxygen at every opportunity; (3) the potential value of awake intubation; and (4) the value of supraglottic airway devices such as the laryngeal mask airway (LMA) as a possible airway rescue maneuver, if failure should occur. Figure 4.1 summarizes the 2003 ASA Difficult Airway Algorithm.

Prediction of intubation difficulty: intubation difficulty scale

Before attempting tracheal intubation it is very helpful for the anesthesiologist to have a means of predicting which patients may have airways difficult to intubate with direct laryngoscopy. While a number of studies and reviews on the topic are available,[5–8] most clinicians will be satisfied with the 11-point airway assessment tool included in the 2003 ASA Difficult Airway Algorithm. This tool is summarized in Table 4.2. In addition, after completion of tracheal intubation, it can sometimes be helpful for the anesthesiologist to describe any difficulties that might have occurred. Here, the Intubation Difficulty Scale (IDS) introduced by Adnet and colleagues[9] can be useful. It is a numerical score indicating overall intubation difficulty based on seven descriptors associated with difficulty of intubation: (1) number of supplementary intubation attempts; (2) number of supplementary operators; (3) alternative techniques used; (4) laryngoscopic grade; (5) subjective lifting force; (6) the use of external laryngeal manipulation; and (7) the characteristics of the vocal cords.

Laryngoscopes

Most intubations for spine surgery are performed using traditional Macintosh and Miller laryngoscopes. When the view at laryngoscopy is suboptimal, the use of introducers such as the Eschmann stylet ("gum elastic bougie") can sometimes be very helpful. It is used as follows. When a poor laryngoscopic view of the glottic

Table 4.2 Components of the preoperative airway physical examination as recommended in the ASA Difficult Airway Algorithm (2003 edition)
In ordinary clinical practice, special emphasis is usually placed on the visibility of the oropharyngeal structures with the tongue protruded when the patient is in the sitting position (Mallampati classification).

Airway examination component	Nonreassuring findings
1. Length of upper incisors	Relatively long
2. Relation of maxillary and mandibular incisors during normal jaw closure	Prominent "overbite" (maxillary incisors anterior to mandibular incisors)
3. Relation of maxillary and mandibular incisors during voluntary protrusion of mandible	Patient cannot bring mandibular incisors anterior to (in front of) maxillary incisors
4. Interincisor distance	Under 3 cm
5. Visibility of uvula	Not visible when tongue is protruded with patient in sitting position (e.g., Mallampati class greater than II)
6. Shape of palate	Highly arched or very narrow
7. Compliance of mandibular space	Stiff, indurated, occupied by mass, or nonresilient
8. Thyromental distance	Less than 3 ordinary finger breadths
9. Length of neck	Short
10. Thickness of neck	Thick
11. Range of motion of head and neck	Patient cannot touch tip of chin to chest or cannot extend neck

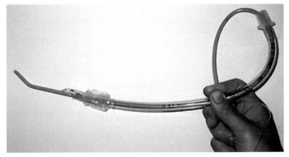

Figure 4.2 Photograph showing a tracheal tube with a preloaded introducer containing a Coudé tip. Intended for situations where the laryngoscopic view is suboptimal, the upturned distal Coudé tip is placed under the epiglottis or, if visible, above the interarytenoid notch, followed by advancement of the tracheal tube into the trachea.

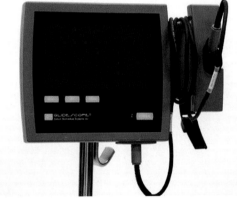

Figure 4.3 The GlideScope video laryngoscope utilizes a color CMOS video camera and LED light source embedded into a plastic laryngoscope blade. The standard (adult) blade is 14.5 mm at its maximum width, and bends 60° at the midline. This configuration provides a view that is frequently superior to that obtained by direct laryngoscopy. The video image is displayed on a liquid crystal display (LCD) monitor, and can also be recorded electronically. An anti-fog mechanism helps ensure that a high-quality image is obtained. In addition to the standard blade, a mid-sized (pediatric) blade and a neonatal blade are also available.

structures is evident, the intubator places the introducer into the patient's mouth and gently advances it through the glottic opening (in the case of a grade II view) or anteriorly under the epiglottis (in the case of a grade III view). Clicks resulting from the introducer passing over the tracheal rings help confirm proper placement of the introducer. With the introducer held steady, one then railroads a tracheal tube over the introducer into the glottis.[10] Some clinicians preload a tracheal tube onto the introducer, as shown in Fig. 4.2.

Special devices such as the McCoy laryngoscope and the Bullard laryngoscope are also popular in some centers. In recent years, however, video laryngoscopes such as the GlideScope, the McGrath video laryngoscope, the Storz video laryngoscope, and the Pentax-AWS have proved to be particularly valuable, especially in patients with an "anterior" larynx or in patients with cervical spine immobilization. Among the available video laryngoscopes, the GlideScope (Fig. 4.3) has the largest market share. Figure 4.4 shows a typical view of the glottis during intubation with the GlideScope.

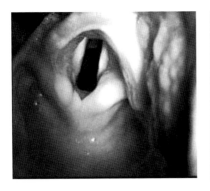
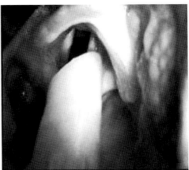
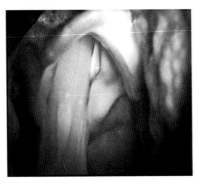
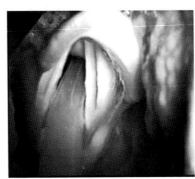

Figure 4.4 Close-up views from the GlideScope, as the endotracheal tube (ETT) passes through the vocal cords. Note that during ETT placement the tube tip often tends to hit against the anterior tracheal wall. This problem is easily solved by pulling back the stylet by about 3 cm and then advancing the ETT. Sometimes it also helps to rotate the ETT 180° to direct the ETT tip more posteriorly (once the stylet has been removed).

Tracheal intubation in patients with cervical spine instability

In patients with confirmed or suspected instability of the cervical spine, special precautions are needed to minimize the likelihood that laryngoscopy and intubation might result in neurologic injury. Airway management in such patients presents an anesthetic challenge; and, for decades, clinicians have debated the safest technique and/or device for securing the airways of these patients. They have usually focused on the association between a particular airway management technique and the degree of neck movement at a given cervical spine location.

In a randomized, controlled, crossover study in cadavers with a posteriorly destabilized third cervical (C3) vertebra, investigators sought to determine the degree of cervical spine motion for six airway management techniques when manual in-line stabilization was applied. They compared face mask ventilation, direct laryngoscopic orotracheal intubation, flexible fiberoptic nasal intubation, use of the Combitube® (Kendall-Sheridan, Neustadt, Germany), use of the intubating laryngeal mask in conjunction with flexible fiberscope-guided tracheal intubation, and laryngeal mask airway (LMA) insertion. The investigators concluded that the

safest method of airway management based on movement criteria was the flexible fiberoptic technique.[11]

In another study the Bullard laryngoscope caused less cervical spine extension than Macintosh and Miller laryngoscopes and resulted in a better view when studied in healthy patients.[12] The Bullard laryngoscope also performed better than the Macintosh laryngoscope, resulting in less neck movement when in the setting of in-line stabilization.[13]

In another study in healthy patients under general anesthesia, investigators compared the Pentax-AWS, the Macintosh laryngoscope, and the McCoy laryngoscope with respect to movement of the upper cervical spine during intubation. The Pentax-AWS produced less movement of the upper cervical spine than did the Macintosh or McCoy laryngoscopes.[14]

When mask ventilation was compared to use of a Macintosh #3 laryngoscope, GlideScope, and use of a lighted stylet with respect to cervical spine movement at the occiput–C1 junction, the C1–2 junction, the C2–5 region, and C5 thoracic region, motion during bag-mask ventilation and lighted stylet intubation was 82% and 52% less, respectively, at the four regions of interest than during Macintosh laryngoscopy. In addition, cervical spine motion was reduced 50% at the C2–5 region with the GlideScope as opposed to direct laryngoscopy but

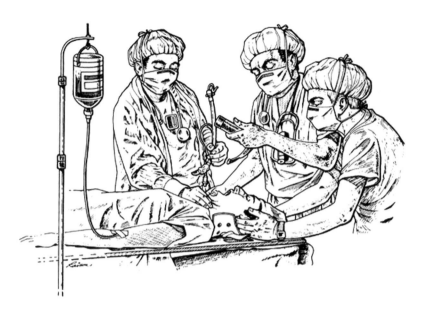

Figure 4.5 Illustration of in-line stabilization (*not* in-line traction!) during laryngoscopy and intubation in a patient with a suspected cervical spine injury. Note also (where appropriate) the application of cricoid pressure to reduce the chance of aspiration. (Image from: http://www.pharmacology2000. com/822_1/inline.jpg and Stene JD, Anesthesia for the critically ill trauma patient. In: Siegel JH, ed. *Trauma: Emergency Surgery and Critical Care.* New York, Churchill Livingstone, 1987.)

was unchanged in the other three regions.[15] Interestingly, even cricothyrotomy resulted in a small, and clinically insignificant, degree of movement across an unstable cervical spine injury in a cadaver model.[16]

Finally, it should be noted that while many clinicians fear untoward consequences from cervical spine movement during intubation in the setting of an unstable neck, cervical spine movements are typically small and their clinical implications have not been well established.[17,18]

In cases where neck movement is deliberately limited via the use of a neck immobilization collar (e.g., Philadelphia collar), airway management becomes even more challenging, as such collars constrict the mouth opening, making direct laryngoscopy much more difficult.[19] In some cases the anterior part of the collar is removed for laryngoscopy (Fig. 4.5). Although many airway devices have been used in such cases, the flexible fiberoptic bronchoscope is the device of choice for many clinicians. More recently, newer-generation video laryngoscopes have been used successfully. For example, the Pentax-AWS has been used successfully for awake nasotracheal intubation in patients using a neck collar for cervical spine stabilization,[20] while the GlideScope provides a better glottic view than does Macintosh direct laryngoscopy in these patients.[21]

Use of succinylcholine in patients undergoing spine surgery

Caution should be exercised with the use of succinylcholine in patients with trauma to the spine, especially those with neurologic symptoms resulting from spinal

cord injury, those experiencing muscle weakness, or individuals who have experienced prolonged inactivity and/or immobility. In such cases the administration of succinylcholine increases the risk of hyperkalemia, potentially severe enough to cause cardiac arrest.[22,23] Patients are susceptible to succinlycholine-induced hyperkalemia for up to two months following massive trauma or until damaged tissues heal.[24] The associated hyperkalemia is believed to stem from the spread of extrajunctional receptors across the muscle membrane upon exposure to succinylcholine. These receptors enter a state of prolonged depolarization characterized by massive potassium release.[23]

Flexible fiberoptic intubation and awake intubation

Whether as a prelude to spine surgery or for other reasons, the use of flexible fiberoptic intubation for the airway management of patients with cervical spine pathology is favored because in contrast with other methods, this technique is associated with minimal movement of the cervical spine. In addition, many clinicians prefer fiberoptic intubation for patients who have limited neck mobility (e.g., ankylosing spondylitis) even when there is no risk of spinal cord injury.[25]

While flexible fiberoptic intubation can usually be easily performed under complete general anesthesia, many clinicians prefer topical anesthesia, with the patient being only lightly sedated ("awake fiberoptic intubation"). However, the decision to go either way (awake versus asleep intubation) depends on the anesthesiologist's level of skill, the extent of the patient's cooperation, and the severity of the neck pathology. A key consideration underlying the choice between "awake" versus "asleep" fiberoptic intubation concerns the safety margin that an awake technique would allow. Specifically, if awake intubation is not successfully accomplished, the patient should be able to maintain his or her own airway.

The awake technique maintains muscle tone that is nearly normal, thus resembling the natural way of splinting the spine and preventing the extension of damage to neural structure.[26] Also, awake intubation allows for a postintubation neurologic check, performed either immediately after intubation, or even after the patient has been positioned for surgery before induction of general anesthesia. Finally, during awake intubation, airway reflexes are generally maintained to a degree sufficient to prevent pulmonary aspiration – an important consideration in a patient at high risk for aspiration, such as a trauma patient having a full stomach. It is not surprising, then, that anesthesiologists in the United States[27] and Canada[28] who were surveyed regarding their preference in airway management of patients with cervical spine disease, favored awake fiberoptic intubation as their first choice.

It should be emphasized that awake intubation is not synonymous with flexible fiberoptic intubation, for awake intubation can be safely accomplished with airway devices other than fiberoptic. These devices include, but are not limited to, direct laryngoscopy with Macintosh and Miller laryngoscopes, blind nasal intubation, the GlideScope, and the lighted stylet. Typically, the airway is anesthetized with gargled and atomized 4% lidocaine. Superior laryngeal and transtracheal blocks are also occasionally employed. In addition, judicious sedation is usually administered. Midazolam, fentanyl, remifentanil, ketamine, propofol, and clonidine have all been used in this setting. Recently, the use of dexmedetomidine,[29] a selective α2 agonist with sedative, analgesic, amnestic,[30] and antisialagogue properties,[31] has been reported. One key advantage of this agent is that it maintains spontaneous respiration with minimal respiratory depression. Another advantage is that patients under dexmedetomidine sedation are generally easy to arouse,[32] a property that has been exploited during awake fiberoptic-assisted intubation.[33] However, these advantages may not hold under very large doses.[34]

Doyle described the successful use of the GlideScope in four cases of awake intubation for nonspinal surgery.[35] The following advantages are noteworthy: (1) The view is generally excellent. (2) In contrast to fiberoptic intubation, the method appears to be less affected by the presence of secretions or blood. (3) All in attendance can see what is going on, while this is the case only with fiberoptic intubation carts that carry a video screen option. (4) There are no special restrictions on the type of ETT that can be placed when using the GlideScope, while this is not the case with fiberoptic methods. (5) The GlideScope is much more rugged than a fiberoptic bronchoscope, and is far less likely to be damaged with use. (6) While it is well known that advancing the ETT into the trachea over the fiberoptic bronchoscope may fail as a result of the ETT impinging on the arytenoid cartilages, this is generally not a problem with the GlideScope.

The above advantages notwithstanding, the use of awake fiberoptic intubation in a patient with cervical spine pathology remains steadfastly preferred because it is gentle to the airway, is generally well tolerated, and does not require the application of force to obtain glottic exposure.

Airway edema in spine cases

Airway edema frequently accompanies prolonged surgery of any kind, especially when vigorous fluid resuscitation has been carried out, or when a patient is undergoing surgery in the prone position. This edema may sometimes make extubation risky. Sagi and colleagues identified hematoma formation and pharyngeal edema as the main reasons for airway complications (2.4%) following anterior cervical spine surgery.[36] Edema is considered an especial contributor to airway complications.[37] More edema is observed to result from upper cervical spine surgery C2–4 than from lower cervical spine surgery C5–6[36,38] and to occur more often in female than in male patients.[36,39] Other risk factors include operative time, administered crystalloid volume, large blood loss, and the need for blood transfusion.[36,40] Massive tongue swelling has been reported as a contributor to airway compromise.[41] Perioperative steroids were reported to be helpful in reducing tongue swelling. However, in a randomized trial, perioperative intravenous steroids were not found to decrease the risk of airway edema, and they delayed postoperative extubation in anterior cervical spine surgery.[39] Many clinicians have used the leak test.[40] (The presence of a leak around the endotracheal tube when the cuff is deflated suggests that the airway is not overly edematous.) However, the test is not without limitations, as the presence of a leak does not guarantee smooth extubation and vice versa.

Spine surgery requiring the use of double-lumen tubes

Many thoracic spine procedures require collapsing a lung to facilitate surgical exposure. Use of a double-lumen tube (DLT) is often preferred in such a setting. While this scenario usually does not mandate any special considerations beyond the usual procedure for placing a double-lumen tube, in patients with a potentially difficult airway, an awake intubation technique is sometimes preferable. Although it is theoretically possible to insert a DLT in an awake patient, most clinicians prefer to initially insert a single-lumen tube utilizing an appropriate awake technique. This is followed by induction of general anesthesia and exchange of the single-lumen tube with a DLT by means of a tube-exchange catheter. However, before attempting the latter step, one should determine the largest diameter of exchange catheter that will fit into the tube in place, and the intended DLT, as a smaller-diameter exchange catheter is prone to kink, creating difficulties when an attempt is made to railroad an endotracheal tube over it. It is helpful to presoak the DLT in warm water to soften it. Many clinicians perform the exchange with the aid of direct laryngoscopy or video laryngoscopy. (Further details are discussed in Chapter 11.)

After the procedure is completed, it is often desirable to reverse the above steps and exchange the DLT with a single-lumen ETT. This is also frequently done by means of an exchange catheter. However, the best time to perform such an exchange might not be immediately postoperatively as it might prove hazardous to reintubate the trachea in a patient with a very swollen airway following extensive prone positioning. It is therefore generally wise to delay this until airway edema has subsided. In the meantime, the endobronchial blue cuff of the DLT should be deflated and the DLT withdrawn approximately 2.5 cm.

Management of accidental extubation

Inadvertent extubation during spine surgery can occur either in the prone or supine position. In the supine position, in which stability of the cervical spine is not a concern, re-intubation is usually straightforward unless the airway has previously been difficult. Mask ventilation with 100% oxygen will be the first step, usually followed by immediate re-intubation with the same device that proved helpful earlier. If ventilation proves difficult, intubation should be attempted immediately.

If both ventilation and intubation are difficult, rescue ventilation via a supraglottic airway is warranted. This would be followed by reevaluation of the situation and deciding whether the procedure could be completed with the use of such an airway, or whether re-intubation is still needed.[42] In desperate cases, transtracheal jet ventilation or a surgical airway might be necessary to regain airway access. In addition, the administration of intravenous anesthesia may be needed to ensure that the patient remains unconscious.

If the cervical spine is unstable, in-line stabilization of the spine may help reduce the likelihood of spinal cord injury. In this case, fiberoptic intubation is usually recommended, although other techniques may also be acceptable.

In the prone position, the challenge is greater. This is a more serious situation because ventilation and intubation in the prone position are much more difficult than in the supine position. Possibly exacerbating such difficulty is the edema that may have developed in the airway.

The traditional teaching about the management of patients who become extubated in the prone position is that they should be promptly flipped into the supine position and then reintubated in that position. For this reason, a gurney should be kept near any patient undergoing anesthesia in the prone position so that the patient may be flipped if necessary. Moreover, an essential precaution is that the surgical wound must be fully covered in a sterile manner before the flip is executed.

An alternate approach often advocated is to first establish a temporary airway through the use of a supraglottic airway device such as the intubating laryngeal mask airway. This provides time to choose between flipping the patient onto a nearby gurney as described above, fiberoptically intubating through the supraglottic airway device in the prone position, or even completing the case using only a supraglottic airway device.

Of course, the importance of preventing inadvertent extubation in the first place cannot be overemphasized. Special care must be taken to firmly secure the tube and to ensure that inadvertent pulling on adjacent tubes such as oral gastric tubes or esophageal temperature probes will not lead to extubation as well.

Spine surgery under spinal anesthesia

Spinal anesthesia for spine surgery offers several advantages. It allows the patient to self-position in prone cases, which will likely reduce the chance of positioning injuries that occasionally occur when general anesthesia is used. Moreover, it reduces intraoperative surgical blood loss; improves perioperative hemodynamic stability; reduces pain in the immediate postoperative period, and therefore the need for analgesics; lowers the incidence of postoperative nausea and vomiting; and lowers the incidence of lower extremity thromboembolic complications. The cumulative effect of these advantages is that patient satisfaction is enhanced and discharge from hospital is expedited.[43]

At Cleveland Clinic Spine Institute, Tetzlaff and colleagues[44] studied 611 cases of elective lumbar spine procedures performed under spinal anesthesia. They found that among perioperative complications, nausea and deep venous thrombosis occurred significantly more often in patients who had undergone general anesthesia than in those who had undergone spinal anesthesia. They also found that the use of plain bupivacaine was associated with the lowest incidence of supplemental local anesthetic use intraoperatively compared with hyperbaric bupivacaine or hyperbaric tetracaine. The authors concluded that for lumbar spine surgery, spinal anesthesia is an effective alternative to general anesthesia and has a lower rate of minor complications.

In a subsequent study at the same institution, a case-controlled analysis of 400 patients compared spinal and general anesthesia in lumbar laminectomy. The authors found that anesthetic and operative times were longer for patients receiving a general anesthetic, and also that these patients experienced more nausea and a greater need for antiemetics and pain medication.[45] The authors also found that complication rates (for instance, the rate of urinary retention) were significantly lower in spinal anesthesia patients. However, neither group experienced neural injuries, and in patients receiving a spinal anesthetic, the incidence of spinal headache was lower. Thus for patients undergoing lumbar laminectomy, spinal anesthesia is not only as safe and effective as general anesthesia but it also offers several advantages.

The utility of supraglottic airway devices in spine surgery

Traditional airway management for patients undergoing surgery under general anesthesia, and in the prone position, is to induce anesthesia in the supine position, secure the airway with a cuffed endotracheal tube, securely tape the tube in place, and then gently shift the patient to the prone position. Since positioning an anesthetized patient from the supine position to the prone position is fraught with potential problems (such as accidental extubation or injury to peripheral nerves), some clinicians have advocated utilizing a supraglottic airway placed in the prone position after the patient has self-positioned and general anesthesia has been induced.

Brimacombe and colleagues[46] conducted a retrospective audit of 245 patients, among whom the ProSeal laryngeal mask airway (PLMA) was used in prone patients. The authors acknowledged that the use of a classic laryngeal mask airway in prone patients is controversial but that the PLMA may be less problematic, since it forms a better seal and provides access to the stomach. Their technique involves the following steps: (1) The patient adopts the prone position with the head to the side and the table tilted laterally; (2) preoxygenation to end-tidal oxygen is >90%; (3) anesthesia is induced with midazolam/alfentanil/propofol; (4) facemask ventilation is used; (5) a single attempt at digital insertion is made, and if unsuccessful a single attempt is made at laryngoscope-guided, gum elastic bougie-guided insertion; (6) a gastric tube is inserted; (7) anesthesia is maintained with sevoflurane-N20; (8) volume-controlled ventilation is maintained at 8–12 ml/kg; (9) emergence from anesthesia occurs in the supine position; and (10) PLMA is removed when the patient is awake.

In their audit, correctable partial airway obstruction occurred in three patients, but there was no hypoxia, hypercapnea, displacement, regurgitation, gastric insufflation, or airway reflex activation. The authors concluded that when used competently, PLMA is feasible for inducing and maintaining anesthesia when the patient is in the prone position.

Sharma and colleagues[47] conducted a prospective audit on the use of the Laryngeal Mask Airway Supreme (SLMA) in 205 consecutive patients undergoing orthopedic surgery in the prone position. Patients positioned themselves in the prone position; afterwards, anesthesia was induced and the SLMA was inserted. The vast majority of patients received positive pressure ventilation (PPV). No failures of SLMA insertion or of maintenance of PPV occurred. The authors concluded that the SLMA is useful for airway management in patients anesthetized in the prone position, and for subsequent airway management with PPV, with or without neuromuscular block. Other studies support the use of supraglottic airway devices in the prone position.[48–51]

We emphasize that all the above studies and case reports are nonrandomized studies; they either assessed feasibility or described a technique, or both. For these reasons, they are subject to patients' selection bias and do not prove superiority over other anesthetic management strategies such as spinal anesthesia and/or general endotracheal anesthesia. These reports simply state that supraglottic airways in prone spine surgery can be done, which is useful information that can be used in case of emergency loss of the airway in the prone position and/or if the anesthesiologist elects to use such a technique as the primary choice. Moreover, these reports apply to procedures performed by users who are expert in LMA; the findings may therefore not apply to infrequent LMA users.

References

1. Practice guidelines for management of the difficult airway. A report by the American Society of Anesthesiologists Task Force on Management of the Difficult Airway. *Anesthesiology* 1993; **78**: 597–602.

2. Practice guidelines for management of the difficult airway: An updated report by the American Society of Anesthesiologists Task Force on Management of the Difficult Airway. *Anesthesiology* 2003; **98**: 1269–77.

3. Frova G. The difficult intubation and the problem of monitoring the adult airway. Italian Society of Anesthesia, Resuscitation, and Intensive Therapy (SIAARTI). *Minerva Anestesiol* 1998; **64**: 361–71.

4. Cook TM. Difficult Airway Society guidelines. *Anaesthesia* 2004; **59**: 1243–4.

5. Randell T. Prediction of difficult intubation. *Acta Anaesthesiol Scand* 1996; **40**: 1016–23.

6. Iohom G, Ronayne M, Cunningham AJ. Prediction of difficult tracheal intubation. *Eur J Anaesthesiol* 2003; **20**: 31–6.

7. Honarmand A, Safavi MR. Prediction of difficult laryngoscopy in obstetric patients scheduled for Caesarean delivery. *Eur J Anaesthesiol* 2008; **25**: 714–20.

8. Khan ZH, Mohammadi M, Rasouli MR, Farrokhnia F, Khan RH. The diagnostic value of the upper lip bite test combined with sternomental distance, thyromental distance, and interincisor distance for prediction of easy laryngoscopy and intubation: a prospective study. *Anesth Analg* 2009; **109**: 822–4.

9. Adnet F, Borron SW, Racine SX, *et al.* The intubation difficulty scale (IDS): proposal and evaluation of a new score characterizing the complexity of endotracheal intubation. *Anesthesiology* 1997; **87**: 1290–7.

10. Nolan JP, Wilson ME. Orotracheal intubation in patients with potential cervical spine injuries. An indication for the gum elastic bougie. *Anaesthesia* 1993; **48**: 630–3.

11. Brimacombe J, Keller C, Kunzel KH, *et al.* Cervical spine motion during airway management: a cinefluoroscopic study of the posteriorly destabilized third cervical vertebrae in human cadavers. *Anesth Analg* 2000; **91**: 1274–8.

12. Hastings RH, Vigil AC, Hanna R, Yang BY, Sartoris DJ. Cervical spine movement during laryngoscopy with the Bullard, Macintosh, and Miller laryngoscopes. *Anesthesiology* 1995; **82**: 859–69.

13. Watts AD, Gelb AW, Bach DB, Pelz DM. Comparison of the Bullard and Macintosh laryngoscopes for endotracheal intubation of patients with a potential cervical spine injury. *Anesthesiology* 1997; **87**: 1335–42.

14. Maruyama K, Yamada T, Kawakami R, *et al.* Upper cervical spine movement during intubation: fluoroscopic comparison of the AirWay Scope, McCoy laryngoscope, and Macintosh laryngoscope. *Br J Anaesth* 2008; **100**: 120–4.

15. Turkstra TP, Craen RA, Pelz DM, Gelb AW. Cervical spine motion: a fluoroscopic comparison during intubation with lighted stylet, GlideScope, and Macintosh laryngoscope. *Anesth Analg* 2005; **101**: 910–15.

16. Gerling MC, Davis DP, Hamilton RS, *et al.* Effect of surgical cricothyrotomy on the unstable cervical spine in a cadaver model of intubation. *J Emerg Med* 2001; **20**: 1–5.

17. Crosby ET. Considerations for airway management for cervical spine surgery in adults. *Anesthesiol Clin* 2007; **25**: 511–33, ix.

18. McLeod AD, Calder I. Spinal cord injury and direct laryngoscopy – the legend lives on. *Br J Anaesth* 2000; **84**: 705–9.

19. Goutcher CM, Lochhead V. Reduction in mouth opening with semi-rigid cervical collars. *Br J Anaesth* 2005; **95**: 344–8.

20. Asai T. Pentax-AWS videolaryngoscope for awake nasal intubation in patients with unstable necks. *Br J Anaesth* 2010; **104**: 108–11.

21. Agro F, Barzoi G, Montecchia F. Tracheal intubation using a Macintosh laryngoscope or a GlideScope in 15 patients with cervical spine immobilization. *Br J Anaesth* 2003; **90**: 705–6.

22. Gronert GA, Theye RA. Pathophysiology of hyperkalemia induced by succinylcholine. *Anesthesiology* 1975; **43**: 89–99.

23. Gronert GA. Succinylcholine-induced hyperkalemia and beyond. 1975. *Anesthesiology* 2009; **111**: 1372–7.

24. Savarese J, Caldwell J, Lien C, Miller R. *Pharmacology of Muscle Relaxants and Their Antagonists.* 5th ed. Philadelphia, PA: Churchill Livingstone; 2000.

25. Langford RA, Leslie K. Awake fibreoptic intubation in neurosurgery. *J Clin Neurosci* 2009; **16**: 366–72.

26. Manninen PH, Jose GB, Lukitto K, Venkatraghavan L, El Beheiry H. Management of the airway in patients undergoing cervical spine surgery. *J Neurosurg Anesthesiol* 2007; **19**: 190–4.

27. Ezri T, Szmuk P, Warters RD, Katz J, Hagberg CA. Difficult airway management practice patterns among anesthesiologists practicing in the United States: have we made any progress? *J Clin Anesth* 2003; **15**: 418–22.

28. Jenkins K, Wong DT, Correa R. Management choices for the difficult airway by anesthesiologists in Canada. *Can J Anaesth* 2002; **49**: 850–6.

29. Avitsian R, Lin J, Lotto M, Ebrahim Z. Dexmedetomidine and awake fiberoptic intubation for possible cervical spine myelopathy: a clinical series. *J Neurosurg Anesthesiol* 2005; **17**: 97–9.

30. Ebert TJ, Hall JE, Barney JA, Uhrich TD, Colinco MD. The effects of increasing plasma concentrations of dexmedetomidine in humans. *Anesthesiology* 2000; **93**: 382–94.

31. Scher CS, Gitlin MC. Dexmedetomidine and low-dose ketamine provide adequate sedation for awake fibreoptic intubation. *Can J Anaesth* 2003; **50**: 607–10.

32. M M. Pharmacology and Use of Alpha-2 Agonists in Anesthesia, European Society of Anesthesiologists Refresher Course, 2003; pp. 37–43.

33. Abdelmalak B, Makary L, Hoban J, Doyle DJ. Dexmedetomidine as sole sedative for awake intubation in management of the critical airway. *J Clin Anesth* 2007; **19**: 370–3.

34. Ebert T, Maze M. Dexmedetomidine: another arrow for the clinician's quiver. *Anesthesiology* 2004; **101**: 568–70.

35. Doyle DJ. Awake intubation using the GlideScope video laryngoscope: initial experience in four cases. *Can J Anaesth* 2004; **51**: 520–1.

36. Sagi HC, Beutler W, Carroll E, Connolly PJ. Airway complications associated with surgery on the anterior cervical spine. *Spine (Phila Pa 1976)* 2002; **27**: 949–53.

37. Emery SE, Smith MD, Bohlman HH. Upper-airway obstruction after multilevel cervical corpectomy for myelopathy. *J Bone Joint Surg Am* 1991; **73**: 544–51.

38. Andrew SA, Sidhu KS. Airway changes after anterior cervical discectomy and fusion. *J Spinal Disord Tech* 2007; **20**: 577–81.

39. Emery SE, Akhavan S, Miller P, *et al.* Steroids and risk factors for airway compromise in multilevel cervical corpectomy patients: a prospective, randomized, double-blind study. *Spine (Phila Pa 1976)* 2009; **34**: 229–32.

40. Kwon B, Yoo JU, Furey CG, Rowbottom J, Emery SE. Risk factors for delayed extubation after single-stage, multi-level anterior cervical decompression and posterior fusion. *J Spinal Disord Tech* 2006; **19**: 389–93.

41. Miura Y, Mimatsu K, Iwata H. Massive tongue swelling as a complication after spinal surgery. *J Spinal Disord* 1996; **9**: 339–41.

42. Avitsian R, Doyle DJ, Helfand R, Zura A, Farag E. Successful reintubation after cervical spine exposure using an Aintree intubation catheter and a Laryngeal Mask Airway. *J Clin Anesth* 2006; **18**: 224–5.

43. Jellish WS, Shea JF. Spinal anaesthesia for spinal surgery. *Best Pract Res Clin Anaesthesiol* 2003; **17**: 323–34.

44. Tetzlaff JE, Dilger JA, Kodsy M, al-Bataineh J, Yoon HJ, Bell GR. Spinal anesthesia for elective lumbar spine surgery. *J Clin Anesth* 1998; **10**: 666–9.

45. McLain RF, Kalfas I, Bell GR, *et al.* Comparison of spinal and general anesthesia in lumbar laminectomy surgery: a case-controlled analysis of 400 patients. *J Neurosurg Spine* 2005; **2**: 17–22.

46. Brimacombe JR, Wenzel V, Keller C. The proseal laryngeal mask airway in prone patients: a retrospective audit of 245 patients. *Anaesth Intensive Care* 2007; **35**: 222–5.

47. Sharma V, Verghese C, McKenna PJ. Prospective audit on the use of the LMA-Supreme for airway management of adult patients undergoing elective orthopaedic surgery in prone position. *Br J Anaesth* 2010; **105**: 228–32.

48. Ng A, Raitt DG, Smith G. Induction of anesthesia and insertion of a laryngeal mask airway in the prone position for minor surgery. *Anesth Analg* 2002; **94**: 1194–8.

49. Dingeman RS, Goumnerova LC, Goobie SM. The use of a laryngeal mask airway for emergent airway management in a prone child. *Anesth Analg* 2005; **100**: 670–1.

50. Weksler N, Klein M, Rozentsveig V, *et al.* Laryngeal mask in prone position: pure exhibitionism or a valid technique. *Minerva Anestesiol* 2007; **73**: 33–7.

51. Lopez AM, Valero R, Brimacombe J. Insertion and use of the LMA Supreme in the prone position. *Anaesthesia*; **65**: 154–7.

Chapter

5

Spine imaging

Doksu Moon, Christian Koopman, and Ramez Malaty

Key points

- Understand the difference between disc disease and facet disease and how they affect the spinal canal and formina.
- Understand the imaging features of infection, especially discitis versus osteomyelitis.
- Understand the key findings in spine trauma and patterns of injury.
- Learn an imaging approach for neoplasms of the spine, including intramedullary lesions versus intradural extramedullary neoplasms.

Introduction

Imaging is integral to the diagnosis of spine disease. This chapter will provide an overview of imaging of spine disease. It will give a brief overview of normal imaging anatomy and illustrate highlights of pathologic processes in the spine. After reviewing this chapter the reader should be able to describe how to determine normal marrow signal in the spine, describe and identify degenerative disc and facet disease, discuss the appearance of pyogenic discitis on MRI, discuss the four types of spinal arteriovenous malformations, and summarize common neoplasms of the spine.

Normal spine

There are typically 7 cervical vertebrae, 12 rib-bearing thoracic vertebrae, 5 lumbar type vertebrae, and 5 fused sacral segments. However, many variants including fusion of the C1 through C3 vertebrae, fusion of C1 with the skull base, cervical ribs, 11 or 13 rib-bearing ribs, and transitional lumbosacral vertebra all combine to add complexity in the counting process. Careful delineation of the spinal levels on imaging is necessary to avoid wrong-level surgery.[1]

The detailed anatomy of the vertebrae and fusion variants is outside the scope of this chapter. However, a brief overview will be provided in the accompanying diagrams. The spinal vertebra can be divided into the vertebral body and posterior elements. The posterior elements consist of the neural ring, transverse process, superior facet joints, inferior facet joints, and spinous process. The neural ring consists of the posterior aspect of the vertebral bodies, pedicles, and laminae. There are multiple excellent textbooks and chapters for study[2,3] (Figs. 5.1 and 5.2).

Marrow

Evaluation of marrow signal abnormalities can be difficult even for the experienced neuroradiologist. Marrow signal on T1 images is typically hyperintense (bright) in the elderly and middle-aged and decreases in younger patients. The reason is that older patients have increased lipid in their marrow.[4] In the very young the T1 marrow signal may be very dark due to the prevalence of red marrow. However, no matter how much red marrow is present, normal marrow is hyperintense to the intervertebral disc signal (Fig. 5.3).

The three main imaging sequences available are T1-weighted (T1W) imaging sequences, T2-weighted (T2W) imaging sequences, and inversion recovery (STIR or IR) sequences. T1 signal is the most useful for evaluating marrow signal abnormalities. Areas of abnormal marrow, whether from a marrow replacement process (e.g., myelodysplasia, sick cell disease, metastasis) or edema (e.g., acute or subacute compression fracture) are of decreased signal compared with normal marrow. Inversion recovery sequences are also very useful. Those sequences typically saturate the fat signal so that fatty structures such as subcutaneous fat and marrow are rendered as decreased signal. T2W and postcontrast sequences are not as useful for evaluating normal marrow. On T2W sequences, for the most part, normal

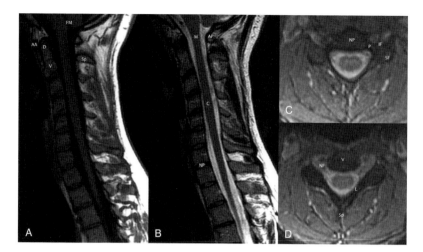

Figure 5.1 Normal cervical spine MRI. (A) Sagittal T1 TR600/TE11. (B) Sagittal T2 TR4000/TE60. (C) and (D) Axial gradient echo TR30/TE15: anterior arch of atlas (AA), posterior arch of atlas (AP), foramen of Magendie (FM), vertebral body (V), spinous process (Sp), medulla (M), cervical spinal cord (C), nucleus pulposus (NP), pedicle (P), inferior facet (IF), superior facet (SF), neuroforamen (NF), lamina (L).

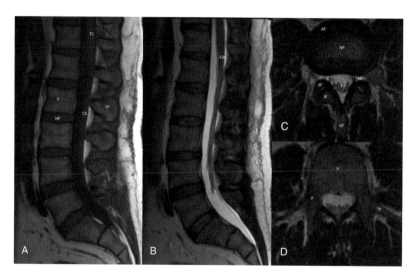

Figure 5.2 Normal lumbar spine MRI: (A) Sagittal T1 TR550/TE11. (B) Sagittal T2 TR4040/TE60. (C) and (D) Axial T2 TR4040/TE60: thoracic cord (TC), spinous process (SP), cauda equina (CE), nucleus pulposus (NP), vertebral body (V), conus medullaris (CM), annulus fibrosus (AF), neuroforamen (NF), inferior facet (IF), superior facet (SF), pedicle (P), transverse process (TP).

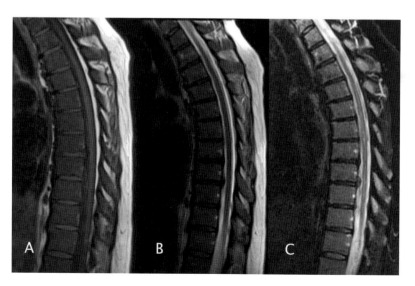

Figure 5.3 Myelodysplasia. (A) T1 sagittal T spine TR500/TE11. (B) T2 sagittal T spine TR2910/TE104. (C) STIR sagittal T spine TR4200/TE60. Note that marrow signal in (A) is diffusely decreased compared with the signal in the disc on T1W images.

marrow signal is hyperintense and pathologic marrow signal also tends to be hyperintense due to the edema associated with it. Postcontrast images are also limited in evaluating marrow signal since pathologic marrow signal enhances as well as normal marrow signal.

Degenerative disease

Degenerative disease is the most common reason for spine imaging and surgery in the United States. There is evidence that genetic factors as well as environmental factors contribute to disc disease.[5] Degenerative disease is diagnosed by imaging. The major pitfall in imaging of degenerative disease is that there may be degenerative disease present in up to one-third of asymptomatic adults, although more severe degenerative changes such as extrusions and sequestration are found rarely in the asymptomatic population.[6,7] We can divide degenerative spine disease anatomically into disc disease and facet disease.

Degenerative disc disease

The primary problem is a defect in the annulus fibrosis, which surrounds the nucleus pulposus. Disc disease can produce spinal canal stenosis and neuroforaminal stenosis via disc bulges, disc protrusions, disc extrusions, and sequestrations.

The weakest point in the annulus fibrosis tends to be dorsal, so the first area affected is the spinal canal and thecal sac.[8] Degenerative disc disease can result in both spinal canal and neuroforaminal stenosis. The classification is complex and has evolved over the years, but there is a common classification system used in North America (Nomenclature and Classification of Lumbar Disc Pathology) which has been recommended by both the North American Spine Society and the American Society of Neuroradiology. According to this system a disc bulge is greater than 50% (180°) of the circumference of the disc; a broad-based disc protrusion is herniation of the disc material greater than 25% and less than 50% of the circumference; a protrusion is displacement of the disc that is less than 25% of the circumference of the disc; and an extrusion is displacement or herniation of the disc in which in at least one plane the edge of the disc material is greater than the distance of the disc material at the base[9] (Figs. 5.4–5.6).

Degenerative end plate changes often accompany degenerative disc disease. Type I end plate changes

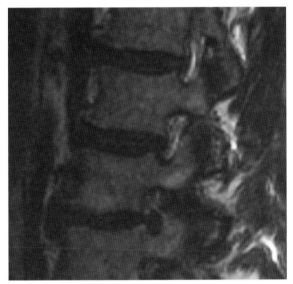

Figure 5.4 Neuroforaminal stenosis. Sagittal T2 shows moderate left L3–4 stenosis due to loss of disc height and lateral extension of disc bulge.

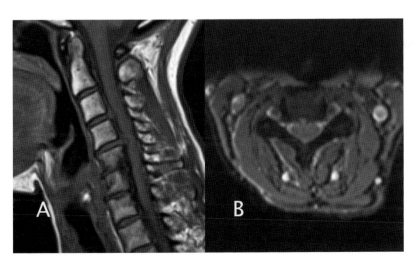

Figure 5.5 (A) Sagittal T1 TR705/TE12. (B) Axial gradient echo TR30/TE14 showing multiple disc extrusions in the cervical spine. The most prominent ones are at C3–4 and C4–5 causing cord compression.

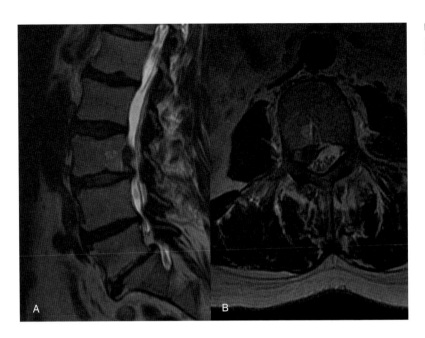

Figure 5.6 T2 images TR4200/TE117 show a disc sequestration (free fragment) in the lumbar spine dorsal to L3.

A   B

(edematous) show decreased T1 signal and increased T2 signal. Type II (fatty) end plate changes show increased T1 and T2 signal in the adjacent end plates. Type III changes (sclerotic) show decreased T1 and T2 end plate signal changes. These types of end plate changes can transition between each other.[10]

Even when there appears to be CSF ventral to the spinal cord and no impingement or compression of the spinal cord by visual inspection, there can be compression of the nerves due to compression on the individual nerve rootlets that exit from the ventral (anterior) aspects of the spinal cord. Even with current imaging the individual nerve rootlets are not usually visualized in a typical MRI scan.

In the most severe cases there is complete effacement of the CSF surrounding the cord or nerve roots. This can be appreciated on both T1 and T2 axial images.

Although many herniations indent the thecal sac, some are more laterally placed and compress the nerve root at the neuroforamen. These are termed lateral or foraminal protrusions or extrusions.

Facet disease

Degenerative facet disease can be a cause of back pain both by itself and also because of direct effects on the spinal canal and neuroforamina. Degenerative facet changes can indirectly cause narrowing of the spinal canal and foramina through spondylolisthesis.

The degenerative facet joints can be a source of pain that is unrelated to radicular pain. The most obvious signs are hypertrophy of the facet joints (most readily visible in the lower lumbar spine). With sufficient degenerative changes, facet hypertrophy alone can result in moderate or several spinal canal stenosis. Facet disease also affects the neuroforamina, causing narrowing due to degenerative changes. Facet effusions are visible on T2W images as areas of increased signal. If facet effusion becomes large enough it can become a synovial cyst which can cause (asymmetric) spinal canal stenosis. Despite the cystic nature of these lesions they may show decreased signal on T2W images depending on the amount of associated calcification.[11]

OPLL

Ossification of the posterior longitudinal ligament (OPLL) occurs most often in patients of East Asian descent, but also in the rest of the population.[12] The exact etiology remains unclear but the process results in spinal canal stenosis and possible cord compression. There is also an association with DISH.[13]

DISH

Diffuse idiopathic skeletal hypertrophy (DISH) happens sporadically. It is identified by four or more levels of contiguously fused vertebral bodies. There is a correlation with increasing age and it is common in the population over the age of 50 years (males 25%, females 15%)[14] (Fig. 5.7).

Baastrup's disease is the close contact of the spinous processes (kissing spine). It results in inflammatory

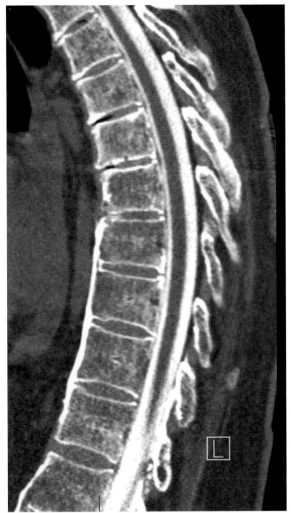

Figure 5.7 Sagittal reconstruction from a thoracic spine CT myelogram showing flowing anterior syndesmophytes in the lower thoracic spine extending to four levels, reflecting DISH (diffuse idiopathic skeletal hypertrophy).

changes between the spinous processes including edema, cyst formation, fluid accumulation, and sclerotic changes. These areas of edema are seen on T2 and inversion recovery as areas of hyperintensity.[15]

Schmorl's nodes. Not significant by themselves in most cases, but in severe cases these are associated with compression fractures. These are "internal" disc herniations, with the nucleus pulposus extending through the cartilaginous end plates rather than the annulus fibrosus. This situation is physiologic since in normal patients the annulus is more resistant to axial loads than the end plates.

Scheuermann's disease. Osteochondrosis of the thoracic spine resulting in a kyphosis. The basic process is interruption of the blood supply and osteonecrosis of the vertebrae resulting in mild kyphosis.

Sarcoidosis

Sarcoidosis is an idiopathic systemic disease. In the head and spine, it presents as thickening and enhancement of the leptomeninges. Spinal sarcoidosis can involve intramedullary, intradural extramedullary, extradural, vertebral, and disc space lesions.

Intramedullary sarcoid is uncommon. Lesions are high in signal intensity on T2 and low on T1 and patchy enhancement after contrast administration.

Leptomeningeal and dural lesions are more common than intramedullary lesions and can be seen on postcontrast T1 weighted images as thin, linear leptomeningeal enhancement or small nodules (Fig. 5.8) Clinical manifestations do not correlate well with MRI findings. Clinical manifestations result from local nerve or spinal cord compression. Surgical resection is usually necessary to relieve the compression, followed by steroids. Differential diagnosis includes

Figure 5.8 Sarcoidosis. Pre- (A) and post- (B) contrast sagittal T1 TR500/TE13 MRI shows nodular enhancement in the conus medullaris.

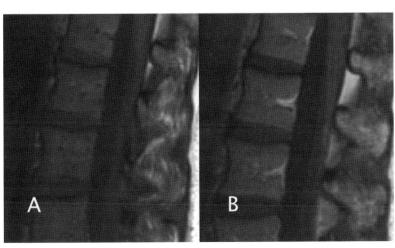

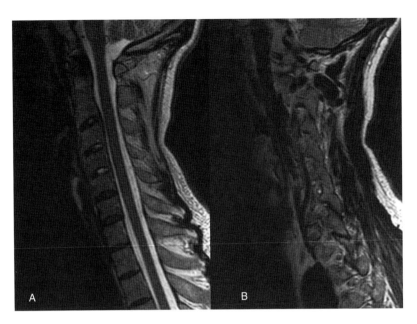

Figure 5.9 Ankylosing spondylitis. Sagittal T2 images TR2780/TE115 show fusion of the vertebral bodies and facet joints. Note the lack of articular cartilage between the facet joints on the parasagittal image (B), which shows that the facet joints are fused. On the midsagittal image (A) the intervertebral discs in the mid- and upper cervical spine do not extend to the margins of the vertebral bodies. The C2–5 vertebrae show body bridging anterior and posterior to the intervertebral discs.

lymphoma and carcinomatous metastasis among other etiologies.[16]

Vertebral involvement is rare with multiple, well-defined lytic lesions with sclerotic margins. Mimicking of metastasis by such lesions is also rare.[16]

Ankylosing spondylitis

Ankylosing spondylitis is a relatively common rheumatologic condition in adults with incidence of 1.4% in the general population. This progressive seronegative spondyloarthropathy results in fusion of the vertebral bodies and sacroiliac (SI) joints. It has an ascending course of progress, with the SI joints and lumbar spine the most commonly and first affected.[17] This disease may result in fractures and dislocations, and spinal stenosis with neurologic compromise[18] (Fig. 5.9).

Rheumatoid arthritis

Rheumatoid arthritis is often associated with its effects on the peripheral joints, but perhaps its most devastating effect is in the cervical spine where inflammatory changes can result in craniocervical subluxation. Oftentimes it is asymptomatic but it can result in myelopathy. The two most common presentations are atlantoaxial subluxation (widening of the anterior atlanto-odontoid distance) and basilar invagination. Atlantoaxial subluxation can also result in C1–2 instability. This can be diagnostic with flexion–extension plain films of the lateral cervical spine (Fig. 5.10). Myelopathy and cord compression can also result

from the presence of inflammatory pannus surrounding the dens.

Infection

Pyogenic discitis and osteomyelitis

This most often involves vertebral bodies (osteomyelitis). However, it may also involve posterior elements, discs (discitis), epidural space, and paraspinous soft tissues.[19] Etiology is most commonly bacterial and usually *Staphylococcus aureus*, although fungi or parasites may be involved. Infection may be due to hematogenous spread, contiguous spread, or direct inoculation in the setting of trauma or surgery. Infections are most commonly hematogenous and usually via the skin, urinary tract, or pulmonary sources.[19] In adults, infection starts in the subchondral portion of the vertebral body and spreads to the disc space and then further along the vertebral body in a subligamentous fashion.[20] In children, however, disc space infection may be the primary site with vertebral body infection secondary.[19,21] Infection most commonly involves the lumbar spine.[21] Symptoms vary, with pain and malaise being common, and patients may be afebrile. Neurologic deficit and cord compression may occur if infection spreads into the epidural space.[21] Plain radiographs are of low sensitivity for detecting this infection. Radionuclide bone scans are sensitive but nonspecific for this infection. CT scans are also less sensitive.[22] Findings on MRI are characteristic, with T1W sequences showing

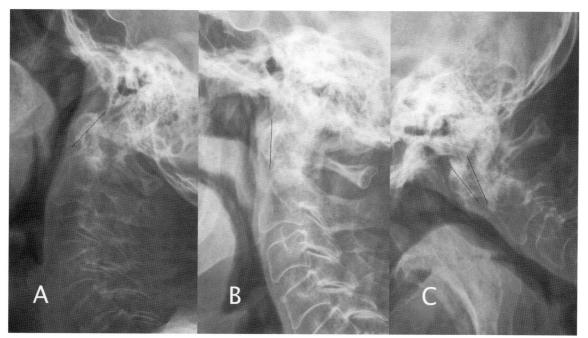

Figure 5.10 Rheumatoid arthritis. (A) Extension view. (B) Neutral view. (C) Flexion view. Note the widening of the anterior atlanto-odontoid distance (AAOD) on the flexion view.

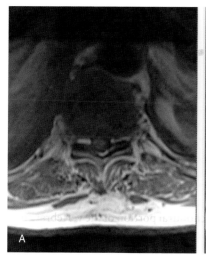
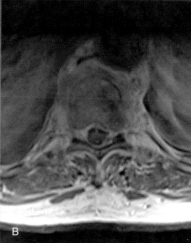

Figure 5.11 Discitis. Pre- (A) and postcontrast (B) axial T1 images through the level of the disc showing circumferential enhancing soft tissue surrounding the vertebral body at the level of discitis. Note the epidural involvement.

a narrowed disc space and decreased signal in adjacent vertebral bodies.[19,22] Subligamentous or epidural soft tissue fluid collections and cortical bone erosion are common. Postcontrast examination demonstrates enhancement of the infected disc and infected bone. Paraspinous abscess, epidural abscess, and meningeal inflammation can all occur and may be detected on MRI imaging.[23,24]

The differential diagnosis includes granulomatous spondylitis, calcium pyrophosphate crystal deposition disease, and in rare circumstances, metastasis[25] (Figs. 5.11 and 5.12).

Granulomatous spondylitis

This is most commonly due to *Mycobacterium tuberculosis* but can be seen in bacterial, viral, parasitic, and fungal etiologies among others, as well as tumors and autoimmune diseases.[19] Other implicated organisms are bacilli of the *Brucella* genus.[26] Tuberculous spondylitis is most prevalent in middle-aged adults with

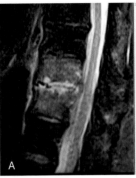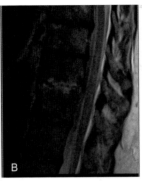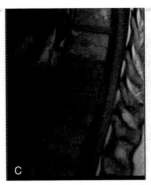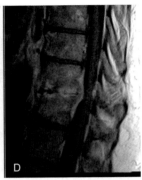

Figure 5.12 Discitis/osteomyelitis. (A) Sagittal STIR TR4350/TE810. (B) Sagittal T2 TR4060/TE120. (C) Sagittal T1 TR500/TE12. (D) Sagittal T1 postcontrast TR500/TE12. Typical appearance showing increased marrow signal on T2 and STIR. Decreased signal on T1 and diffuse end plate enhancement on postcontrast images.

predisposing factors including debilitation, immuno-suppression, alcoholism, and drug addiction.[19] The lumbar spine is also the most common level of involvement, with nearly 90% of cases having at least two affected vertebral bodies with skip lesions commonly occurring.[19,27,28] Paraspinous abscesses occur in more than 50% of cases.[27] Tuberculosis can affect only part of the vertebral body, with transverse processes and posterior elements involved only some of the time.[19] Tuberculous spondylitis is typically more indolent than pyogenic osteomyelitis, with insidious onset and symptoms lasting months to years and with untreated patients developing progressive vertebral body collapse and gibbus formation.[27,29] CT imaging demonstrates extensive bony destruction and large paraspinous abscesses that are disproportionate to the amount of bone destruction. Epidural extension and subligamentous spread are also frequently present.[19,27] MRI shows loss of cortical definition of vertebral bodies involved. Infection spreads beneath longitudinal ligaments to involve adjacent vertebral bodies, with discs sometimes relatively spared. Posterior elements are commonly involved.[27]

Epidural abscess

Again infection is typically hematogenous from skin, pulmonary, or urinary tract sources, with *S. aureus* being by far the most common organism.[20,30] Two basic stages are observed. The first stage demonstrates thickened and inflamed tissue with granulomatous material and embedded microabscesses that represent a phlegmonous stage.[31] The second stage demonstrates a collection of liquid pus material with frank abscess formation.[30] Epidural abscesses are uncommon, with incidence on the rise and mean age being 50–55 years[31–33] They are commonly extensive and can extend along multiple vertebral body levels with concomitant discitis

or osteomyelitis seen in 80% of cases.[30] Fever and localized tenderness are early symptoms but symptoms are often nonspecific. Predisposing conditions include diabetes, intravenous drug abuse, multiple medical illnesses, and trauma. Epidural abscess may result in severe neurologic deficit or even death in untreated cases.[31,32] Myelography and CT myelography demonstrate extradural soft tissue mass with blockage of normal CSF flow.[32] MRI scans show extradural soft tissue mass that is isointense to hypointense compared with spinal cord on T1W images and hyperintense on proton density and T2W images[31] Coexisting signal changes in adjacent vertebral bodies are often seen. Three patterns are observed after contrast administration. One is of diffuse homogeneous enhancement seen in 70% of the cases, likely representing a phlegmonous stage. The second most common finding is a thick or thin enhancing rim surrounding a liquefied, low-signal pus collection, representing frank necrotic abscess. Finally, a combination of both patterns can be observed.[31,32]

Subdural abscess

Subdural abscesses are rare and the rarity is due to absence of venous sinuses in the spine, wide epidural space acting as a filter, and centripetal direction of spinal blood flow.[34] Clinical presentation is nonspecific, with symptoms mimicking acute transverse myelitis and spinal epidural abscess among other pathologies. Imaging studies reveal an intraspinal space-occupying mass with features that would localize the lesion to the subdural compartment.

Meningitis

The cause of meningitis is fungal, parasitic, or viral, with pyogenic leptomeningitis being the most common bacterial infection. The majority of cases occur

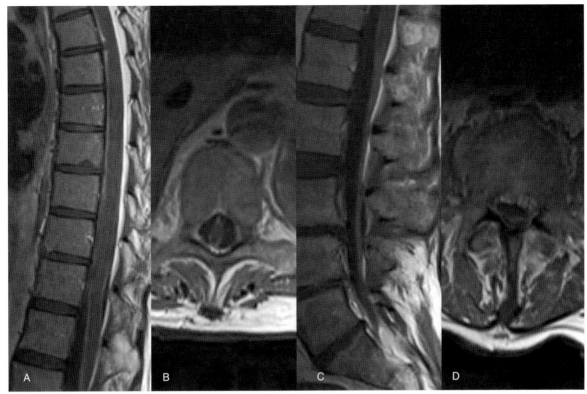

Figure 5.13 Syphilis. Postcontrast T1 (TR500/TE12) images through the thoracic and lumbar spine demonstrate diffuse leptomeningeal enhancement throughout the spinal cord (A) and clumped enhancing nerve roots (C and D) reflecting adhesive arachnoiditis. Note the narrowing of the lateral diameter of the thoracic cord (B) on the axial images.

as manifestation of cerebral meningitis.[19] Infection is seen as contrast-enhancing tissue that surrounds the spinal cord and nerve roots. Three patterns are seen: one pattern is delicate, smooth, linear enhancement outlining the cord and nerve roots; another is discrete nodular foci on the surface; a third pattern is of diffusely thickened soft tissues appearing as an intradural filling defect. There is no correlation between the pattern of enhancement and etiology of the organism or disease severity[35] (Fig. 5.13).

Paraspinous abscess

Instrumented patients can have seeding of the hardware by hematogenous spread of organisms (Fig. 5.14). Hematogenously spread pyogenic organisms can often seed the paravertebral muscles unless the scan is carefully examined (Fig. 5.15).

Myelitis

The term myelitis is restricted to inflammatory diseases of the spinal cord, with myelopathy being a general term applied to cord dysfunction from noninflammatory

sources.[36] Infectious agents can cause myelitis. Viral infections typically affect the gray matter with herpes, coxsackie, and HIV being the more common infections.[36] Epidural abscess and chronic meningeal infection such as tuberculosis and fungal meningitis can also cause a secondary myelitis.[21,35] Imaging findings are nonspecific, with focal or diffuse increased intramedullary signal on T2W images with or without mass effect and with or without enhancement following contrast administration.[35]

Intramedullary abscess

Frank pyogenic spinal cord abscesses are extremely rare compared with brain abscesses. There are only a few reported cases.[19]

Demyelinating diseases

Multiple sclerosis

Multiple sclerosis is a disease of the central nervous system. There are plaques that occur in the brain and spinal cord. Spinal cord plaques are almost universal

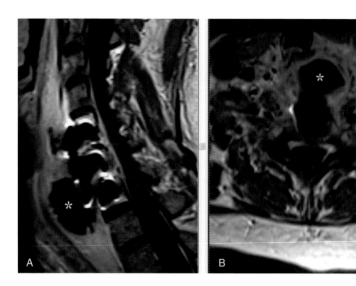

Figure 5.14 Postcontrast T1 images TR427/TE11 through the cervical thoracic junction show a prevertebral abscess (asterisk) anterior to the area of fusion. There is also epidural enhancement at C3 through C7 causing narrowing of the spinal canal without evidence for an epidural abscess.

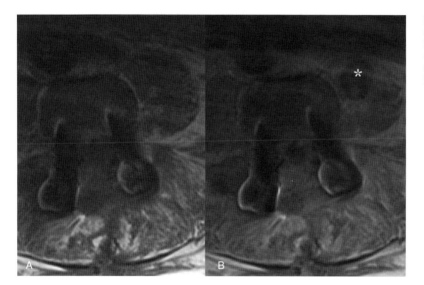

Figure 5.15 Psoas abscess. Pre- (A) and postcontrast (B) axial T1 TR682/TE12 images showing a rounded peripherally enhancing abscess which was not apparent on precontrast images in the left iliopsoas muscle.

at autopsy findings. Plaques occur preferentially in the dorsal lateral cord and do not respect boundaries between specific tracts or between gray and white matter. Multiple sclerosis demonstrates disease onset typically between 15 and 50 years of age, with the peak in the third and fourth decades and with distinct female predominance. In early disease, there is distinct cervical spinal cord predilection.[37] Initial imaging evaluation in suspected multiple sclerosis is by brain MRI. Spinal MRI is not required for confirmation when definitive diagnosis of multiple sclerosis is made on clinical grounds. In patients suspected to have multiple sclerosis, if brain MRI is normal, MRI examination of the spinal cord is appropriate. Imaging of the spinal cord

most commonly reveals one or more elongated, poorly marginated hyperintense intramedullary lesions on T2W images. Focal or generalized cord atrophy can be seen on T1W images. Acute demyelinating lesions may have mass effect and enhance following contrast administration.[38,39]

Acute transverse myelopathy

Sometimes termed acute transverse myelitis, this is characterized by an acutely developing, rapidly progressing lesion affecting both sides of the cord. This is not a true disease but a clinical syndrome with many causes.[40] Causes include active infection, postinfectious demyelinating disorder (acute disseminated encephalomyelitis or ADEM), immune disorders such as systemic lupus erythematosus, multiple sclerosis, vascular occlusion with resultant cord infarction; it may occur following vaccination and as a complication of systemic malignancy similar to limbic encephalitis, and often the etiology is unknown. Annual incidence is 1 case per million without age or sex predilection. In the typical case, there is no prior history of neurologic abnormality, with time from symptom onset to maximum deficit ranging from 1 hour to 17 days. Prognosis is poor in most cases, with severe residual neurologic deficit being common. Imaging is to exclude treatable conditions that can mimic acute transverse myelitis. These may include acute disc herniation, hematoma, epidural abscess, or compression myelopathy. Imaging findings are nonspecific, with focal cord enlargement on T1W and poorly delineated hyperintensities on T2W images, and enhancement occurring in some cases.[36,40,41]

Miscellaneous myelopathies and conditions

Radiation myelopathy

This is a rare complication of therapeutic irradiation. Three criteria exist to establish the diagnosis. These include that the spinal cord must have been included in the radiation field, that the neurologic deficit must correspond to the cord segment that was irradiated, and that metastasis or other primary spinal cord lesions must be ruled out.[42] Four distinct clinical syndromes exist in irradiated spines, with chronic progressive radiation myelopathy (CPRM) being the most common form identified on imaging studies.[41–43] Most cases are seen following radiotherapy of nasopharyngeal carcinoma, with the area most commonly affected accordingly being cervical spinal cord. The latent period between termination of irradiation and onset of symptoms varies from 3 to 40 months, with most cases occurring between 9 and 20 months.[43] Imaging findings vary. If MRI scans are observed more than 3 years after symptom onset, cord atrophy without abnormal signal is seen. Scans performed within 8 months of symptom onset typically demonstrate long segment hyperintense lesions on T2W images with or without associated cord swelling and enhancement following contrast administration.[44]

AIDS-related myelopathy

This is probably related to direct injury of neurons by HIV, although secondary demyelination of posterior and lateral columns also occurs.[36]

Compressive myelopathy

Intramedullary high signal intensity foci on proton density or T2W MRI scans in cases of moderate to marked spinal stenosis have been observed.[45] This can be due to degenerative disc disease or spondyloarthropathy and is probably related to focal cord ischemia. Some cases resolve following decompressive surgery.[45] Other causes of compressive myelopathy can be due to mass effect from primary or secondary spine tumors or other epidural lesions such as epidural abscess.[36]

Degenerative and toxic myelopathies

Inherited and acquired degenerative disorder such as Friedrich ataxia and other spinocerebellar degenerations, amyotrophic lateral sclerosis, toxic diseases such as chronic alcoholism, and metabolic disorders such as vitamin B_{12} deficiency are miscellaneous causes of spinal cord dysfunction.[36]

Superficial siderosis

This is due to previous episodes of hemorrhage in the subarachnoid space. The pathognomonic appearance is diffuse decreased signal surrounding the cord and brainstem. Hemosiderin is toxin to the neuronal tissue causing volume loss of the CNS. Patients most commonly present with hearing loss, ataxia, and myelopathy[46] (Fig. 5.16).

Postoperative arachnoiditis

Postoperative arachnoiditis is a chronic inflammatory condition causing formation of scar tissue. This results in clumping of the nerve roots. The nerve roots may adhere to the dura, which results in a false "empty sac"; they may clump together to form what appears to be a few but very thick nerve roots; or they may adhere to each other in an irregular fashion. Enhancement of the nerve roots may also occur in postoperative arachnoiditis[47] (Fig. 5.17).

Vascular diseases

Aneurysms

Spinal aneurysms are localized saccular dilatations of spine or spinal cord arteries that are frequently associated with intramedullary spinal cord arteriovenous malformations. These are extremely rare. Most commonly they are seen in the cervical and thoracic spinal cord. They are almost always located on one of the main high-flow vessels feeding the arteriovenous malformation, with nearly 70% found on the anterior spinal

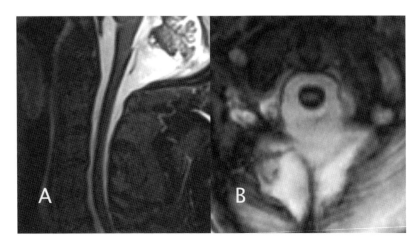

Figure 5.16 Superficial siderosis. (A) Sagittal STIR TR4000/TE60. (B) Axial gradient echo TR30/TE15. There is diffuse circumference-decreased signal surrounding the cervical cord and brainstem due to the susceptibility artifact from the hemosiderin deposition. Also note the diffuse volume loss in the cord, which is also a feature of siderosis.

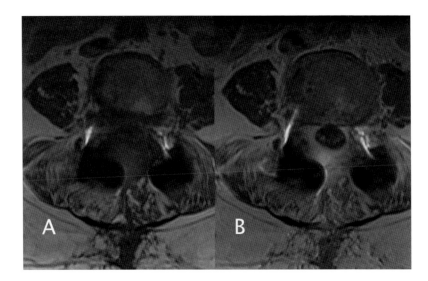

Figure 5.17 Pre- (A) and postcontrast (B) axial T1 TR580/TE11 images through the lumbar spine showing enhancement of the nerve roots reflecting arachnoiditis.

artery. In contrast to intracranial aneurysms, spinal aneurysms do not usually occur at bifurcation points. Symptoms are due to subarachnoid hemorrhage in the majority of cases. Angiography is the definitive imaging study.[36]

Vascular malformations

These are uncommon lesions. Most are arteriovenous malformations or arteriovenous fistulas. Cavernous angiomas and capillary telangiectasias are less common, with venous angiomas being rarely seen.

Arteriovenous malformations and arteriovenous fistulas

Arteriovenous malformations (AVMs) have a true nidus of pathologic vessels interposed between feeding

arteries and draining veins that are both enlarged. In contrast, arteriovenous fistulas drain directly into an enlarged venous outflow tract.[47,48]

Spinal AVMs are subdivided into four general categories. Type I is a dural arteriovenous fistula that is primarily found in the dorsal aspect of the lower thoracic cord and conus medullaris. Most consist of a single transdural arterial feeder that drains into an intradural arterialized vein. The draining vein often extends over multiple segments. Nearly 60% are spontaneous and approximately 40% are posttraumatic. Progressive neurologic deterioration likely due to chronic venous hypertension is typical[49-51] (Fig. 5.18). Type II AVMs called glomus malformations are intramedullary AVMs in which a localized compact vascular plexus is supplied by multiple feeders from anterior or posterior spinal arteries. Type II AVMs drain into a tortuous arterialized

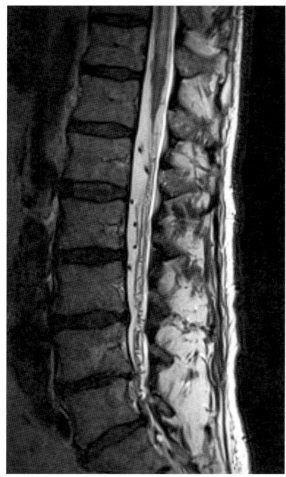

Figure 5.18 Sagittal T2 image (TR7660/TE79) shows increased signal in the conus medullaris as well as flow voids associated with the cauda equina in a patient with a dural AV fistula.

AVMs are the most common spinal vascular anomaly. The most common AVM is type I, with type III being least common. The thoracolumbar area is the most common location overall.[48,52] Paresis, sensory changes, bowel and bladder dysfunction, and impotence are common symptoms. Hemorrhage is seen frequently. Venous hypertension may be important in the development of cord symptoms.[48] Imaging findings include filling defects of enlarged vessels seen on myelography. Cord atrophy is common. MRI may show flow voids with enlarged vessels. High signal intensity is often seen on T2W images, with the cord sometimes being atrophic. Hemorrhagic byproducts may be present. Spinal angiography is the definitive diagnostic procedure for evaluation of spinal AVMs.[51,52]

Cavernous angiomas

These are similar to intracranial cavernous angiomas, with imaging findings demonstrating well-circumscribed masses. Microscopically they consist of blood-filled, endothelium-lined spaces. There are localized hemorrhages of different ages. Calcification is rare. These are, however, extremely rare lesions. Spinal angiography is typically normal since these are slow-flow vascular lesions. Findings on MRI scans demonstrate blood products of subacute and chronic ages with mixed high- and low-signal components. Typical appearance is a small, high-signal focus on both T1W and T2W images and typical imaging characteristics on gradient-refocused scans. If a typical spinal cord lesion is identified on MRI scan, the brain should be studied using gradient-refocused sequences to screen for asymptomatic intracranial lesions.[53–55]

Cord infarction

Arterial infarction: Blood supply to the cord depends on three longitudinal arterial trunks: a single anterior spinal artery and paired posterior spinal arteries with collateral flow comparatively limited. The anterior spinal artery gains its supply in most individuals from the artery of Adamkiewicz, which usually originates from the left-sided spinal arteries directly off the aorta at the T10–12 level. It sports a characteristic "hairpin" curve. Spontaneous anterior spinal cord infarction primarily affects individuals with severe atherosclerotic disease or aortic dissection, with other reported etiologies including vasculitis and hypertension.[56,58–59] Arterial infarction is extremely rare and is most often seen after aortic surgery. Most cord infarctions occur at the upper thoracic or thoracolumbar junction, with extensive involvement ranging from a single segment to multiple levels.[56,57]

venous plexus that surrounds spinal cord. These AVMs are located dorsally in the cervicomedullary region, with most occurring in younger patients with acute onset of neurologic symptoms due to intramedullary hemorrhage.[49] Type III AVMs, called juvenile type, are large, complex vascular masses that involve the cord and often have extramedullary or even extraspinal extension. Multiple arterial feeders from several different vertebral levels are common. Type IV AVMs are intradural extramedullary arteriovenous fistulas that are fed by the anterior spinal artery and lie completely outside the spinal cord and pia matter. There is no intervening small-vessel network and the fistula drains directly into an enlarged venous outflow tract. Most are anterior to the spinal cord and fed by the anterior spinal artery and most occur near the conus medullaris. Progressive neurologic deficits are typical.[49]

Clinical symptoms vary with classic presentation including sudden onset of flaccid paraparesis or quadriparesis. Associated sensory loss with preserved touch, vibration, and position sense is common.[58] Imaging demonstrates enlargement of the cord on T1W images with central or anterior intramedullary high signal on T2W images. Enhancement following contrast administration may be initially absent but occurs a few days to a few weeks after symptom onset. Follow-up scans may show cord atrophy focally and residual high signal intensity on T2W images.[58,60] In terms of imaging, chronic cord infarct is indistinguishable from myelomalacia of other causes. In acute cases, diffusion imaging may be performed, which shows increased signal on the diffusion-weighted images and decreased signal on the apparent diffusion coefficient maps. (Figs. 5.19, 5.20).

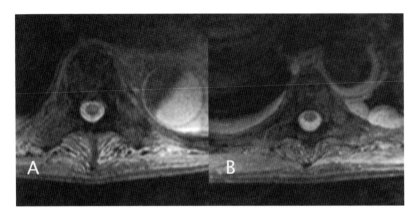

Figure 5.19 Infarct. Axial gradient echo images. Note the increased signal along the ventral aspect of the cord in (A) reflecting infarction of the cord. (B) Shows the normal appearance of the cord above the level of spinal cord infarction. Also note the descending aortic dissection.

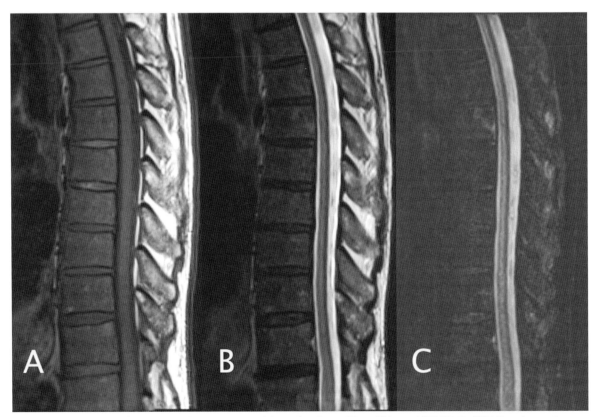

Figure 5.20 Spinal cord infarct. (A) Sagittal T1 TR500/TE12. (B) Sagittal T2 TR4620/TE117. (C) Sagittal STIR TR3830/TE82. Note that on the sagittal T1 image the spinal cord looks normal but on the sagittal T2 and STIR there is a band of hyperintensity in the ventral aspect of the cord reflecting the area of infarction in the cord.

Venous infarction, also known as subacute necrotic myelitis, is a less well known entity. Pathologic studies demonstrate enlarged, thick-walled often thrombosed veins with necrosis involving both gray and white matter. MRI suggests vascular malformation with serpentine filling defects, thrombosed veins, and cord edema.[43,61]

Spine trauma

A standardized approach to sensitive and efficient assessment of the spine is essential, with nearly 11 000 spinal cord injuries occurring in the United States annually, and total lifetime treatment and rehabilitation costs in the range of $200 000 to $800 000 per patient.[62,63] In the rare absence of CT, initial plain film evaluation may be warranted, with inclusion of no fewer than three standard views: anteroposterior, lateral, and open mouth odontoid. With missed fracture rates between 23% and 57% and delays in diagnosis ranging from 5% to 23%, there has been a global transition to CT evaluation of the spine in those patients clinically deemed high-risk as the preferred initial modality of choice.[64-66]

The isotropic nature of data acquisition allows for accurate sagittal and coronal reformatted sequences, avoiding the axial limitations of decreased sensitivity to subluxation, increased intervertebral distance, angulations, and horizontally oriented fractures. The strength of CT remains in detection of the full spectrum of fracture patterns, facet injuries, and vertebral body subluxations and malalignment.[67] Addition of intravenous contrast in combination with CT angiography (CTA) protocols is also commonly used to evaluate for acute vascular injury when suggested by the pattern of osseous injury. Typical MDCT (multidetector CT) technique consists of 0.75 mm axial acquisitions with subsequent axial, sagittal, and coronal reformats utilizing both bone and soft tissue algorithms.

Magnetic resonance imaging, subsequently discussed, is the only modality capable of identifying cord edema, cord hemorrhage, disc injury, and canal compromise in the presence or absence of osseous injury in the setting of focal neurologic deficit.

Spinal injury patterns: stability and mechanism

The most widely accepted spinal stability assessment model is a three-column classification system proposed by Denis.[68,69] The basis of the model is the sagittal designation of anterior, middle, and posterior osteoligamentous columns. The anterior column is composed of the anterior longitudinal ligament and anterior 2nd/3rd vertebral body and disc. The middle column is composed of the posterior longitudinal ligament and posterior 1st/3rd vertebral body and disc. The posterior column is composed of the posterior arch, articular processes, and posterior ligamentous complex (supraspinous ligament, interspinous ligament, ligamentum flava, articular pillar capsular ligaments). The basic premise is that injuries isolated to the middle column and injuries involving two or more columns are considered unstable. This classification system was designed to be applied to the thoracic and lumbar spine, but allowing for certain modifications, the model may be applied to the cervical spine.

Classification schemes based on injury mechanism are also proposed as an aid to characterization of not only fracture patterns but anticipated ligamentous disruption and subsequent instability. These mechanisms include axial loading, flexion, lateral compression, flexion–rotation, flexion distraction, extension, and shear.

Cervical spine injuries

While an all-inclusive review of cervical spine injuries is beyond the scope of this chapter, several classic patterns of injury are discussed.

The "Jefferson" fracture typically occurs in conjunction with axial loading, such as with a blow to the top of the head, resulting in disruption of the osseous ring of C1 with lateral displacement of the lateral masses, best evaluated in coronal reformatted sequences. The classic form is considered stable.[70,71]

Atlantoaxial dissociation is a generic term applied to injuries in which the C1 ring is displaced by rotation about the odontoid peg or articular mass. Concomitant fractures, transverse atlantal ligamentous injury, and vertebral artery injury may result. Diagnosis is suggested by asymmetry of the atlantodental space and anterior or posterior displacement of lateral mass(es); stability is variable. Three-dimensional CT reformats often aid in confirmation of the diagnosis.[72]

Odontoid fractures are commonly classified as types I, II, or III. Type I injury is an oblique fracture through the tip; type II, or "high odontoid fracture," is a horizontal fracture through the base; and type III, or "low odontoid fracture," is generally an oblique fracture through the base with extension into the body of C2. Type I fractures generally involve avulsion of portions of the alar ligament as may result from atlantooccipital dislocation and thus should be treated as unstable.[73]

Traumatic spondylolisthesis as a result of hyperextension distraction in the upper cervical spine results in a "hangman's" fracture. Classically there is fracture

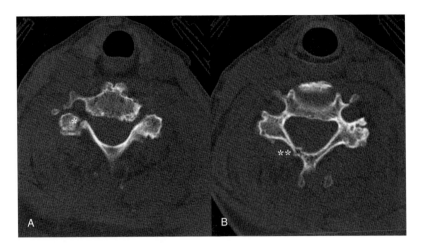

Figure 5.21 Two axial images from a cervical spine film in a patient post fall demonstrates a fracture through the right pars interarticularis (*) and lamina (**).

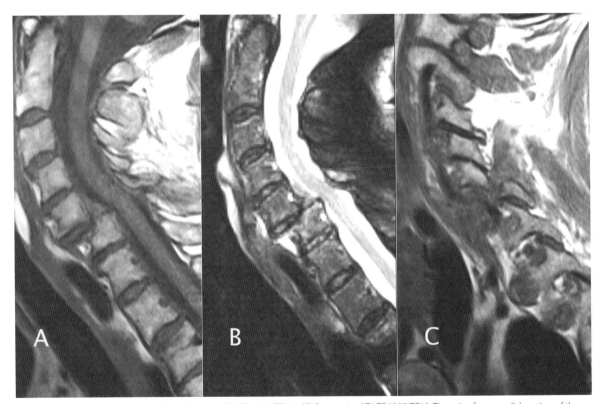

Figure 5.22 (A) Sagittal T1 TR687/TE10. (B) Sagittal T2 TR 2693/TE110. (C) Parasagittal T1 TR6887/TE10. There is a fracture dislocation of the cervical spine due to a suboptimally treated pedicle fracture. Despite the grade III anterolisthesis there is just mild cord compression. Also note the dislocation of C6–7 due to a pars fracture and a "jumped" facet joint.

of the C2 pars interarticularis bilaterally, with variable degrees of extension into the posterior elements and anterior displacement of the C2 vertebral body relative to the C3 vertebral body; it is unstable[74,75]

Flexion-teardrop fractures are severe injuries that are a product of hyperflexion. A constellation of findings is demonstrated: compression of the anterior vertebral body with small anterior avulsion fragment; retropulsion of the posterior vertebral body fragment; narrowing of the intervertebral disc space; and widening of the interlaminar and interspinous distances compatible with extensive posterior ligamentous disruption; it is unstable. Resultant cord contusion and hemorrhage are common.[76–78]

Hyperflexion with rotation may result in a unilaterally locked facet as a result of apophyseal joint ligamentous rupture and facet joint dislocation, generally considered stable. Bilateral locked facets occur in the setting of extreme flexion and distraction forces. The result is anterior dislocation of the bilateral inferior facets in relation to subjacent superior facets with ligamentous and capsular rupture; it is unstable.[79] (Figs. 5.21, 5.22)

Thoracolumbar spine injuries

The most commonly encountered thoracic and lumbar spine fracture is the compression or wedge fracture. Making up nearly 50% of all thoracolumbar fractures, these injuries are considered stable.[80]

"Seat belt" injuries are the result of forceful flexion about a fulcrum, i.e., seat belt, with associated vertebral body compression fracture and variable degrees of posterior element. Type I ("Chance" fracture) involves posterior osseous elements; type II ("Smith" fracture) involves posterior ligaments; and type III involves rupture of the annulus fibrosis.[80]

Spondylolysis is a special scenario, encountered in the lower lumbar spine in which there is a defect in the pars interarticularis. When bilateral, instability may result in anterior displacement or spondylolisthesis of the vertebral body. The specific etiology remains a subject of debate, with speculation about congenital origin versus sequela of recurrent trauma.

Pedicle fractures are among the least common injury to the spine. They can be the result of chronic or acute trauma and they can be unilateral or bilateral. Depending on their age they may show edema or fatty marrow change. Like spondylolisthesis they result in instability[81] (Fig. 5.23)

Sacral insufficiency fractures can be difficult to diagnose because they can present as hip pain or lower back pain. MRI is very sensitive on T1W sequences (Fig. 5.24), where the dark marrow edema is outlined by the normal bright fatty marrow.

MRI and spine trauma

Specific imaging protocols vary to some degree between institutions. In general, commonly used pulse sequences include: sagittal SE T1 (spin echo) for definition of anatomy and identification of disc herniations, epidural fluid collections, subluxations, vertebral body fractures, cord swelling, and cord compression; sagittal FSE/TSE T2 (fast-spin echo/turbo-spin echo) with fat saturation allowing for characterization of spinal cord edema, cord hemorrhage, ligamentous injury, disc herniation, and epidural fluid; sagittal T2*GRE (gradient

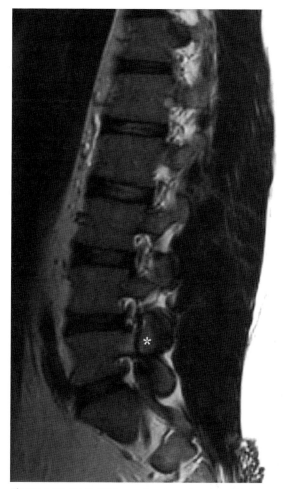

Figure 5.23 Sagittal T2 image showing a chronic pedicle fracture at L5 with a small amount of edema in the adjacent bone.

echo) for identification of cord hemorrhage, fractures, and disc protrusions; axial T2*GRE for evaluation of gray–white differentiation. STIR (short tau inversion recovery) may also be used to increase the conspicuity of edema.

Extensive investigation has been performed into spinal cord injury (SCI) patterns presenting neurologic deficit on MRI and clinical outcomes. Kulkarni et al. first proposed an approach to predicting neurologic outcomes based on three patterns of acute SCI on MRI including spinal cord hemorrhage (type I), spinal cord edema (type II), and mixed edema and hemorrhage (type III).[82] Subsequently, Schaefer et al. added the assessment of injury segment size.[83] Additional features of cord compression, cord swelling, and persistent cord signal abnormality in follow-up evaluation were found to be of prognostic significance by Yamashita et al.[84,85] In general, the presence and extent of cord

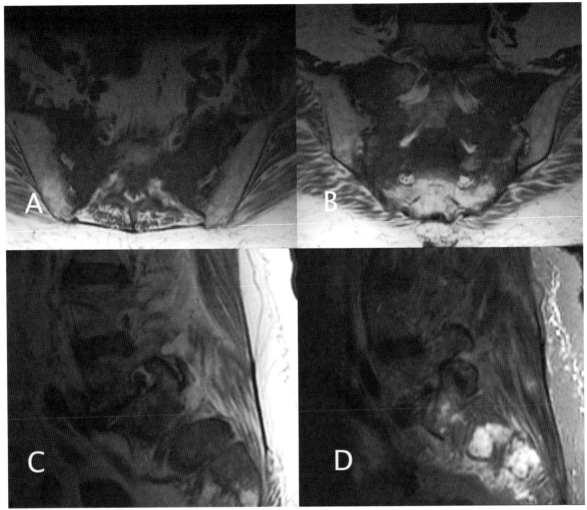

Figure 5.24 Sacral insufficiency. (A) Axial T1 TR400/TE13. (B) Coronal T1 TR425/TE13. (C) Sagittal T1 TR529/TE11. (D) Sagittal STIR TR4820/TE90. The T1 weighted sequences show the edema from the acute bilateral sacral insufficiency fracture as areas of decreased signal in this osteoporotic 79-year-old patient. The parasagittal STIR shows the edema as an area of hyperintensity.

hemorrhage is a good indicator of prognosis. Less predictable is the secondary cord injury that results from a cycle of edema and ischemia.[86]

Spinal cord edema as a result of contusion is characterized by T1 isointentsity to hypointensity with concomitant T2 hyperintensity. Spinal cord hemorrhage, most commonly localizing to the central gray matter at the level of injury, is initially T1 isointense with T2 and GRE relative hypointensity to the surrounding cord signal. Subsequently, intramedullary hemorrhage of the spinal cord undergoes a typical pattern of degradation similar to that of intracranial hemorrhage, but over a greater period of time due to differences in cord perfusion and hypoxia. Cord transection may have intercalated hemorrhage.

Careful evaluation of the anterior and posterior longitudinal ligaments, supraspinous, nuchal, and interspinous ligaments, as well as the ligamentum flavum, should be performed on all trauma patients. Ligamentous tear is depicted as discontinuity of the anticipated normal linear T1 signal hypointensity with associated soft tissue changes. Adjacent T2-hyperintense edema and hemorrhage should prompt ligamentous scrutiny. Partial and intrasubstance tears may appear as linear T2 signal hyperintensity.

Traumatic disc extrusions are variable in appearance based on the presence or absence of associated hemorrhage. If no associated hemorrhage is present, the fragment will have signal intensity similar to the native disc, whereas, hemorrhage may result in T2

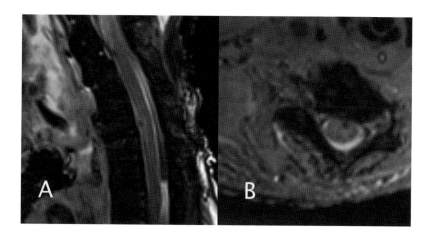

Figure 5.25 Cord hemorrhage. (A) Sagittal STIR TR4040/TE95. (B) Axial gradient echo TR30TE15. Note the punctate susceptibility artifact (dark) in the anterior aspect of the cord with surrounding edema on both sagittal and axial images in this anticoagulated patient presenting with paraplegia.

signal hyperintensity of the fragment in comparison with the native disc. Identification is important as open reduction may be necessary in the setting of cervical facet dislocations to prevent increased neurologic compromise.

Epidural hematoma presents as a hypointense T2*GRE focus adjacent to the cord with isointense T1 signal. It may complicate cord injury or lead directly to cord ischemia as a result of mass effect.

Cord hemorrhage can be best detected using a gradient echo sequence or T2W image in the acute stage, where the hemorrhage appears as a dark area. In subacute stage the hemorrhage is bright on T1 and T2 (Fig. 5.25).

Insensitivity of MRI to acute fracture makes it inappropriate as the initial imaging modality in the setting of suspected osseous injury. A solitary exception is the utility of MRI in the characterization of vertebral body fractures as acute or chronic. Hemorrhagic blood products and marrow edema are relatively conspicuous in the trabecular bone of the vertebral body.

Carotid dissection and vertebral artery thrombosis occur to some degree in the setting of significant trauma and should be considered. Cervical vascular injury evaluation with CTA, MRA, Doppler sonography, or catheter angiography may be considered.

Congenital anomalies of the spine and spinal cord

Congenital anomalies of the spine and spinal cord are generically classified as spinal dysraphisms. The dysraphisms, or "defective fusion of parts that normally unite," comprise a group of anomalies that result from specific aberrations of the embryologic stages of spinal development: gastrulation (weeks 2–3), primary neurulation (weeks 3–4), and secondary neurulation (weeks 5–6). These anomalies were classically characterized specifically by developmental embryologic origin. This is a complex strategy with limited clinical application. The current widely accepted model, developed and introduced by Tortori-Donati and Rossi, is a clinical-neuroradiological classification strategy relying upon only a few fundamental key features: (1) clinical classification of the dysraphism as open (exposed to environment through osseous and skin defect) or closed (covered with skin); (2) closed dysraphisms are subsequently divided into those entities with an associated subcutaneous mass versus those without a mass; and (3) finally, those closed defects without associated mass are further divided into simple and complex.[87]

Open spinal dysraphisms (OSD)

Open dysraphic defects account for 85% all cases and are commonly diagnosed by ultrasound (US) or fetal MRI following identification of elevated maternal alpha fetoprotein. Nearly all are associated with Chiari II malformations and all exhibit neural placodes. Neural placodes are a splayed-out segment of embryonal neural tissue which fails to transform through a process of bending and folding (neurulation) into the neural tube. Myelomeningoceles make up the overwhelming majority of open defects at 98%, characterized by protrusion portions of spinal cord and nerve roots (neural placode) beyond the skin. Myeloceles are second most common, exhibiting a placode that is flush with the skin. Hemimyeloceles and hemimyelomeningoceles are rare entities with features similar to those above but associated with diastematomyelia or "cord splitting."[88]

Closed spinal dysraphisms (CSD) with a mass

Defined as a closed dysraphic defect with associated subcutaneous mass. The majority of masses are localized to the lower lumbar spine above the intergluteal fold. Lipomyeloceles and lipomyelomeningoceles exhibit a placode-lipoma morphology. The result of invasion the neural tube defect by mesenchymal tissue that is subsequently induced to form adipose tissue. The lipomyelocele placode–lipoma interface resides within the spinal canal, whereas the lipomyelomeningocele placode–lipoma interface is outside of the canal. Meningoceles are CSF-filled herniated meningeal sacs without cord protrusion. Terminal myelocystoceles are meningoceles that contain a herniated terminal syrinx. Myelocystoceles (nonterminal) are meningoceles that contain a dilated herniated central canal and occur more commonly in the cervicothoracic region.

Closed spinal dysraphisms (CSD) without a mass: simple

Intradural lipoma is simply a lipoma dorsally located within the dural sac. Their presence should prompt close inspection for tethered cord. Tethered cord is defined as low-lying conus medullaris below L2–3 with associated shortened and thickened filum terminale >2 mm. The persistent terminal ventricle is a cystic cavity immediately above the filum terminale that does not enhance and is generally incidental, with no clinical significance. The dermal sinus is an epithelium-lined tract connecting neural tissues/meninges with skin surfaces.[88]

Closed spinal dysraphisms (CSD) without a mass: complex

A dorsal enteric fistula is the result of abnormal persistent communication between skin and bowel. The neurenteric cyst occurs anterior to the cervicothoracic spinal cord and is a mucin-secreting lined cyst similar to gastrointestinal tract elements. Disorders of notochordal formation include segmental spinal dysgenesis and caudal agenesis. Misallocation of notochord cells results in varying degrees of segmental deficits and less commonly dysgenesis. Wedge vertebra, bony bars/block vertebra, butterfly vertebra, and hemivertebra represent a few of the osseous abnormalities encountered. When associated with pathologic curvature and alignment of the spine, the phenomena may be classified as congenital scoliosis. Segmental spinal dysgenesis is a less common entity in which an isolated level, usually lumbar or thoracic, is affected by the failure of osseous, central cord, and nerve root development. Caudal regression represents a similar total or partial failure of spinal column development, often with associated developmental anomalies of multiple systems.[88]

Down's syndrome and spinal abnormalities

Down's syndrome is associated with several spinal abnormalities. These include atlanto-occiptal instability, scoliosis, and cervical spondylosis.[89] The most prevalent is atlanto-occipital instability. This can be identified radiographically in children as widening of the anterior atlanto-odontoid distance (AAOD) greater than 5 mm. This is felt to be caused by posterior transverse ligament laxity.[90] This widening of the AAOD can cause compression of the brainstem by the dens. The frequency is reported as high as 30% in patients with Down's syndrome.[91] However, the percentage of patients who are clinically symptomatic is much lower. Given the large percentage of patients who have radiographic instability and yet the paucity of Down's syndrome patients who are clinically symptomatic, there has been controversy whether there is a need to screen patients who might be engaged in sports or the Special Olympics.[92,93] Cervical plain films are currently a recommended part of the childhood screening by the American National Down Syndrome Society (1999), but are deemed to be too unreliable for screening purposes by the UK and Ireland Down's Syndrome Medical Interest Group.[94,95]

Scoliosis

Scoliosis is curvature of the spine in the coronal plane. Scoliosis is a three-dimensional phenomenon and has a rotatory component associated with it that can be determined by observing the placement of the pedicles in relation to the vertebra. It can be subdivided by cause (idiopathic, congenital, developmental, neuromuscular, and tumor associated) as well as age. Idiopathic scoliosis accounts for 80% of the cases of scoliosis.[96]

Scoliosis is described by the apex of the curvature and the degree of curvature. The apex is given as the level (vertebral body) and the side to which it is pointed (left or right). Cobb angle is the measurement used to characterize scoliosis. A Cobb angle of 10° or greater is typically used as the cut-off for determining scoliosis.

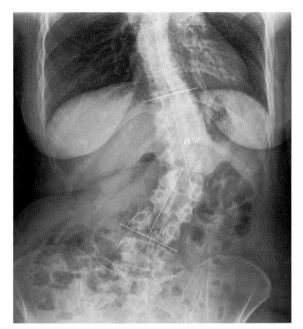

Figure 5.26 AP scoliosis film measuring the Cobb angle. This patient has a levoscoliosis with the apex at L1. Note the lines overlying the end plates of L4 and T11. These are drawn on the end vertebrae, which are the vertebrae demonstrating maximum tilt in relation to the horizontal plane. The angle α formed by the lines perpendicular to the end vertebrae is the Cobb angle.

The Cobb angle is obtained from an AP film by drawing lines parallel to the end plates of the end vertebral bodies which are at the inflection points of the superior and inferior curves (the end plates which produce the greatest tilt in relation to horizontal.) These end vertebrae also show the least rotation. If the end plates are difficult to see, a line can be drawn through the pedicles and that can be used to determine what are the end vertebrae. The angle formed from the lines drawn along the superior and inferior end vertebra (or lines perpendicular to them) is the Cobb angle (Fig. 5.26)

Neoplastic disease of the spine

High-contrast sensitivity and multiplanar capability make MRI the study of choice when evaluating neoplastic disease of the spinal cord. Standard T1W precontrast, T1W postcontrast with fat saturation, and T2W pulse sequences are acquired. Addition of GRE increases the conspicuity of cord hemorrhage and STIR allows for sensitive assessment of sites of edema. Osseous spinal abnormalities continue to be best evaluated by CT due to the inherent high sensitivity to alterations of bone mineralization.

Features common to nearly all spinal cord neoplasms include: a tendency to enlarge the cord focally or diffusely, T2/PD signal hyperintensity, and enhancement. Once a mass is identified, subsequent classification using location allows for greater accuracy in generating a practical differential diagnosis: specifically, intramedullary (within the spinal cord), intradural/extramedullary, and extradural.

Intramedullary neoplasms

Intramedullary neoplasms directly involve/originate from the spinal cord and account for nearly 25% of all tumors of the spine. The majority (90–95%) of intramedullary neoplasms are malignant.[97] Adults most commonly develop ependymomas and children astrocytomas. These two cell types alone make up more than 70% of intramedullary malignancies.

Ependymoma

Ependymomas account for 60% of all glial-based intramedullary/filum tumors.[97] Multiple histologic subtypes exist; most common overall is the "cellular" type, arising from ependymal cells lining the central canal as well as nests of ependymal cells at the filum and sacral regions and occurring with greatest frequency in the cervical spine. The filum terminale is affected by the "myxopapillary" subtype, which is complicated more commonly by hemorrhage, and by definition intradural extramedullary. Ependymomas are glial in origin, tend to be central in position, and exhibit sharp margins. Cystic changes and hemorrhage are also observed with moderate frequency. Generally T1 iso/hypointense, patchy heterogeneous T2 hyperintense, T2 hypointense; "cap sign" is occasionally noted, the result of hemosiderin staining and development of a pseudocapsule on gross specimen. Both homogenous and heterogeneous contrast enhancement occur commonly, sometimes in the typical "cyst with mural nodule" configuration (Fig. 5.27).

Astrocytoma

Astrocytomas are the second most common adult intramedullary tumor and the most common intramedullary tumor in children.[98] Generally low grade and infiltrative, astrocytomas demonstrate more ill-defined margins and eccentric orientation in the cord as opposed to the sharply delineated central morphology of ependymomas. Intratumoral cysts are not uncommon and are sometimes associated with proximal or distal syrinx in the pilocytic type. Thoracic

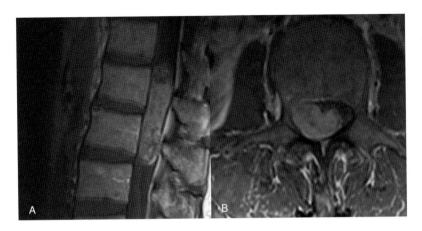

Figure 5.27 Ependymoma. Postcontrast sagittal (A) and axial (B) T1 TR773/TE10 MRI showing diffuse enhancement and compression of the conus medullaris which is displaced anterior on the axial images.

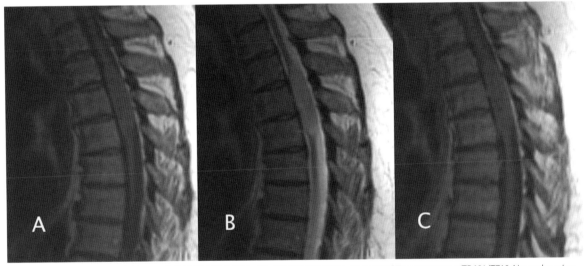

Figure 5.28 Astrocytoma. (A) Sagittal T1 TR681/TE10. (B) Sagittal T2 TR3770/TE113. (C) Sagittal T1 postcontrast TR681/TE10. Nonenhancing expansile mass on postcontrast image (C) reflects a low-grade thoracic spine astrocytoma. Note the increased signal on T2 weighted images.

spine is involved only slightly more frequently than cervical spine. There is a minimal male predominance. MRI examination reveals mild fusiform widening of the cord, T1 iso/hypointensity, avid enhancement, and T2 signal hyperintensity (Figs. 5.28, 5.29).

Hemangioblastoma

Although predominantly intramedullary and involving the dorsal spinal cord and posterior fossa, hemangioblastomas may also infrequently involve extramedullary structures. Overall, they account for less than 1–7.2% of cord tumors. The thoracic spine is affected slightly more frequently than the cervical spine. The vast majority of lesions are solitary, as many as 80%. Approximately 1/3 of cases are associated with von Hippel–Lindau syndrome. MRI appearance: T1

isointensity, T2 hyperintensity, avid enhancement, flow voids [99] (Fig. 5.30)

Metastatic disease

Lung, breast, colon, lymphoma, and kidney carcinomas may all infrequently metastasize to the intramedullary spinal cord but are found in only 2% of cancer patients at autopsy. MRI appearance: T1 hypointense, T2 hyperintense, avidly enhancing.[97] They can appear as enhancing intramedullary lesions, intradural extramedullary masses. or as leptomeningeal disease (Figs. 5.31, 5.32)

Ganglioglioma

Gangliogliomas represent neoplastic ganglion and glial cell proliferation resulting in long segment expansion

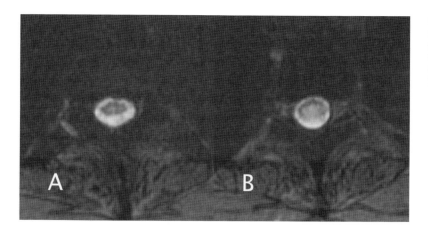

Figure 5.29 Two axial gradient echo (TR94TE34) images from astrocytoma above the level of the tumor (A) and at the level of the tumor in the thoracic spine (B). Note the marked difference in the caliber of the cord.

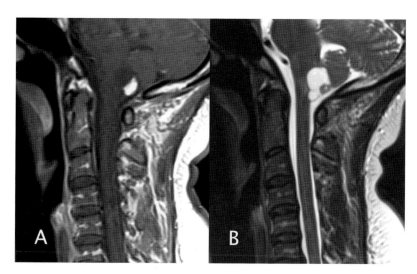

Figure 5.30 Hemangioblastoma. (A) Sagittal T1 TR700/TE9 postcontrast. (B) Sagittal T2 TR3000/TE87. Cystic mass at the craniocervical junction with enhancing mural nodule.

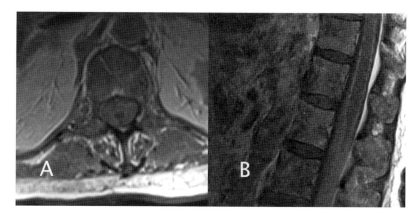

Figure 5.31 Postcontrast T1 images TR769/TE12 through the thoracolumbar junction showing diffuse enhancement in the subarachnoid space reflecting leptomeningeal metastasis. The axial image (A) shows diffuse enhancement outlining the conus medullaris.

of the cord with associated cystic components. The intramedullary tumor predominantly affects children and young adults. Commonly affecting the cervical and upper thoracic cord, the tumor exhibits slow, expansive growth resulting in osseous erosions/remodeling and scoliosis. MRI features demonstrated are typically mixed isohypointensity T1 signal, heterogeneous isohyperintensity T2, patchy enhancement, and cystic changes. Calcifications, when present help in distinguishing from astrocytoma.[97–99]

Intradural extramedullary neoplasms

Meningioma

Meningioma is the second most common primary "intraspinal" tumor.[97] It most commonly affects the thoracic spine followed by the cervical spine. MRI demonstrates T1 isointensity, T2 isointensity, and intense homogeneous enhancement. Dural tail and/or adjacent dural thickening are classic features. Those

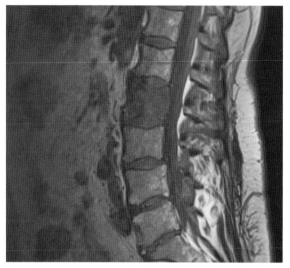

Figure 5.32 Noncontrast sagittal T1 TR500/TE11 image showing pathologic compression fracture from endometrial carcinoma metastatic disease. Note that there is mild dorsal displacement of the posterior wall and a small amount of epidural tumor dorsal to L2.

meningiomas that occur below the level of C7 are most commonly posterior to the cord. An association with neurofibromatosis II should prompt evaluation for other abnormalities (Fig. 5.33).

Schwannoma

Schwannoma is the most common "intraspinal" tumor.[97] It is an eccentric, exophytic, nerve sheath tumor of Schwann cell origin. Generally affecting the cervical region, schwannomas often have both extradural and intradural components in a so-called "dumbbell" shape. MRI findings include: T1 isohypointensity, T2 isohyperintensity, moderate to marked homogenous enhancement, occasionally "target" enhancement with lower central intensity (Fig. 5.34).

Neurofibroma

Neurofibromas are an infiltrative mixture of Schwann cells and fibroblasts and are associated neurofibromatosis I. MRI findings include: T1 isohypointensity, T2 hyperintensity, and marked homogenous enhancement.[76] Neurofibromas may be solitary or multiple nodular masses.

Myxopapillary ependymoma

Myxopapillary ependymomas account for 83% of filum tumors.[99] They are generally slow growing, leading to vertebral scalloping and canal enlargement. MRP findings include: isointense T1W and hyperintense T2W with avid enhancement. Their highly vascular nature

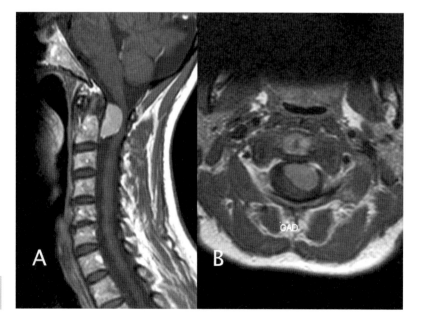

Figure 5.33 Sagittal (A) and axial (B) postcontrast T1 MRI images through the cervical spine showing an enhancing dural-based meningioma compressing the cord at the level of the craniocervical junction.

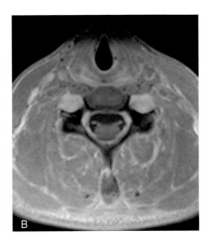

Figure 5.34 Postcontrast T1 images TR700/TE9 in the lower cervical spine showing enhancing paraspinous masses following the nerve roots consistent with diffuse schwannoma.

commonly leads to hemorrhage. Classic "cap" type T2 hypointensity from hemosiderin and formation of a pseudocapsule are occasionally demonstrated.

Intrathecal metastases: "drop mets"

Drop metastases represent seeding of the subarachnoid space, classically as the result of migration of exfoliated tumor cells from primary CNS tumors such as astrocytoma, medulloblastoma, ependymoma, and pineal neoplasms. Non-CNS primary malignancy such as breast, lung, leukemia, and lymphoma also metastasize to the leptomeninges. MRI will demonstrate either multiple enhancing nodules or diffuse thickening and enhancement of the meninges.

Extradural neoplasms

The majority of extradural neoplasms are metastatic in etiology with less than 5% being primary bone tumors.[87] While discussion of primary bone tumors is beyond the scope of this chapter, brief discussion of metastatic marrow replacement is in order. As the marrow of the vertebral bodies is exposed to a large volume of blood flow, implantation of malignant cells is common. Growth and proliferation of the metastatic foci ultimately results in replacement of the normal T1 bright fatty marrow signal with T1 signal hypointensity. The accompanying T2 signal is generally hyperintense but may be variable. Postcontrast imaging is of minimal benefit, but addition of inversion recovery sequences has great utility in exaggerating the conspicuity of pathologic marrow signal.

References

1. Mody MG, Nourbakhsh A, Stahl DL, *et al.* The prevalence of wrong level surgery among spine surgeons. *Spine* 2008; **33**(2): 194–8.

2. Harnsberger HR, Osborn A, Macdonald AJ. *Diagnostic and Surgical Imaging Anatomy Brain, Head & Neck, Spine.* Salt Lake City, UT: Amirsys; 2006.

3. Modic MT, Masaryk TJ, Ross JS. *Magnetic Resonance Imaging of the Spine.* 2nd ed. St. Louis, MO: Mosby Year Book; 1994.

4. Fox MW, Ootrio BM, Kilgore JE. Neurologic complications of ankylosing spondylitis. *J Neurosurg* 1993; **78**: 871–8.

5. Matsui H, Kanamori M, Ishihara H, *et al.* Familial predisposition for lumbar degenerative disc disease: a case–control study. *Epidemiology* 1998; **23**: 1029–34.

6. Powell M, Szypryt P, Wilson M, *et al.* Prevalence of lumbar disc degeneration observed by magnetic resonance in symptomless women. *Lancet* 1986; **328**: 1366–7.

7. Weishaupt D, Zanetti M, Hodler J, *et al.* MR imaging of the lumbar spine: prevalence of intervertebral disk extrusion and sequestration, nerve root compression, end plate abnormalities, and osteoarthritis of the facet joints in asymptomatic volunteers. *Radiology* 1998; **209**: 661–6.

8. Kramer J. Intervertebral disc disease, causes, diagnosis, treatment and prophylaxis. 2nd ed. New York: George Thieme Verlag; 1990: 14–47.

9. Nomenclature and Classification of Lumbar Disc Pathology. http://www.asnr.org/spine_nomenclature/ (accesssed December 1, 2011).

10. Modic MT, Steinberg PM, Ross JS, *et al.* Degenerative disk disease: assessment of changes in vertebral body marrow with MR imaging. Radiology 1988; **166**: 193–9.

11. Liu SS, Williams KD, Drayer BP, Spetzler RF, Sonntag VK: Synovial cysts of the lumbosacral spine: diagnosis by MR imaging. *AJR* 1990; **154**: 163–9.

12. Hiramatsn Y, Nobechi T. Calcification of posterior longitudinal ligament of spine among Japanese. *Radiology* 1971; **100**: 307–12.

13. Resnick D, Guerra Jr J, Robinson CA, Vint VC. Association of diffuse idiopathic skeletal hyperostosis (DISH) and calcification and ossification of the posterior longitudinal ligament. *AJR* 1978; **131**(6): 1049–53.

14. Weinfeld RM, Olson PN, Maki DD, Griffiths HJ. The prevalence of diffuse idiopathic skeletal hyperostosis (DISH) in two large American Midwest metropolitan hospital populations. *Skeletal Radiol* 1997; **26**(4): 222–5.

15. Resnick D. Degenerative diseases of the vertebral column. *Radiology* 1985; **156**: 3–14.

16. Smith JK, *et al.* Imaging manifestations of neurosarcoidosis. *AJR Am J Roentgenol* 2004; **182**(2): 289–95.

17. Braun J, Bollow M, Sieper J. Radiologic diagnosis and pathology of the spondyloarthropathies. *Rheum Dis Clin North Am* 1998; **24**: 697–703.

18. Fox MW, Ootrio BM, Kilgore JE, Neurologic complications of ankylosing spondylitis, *J Neurosurg* 1993; **78**: 871–8.

19. Sharif HS. Role of MR imaging in the management of spinal infections. *AJR* 1992; **158**: 1333–45.

20. Mark AS. MRI of infections and inflammatory diseases of the spine. *MRI Decisions* 1991 March/April: 12–26.

21. Brant-Zawadzki M. Infections. In: Newton TH, Potts DG, eds. *Modern Neuroradiology, vol. 1: Computed Tomography of the Spine and Spinal Cord.* San Anselmo, CA: Clavedel Press; 1983: 205–29.

22. Thrush A, Enzmann D. MR imaging of infectious spondylitis. *AJNR* 1990; **11**: 1171–80.

23. Sklar EML, Post MJD, Lebwohl NH. Imaging of Infection of the lumbosacral spine. *Neuroimaging* 1993; **3**: 577–90.

24. Post MJD, Sze G, Quencer RM, *et al.* Gadolinium-enhanced MR in spinal infection. *J Comput Assist Tomogr* 1990; **14**: 721–9.

25. Resnick D. Inflammatory diseases of the vertebral column. *Categorical course on Spine and Cord imaging.* American Society of Neuroradiology; 1988: 51–49.

26. Sharif HS, Aideyan OA, Clark DC, *et al.*. Brucellar and tuberculosis spondylitis: comparative imaging features. *Radiology* 1989; **171**: 419–25.

27. Smith AS, Weinstein MA, Mizushima A, *et al.* MR imaging of characteristics of tuberculosis spondylitis vs. vertebral osteomyelitis. *AJNR* 1989; **10**: 619–25.

28. Arabi KM, Al Sebai MW, Al Chakaki M. Evaluation of radiological investigations in spinal tuberculosis. *Int Orthop (SICOT)* 1992; **16**: 165–7.

29. Boxer DI, Pratt C, Hine AL, McNicol M. Radiological features during and following treatment of spinal tuberculosis. *Br J Radiol* 1992; **65**: 476–9.

30. Numaguchi Y, Rigamonti D, Rothman MI, *et al.* Spinal epidural abscess: evaluation with gadolinium-enhanced MR imaging. *Radiographics* 1993; **13**: 545–59.

31. Sandhu FS, Dillon WP. spinal epidural abscess: evaluation with contrast-enhanced MR imaging. *AJNR* 1991; **12**: 1087–93.

32. Nussbaum ES, Rigamonti D, Standiford H, *et al.* Spinal epidural abscess: a report of 40 cases and review *Surg Neurol* 1992; **38**: 225–31.

33. Kricun R, Shoemaker EI, Chovanes GI, Stephens HW. Epidural abscess of the cervical spine: MR findings in five cases. *AJR* 1992; **158**: 1145–9.

34. Bartels RH, deJong TR, Grotenhuis JA. Spinal subdural abscess. *J Neurosurg* 1992; **76**: 307–11.

35. Gero B, Sze G, Sharif H. MR imaging of intradural inflammatory diseases of the spine. *AJNR* 1991; **12**: 1009–19.

36. Scotti G, Righi C, Campi A. Myelitis and myelopathies. *Riv di Neuroradiol* 1992; **5**(suppl 2): 49–52.

37. DeLaPaz R. Demyelinating disease of the spinal cord. In: Enzmann D, DeLaPaz R, Rubin J, eds. *Magnetic Resonance of the Spine.* St. Louis: Mosby; 1990; 423–36.

38. Osborn AG, Harnsberger HR, Smoker WRK, Boyer R. Multiple sclerosis in adolescents: CT and MR findings, *AJNR* 1990; **12**: 521–4.

39. Larsson E-M, Holtas S, Nilsson O. Gd-DTPA-enhanced MR of suspected spinal multiple sclerosis. *AJNR* 1989; **10**: 1071–6.

40. Holtas S, Basibuyuk N, Frederiksson K. MRI in acute transverse myelopathy, *Neuroradiol* 1993; **35**: 221–6.

41. Austin SG, Zee C-S, Walters C. The role of magnetic resonance imaging in acute transverse myelitis. *Can J Neurol Sci* 1992; **19**: 508–11.

42. Zweig G, Russell EJ. Radiation myelopathy of the cervical spinal cord: MR findings. *AJNR* 1990; **11**: 1188–90.

43. Michikawa M, Wada Y, Sano M, *et al.* Radiation myelopathy: significance of gadolinium-DTPA enhancement in the diagnosis. *Neuroradiol* 1991; **33**: 286–9.

44. Wang P-Y, Shen W-C, Jan J-S. MR imaging in radiation myelopathy. *AJNR* 1992; **13**: 1049–55.

45. Takahashi M, Yamashita Y, Sakamoto Y, Kojima R. Chronic cervical cord compression: clinical significance of increased signal intensity on MR images. *Radiol* 1989; **173**: 219–224.

46. Levy M, Turtzo C, Llinas RH. Superficial siderosis: a case report and review of the literature. *Nat Clin Pract Neurol* 2007; **3**: 54–8.

47. Ross JS, Masaryk TJ, Modic MT, *et al.* MR imaging of lumbar arachnoiditis. *AJR* 1987; **149**: 1025–32.

48. Rodesch G, Lasjaunias P, Berenstein A. Embolization of spinal cord arteriovenous malformations. *Riv di Neuroradiol* 1992; **5**(suppl 2): 67–92.

49. Anson JA, Spetzler RF. Classification of spinal arteriovenous malformations and implications for treatment. *BNI Quarterly* 1992; **8**: 2–8.

50. Nichols DA, Rufenacht DA, Jack CR Jr, Forbes GA. Embolization of spinal dural arteriovenous fistula with polyvinyl alcohol particles: experience in 14 patients. *AJNR* 1992; **13**: 933–40.

51. Beaujeux RL, Reizine DC, Casasco A, *et al.* Endovascular treatment of vertebral arteriovenous fistula. *Radiology* 1992; **183**: 361–7.

52. Naidich TP, McLone DG, Harwood-Nash DC. Vascular malformations. In: Newton TH, Potts DG, eds. *Modern Neuroradiology, vol 1: Computed Tomography of the Spine and Spinal Cord.* San Anselmo, CA: Clavedel Press; 1983: 397–400.

53. Ogilvy CS, Louis DN, Ojemannn RG. Intramedullary cavernous angiomas of the spinal cord: clinical presentation, pathologic features, and surgical management. *Neurosurgery* 1992; **31**: 219–30.

54. Anson JA, Spetzler RF. Surgical resection of intramedullary spinal cord cavernous malformations. *J Neurosurg* 1993; **78**: 446–51.

55. Bourgouin PM, Tampieri D, Johnston W, *et al.* Multiple occult vascular malformations of the brain and spinal cord: MRI diagnosis. *Neuroradiology* 1992; **34**: 110–11.

56. Friedman DP, Flanders AE. Enhancement of gray matter in anterior spinal infarction. *AJNR* 1992; **13**: 983–5.

57. Yuh WTC, March EE, Wang AK, *et al.* MR Imaging of spinal cord and vertebral body infarction. *AJNR* 1992; **13**: 145–54.

58. Takahashi S, Yamada T, Ishii K, *et al.* MRI of anterior spinal artery syndrome of the cervical spinal cord. *Neuroradiology* 1992; **35**: 25–9.

59. Mikulis DJ, Ogilvy CS, McKee A, *et al.* Spinal cord infarction and fibrocartilagenous emboli. *AJNR* 1992; **13**: 155–60.

60. Hirono H, Yamadori A, Komiyama M, *et al.* MRI of spontaneous spinal cord infarction: serial changes in gadolinium-DTPA enhancement. *Neuroradiol* 1992; **34**: 95–7.

61. Enzmann DR. Vascular diseases. In: Enzmann DR, DeLaPaz R, Rubin J, eds. *Magnetic Resonance Imaging of the Spine.* St. Louis, MO: Mosby; 1990: 510–37.

62. [No authors listed]. Spinal cord injury: facts and figures at a glance. *J Spinal Cord Med* 2000; **23**(1): 51–3.

63. Pope A, Tarlov AR. *Disability in America: Toward a National Agenda for Prevention.* Washington, DC: National Academy Press; 1991.

64. Blackmore CC, Ramsey SD, Mann FA, *et al.* Cervical spine screening with CT in trauma patients: a cost effectiveness analysis. *Radiology* 1999; **212**: 117–25.

65. Nunez DB, Quencer RM. The role of helical CT in the assessment of cervical spine injuries. *Am J Roentgenol* 1998; **171**: 951–7.

66. Nunez DB, Zuluaga A, Fuentes Bernardo DA, *et al.* Cervical spine trauma; how much do we learn by routinely using helical CT? *Radiographics* 1996; **16**: 1307–18.

67. Woodring JH, Lee C. The role and limitations of computed tomography scanning in the evaluation of cervical trauma. *J Trauma* 1992; **33**(5): 698–708.

68. Denis F. The three column spine and its significance in the classification of acute throacolumbar spinal injuries. *Spine* 1983; **8**: 817.

69. Denis F. Spinal instability as defined by the three column spine concept in acute spinal trauma. *Clin Orthop* 1984; **189**: 65.

70. Han SY, Witten DM, Mussleman JP. Jefferson fracture of the atlas. Report of six cases. *J Neurosurg* 1976; **44**: 368.

71. Keterson L, Benzel E, Orrison W, Coleman J. Evaluation and treatment of atlas burst fractures (Jefferson fractures). *J Neurosurg* 1991; **75**: 213.

72. Moore KR, Frank EH. Traumatic atlantoaxial rotatory subluxation and dislocation. *Spine* 1995; **20**: 1928.

73. Anderson LD, D'Alonzo RT. Fractures of the odontoid process of the axis. *J Bone Joint Surg Am* 1974; **56**: 1663.

74. Fielding JW, Francis WR Jr, Hawkins RJ, *et al.* Traumatic spondylolisthesis of the axis. *Clin Orthop* 1989; **239**; 47.

75. Mirvis SE, Young JW, Lim C, Greenberg J. Hangman's fracture: radiologic assessment in 27 cases. *Radiology* 1987; **163**: 713.

76. Scher AT. "Tear-drop" fractures of the cervical spine – radiological features. *S Afr Med J* 1982; **61**: 355.

77. Schneider R, Kahn E. Chronic neurologic sequelae of acute trauma to the spine and spinal cord. Part 1: the significance of the acute flexion or "tear-drop" fracture-dislocation of the cervical spine. *J Bone Joint Surg Am* 1956; **38**: 985.

78. Kim KS, Chen HH, Russell EJ, Rogers LF. Flexion teardrop fracture of the cervical spine: radiographic characteristics. *Am J Roentgenol* 1989; **152**: 319.

79. Shanmuganathan K, Mirvis SE, Levine AM. Rotational injury of cervical facets: CT analysis of fracture patterns with implications for management and neurologic outcomes. *Am J Roentgenol* 1994; **163**: 1165.

80. Rogers LF. The roentgenographic appearances of transverse or chance fractures of the spine: the seat belt fracture. *Am J Roentgenol* 1971; **111**: 844–9.

81. Guillodo Y, Botton E, Saraux A, *et al.* Contralateral spondylolysis and fracture of the lumbar pedicle in an elite female gymnast: a case report. *Spine* 2000; **25**(19): 2541–3.

82. Kulkarni MV, McArdle CB, Kopanicky D, *et al.* Acute spinal cord injury: MR imaging at 1.5 T. *Radiology* 1987; **164**: 837–43.

83. Schaefer DM, *et al.* Magnetic resonance imaging of acute cervical spine trauma. Correlation with severity of neurologic injury. *Spine* 1989; **14**(10): 1090–5.

84. Yamashita Y, *et al.* Acute spinal cord injury: magnetic resonance imaging correlated with myelopathy. *Br J Radiol* 1991; **64**(759): 201–9.

85. Yamashita Y, *et al.* Chronic injuries of the spinal cord: assessment with MR imaging. *Radiology* 1990; **175**(3): 849–54.

86. Leypold BG, Flanders AE, Burns AS. The early evolution of spinal cord lesions on MR imaging following traumatic spinal cord injury. *AJNR* 2008; **29**: 1012–16.

87. Tortori-Donati P, Rossi A, Cama A. Spinal dysraphism: a review of neuroradiological features with embryological correlations and proposal for a new classification. *Neuroradiology* 2000; **42**: 471–91.

88. Rufener SL, Ibrahim M, Raybaud CA, *et al.* Congenital spine and spinal cord malformations – pictorial review. *AJR* 2010; **194**: S26–S37.

89. Bosma GP, van Buchem MA, Voormolen JH, van Biezen FC, Brouwer OF. Cervical spondylarthrotic myelopathy with early onset in Down's syndrome: five cases and a review of the literature. *J Intellect Disabil Res* 1999; **43**(4): 283–8.

90. Merrick J, Ezra E, Josef B, *et al.* Musculoskeletal problems in Down Syndrome European Paediatric Orthopaedic Society Survey: the Israeli sample. *J Pediatr Orthop B.* 2000; **9**(3): 185–92.

91. Alvarez N, Rubin L. Atlantoaxial instability in adults with Down syndrome: a clinical and radiological survey. *Appl Res Ment Retard* 1986; **7**(1): 67–78.

92. American Academy of Pediatrics. Committee on Sports Medicine. Atlantoaxial instability in Down syndrome. *Pediatrics* 1984; **74**(1): 152–4.

93. Pueschel SM, Scola FH, Perry CD, Pezzullo JC. Atlantoaxial instability in children with Down syndrome. *Pediatr Radiol* 1981; **10**(3): 129–32.

94. Down Syndrom Health Care Guidelines. http://www.dsacc.org/downloads/healthcare/dshealthcareguidelines.pdf. New York: National Down Syndrome Society (accessed December 1, 2011).

95. Basic Medical Surveillance Essentials for People with Down's Syndrome. http://www.dsmig.org.uk/library/articles/guideline-cervsp-4.pdf. Nottingham, UK: Down's Syndrome Medical Information Services (accessed December 1, 2011).

96. Kim H, Kim HS, Moon ES, *et al.* Scoliosis imaging: what radiologists should know. *Radiographics* 2010; **30**(7): 1823–42.

97. Bloomer CW, Ackerman A, Bhatia R. Imaging for spine tumors and new applications. *Top Magn Reson Imaging* 2006; **17**: 69–87.

98. Karagianis A, Klufas R, Schwartz R. MRI of cervical spine neoplasms. *Appl Radiol* 2003; **12**: 26–38.

99. Koeller K, Rosenblum R, Morrison AL, *et al.* Neoplasms of the spinal cord and filum terminale: radiologic-pathologic correlation. *Radiographics* 2000; **20**(6): 1721–49.

Chapter

6

Evoked potential monitoring

Chakorn Chansakul and Dileep R. Nair

Key points

- Neurophysiologic intraoperative monitoring is the use of electrophysiological techniques to assess functional integrity of the nervous system during surgery, to prevent iatrogenic injuries to the neural structures.
- Somatosensory evoked potentials are used primarily for spinal cord monitoring. This technique mainly assesses the function of the proprioceptive sensory pathway in the dorsolateral funiculus of the spinal cord; hence, injury to the motor pathway may at times be missed.
- Motor evoked potential monitoring is a very efficacious modality to evaluate the function of the motor pathways during surgery.
- Continuous electromyography monitoring is a sensitive technique that can be used during operations to detect potential damages to the nerve roots and peripheral nerves.
- Triggered EMG monitoring can be beneficial in assessing the accuracy of pedicle screw placement.

Introduction

Spine surgery risks injury to spinal cord, nerve roots, plexuses, as well as peripheral nerves. Although the overall incidence of neurological complications after spine surgery is low, the sequelae of such injuries can be debilitating and create tremendous burdens for individuals and their families. The potential number of patients who are at risk for such complications has increased significantly over the past few decades as the number and complexity of spine operations has increased dramatically.

Neurophysiologic intraoperative monitoring (NIOM) is the use of electrophysiological techniques to monitor the functional integrity of neural structures

during surgery. The purpose of NIOM is to minimize the risks of iatrogenic neurological deficits when clinical examination is not possible by detecting early changes in the neural structures prior to irreversible damage.

Various electrophysiological methods can be used intraoperatively during spine surgery. Somatosensory evoked potential monitoring and motor evoked potential monitoring are used primarily to monitor the functional integrity of the spinal cord, although both techniques also assess the entire neuraxis from the peripheral nerve level to the cerebral hemisphere. Continuous electromyography (EMG) monitoring is effective in detecting injury to the peripheral nervous system. Triggered EMG (tEMG) monitoring or pedicle screw stimulation can prevent neurological impairments related to misplaced hardware in surgery for spine deformities.

Somatosensory evoked potential monitoring

Background

Somatosensory evoked potentials (SSEPs) are responses recorded over the limbs, spine, and scalp following stimulation of peripheral nerves. These potentials are believed to represent activity in the proprioceptive sensory pathway when low-intensity electrical stimulation is used. Stimuli are conducted peripherally by large-diameter, heavily-myelinated, fast-conducting nerve fibers, and conducted centrally by the dorsal column–medial lemniscal system.

There are several synapses in the proprioceptive sensory pathway. The first-order neurons in the dorsal root ganglion receive sensory input from peripheral nerve fibers and extend their central processes into the spinal cord. The central axons of the dorsal root ganglion travel within the ipsilateral fasciculus gracilis and fasciculus cuneatus to the caudal medulla, where they synapse on the second-order neurons in perspective nucleus gracilis and nucleus cuneatus. The second-order axons decussate as internal arcuate fibers and ascend as the medial lemniscus to the third-order neurons in the ventral posterolateral (VPL) nucleus of the thalamus. The third-order axons project into the primary somatosensory cortex in the contralateral postcentral gyrus. The traveling volley of the action potentials propagating along these pathways, or the responses generated at the sites of the synapses or within the sensory pathway nuclei, can be recorded at different sites in the limb, spine, and scalp as somatosensory evoked potentials.

SSEP monitoring has been used widely for NIOM during a wide variety of surgical procedures. It has been the primary spinal cord monitoring modality for several decades. Several animal models have demonstrated that the duration and severity of damage to the spinal cord correlate with the degree of changes in the SSEP findings.[1] One large multicenter survey showed that the incidence of postoperative neurologic deficits after scoliosis surgery was 0.46% with SSEP monitoring and 1.04% without.[2]

SSEPs are appropriate for NIOM for several reasons. First, SSEP waveforms have a definable latency and amplitude that can be quantified for comparison throughout the surgical procedure. Second, the responses are reproducible with reasonable stability, so changes related to injury can be identified with confidence. Third, stimulation can be performed at almost every nerve that contains the sensory fibers. Fourth, the entire somatosensory pathway can be assessed along the course of surgery. Finally, the neural generators for each waveform are known within practical precision, so localization of the damage to the nervous system is possible and this allows the appropriate corrective measures to be taken.[3] However, an important caveat is that SSEP monitoring alone does not directly assess the motor function carried by the pyramidal pathway. Postoperative motor deficits can occur, although infrequently, with no associated changes in SSEP intraoperatively.[4] In addition, although SSEPs are good basic indicators of the functional integrity of the spinal cord, limited information is provided regarding the function of nerve roots, because SSEPs are a composite of multiple action potentials that enter the spinal cord through several segments.[5]

Methodology

SSEPs are typically obtained with electrical stimulation of a peripheral nerve because responses generally have high amplitude and are reliably reproducible. Stimulation can be performed on any major peripheral nerves and can be either unilateral or bilateral. However, it is good practice to monitor all four extremities since the responses in other limbs can be used as controls to differentiate focal injury from systemic factors, such as anesthetic effects, hypothermia, or hypotension. Commonly stimulated nerves include the median and ulnar nerves at the wrist, common peroneal nerve at the knee, and posterior tibial nerve at the ankle. The selection of the peripheral nerve to be stimulated is determined by the segmental level of the spine surgery. Upper limb SSEPs are generally required for cervical spinal cord monitoring. Median nerve stimulation is commonly used for upper limb SSEPs. When the surgery involves the lower cervical segments (C7–8), ulnar nerve SSEP monitoring is suggested instead as the damage can be missed by median SSEPs. Posterior tibial or common peroneal nerve SSEPs are necessary for thoracic spinal cord monitoring.

Several types of electrodes can be used for stimulation. Transcutaneous stimulation can be performed through the use of standard metal disc electroencephalography (EEG) electrodes, or bar electrodes. These electrodes should be applied firmly to the skin over the selected nerve with collodion and sealed with plastic tape or sheet to prevent drying and contamination with blood or other fluids and to ensure stable SSEP responses. Adhesive surface electrodes can also be applied, but carry the risk of dislodgement. Contact impedance of less than 5 kΩ is recommended for transcutaneous stimulation. Subdermal needle electrodes can be useful in the operating room setting, in certain conditions producing excessive adipose tissue, edema, or unusually thick skin, and when neuropathy is present. The electrodes need to be secured in a similar fashion as disc and bar electrodes. The operating room personnel should be informed of the needle electrode locations, so that necessary care can be observed to avoid needle sticks.

The electrical stimulus should be monophasic rectangular pulses delivered using either a constant-voltage or a constant-current stimulator. The pulse width should be between 100 and 300 μs (optimally 200–300 μs). The stimulus intensity should be sufficient to produce a small visible twitch of the muscle, typically 30–40 mA.

SSEPs can be recorded with standard surface electrodes on the scalp, or subdermal needle electrodes. Contact impedance should be maintained at less than

Table 6.1 Electrode designation for recording SSEPs

Electrode designation	Location
Cc, Ci	Contralateral and ipsilateral central (C3 and C4 of the international 10/20 system)
CPc, CPi	Contralateral and ipsilateral centroparietal (half way between C3 or C4 and P3 or P4)
Fpz	Frontopolar, midline
CPz	Midway between Cz and Pz
C2S	2nd cervical spine
C5S	5th cervical spine
T10S	10th thoracic spine
T12S	12th thoracic spine
L2S	2nd lumbar spine
Epc, Epi	Contralateral and ipsilateral Erb's point (2 cm superior to the midpoint of the clavicle)
AC	Anterior cervical above thyroid cartilage
Pf	Popliteal fossa
REF	Noncephalic reference

Table 6.2 Recommended montages for SSEP recording

Generator	Median or ulnar nerve	Posterior tibial nerve
Peripheral nerve	Epi-Epc	Popliteal fossa
Spinal cord	C5S-Fpz	T12S-REF
Subcortical	Cpi-REF	Fpz-C5S
Cortical	CPc-CPi	CPz-FPz

5 kΩ. Electrodes are placed at standard sites over the peripheral nerve, lumbar or cervical spine, and scalp. The standard designation and the recommended montage are listed in Tables 6.1 and 6.2, respectively. The recommended bandpass is typically 30–100 Hz and 2000–3000 Hz for the low- and high-frequency filter, respectively. Sensitivity of 5–10 μV/cm and sweep of 2–10 ms/cm are usually adequate to identify the SSEP waveforms.[6]

One of the major technical limitations to recording SSEPs is that the sensory response amplitude is low compared with the noise, such as muscle and motion artifacts and electrocardiograph, electroencephalograph, or electromagnetic activity in the environment. The use of averaging improves signal-to-noise ratio by summing the activity that is time-locked to the stimulus trigger, and iteratively subtracting random background noises. There is no specific number of stimuli required to be averaged. The larger the signal and the smaller the noise, the fewer trials will be required. The number of averaging trials should be just enough to obtain reliable recordings in order to give the surgeon feedback as quickly as possible. In general, 200–600 stimuli are usually required to display high-quality, well-defined, reproducible SSEP waveforms of 1–10 μV. The baseline responses must be obtained prior to critical stages and then followed continuously when critical structures are at risk.

Significant findings

Following the stimulation of a peripheral nerve, SSEP responses can be recorded along the proprioceptive somatosensory pathway. The nomenclature of SSEP waveforms is according to the direction of peak deflection (N = negative, P = positive) and the latencies of the peak response in milliseconds. The number following the N and P derives from the average latency at which the particular waveform is recorded in normal healthy controls. For example, an N20 response is an SSEP waveform with upward deflection recorded at approximately 20 ms after the median nerve is stimulated at the wrist. The nomenclature of SSEP responses has not been standardized, so the peak nomenclature may vary slightly between different institutions.

SSEPs following the median or ulnar nerve stimulation include the following waveforms (Fig. 6.1):

Erb's point potential (EP). EP is the response recorded with an electrode placed over Erb's point referenced to an electrode in the same location contralaterally. EP represents the volley of action potentials in sensory fibers traveling through the brachial plexus.

N13. N13 is the waveform recorded with an electrode at the fifth cervical spine referred to Fpz. N13 probably represents a dorsal horn postsynaptic potential generated by collaterals of the primary afferent fibers in the lower cervical cord. Some investigators suggest that N13 can be a far-field potential that originates in the ipsilateral dorsal column pathway at the cervicomedullary junction.[7]

P14. P14 is a subcortically generated, far-field potential, best obtained referentially from scalp electrodes. Its neural generators remain controversial. Some believe that this waveform originates from the thalamus, while some evidence suggests that it probably reflects activity in the caudal medial lemniscus.

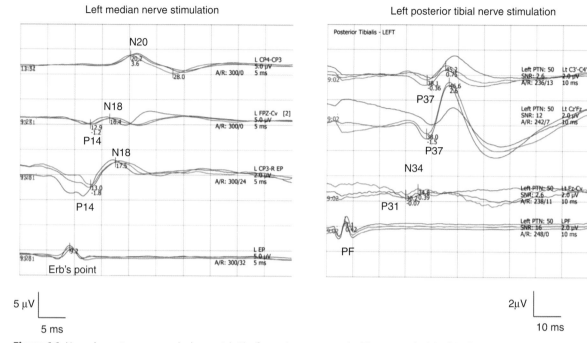

Figure 6.1 Normal somatosensory evoked potentials. The figure shows two graphs. The one on the left of the figure shows normal somatosensory evoked potential waveforms obtained in the operating room after left median nerve stimulation. The graph on the right shows a normal somatosensory evoked potential following left posterior tibial nerve stimulation. The traces colored in red are obtained at the beginning of monitoring (also called baseline recordings). The green traces are the most current obtained waveforms at the time of surgery.

N18. N18 is a subcortically generated, far-field potential, recorded referentially from scalp electrodes ipsilateral to the stimulated nerve. It may occur as early as 16 ms after stimulation of the peripheral nerve, and can persist for 6 ms or more. N18 likely represents postsynaptic activity from multiple generator sources in the brainstem and perhaps the thalamus. The precise location of the neural generators remains to be determined.

N20. N20 is a near-field potential, recorded from a scalp electrode contralateral to the stimulus. It represents the response arising from the primary somatosensory cortex in the postcentral gyrus. This is the most important waveform of the upper limb SSEP monitoring.

The SSEP responses after the stimulation of the posterior tibial nerve consist of the following (Fig. 6.2):

Popliteal fossa potential (PF). PF is the waveform recorded with an electrode placed over the popliteal fossa. This response reflects the volley of action potentials in sensory fibers of the posterior tibial nerve.

Lumbar potential (LP). LP is the response recorded referentially over the dorsal lower thoracic (T10S, T12S) or upper lumbar spines (L2S). It mainly represents postsynaptic activity generated in the dorsal horn of the lumbar spinal cord, analogous to the N13 response of the median nerve SSEP.

N34. N34 is a subcortically generated, far-field potential recorded referentially from the Fpz electrode. It is analogous to the N18 response following median nerve stimulation. The neural generator of this potential is controversial, and it may represent postsynaptic activity from many generator sources in the brainstem, and perhaps, the thalamus.

P37. P37 is the response which is generally recorded by scalp electrodes placed somewhere between the midline and the centroparietal locations. This potential represents the activation of the primary cortical somatosensory area of the leg, contralateral to the stimulus. As the cortical representation of the leg is in the midline, the orientation of the P37 dipole can be variable, and at times may cause paradoxical lateralization, i.e., maximal P37 activity is recorded over the ipsilateral scalp. As a result, it is crucial to record from both midline and ipsilateral scalp locations to be certain that the P37 response is absent.

The SSEP responses are recorded as a baseline prior to the operation, and continuously monitored throughout the surgery especially during critical stages. The most commonly used "warning criteria" by most centers for identifying a significant change of the SSEPs is a 50% decrement in amplitude from the baseline and/or a latency prolongation of 5–10% over the baseline value. These cutoffs are generally guidelines for high likelihood of damage and are supported by several animal and clinical studies as warning criteria that predict neurological deficits if uncorrected, but are also reversible if appropriate actions are taken. It is also important to note trends during monitoring so that early warning can be given to the surgeon in order to prevent any impending damage to neural structures.

However, several factors beside injury to the nervous system can affect SSEP waveforms. These factors include the following:

1. *Anesthesia*

   Anesthetic agents, especially inhalational agents, generally result in a reduction in amplitude and a prolongation of the interpeak latency of the SSEP responses, particularly the cortical potentials (N20 and P37). Subcortical and spinal responses tend to be less affected by anesthesia; thus, this can be a helpful clue to guide that the changes in SSEP waveforms may result from systemic factors and permit continued monitoring. The reduction in SSEP amplitude directly correlates with the depth of anesthesia, so the level of anesthesia should be kept as light as possible. However, this may not always be possible, and conflicts between the needs of the surgeon, the anesthesiologist, and the neurophysiologist are sometimes unavoidable. Hence, effective communication is necessary so that compromises can be reached. Generally SSEP monitoring can be successful with almost every anesthetic technique.

   The effects of commonly used anesthetic agents are listed in Table 6.3.

2. *Blood pressure*

   A certain amount of perfusion to neural tissue is required to meet the metabolic demands. If the demands are not met, electrical activity of neural tissue will start to shut down. When cortical blood flow is reduced below 18 ml/100 g/min,

Table 6.3 Effects of commonly used anesthetic agents on SSEP responses

Agents	Latency	Amplitude
Inhalational anesthetic agents		
Nitrous oxide	Increase	Decrease
Halothane	Increase	Decrease
Enflurane	Increase	Decrease
Isoflurane	Increase	Decrease
Desflurane	Increase	Decrease
Sevoflurane	Increase	Decrease
Intravenous anesthetic agents		
Barbiturates		
Low dose	No change	No change
High dose	Increase	Decrease
Benzodiazepines	Increase	Decrease
Opioids	Increase	Decrease
Etomidate	Increase	Increase
Ketamine	Increase	Increase
Propofol	Increase	Decrease

cortical SSEPs begin to change with a drop in amplitudes and a prolongation in latency. A loss of cortical SSEPs occurs if cerebral blood flow drops below 15 ml/100 g/min. This rate of flow is not adequate to maintain cortical electrical activity but is just above the critical threshold for permanent neuronal injury. Therefore, a loss of cortical SSEP responses is an early warning sign for decreased cerebral perfusion and, if not corrected, may result in permanent neurological deficits. Subcortical and spinal SSEP responses tend to be more resistant to ischemia, and measurable electrical signals may be recorded even after blood flow to the generator sites has ceased for several minutes.

Generally, SSEP waveforms are minimally affected if mean arterial pressure is kept more than 70 mmHg due to cerebral autoregulation. However, the degree of SSEP degradation with decreases in blood pressure varies between individuals, especially among patients with underlying cardiovascular and cerebrovascular diseases.

3. *Temperature*

   Diminished body temperature results in a decrease in neural conduction velocity and can cause a prolongation of SSEP peak latencies. For every 1°C decrease in body temperature, the latency of the N20 response increases every 0.75–1.0 ms. Cortical

Table 6.4 Localization of neural dysfunction based on the pattern of changes in SSEP responses

Locus of neural injury	Pattern of SSEP degradation
Peripheral nerve e.g., limb malpositioning	Unilateral loss of Erb's point, subcortical, and cortical signals
Spinal cord dysfunction	Intact Erb's point potential Prolongation or loss of subcortical and cortical signals
Cerebral dysfunction e.g., cerebral ischemia	Intact Erb's point potential and subcortical signal Unilateral loss of cortical responses
Systemic factors e.g., anesthetic effect, hypotension	Global cortical loss Intact subcortical signals

SSEP signal disappears when the temperature is less than 22°C. Subcortical and spinal responses are generally more resistant to hypothermia and can provide a clue to systemic etiology of SSEP changes. In addition, alteration in temperature affects the metabolism of anesthetic agents, which can also contribute to the changes in SSEP responses.

When there is a "significant" change in SSEP responses consistent with the warning criteria, it must be interpreted within its clinical context and several systemic factors mentioned above must be considered. Localization of the neural insult based on the pattern of SSEP degradation allows appropriate measures to be taken, and may help guide the surgeon to the most appropriate course of action to correct the dysfunction related to surgical complications. Some important patterns of SSEP changes and the localization of the neural insult are demonstrated in Table 6.4.

Outcomes

In addition to merely predicting the neurological deficits, in order to be clinically useful NIOM must be able to cost-effectively alter operative morbidity. Ethical considerations prevent the use of prospective, randomized controlled trials on surgical outcome of intraoperative SSEP monitoring. As a result, the evidence on the efficacy of SSEP monitoring mostly is from case series and historical controls.

The largest multicenter study to assess the efficacy of SSEP monitoring during spine surgery to date is that of Nuwer et al.[2] In this study, questionnaires were sent to the US members of the Scoliosis Research Society (SRS). Surgeons were questioned about the morbidity and the use of SSEP monitoring. The neurophysiologists involved were questioned about monitoring techniques and the warning criteria for significant SSEP changes. Responses were obtained from 153 surgeons and 90 neurophysiologists. SSEP monitoring was performed in 51 263 cases of spine surgery (53% of 97 586 total cases). The majority (60%) of the cases were scoliosis surgery. Compared with the historical data, the rate of neurological deficits reduced from 0.72% to 0.55%. The incidence of persistent neurological deficits decreased from 0.46% to 0.31%. The rate of major neurological deficits (e.g., paraplegia) dropped significantly from 0.61% to 0.24%. All these changes are statistically significant ($p < 0.001$). The false-negative rate was 0.127%, while the false-positive rate was 1.51%. The negative predictive value was 99.93%, signifying that the monitoring is likely to be accurate if SSEPs remain stable throughout the surgery. The positive predictive value was 42%, suggesting a tendency to false alarm. However, as surgeons may have prevented the neurological deficits based on the intraoperative monitoring information, the "false positive" may not be truly false. SSEP monitoring is estimated to prevent one neurological deficit for every 200 cases monitored. The cost to prevent one complication is estimated to be around $120 000, which is still less than the lifetime cost of medical care for a young paraplegic.

According to a systematic review by Fehlings et al.,[8] eight studies evaluating the diagnostic characteristics of SSEP monitoring were identified. The sensitivity and specificity of unimodal SSEP monitoring ranged from 0% to 100% and 27% to 100%, respectively. The positive predictive value was 15–100%, and the negative predictive value was 95–100%. The investigators concluded that the overall strength of the evidence for unimodal SSEP monitoring was "very low," signifying uncertain estimates of effect. The quality of studies was "poor." The quantity was "high," and the consistency was "poor." However, when SSEP monitoring is used in combination with other neurophysiologic modalities, such as motor evoked potential monitoring, the overall strength of evidence with respect to sensitivity and specificity is "high." This systematic review recommends the use of SSEP monitoring together with other neurophysiologic modalities for spine surgery where the spinal cord or nerve roots are deemed to be at risk.

Motor evoked potential monitoring

Background

Although SSEP monitoring has been proven to be useful for neurophysiologic intraoperative monitoring and had been a primary modality for monitoring the functional integrity of the spinal cord over the past several decades, it is not always accurate at predicting damage to the motor pathways. In the past, neurophysiologists assumed that a significant injury to the nervous system that results in motor deficits would be sufficient to cause changes in the SSEP responses. However, it is well documented that a damage sparing the posterior columns can cause debilitating motor deficits but may not significantly alter the SSEP recording.[4] This is due to the fact that the main motor pathways of the spinal cord are located in the dorsolateral funiculus, separated from the somatosensory pathways which are in the dorsal columns. Furthermore, the anterior spinal artery supplies the motor pathway and a significant portion (approximately 75%) of the arterial supply to the spinal cord, while the dorsal columns are mainly supplied by the posterior spinal arteries. Therefore, SSEP responses do not accurately represent the vascular state of the spinal cord. In addition, neurons in the motor gray matter of the spinal cord are more vulnerable to ischemia than axons in the dorsal column sensory white matter. Thus, assessment of the pyramidal pathway would be more sensitive to vascular events of the spinal cord than SSEP monitoring.

Because prevention of motor deficits is always the main objective of NIOM, monitoring the integrity of the corticospinal tract has always been an issue of interest. Prior to the widespread use of motor evoked potential monitoring, the only way to evaluate the function of the motor pathway during surgery was the Stagnara wake-up test.[9] Patients are awakened during the operations and asked to move their feet. This technique possesses several drawbacks. First, it causes significant delay to the surgery. Furthermore, monitoring certain patient populations, such as those with cognitive or hearing impairments, would be technically challenging. Additionally, this test cannot assess the motor pathway continuously, and, thus, when positive, it is possible that a substantial period of time has elapsed from the onset of injury.

Motor evoked potential (MEP) monitoring was developed in 1980, and has since emerged as an extremely effective way to assess the functional integrity of the corticospinal tract. Changes in MEPs are sensitive in detection of postoperative neurological deficits. MEP monitoring has become the gold standard for neuromonitoring of the motor pathways, especially since the advent of multipulse technique for transcranial electrical stimulation of the motor pathways.

MEPs are the responses recorded after stimulation of the motor pathways of the central nervous system (cerebral hemispheres or spinal cord). MEPs assess the functional integrity of the descending motor pathway at various levels. The purpose of MEPs in NIOM is to stimulate rostral to the structure at risk and record the responses at a distal site.

There are several types of MEPs depending on where the stimulation occurs and where the responses are recorded. Transcranial MEPs (TcMEPs) can be attained by stimulation through the skull, activating the primary motor cortex which is located at the precentral gyrus. The signal recording is possible at the level of muscle (compound muscle action potential, or myogenic MEPs), nerve (neurogenic MEPs), or spinal cord (D wave recording). Stimulation can also be performed directly in the spinal cord during operations and signals are recorded distally from peripheral nerves or muscles. The spinal stimulation has drawbacks including the potential for antidromic stimulation of sensory pathways leading to a motor evoked response.[10] At each location, either electrical or magnetic stimulation can be performed.

Stimulation of the primary cortex produces activation of contralateral muscles. A propagated action potential travels down the corticospinal tract to the spinal cord where it activates the anterior horn cells. The signal then travels along the peripheral nerve, traverses the neuromuscular junction, and stimulates the muscle fibers leading to muscular contraction.

Methodology

MEPs can be elicited with either electrical or magnetic stimulation. In awake subjects, magnetic stimulation is generally the preferred technique because a magnetic pulse is painless while an electric shock is painful. In anesthetized patients, however, magnetic stimulation has no advantage over electric stimulation, and indeed possesses several major drawbacks. For example, equipment used for magnetic stimulation is more expensive and more cumbersome in the operating room setting, and magnetic MEPs are more sensitive than electric MEPs to anesthetic agents. Therefore, intraoperative MEP monitoring is most commonly performed by electrical stimulation.

Transcranial stimulation of the motor cortex is minimally invasive and allows monitoring of the entire motor neuraxis. The techniques of transcranial electrical stimulation vary among institutions. The single-pulse stimulation technique is highly sensitive

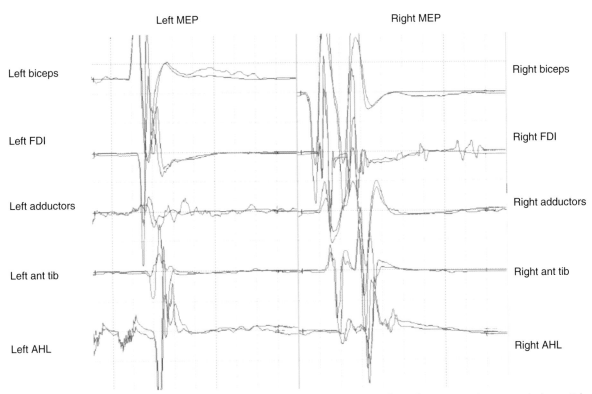

Figure 6.2 Myogenic motor evoked potentials after transcranial electrical stimulation. The figure shows myogenic motor evoked potentials obtained in the operating room following multipulse transcranial electrical stimulation. The traces on the left are from the muscle groups listed from the left side of the body, whereas the traces on the right are from the muscle groups on the right. The red traces are the baseline recordings while the green are the most recently obtained motor evoked potentials.

to anesthetic effects, so multipulse stimulation is generally performed. Anodal stimulation with a short duration (0.05 ms), rapid rise time pulses to subcutaneously placed EEG electrodes at C3 and C4 is commonly used. The output current range is 0–1000 mA, from a source voltage as high as 200–800 V. The pulse width range can be varied from 50 to 500 μs, and the interstimulus interval is typically between 1 and 4 ms. These parameters are adjusted until reproducible responses can be observed in all the muscles examined. Transcranial electrical stimulation is relatively contraindicated in patients with epilepsy, due to the theoretical possibility of seizure kindling effect. Other relative contraindicationa are the presence of a pacemaker, infusion pumps, cochlear implants, aneurysm clips and other retained metal fragments, a history of skull fracture, or other intracranial diseases. The risk–benefit ratio for use of this modality in these scenarios should be assessed prior to its use.

Spinal cord stimulation of the motor system can be achieved through the use of a nasopharyngeal/esophageal active and laminar needle electrode (needle electrodes placed in the interlaminar space). In addition, electrical stimulation can be performed in the operative field with interspinous or epidural electrodes using a distant anode in the subcutaneous tissue, but this is more technically challenging. Although this technique is less sensitive to anesthetic agents, MEP responses obtained via direct spinal cord stimulation are less likely to represent motor function because, in addition to the anterograde activation of the motor pathways, spinal cord stimulation produces antidromic sensory responses via retrograde activation of the dorsal column, similar to traditional SSEP recordings.[10]

Stimulation of the motor system at either the cortical or the spinal cord level results in activation of multiple descending tracts and causes contraction of several muscles. Therefore, theoretically, recording electrodes can be placed anywhere along the descending pathway.

MEPs are generally recorded from muscles (myogenic MEPs) in most institutions with surface, subdermal, or intramuscular electrodes as a compound muscle action potential (CMAP). The potentials can be obtained from most limb muscles relatively easily, and recording techniques are not invasive. The selection of the muscles for recording is determined by the clinical question. Typically, the ankle extensor and flexor muscles and the quadriceps muscles are used in the lower limbs, while the intrinsic hand muscles, forearm extensors, and arm flexors are monitored in the upper extremities. Unilateral dysfunction of the motor pathway can be identified with the CMAP recording. MEP responses have high signal-to-noise ratio, so no averaging is required, and feedback can be instantaneous. Disadvantages of recording from muscles include variability in the CMAP responses with the level of neuromuscular blockade. Cortically evoked CMAPs are more variable and more sensitive to anesthesia than spinally evoked CMAPs.

MEPs can be recorded from the spinal cord with transcranial stimulation (D wave recording). This has the advantage of being relatively insensitive toward anesthetic agents and not affected by full neuromuscular blockade. Moreover, SSEPs can be recorded reliably if the cerebral cortex and peripheral nerve are stimulated at the same time. The disadvantages of the spinal cord recordings are that they require insertion of epidural leads, which usually requires a posterior approach to the spinal cord, and the recordings are limited to the level above T11. Although rare, there is a risk of hematoma from placement of the recording electrodes. The recordings from the lumbar cord are generally not as reliable. Importantly, the side responsible for deterioration in the recorded volleys cannot be readily identified as the epidural electrode may move during surgery, such as during spinal distraction.

MEP responses can also be obtained from the peripheral nerves (neurogenic MEPs). Neurogenic MEPs are relatively immune to the effects of muscle relaxants compared with myogenic MEPs. However, neurogenic MEPs are technically challenging. Only a few nerves supplying upper and lower extremities are suitable for recording. The responses have low signal-to-noise ratio, so averaging of more than 100 responses is necessary.

Significant findings

When recording MEP responses from the muscle (myogenic MEPs), the compound muscle action potentials will be obtained (Fig. 6.2).

There are four routinely used warning criteria for interpretation of TcMEP responses: (1) the all-or-none criterion, (2) the amplitude criterion, (3) the threshold criterion, and (4) the morphology criterion.

The all-or-none criterion is the method that is used widely in most institutions, because TcMEP CMAP responses are exceptionally variable in size and configuration. A complete loss of the MEP waveform is considered significant and indicative of potential damage to the motor pathways. However, given the all-or-none nature of this approach, there is a concern that this method is not sensitive enough in detecting subtle injury to the corticospinal tract, and postoperative motor deficits are possible.[11]

A modification of the all-or-none criteria includes measuring the CMAP amplitude preoperatively as a baseline value, then measuring relative changes in amplitude during surgery to determine whether a significant change has occurred. Due to significant variability in CMAP signals, an 80% reduction in amplitude from baseline in at least one out of six recording sites is required for a significant change. When this criterion was used in a study of 142 patients who underwent corrective surgery for spinal deformity, a sensitivity of 100% and a specificity of 91% were achieved.[12]

The threshold criterion is another approach that has been proposed in an attempt to improve the sensitivity in detecting damage to the motor tracts. According to the study by Calancie and Molano involving 903 patients who underwent spinal surgery at either cervical, thoracic, or lumbar levels, the increase in the threshold required for obtaining CMAP responses of 100 V or more that persists for more than one hour and is not due to systemic factors is highly correlated with postoperative motor deficits.[11]

Finally, the morphology criterion has also been proposed. This approach detects impairment of motor conduction in the corticospinal tract by tracking changes in the morphology of MEP signals, such as reduction in complexity of the MEP waveforms. In particular, Quiñones-Hinojosa and colleagues observed changes in the CMAP responses from a polyphasic to a biphasic waveform, or from polyphasic to biphasic and ultimately to loss of signal, in 28 patients who underwent intramedullary spinal cord tumor resection. The alterations in morphology persisted despite significant raise in the threshold voltage. The reduction in the complexity and/or loss of the MEP waveforms significantly correlated with postoperative motor deficits.[13]

TcMEP responses can at times fluctuate extremely strongly. Abrupt loss or marked attenuation of the CMAP amplitude can occur immediately after recording a robust response. This may result from spontaneous fluctuation of excitability of the anterior horn cells. Therefore, significant changes of CMAP response must be verified before deciding that the changes are "real."

Table 6.5 Effects of commonly used anesthetic agents on CMAP responses

Agents	Latency	Amplitude
Inhalational anesthetic agents		
Nitrous oxide	Increase	Decrease
Halothane	Increase	Decrease
Enflurane	Increase	Decrease
Isoflurane	Increase	Decrease
Desflurane	Increase	Decrease
Sevoflurane	Increase	Decrease
Intravenous anesthetic agents		
Barbiturates		
Low dose	Increase	Decrease
High dose	Increase	Decrease
Benzodiazepines	Increase	Decrease
Opioids	No change	No change
Etomidate	No change	No change
Ketamine	No change	No change
Propofol	Increase	Decrease

Similarly to the SSEP monitoring, several systemic factors can affect CMAP signals. These factors include the following:[3]

1. *Anesthesia*

    MEPs can be significantly affected by anesthetic agents. These agents can abolish the response at multiple sites that involve synaptic transmission, particularly at the level of the cerebral cortex and anterior horn cells and less so at the neuromuscular junction. Halogenated inhalational anesthetic agents can easily reduce the CMAP responses by blockade at the cortex and anterior horn cells. If these agents are necessary, the concentration must remain very low (<0.5%).

    The effects of commonly used anesthetic agents are listed in Table 6.5.

2. *Paralytics*

    Since CMAPs are motor responses, the use of neuromuscular blocking agents will suppress or eliminate these potentials. However, partial neuromuscular blockade is sometimes beneficial for the surgery and the MEP monitoring since it improves surgical retraction and can lead to substantial reduction in patient movements following the stimulation, thus lessening the risk of injuries. A neuromuscular blockade up to 50% may be used during MEP monitoring with CMAP. MEP stimulation must be performed at times when the patient movement is acceptable, and the surgeon should be notified before the stimulus is applied.

3. *Temperature*

    MEP responses are generally less affected by changes in temperature than are SSEP responses. Hypothermia may result in a gradual increase in stimulation threshold.

When the MEP signals are recorded from the spinal cord, two types of waveforms are obtained: D (direct) and I (indirect) waves. Cortical stimulation generates a series of descending action potentials in the corticospinal tracts. The D wave is generated by depolarization of the axon hillocks of the large motor neurons. It is followed by a series of I waves that result from synaptic depolarization of interneurons within the cortical gray matter.

Compared with CMAP recordings, the D wave is relatively resistant to anesthesia because there are no synapses involved between the stimulating and the recording sites. The I waves, in contrast, are severely affected by inhalational anesthetic agents. The D wave is also immune to neuromuscular blockade as the recording does not involve the activation of muscle fibers. The latency of the D wave may be temporarily prolonged if the exposed spinal cord is cooled, either by cold saline irrigation or by a low operating room temperature.

The warning criteria used by most institutions for identifying a significant change of the D wave are a 50% reduction in amplitude from the baseline and/or a latency prolongation of 10% over the baseline value. D wave monitoring has been shown to be correlated with the postoperative motor functions. A complete loss of TcMEP CMAP responses with at least 50% preservation of the D wave amplitude generally corresponds to transient paraplegia after the operation. Patients with complete loss of the D wave during surgery are likely to have permanent postoperative motor deficits.[14] Caveats for the D wave monitoring are that epidural D waves can produce false positive results during a scoliosis surgery. A decrease of up to 75% or an increase of D wave amplitude can be found in a number of patients despite unchanged muscle CMAP responses and neurologic outcomes.[15]

Outcomes

As discussed above, it had been assumed in the past that the motor tracts should be spared if the SSEP responses are stable during surgery. Although this is true in the majority of cases, motor deficits in the setting of normal SSEP can occur. The development of reproducible MEP recording techniques has enabled the monitoring of motor pathways during spine surgery.

Several studies have evaluated the utility of MEP monitoring during surgery. In these reports, there were no patients with intraoperative preservation of MEPs who developed new motor deficits postoperatively. Overall, there is a good correlation between changes in the MEP and postoperative motor function. All patients with new postoperative deficits had at least a 50% reduction in the amplitude of the MEP responses.[16,17] The false positive rate of MEP monitoring has varied among the studies because different warning criteria were used. When relatively strict criteria, such as an all-or-none response of the CMAPs, are employed, there is a reduction in the number of false-positive cases. In addition, the false-positive cases may not be "truly false" because surgeons may be able to prevent postoperative neurological deficits based on the intraoperative monitoring information.

According to a systematic review by Fehlings *et al.*, two studies evaluating the diagnostic characteristics of MEP monitoring were determined to be adequate to undergo further evaluation. The sensitivity and specificity of MEP monitoring varied due to different warning criteria being used. In summary, both the sensitivity and the specificity of MEP monitoring varied from 81% to 100%. The positive predictive value and the negative predictive value ranged from 17% to 96% and 97% to 100% respectively. The overall strength of evidence for unimodal MEP monitoring is "very low," so any estimates of effect are very uncertain. The quality of studies was "poor." The quantity was "poor," and the consistency was "high." When MEP monitoring is used in combination with other neurophysiologic modalities, the overall strength with respect to sensitivity and specificity is "high." MEP monitoring together with other neurophysiologic modalities is recommended in spine surgery where the spinal cord or nerve roots are deemed to be at risk.[8]

Continuous electromyography monitoring (free-running electromyography)

Background

Electromyography (EMG) is a neurophysiologic technique for evaluating and recording the electrical potentials generated by muscle fibers. When nerve roots or peripheral nerves are at risk, such as during spine surgery, EMG monitoring can be utilized to minimize the chance of injury to these structures, by detecting impending damages to the peripheral nerve caused by manipulation, traction, compression, or vascular events.

Each muscle fiber is innervated by an alpha motor neuron in the spinal cord. Conversely, an axon of a single motor neuron may innervate from a few muscle fibers (as in ocular muscles) to more than 500 fibers (as in the gastrocnemius). A motor neuron plus all corresponding muscle fibers that it innervates comprise a motor unit. When the mechanical irritation of the nerve roots or peripheral nerves during the surgery is sufficient, there will be axonal depolarization that results in the activation of the corresponding musculature, which can be recorded by EMG. The consequent EMG findings provide immediate feedback to the surgeon regarding the effects of his or her actions.

EMG can be recorded from any muscle accessible to needle, wire, or surface electrodes. The selection of the muscles for recording is determined by the structures at most risk. Commonly used spinal nerve-innervated muscles are listed in Table 6.6. Each spinal nerve root innervates a group of muscles, which is termed the "myotome" for that nerve root. On the other hand, most muscles are innervated by several spinal nerve roots.

Methodology

A variety of electrodes can be used to record EMG activity intraoperatively. Surface and subcutaneous electrodes can capture some muscle activities of interest, but generally these electrodes are inadequate since they cannot reliably record activity deep in a muscle nor can they precisely identify the specific responsible muscle. Standard concentric and monopolar needle electrodes can record EMG activity with excellent quality, but have limitations related to their being bulky and difficult to keep in place and out of the way of the surgeon and anesthesiologist. Subcutaneous EEG needle electrodes are commonly used; when a record from deeper muscles is required, fine Nichrome wires can be inserted with a hollow-bore needle.

EMG monitoring is generally recorded with standard gains of 100–500 µV, and a sweep speed of 10–200 ms/division. The commonly used bandpass is 20–30 Hz and 20 000 Hz for the low- and high-frequency filter, respectively. EMG recording is typically presented on a monitor as well as over a speaker, and the activity of interest can be printed or stored for later review.

Table 6.6 Commonly used muscles in EMG monitoring

Root	Muscles
Cervical myotomes	
C1	None
C2	Sternocleidomastoid
C3	Sternocleidomastoid, trapezius
C4	Trapezius, rhomboids, levator scapulae
C5	Deltoids, biceps brachii
C6	Biceps brachii, brachioradialis, pronator teres, flexor carpi radialis
C7	Triceps brachii, forearm extensors
C8	Forearm flexors, pronator quadratus
Thoracic myotomes	
T1	Intrinsic hand muscles
T2–12	Intercostal and paraspinal muscles
T6–8	Upper rectus abdominis
T8–10	Middle rectus abdominis
T10–12	Lower rectus abdominis
Lumbosacral myotomes	
L1	Quadratus lumborum, paraspinal muscles
L2	Iliopsoas
L3	Quadriceps femoris, adductor longus, adductor magnus
L4	Quadriceps femoris, adductor longus, adductor magnus
L5	Tibialis anterior, gluteus medius
S1	Gastrocnemius, biceps femoris, gluteus maximus
S2–5	Anal sphincter, urethral sphincter

Significant findings

The potentials of major interest for intraoperative EMG monitoring are neurotonic discharges (Fig. 6.3). Neurotonic discharges are distinctive, high-frequency bursts of motor unit potentials recorded from a muscle when the nerve is mechanically or metabolically stimulated.

Neurotonic discharges may appear as rapid, irregular "bursts" lasting several milliseconds or prolonged "trains" lasting up to one minute. An EMG burst represents near-simultaneous activation of multiple axons, while an EMG train is repetitive firing of one or more motor units.

When neurotonic discharges are present, the cause of such EMG activity needs to be identified immediately. The most important etiology to be considered is trauma to the nerve roots or peripheral nerves, particularly blunt mechanical irritation/injury. Additionally, nonmechanical irritation including temperature (such as cold saline or heat from electrocautery) and osmotic irritation can produce intense EMG activity. Recognition of these nonmechanical etiologies is important, because they generally do not have clinical implications. Mechanical irritation, however, is associated with a risk of damage to the corresponding nerve either immediately or with repetitive trauma.

Neurotonic discharges must be distinguished from several electromyographic activities including semi-rhythmic voluntary motor unit action potentials if the patient is not deeply anesthetized, fibrillation potentials if the muscle has been partially denervated, end plate potentials, complex repetitive discharges, and

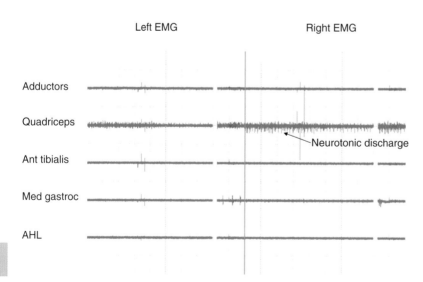

Figure 6.3 Neurotonic discharges on EMG. The figure shows a neurotonic discharge recorded from free running EMG arising from the right quadriceps muscle. This would implicate potential irritation of the right L2–4 nerve root.

myokymic discharges. These activities can be differentiated by typical firing patterns and action potential characteristics.

The most important feature suggesting clinical significance of neurotonic discharges is a relation to surgical events. The onset of EMG discharges with a surgical activity suggests a causative role. The activity that does not correspond with surgical actions tends to be of benign etiology, such as return of muscle tone and voluntary muscle contraction. Some muscles, such as the anal sphincter, are more likely to demonstrate return of tone than others, and this can be seen during low levels of neuromuscular blockade and low anesthetic depth. Voluntary muscle contraction can rarely occur in the case of low anesthetic depth, and electrical activity typically precedes gross clinical movement. Moreover, EMG activity can be observed prior to incision in some patients. This usually relates to the reason for surgery (e.g., radiculopathy) and in such cases only increased EMG activity over the preincision baseline would reflect further nerve irritation.

The intensity of EMG activity correlates roughly with the degree of irritation. Since each motor unit potential represents a separate depolarizing axon, an increase in the number of axons affected by any irritative sources would result in a larger number of distinct motor unit potentials, and thus a greater intensity of recorded EMG activity. EMG activity that persists after the end of the offending surgical action indicates a relatively intense initial irritation, and is often described as "significant." Its presence often suggests some level of ongoing insult or injury. EMG activity that appears as short bursts or low-frequency trains is relatively more benign, and commonly is a physiological phenomenon resulting from the excitation of mechanoreceptors of the axon. Its presence, at worst, poses a low risk for persisting injury.

EMG monitoring can produce a false negative result for sharp nerve transection.[18] Furthermore, in patients with underlying abnormal motor nerves, EMG monitoring may fail to detect additional intraoperative damage even though such injury is blunt mechanical trauma.[19] EMG monitoring is more likely to yield false-negative findings in patients with some underlying neurological diseases, particularly in those with disorders of the neuromuscular junction or the muscle. Classic examples of these conditions include myasthenia gravis, botulinum toxin treatment for dystonia, and muscular dystrophy.

Because EMG monitoring detects the activity in the skeletal muscles, neuromuscular blocking agents will significantly attenuate the EMG and CMAP activity and should be avoided as much as possible. Inhalational anesthetic agents or narcotic anesthesia are usually preferred when EMG monitoring is necessary, although short-acting, nondepolarizing neuromuscular blocking agents titrated to produce a 50% reduction of the baseline motor action potentials still allow neurotonic discharges to be recorded. While such a level of muscle relaxation increases the likelihood of undesired movements during the surgery, movements of the patient can be prevented with adequate levels of narcotics or inhalational anesthesia. Additional agents such as fentanyl or midazolam may be necessary to lessen background muscle contractions and associated motor unit potentials. A continuous monitor of the degree of blockage is recommended if partial neuromuscular blockade is used.

Outcomes

Although EMG was one of the first neurophysiologic modalities to be used for intraoperative monitoring, there are still limited studies to determine the outcome of patients undergoing EMG monitoring during spine surgery.

In a case series reported by Beatty and colleagues, EMG monitoring was performed in a total of 150 patients who underwent spinal surgery for radiculopathy (120 had lumbar surgery, and 30 underwent cervical operations). All surgeries were performed to relieve symptoms due to disc herniation, spondylosis, or both. During the operations, continuous intraoperative EMG recordings were obtained from the muscle corresponding to the involved nerve root. In baseline recordings acquired in the operating room 10 minutes prior to the lumbar surgery, electrical discharge or firing was detected from the corresponding muscle in 22 of 120 patients (18% of the cases). Once the nerve was decompressed, electrical activity diminished. These electrical discharges were produced with regularity on nerve root retraction. The authors concluded that continuous EMG monitoring can be easily accomplished and yields valuable information that indicates when the nerve root is adequately decompressed or when undue retraction is exerted on the root.[20]

Jimenez et al. reported that the incidence of postoperative C5 palsies reduced from 7.3% to 0.9% as a consequence of continuous intraoperative EMG monitoring. The authors also noted that no patient suffered a postoperative C5 palsy when there was no intraoperative evidence of root irritation.[21]

Continuous intraoperative EMG plus SSEP monitoring has been used commonly in spinal surgery to prevent postoperative neurological deficits. However, only limited data are available on the sensitivity, specificity, and predictive values of multimodality techniques. Gunnarsson *et al.* retrospectively analyzed a prospectively accumulated series of patients who underwent intraoperative monitoring with SSEP and EMG during thoracolumbar spine surgery. The analysis focused on the correlation of intraoperative electrophysiological findings with the development of postoperative neurological deficits. There were 213 patients who underwent surgery on a total of 378 levels; 32.4% underwent an instrumented fusion. Significant EMG activity was noted in 77.5% of the patients and significant SSEP changes were seen in 6.6%. Fourteen patients (6.6%) developed new postoperative neurological symptoms. Of those patients, all had significant EMG activation while only four had significant SSEP changes. Intraoperative EMG activation had a sensitivity of 100% and a specificity of 23.7% for the detection of a new postoperative neurological deficit, whereas SSEP had a sensitivity of 28.6% and specificity of 94.7%. The authors concluded that intraoperative EMG monitoring has a high sensitivity for the detection of a new postoperative neurological deficit but a low specificity. On the other hand, SSEP has a low sensitivity but a high specificity. The authors also noted that combination of intraoperative EMG and SSEP monitoring is helpful for predicting and possibly preventing neurological injury during thoracolumbar spine surgery.[22]

Triggered EMG monitoring (pedicle screw stimulation)

Background

Spinal instrumentation and fusion has become the standard procedure for spinal stabilization over the past few decades because it provides a permanent solution to spinal instability. Spinal instrumentations are usually anchored to the vertebral column with screws placed in the pedicles to provide support and allow bony fusion. Malpositioned screws that have breached the medial or inferior pedicle wall may impinge on exiting nerve roots, causing radiculopathy of the corresponding level. The incidence of such complications has been estimated to be between 2% and 10%.[23]

Triggered EMG monitoring or pedicle screw stimulation is a technique that can be used to determine whether screws have breached the pedicle wall and thus pose a risk of injury to the exiting nerve root. When a screw is accurately placed in the pedicle, the surrounding bone serves as an insulator to electrical conduction. Thus, a higher amount of electrical current is required to activate the surrounding nerve roots. On the other hand, if the screw perforates the pedicle wall, a low-impedance pathway will be created between the hole and nearby exiting nerve roots, and the stimulation threshold will be significantly reduced. As a result, evaluation of the integrity of the pedicles can be based on the minimum level of electric current required to activate nearby nerve roots.

Methodology

Triggered EMG monitoring can be performed by using an electrode to directly stimulate the pedicle screw at increasing current intensities. Monopolar electrodes such as nasopharyngeal electrodes are commonly used, and are placed within the pedicle screw holes and/or on hardware. Responses are recorded with needle electrodes that are typically placed in the appropriate muscle group corresponding to the level of spinal surgery (Table 6.6).

Direct nerve root stimulation using <2 mA can be tried prior to pedicle screw stimulation to ensure that the stimulus current is accurately delivered. CMAP responses that are time locked to the stimulation can be recorded from the monitored muscle innervated by that nerve.

Several stimulation parameters and techniques of pedicle screw stimulation have been described in the literature. The rates of pulsatile stimulation range from 1 to 5 Hz with pulse durations between 50 and 300 ms. The intensity of the stimulation is gradually increased from zero until a reliable and repeatable EMG response is obtained from corresponding muscle groups or a predetermined maximum stimulus intensity is achieved. It is generally recommended that the maximum stimulation intensity is 50 mA.

The EMG activity is typically recorded with standard gains of 100–500 µV, and a sweep speed of 10–200 ms/division. The bandpass is generally set at 20–30 Hz and 20 000 Hz for the low- and high-frequency filter, respectively. The CMAP responses are presented on a monitor for review (Fig. 6.4).

Significant findings

There are several "warning thresholds" described in the literature and each institution may use slightly different cut-off values. In general, pedicle screw placements that are associated with stimulation thresholds greater than 10 mA suggest that the pedicle wall is intact, and are unlikely to represent a risk of postoperative neurological

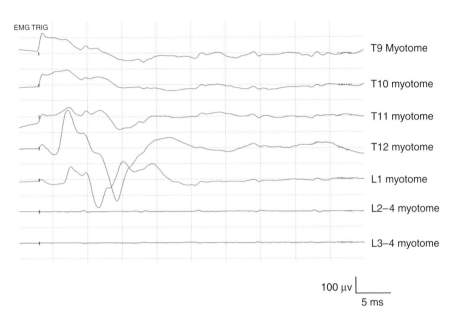

EMG TRIG

T9 Myotome

T10 myotome

T11 myotome

T12 myotome

L1 myotome

L2–4 myotome

L3–4 myotome

100 μv

5 ms

Figure 6.4 Pedicle screw stimulation triggered EMG. The figure shows triggered EMG obtained following stimulation of a pedicle screw at an intensity of 3 mA. This result would suggest the possibility of perforation of the medial pedicle wall.

deficits. A stimulation threshold between 10 and 20 mA reasonably implies that no breach of the medial wall has occurred, while a threshold response of >15 mA indicates a 98% chance of accurate screw positioning on postoperative CT scan.[24] Stimulation thresholds greater than 20 mA signify a strong probability that there is no breach of the medial pedicle wall.

A perforation of the pedicle wall is possible if pedicle screws stimulate nearby exiting nerve roots at less than 7 mA. In such cases, the surgeon may choose to remove or adjust the screw at the corresponding site. In a situation where redirection is not feasible or the screw is a keystone to the success of spinal fusion, the surgeon may opt to leave that screw in place after determining that the pedicle wall is unlikely to be perforated in a clinically significant manner. This is typically confirmed by probing the pedicle hole and/or obtaining a fluoroscopy to look for a potential impingement on a nerve root. The presence of neurotonic discharges on spontaneous EMG monitoring corresponding to screw placement or probing strongly suggests that a perforation with nerve impingement is present.

Because the low-threshold stimulation intensities only implies a low-impedance pathway between the pedicle hole and exiting nerve roots, false-positive results can be seen in patients with osteoporosis resulting in thin pedicle walls or cracked pedicles. Nonetheless, there is a relationship between threshold stimulation intensities and the exposure of a pedicle screw. Cracked pedicles, osteoporotic bone, or a minimally exposed screw are likely to be associated

with stimulation threshold greater than 7 mA, while exposed screws near a nerve root tend to have stimulation thresholds of less than 5 mA.

False-negative results can occur due to various factors, such as the use of muscle relaxants, current spread, or preexisting nerve damage. These factors need to be kept in mind to ensure the accuracy of pedicle screw stimulation. The degree of muscle relaxation can be assessed by a train-of-four test. Triggered EMG monitoring is best performed when no paralytics are used and four of four twitches are optimal for reliable recording. Excessive fluid, blood, or soft tissue around the head of the screw at the time of stimulation can potentially shunt current away from the screw, and thus result in no activation of the nerve roots. Lastly, chronically compressed nerve roots have higher stimulation thresholds, with literature reports ranging from 6 to >10 mA, compared with 2 mA for a normal nerve root.[19] As a result, in nerve roots where there is known or suspected damage, direct nerve root stimulation threshold is essential to establish a baseline value.

Outcomes

The data on postoperative outcomes in patients who underwent pedicle screw stimulation or triggered EMG monitoring are conflicting in the literature. In a prospective study conducted by Raynor and colleagues, the sensitivity of rectus abdominis-triggered EMG to assess the placement of thoracic screw was evaluated. A total of 677 thoracic screws were placed into 92 patients. Screws were inserted between T6 and T12 and were stimulated with a CMAP recorded from the rectus abdominis muscle. Threshold values were compared both in absolute values and relative to other locations in the same patient. The stimulation thresholds can be divided into three groups: group A ($n = 650$ screws) had thresholds greater than 6.0 mA with intraosseus placement confirmed radiographically; group B ($n = 21$) had thresholds less than 6.0 mA but with an intact medial pedicle border on reexamination and radiographic confirmation; and group C ($n = 6$) had thresholds less than 6.0 mA with medial pedicle wall perforations confirmed by tactile and/or visual inspection. Therefore, the positive predictive value of triggered EMG monitoring is 22% (6 of 27 patients with threshold less than 6.0 mA). There were no postoperative neurological deficits. Group B screws averaged a 54% decrease of stimulation thresholds, while group C had a 69% reduction in threshold from baseline ($p = 0.016$). The authors concluded that for assessment of thoracic pedicle screw placement, triggered EMG thresholds of less than 6.0 mA, together with 60–65% reduction of stimulation threshold from the mean of all other thresholds in a given patient, should alert the surgeon to suspect a medial pedicle wall breach.[25]

However, the above data were contradictory to the study by Reidy et al., which was a prospective study that determined the use of intercostal EMG monitoring as an index of the accuracy of the placement of pedicle screws in the thoracic spine. A total of 95 thoracic pedicle screws were placed into 17 patients. A CMAP was recorded from the corresponding intercostal or abdominal muscles. Postoperative CT was performed to determine the position of the screw. The stimulus thresholds were correlated with the position of the screw on the CT scan. Using 7.0 mA as a warning threshold, the sensitivity of EMG was 50% in detecting a breached pedicle and the specificity was 83%. There were eight unrecognized breaches of the pedicle based on triggered EMG results alone. Thoracic pedicle screws were placed accurately in more than 90% of patients. These authors concluded that triggered EMG monitoring did not significantly improve the reliability of pedicle screw placement.[26]

Regarding the cost-effectiveness of pedicle screw stimulation, the experience of Toleikis over 1000 cases suggests that triggered EMG monitoring is worthwhile. The cost of monitoring for a typical instrumented fusion involving pedicle screw placement with continuous and triggered myogenic techniques was estimated to be $1000 or less. Therefore, the cost for monitoring 1000 patients would be approximately $1 million. Since the estimated incidence of postoperative neurological deficits resulting from the placement of pedicle screws is around 2–10%, at least 20 patients would develop some neurological complications after the operations. The average medical costs to correct a patient's postoperative outcome and to rehabilitate that patient are usually more than $50 000. Thus, the use of triggered EMG monitoring during spine surgery is cost-effective.[23]

Conclusion

NIOM can minimize potential neurological deficits that may result from spine surgery. SSEPs are the most commonly used modality for monitoring spinal cord function and have had the widest application. SSEP monitoring can identify the injury early enough to alert the surgeon in most cases. However, anterior spinal cord injury that may result from a vascular accident or direct trauma can be missed, and addition of MEP monitoring in some spinal procedures may better protect the motor pathways. Neurotonic discharges recorded from peripheral muscle during spontaneous EMG monitoring are sensitive to irritation of the nerve root. Triggered EMG monitoring is helpful to assess the accuracy of pedicle screw placement and, thus, can alert the surgeon when the damage may be occurring. A thorough familiarity with these monitoring techniques, as well as knowledge of the benefits and limitations of each modality, enhance the value of NIOM and the neurological and functional outcomes during spinal procedures.

References

1. Daube JR, Rubin DI, eds. *Clinical Neurophysiology*. Oxford: Oxford University Press; 2009.

2. Nuwer MR, Dawson EG, Carlson LG, *et al.* Somatosensory evoked potential spinal cord monitoring reduces neurologic deficits after scoliosis surgery: results of a large multicenter survey. *Electroencephalogr Clin Neurophysiol* 1995; **96**: 6–11.

3. Husain AM, ed. *A Practical Approach to Neurophysiologic Intraoperative Monitoring*. New York: Demos Medical Publishing; 2008.

4. Lesser RP, Raudzens P, Lüders H, *et al.* Postoperative neurological deficits may occur despite unchanged intraoperative somatosensory evoked potentials. *Ann Neurol* 1986; **19**: 22–5.

5. Tsai TM, Tsai CL, Lin TS, *et al.* Value of dermatomal somatosensory evoked potentials in detecting acute

nerve root injury: an experimental study with special emphasis on stimulus intensity. *Spine* 2005; **30**: E540–6.

6. American Clinical Neurophysiology Society. *Guideline 11B: Recommended standards for intraoperative monitoring of somatosensory evoked potentials.* Bloomfield, CT: American Clinical Neurophysiology Society; October, 2009.

7. Lueders H, Lesser R, Hahn J, *et al.* Subcortical somatosensory evoked potentials to median nerve stimulation. *Brain* 1983; **106**: 341–72.

8. Fehlings MG, Brodke DS, Norvell DC, *et al.* The evidence for intraoperative neurophysiological monitoring in spine surgery: does it make a difference? *Spine* 2010; **35**: S37–46.

9. Vauzelle C, Stagnara P, Jouvinroux P. Functional monitoring of spinal cord activity during spinal surgery. *Clin Orthop Relat Res* 1973; **93**: 173–8.

10. Toleikis JR, Skelly JP, Carlvin AO, Burkus JK. Spinally elicited peripheral nerve responses are sensory rather than motor. *Clin Neurophysiol* 2000; **111**(4): 736–42.

11. Calancie B, Molano MR. Alarm criteria for motor-evoked potentials: what's wrong with the "presence-or-absence" approach? *Spine* 2008; **33**: 406–14.

12. Langeloo DD, Lelivelt A, Louis Journée H, *et al.* Transcranial electrical motor-evoked potential monitoring during surgery for spinal deformity: a study of 145 patients. *Spine* 2003; **28**: 1043–50.

13. Quiñones-Hinojosa A, Lyon R, Zada G, *et al.* Changes in transcranial motor evoked potentials during intramedullary spinal cord tumor resection correlate with postoperative motor function. *Neurosurgery* 2005; **56**: 982–93.

14. Morota N, Deletis V, Constantini S, *et al.* The role of motor evoked potentials during surgery for intramedullary spinal cord tumors. *Neurosurgery* 1997; **41**: 1327–36.

15. Ulkatan S, Neuwirth M, Bitan F, *et al.* Monitoring of scoliosis surgery with epidurally recorded motor evoked potentials (D wave) revealed false results. *Clin Neurophysiol* 2006; **117**: 2093–101.

16. Levy WJ, York DH, McCaffrey M, Tanzer F. Motor evoked potentials from transcranial stimulation of the motor cortex in humans. *Neurosurgery* 1984; **15**: 214–27.

17. Kitagawa H, Itoh T, Takano H, *et al.* Motor evoked potential monitoring during upper cervical spine surgery. *Spine* 1989; **14**: 1078–83.

18. Nelson KR, Vasconez HC. Nerve transaction without neurotonic discharges during intraoperative electromyographic monitoring. *Muscle Nerve* 1995; **18**: 236–8.

19. Holland NR. Intraoperative electromyography. *J Clin Neurophysiol* 2002; **19**: 444–53.

20. Beatty RM, McGuire P, Moroney JM, *et al.* Continuous intraoperative electromyographic recording during spinal surgery. *J Neurosurg* 1995; **82**: 401–5.

21. Jimenez JC, Sani S, Braverman B, *et al.* Palsies of the fifth cervical nerve root after cervical decompression: prevention using continuous intraoperative electromyography monitoring. *J Neurosurg Spine* 2005; **3**: 92–7.

22. Gunnarsson T, Krassioukov AV, Sarjeant R, *et al.* Real-time continuous intraoperative electromyographic and somatosensory evoked potential recordings in spinal surgery: Correlation of clinical and electrophysiologic findings in a prospective, consecutive series of 213 cases. *Spine* 2004; **29**: 677–84.

23. Toleikis RJ. Neurophysiological monitoring during pedicle screw placement. In: Deletis V, Shils JL, eds. *Neurophysiology in Neurosurgery.* New York: Academic Press; 2002: 231–64.

24. Shi YB, Binette M, Martin WH, *et al.* Electrical stimulation for intraoperative evaluation of thoracic pedicle screw placement. *Spine* 2003; **28**: 595–601.

25. Raynor BL, Lenke LG, Kim Y, *et al.* Can triggered electromyograph thresholds predict safe thoracic screw placement? *Spine* 2002; **27**: 2030–5.

26. Reidy DP, Houlden D, Nolan PC, *et al.* Evaluation of electromyographic monitoring during insertion of thoracic pedicle screws. *J Bone Joint Surg Br* 2001; **83**: 1009–14.

Chapter

7

Pharmacology of adjunct anesthetic drugs

John E. Tetzlaff

Key points

- Pharmacologic choices for major spine surgery are dictated by the severity of the surgery, patient comorbidity, and the techniques of spinal cord monitoring.
- The approaches to spinal cord monitoring require anesthetic choices compatible with the specific monitoring technique.
- When the "wake-up" test is planned, intraoperative emergence and focused neurologic examination require agents with predictable recovery.
- When evoked potentials are selected, agents with predictable impact on the amplitude and latency of the evoked signal are required.
- Continuous infusion of intravenous agents has an important role in the anesthetic technique when evoked potential monitoring is part of the surgical plan.

Introduction

Surgery of the spine can be elective – in the case of spinal stenosis, nerve root entrapment, or disc herniation; urgent – as in the case of metastatic disease with developing neurologic deficit; or an acute emergency – as in the case of fracture or fracture-dislocation. The anesthetic techniques are dictated by the degree of urgency involved, the indication for the surgery, and the level of the spine to be operated on. Spine surgery has a wide range of acuity from relatively minor surgical procedures to some of the most invasive procedures performed. The anesthetic drugs selected for major spine surgery are dictated by the comorbidities in the patient's health history, the severity of the surgery, and the preference of the anesthesiologist. As with almost everything in anesthesia, there is always more than

one pharmacologic option for the elements of the anesthetic for major spine surgery. One unique element of major spine surgery that dictates the choice of various adjunct drugs is central nervous system (CNS) monitoring. The pharmacologic options for spine surgery will be presented in the context of requirements imposed by this monitoring.

Advanced neurophysiologic monitoring

With the continued evolution of spine surgery and the development of better instrumentation options, more and more aggressive surgical procedures are being performed from the sacrum to the foramen magnum. A common element for all of these procedures is risk of injury to the spinal cord and/or nerve roots, and complex spinal cord monitoring has become a routine part of prevention of injury to the CNS. With the application of these monitoring techniques to major surgery comes the requirement to adjust the anesthetic drug selection to allow the early detection of potential risk to the spinal cord. Two broad categories for strategy are the "wake-up test" and neurophysiologic monitoring of the spinal cord. The approach to the pharmacologic choices is different for these two options.

Anesthetic approach for the wake-up test

The wake-up test[1] was first introduced for scoliosis surgery to prevent catastrophic spinal cord injury and involves awakening the patient after completion of key phases of instrumentation and performing a focused neurologic examination prior to completing the surgery. Any motor or sensory deficit not present prior to the start of surgery is taken as a sign that spinal cord function is impaired (distraction, kinking, vascular compromise) as a result of instrumentation, and

Anesthesia for Spine Surgery, ed. Ehab Farag. Published by Cambridge University Press. © Cambridge University Press 2012.

removal of some or all of the rods, screws, and/or wires to decrease distraction on the spinal cord is indicated to prevent irreversible injury. After the adjustment of instrumentation, the wake-up test is repeated to determine whether the correction has restored normal neurologic function. Clinical experience confirms that adjustment of instrumentation after an abnormal wake-up test can result in reversal of the neurologic deficit.[2]

The anesthetic technique for major spine surgery using a wake-up test is focused around agents that allow for a reasonably rapid return of consciousness. Volatile agents have a role in this anesthetic technique, although when used as the primary agents they can result in slow emergence. As a result, a volatile agent is often used with one or more other classes of agents to reduce the time to responsiveness. The options include injection or infusion of members of the fentanyl family, propofol, and/or dexmedetomidine. Neuromuscular blockade must either be avoided or maintained at a level where reversal is possible. If the neurologic examination has changed when there is an abnormal wake-up test, the anesthetic is deepened using the same strategy, the instrumentation is adjusted by the surgeon, and the patient is awakened again. If the neurologic examination reverts to baseline, the risk of spinal cord injury is greatly reduced. The limitations of this technique are the time involved, the preparation of the patient to ensure they are aware that they will be awakened intraoperatively, and the potential to lose the airway or lines during the emergence if agitation occurs. In extreme cases, patient movement could potentially cause injury to the spinal cord or nerve roots related to excessive movement. Although both options are effective, the combination of desflurane with remifentanil provided more rapid emergence for a wake-up test than propofol and remifentanil.[3]

Anesthetic options for neurophysiologic monitoring

An alternative to the wake-up test is neurophysiologic monitoring of spinal cord function. A small number of centers used neurophysiologic monitoring of spinal cord function in addition to using the wake-up test. The two options are somatosensory evoked potentials (SSEPs) and motor evoked potentials (MEPs). Each imposes different conditions on the anesthetic drug selection. In contrast to the wake-up test approach, there is no need to plan for intraoperative emergence, and the strategy focuses on selecting an anesthetic technique compatible with evoked potential monitoring, and a steady level of

anesthesia to ensure that any changes in evoked potentials can be attributed to the surgical procedure and not to changes in the depth of anesthesia.[4,5] When significant changes in the evoked potentials are detected, adjustment of the instrumentation has been shown to preserve neurologic function.[6] The basal anesthetic can include a volatile agent, but not to exceed one-half MAC, because the volatile agents at higher doses suppress the evoked potential signs in a dose-related manner. The choice of which evoked potential monitoring approach (SSEP, MEP, or both) depends on the specific spine surgery procedure and the preferences of the surgical team. The choice selected has direct impact on the anesthetic drug selection. For SSEP alone, the anesthetic choice can include one-half MAC volatile agents, a nondepolarizing muscle relaxant to prevent gross movement and motion artifact on the SSEP recording, and additional anesthetic agents to deepen the anesthesia and ensure amnesia. The options to deepen the anesthesia include intermittent injection or infusion from the fentanyl family, infusion of propofol or infusion of dexmedetomidine. When MEP monitoring is selected, there are similar requirements to SSEP monitoring, except nondepolarizing muscle relaxants must be avoided to allow measurement of motor evoked activity. This, in turn, imposes a greater burden on the additional agents because they must deepen the anesthetic sufficiently to ensure that sudden movement does not disrupt the surgery during intervals of critical instrumentation in the absence of neuromuscular blockade. The same options include infusions of the fentanyl family, propofol, and/or dexmedetomidine, with combinations of two or more being more common because of the need to withhold neuromuscular blockade. Because the volatile agent dose is fixed, the depth of anesthesia can be adjusted to the surgical stimulus using these intravenous agents with minimal impact on the evoked potential signals.

Pharmacologic implications of anesthetic agents used during major spine surgery

Inhaled anesthetic agents

The volatile anesthetic agents and nitrous oxide have been used successfully in virtually every kind of major spine surgery. All of the volatile agents cause a dose-dependent decrease in signal amplitude of evoked potentials with an increase in signal latency,[7] although there are differences in this impact among the volatile

Table 7.1 Intravenous agents used for spine surgery

Agent	Elimination	Dose range	Issues with use	Contraindications
Thiopental	Hepatic	3–5 mg/kg	Hypotension	Porphyria
Methohexital	Hepatic	0.5–1.0 mg/kg	Hypotension	Porphyria
Etomidate	Hepatic	0.1–0.2 mg/kg or 5–10 µg/kg/min	Nausea, myoclonus, adrenal suppression	? Prolonged infusion for sedation (adrenal suppression)
Propofol	Hepatic	1–2 mg/kg (induction) 50–100 µg/kg/min (sedation) 100–200 µg/g/min (primary anesthetic)	Pain with injection, mild antiemetic	
Dexmedetomidine	Hepatic	1 µg/kg loading over 20 min 0.2–0.7 µg/kg/h maintenance	Hypotension with rapid infusion of loading dose Hypertension with high doses	
Ketamine	Hepatic	0.5–2.0 mg/kg induction 25–100 µg/kg/min maintenance infusion	Increased oral secretion, sympathomimetic properties, bronchodilator	Preexisting dysphoria
Midazolam	Hepatic	0.1 mg/kg for anxiolysis, less when used as adjunct	Reduced dose with advanced age or renal impairment	

agents that have been studied.[8] Isoflurane and enflurane have less impact on evoked potentials than halothane at MAC equivalent doses.[9] Although these differences can be measured reproducibly, there is no clinically significant difference. The newer inhaled agents, sevoflurane and desflurane have a similar impact to isoflurane.[10–12] When brainstem integrity must be monitored, high doses of volatile agents probably should be avoided.[13] Nitrous oxide causes a dose-related reduction in the amplitude of evoked potentials which must be considered if nitrous oxide is part of the anesthetic plan.[14] At 70%, nitrous oxide reduced the amplitude of SSEPs by 50% in adults[15] and children.[16] Desflurane, combined with remifentanil, may provide appropriate conditions for rapid emergence if a wake-up test for critical neurologic examination is required intraoperatively.[17]

Table 7.1 shows intravenous agents used for spine surgery, which are discussed separately below.

Barbiturates

The best-studied class of drugs for impact on evoked potentials is the barbiturate induction drugs. The most commonly used barbiturate during spine surgery is thiopental. The most common use would be for induction. Enthusiasm for continuous infusion is limited by the hemodynamic consequences (afterload reduction causing hypotension) and the cumulative effects. Thiopental (3–5 mg/kg) produces unconsciousness within 1 minute with a duration, if not dosed, of 5–8 minutes. Methohexital (0.5 mg/kg) is an infrequently chosen alternative. Neither should be selected in

patients with poryphyria, as they may induce fatal attacks of porphyria.

Thiopental causes a dose-related decrease in amplitude and increase in signal latency of short duration with modest doses.[7] Evoked potential monitoring is possible shortly after administration of thiopental,[18] although bolus administration during critical surgical instrumentation could create changes that would appear the same as spinal cord ischemia. Continuous infusion of thiopental allows the measurement of somatosensory evoked potentials and detection of spinal cord pathology.[19]

Etomidate

Etomidate as a single-dose induction agent has a role in major spine surgery when hemodynamic stability during induction is important, and when used in this manner it will have little impact on evoked potential recording. Etomidate can be used as an induction agent at 0.2–0.4 mg/kg and can be used for maintenance of short cases at 10 µg/kg/min, although this has limited application to spine surgery. Termination of action is by redistribution, and the short redistribution half life (2–5 minutes) limits the duration of action of a single dose to about 5 minutes. Injection can be painful, and myoclonus is frequently observed shortly after injection. Etomidate inhibits adrenal enzymes that produce cortisol, and even single doses have been reported to produce adrenal suppression. Sustained infusion of etomidate for sedation in the intensive care setting has been highly associated with adrenal suppression

In contrast with the barbiturates, etomidate causes an acute increase in the amplitude of evoked potentials with minimal increase of latency.[7,20] Under certain circumstances, etomidate infusion has been reported to improve intraoperative SSEP monitoring[21] and detection of potential spinal cord ischemia during instrumentation. Conversely, by comparison with infusion of fentanyl, the accentuation of scalp electrode signals from etomidate could make detection of acute changes more difficult.[22]

Propofol

Propofol can be used in spine surgery for induction or maintenance of anesthesia. When administered as a bolus at 1.0–2.0 mg/kg, propofol induces unconsciousness within 1 minute, with a duration of 7–8 minutes. It can be used as an adjunct to ensure continuous unconsciousness and amnesia with an infusion rate of 50–100 µg/kg/min or as a sole anesthetic at 100–200 µg/kg/min. Injection is generally preceded by lidocaine due to the pain with injection of propofol. The high clearance rate ensures rapid emergence even after prolonged infusions of propofol. The respiratory depressant properties of propofol during sedation should be considered and airway management equipment and personnel should be immediately available. An attractive part of the profile of propofol is its mild antiemetic properties. When propofol is used as a sole agent, vivid dreaming has been reported.

The impact of propofol on evoked potential signals is clinically insignificant as long as boluses are avoided during critical instrumentation.[23–25] Continuous infusion of propofol mixed with opioids allows for satisfactory monitoring of spinal cord function during scoliosis and vertebral fracture.[15] Targeted controlled infusion of propofol for a wake-up test provides a smoother, more rapid intraoperative emergence than manual adjustment based on dose and observation.[26] At high doses, propofol has been reported to decrease the amplitude of transcranial electrical motor evoked potentials.[27] Interestingly, peripheral blood flow was increased and blood loss decreased[28] due to selective vasodilation from propofol[29]) compared with sevoflurane during major spine surgery.

The fentanyl family

Fentanyl can be used during spine surgery as a component of induction (2–5 µg/kg) combined with another induction agent, or as an element of balanced anesthesia with intermittent boluses at 25–50 µg every

Table 7.2 Elimination half-life (EHL) and context-sensitive half-time (CSHT) for opioids

Agent	EHL (min)	CSHT (min)
Fentanyl	475	>100 [a]
Sufentanil	562	26 [a]
Alfentanil	111	51 [a]
Remifentanil	48	<5 [b]

[a] After 200 minutes or longer infusion.
[b] After any infusion.

30 minutes, or as an infusion at 1–2 µg/kg/h. At lower doses, fentanyl infusion can be used to reduce the need for either propofol or inhalation agent. Sufentanil can use used in a similar manner with loading doses of 0.1–0.3 µg/kg and maintenance infusion at 0.5–2.0 µg/kg/h. The slightly longer duration of action requires termination of sufentanil earlier in the procedure (45–60 minutes prior to emergence) to avoid delayed awakening. Alfentanil is generally used as an adjunct to other infused anesthetics, achieving analgesia with a short half-life at 0.5–2.0 µg/kg/min. Remifentanil is unique within the fentanyl family because of the ester linkage in its molecular structure, rendering it susceptible to rapid ester hydrolysis. This results in rapid termination of action. It is not used as a sole anesthetic, and when used as an adjunct for balanced anesthesia during spine surgery (0.1–1.0 µg/kg/min) it provides analgesia and sparing of other agents that is rapidly resolved when the infusion is stopped. The elimination half-life (EHL) and the context-sensitive half-time (CSHT, defined as the time for the central compartment to decrease by 50% from termination of infusion) can be used to determine when to end an infusion to allow for emergence (Table 7.2), especially if the CSHT is considered as the time for termination of brain action of the opioid.

Continuous infusion of fentanyl is consistent with deepening anesthesia while allowing THE recording of somatosensory evoked potentials.[30] Infusions of fentanyl or morphine were equivalent in the impact on evoked potential recording, allowing for clinical spinal cord monitoring, although more impact was noted with bolus injection compared with infusion.[31] Remifentanil is an excellent addition to either desflurane or propofol to facilitate intraoperative emergence for a wake-up test.[3] Remifentanil combined with less than half-MAC of isoflurane allowed for emergence during surgery to facilitate intentional fracture of the cervical spine in two patients with chin-on-chest consequences of ankylosing spondylitis.[32] Among the rapid-emergence opioid combinations, intraoperative emergence for wake-up testing was more rapid with remifental than with alfentanil.[33]

Dexmedetomidine

Dexmedetomidine can be used to achieve sedation and analgesia with alpha adrenergic agonist action when administered as an infusion. The loading dose is 1 µg/kg and is administered slowly over 20 minutes. The sedation and analgesia achieved by the loading dose can be maintained with an infusion at 0.2–0.7 µg/kg/h. Rapid administration of the loading dose can activate vasoconstriction and cause significant hypertension.

Dexmedetomidine can be used an additive to virtually any basal anesthetic, and has demonstrated the ability to allow lower doses of the primary agents and rapid emergence either during or at the conclusion of surgery. The total propofol was reduced and emergence was more rapid when dexmedetomidine was added to remifentanil plus propofol than with propofol and remifentanil alone.[34] When dexmedetomidine infusion was introduced during desflurane/remifentanil anesthesia, SSEP and MEP recording was not disturbed.[35] This was also reported during total intravenous anesthesia.[36,37] Although not an issue at lower doses, high doses of dexmedetomidine decreased the amplitude of transcranial motor evoked potentials compared with propofol/remifentanil anesthesia in children.[38] This attenuation did not occur when the dexmedetomidine was left at the lower level and the propofol concentration was increased. Clinical experience with higher doses of dexmedetomidine has been associated with compromise of intraoperative spinal cord monitoring using transcranial motor evoked potentials.[39]

Ketamine

Ketamine has its most common application in spine surgery as an induction agent. An induction dose of 0.5–1.5 mg/kg produces amnesia, analgesia, and unconsciousness. At lower doses, amnesia and analgesia can be achieved with minimal respiratory depression. The unconsciousness is different from other induction agents, being more like catalepsy, and eye opening or involuntary motor activity may occur if other agents or nondepolarizing muscle relaxants are not coadministered. An unattractive aspect of ketamine is the dysphoria and psychomimetic properties reported after ketamine use as a sole agent. These events are much less likely when benzodiazepines or propofol are also administered. Ketamine can have a role in the induction

of anesthesia if there is hypovolemia or bronchospasm, and as an induction agent only would have minimal impact on spinal cord monitoring.

Low-dose ketamine infusion (1 µg/kg/min) has been used as an additive during major spine surgery to achieve hemodynamic stability and to reduce the amount of other agents needed to maintain anesthesia.[40] Motor evoked potential monitoring is not significantly altered by the use of ketamine.[41,42]

Benzodiazepines

The most common benzodiazepine used for major spine surgery is midazolam. Midazolam is selected as a short-acting sedative as a premedicant, or as part of a balanced anesthetic regimen to ensure amnesia. When injected intravenously, anxiolysis peaks at 1.5–2.0 minutes. Midazolam is arguable the best sedative agent to achieve amnesia.

Benzodiazepines have a role during major spine surgery to ensure amnesia during times when anesthetic doses must be kept low. However, there is impact on amplitude and latency with diazepam[43] and with amplitude after midazolam with no impact on latency.[20] This would make bolus injection of either benzodiazepine unwise during intervals of critical surgical instrumentation.

References

1. Vauzella C, Stagnara P, Jouvinroux P. Functional monitoring of spinal cord activity during spinal surgery. *Clin Orthop* 1973; **93**: 73–8.

2. Hall JE, Levine CR, Sudhir HG. Intraoperative awakening to monitor spinal cord function during Harrington rod instrumentation and spinal fusion. *J Bone Joint Surg* 1978; **60A**: 533–6.

3. Grottke O, Dietrich PJ, Wiegels S, Wappler F. Intraoperative wake up test and postoperative emergence in patients undergoing spinal surgery: a comparison of intravenous and inhaled anesthetic techniques using short acting anesthetics. *Anesth Analg* 2004; **99**: 1521–7.

4. McTaggart Cowan RA. Somatosensory evoked potentials during spinal surgery. *Can J Anaesth* 1998; **45**: 387–92.

5. Grundy BL. Intraoperative monitoring of somatosensory evoked potentials. *Anesthesiology* 1983; **58**: 72–87.

6. Lyon R, Lieberman JA, Grabovac ME, Hu S. Strategies for managing decreased motor evoked signals while distracting the spine during correction of scoliosis. *J Neurosurg Anesthesiol* 2004; **16**: 167–70.

7. Banoub M, Tetzlaff JE, Schubert A. Pharmacologic and physiologic influences affecting sensory evoked potentials. *Anesthesiology* 2003; **99**: 716–23.

8. Pathak KS, Ammadio BS, Scoles PV. Effects of halothane, enflurane, and isoflurane in nitrous oxide on multi-level somatosensory evoked potentials. *Anesthesiology* 1989; **70**: 207–14.

9. Pathak KS, Ammadio M, Kalamchi A, *et al.* Effects of halothane, enflurane, and isoflurane on somatosensory evoked potentials during nitrous oxide anesthesia. *Anesthesiology* 1987; **66**: 753–7.

10. Scholz J, Bischoff P, Szafarczyk W. Comparison of sevoflurane and isoflurane in ambulatory surgery; Results of a multicenter study. *Anesthetist* 1996; **45**: 580–6.

11. Haghighi SS, Sirintrapun SJ, Johnson JC. Suppression of spinal and cortical somatosensory evoked potentials by desflurane anesthesia. *J Neurosurg Anesthesiol* 1996; **8**: 148–53.

12. Vaugha DJ, Thornton C, Wright DR. Effects of different concentrations of sevoflurane and desflurane on subcortical somatosensory evoked potentials in anesthetized, non-stimulated patients. *Br J Anaesth* 2001; **86**: 59–67.

13. Samra SK, Vanderzant CW, Domer PA, Sackellares JC. Differential effects of isoflurane on human median nerve somatosensory evoked potentials. Anesthesiology 1987; **66**: 29–35.

14. Sebel PS, Flynn PJ, Ingram DA. Effect of nitrous oxide on visual, auditory and somatosensory evoked potentials. *Br J Anaesth* 1984; **56**: 1403–7.

15. Kalkman CJ, Traast H, Zuurmond WA, Bovill JG. Differential effects of propofol and nitrous oxide on posterior tibial nerve somatosensory cortical evoked potentials during alfentanil anaesthesia. *Br J Anaesth* 1991; **66**: 483–9.

16. Schaney CR, Sanders J, Kuhn P, LaJohn S, Heard C. Nitrous oxide with propofol reduces somatosensory evoked potential amplitude in children and adolescents. *Spine* 2005; **30**: 689–93.

17. Rodola F, D'Avolio R, Chierichini, *et al.* Wake-up test during major spinal surgery under remifentanil balanced anaesthesia. *Eur Rev Med Pharmacol Sci* 2000; **4**: 67–70.

18. Shimoji K, Kano T, Nakashima H. The effects of thiamylal sodium on electrical activities of the central and peripheral nervous system in man. *Anesthesiology* 1974; **40**: 234–9.

19. Ganes T, Lundar T. The effect of thiopentone on somatosensory evoked responses and EEGs in comatose patients. *J Neurol Neurosurg Psychiatry* 1983; **46**: 509–14.

20. Koht A, Schutz W, Schmidt G. Effects of etomidate, midazolam, and thiopental on median nerve somatosensory evoked potentials and the additive effect of fentanyl and nitrous oxide. *Anesth Analg* 1988; **67**: 582–9.

21. Sloan TB, Ronai AK, Toleikis JR. Improvement of somatosensory evoked potentials by etomidate. *Anesth Analg* 1988; **67**: 582–9.

22. McPherson RW, Sell B, Traystman RJ. Effects of thiopental, fentanyl, and etomidate on upper extremity somatosensory evoked potentials in humans. *Anesthesiology* 1986; **65**: 584–8.

23. Nathan N, Tabaraud F, Lacroix F. Influence of propofol concentrations on multiple transcranial motor evoked potentials. *Br J Anaesth* 2003; **91**: 493–9.

24. Pechstein U, Nadstawek J, Zentner J. Isoflurane plus nitrous oxide versus propofol for recording of motor evoked potentials after high frequency repetitive electrical stimulation. *Electrocephalogr Clin Neurophysiol* 1998; **108**: 175–83.

25. Kajiyama S, Sanuki M, Kinoshita H. Effect of bolus propofol administration on muscle evoked potential (MsEP) during spine surgery. *Masui* 2001; **50**: 867–73.

26. Russell D, Wilkes MP, Hunter SC, *et al.* Manual compared to targeted infusion of propofol. *Br J Anaesth* 1995; **75**: 562–6.

27. Nathan N, Tabaraud F, Lacroix F, *et al.* Influence of propofol concentrations on multipulse transcranial motor evoked potentials. *Br J Anaesth* 2003; **91**: P3493–7.

28. Albertin A, LaColla L, Gandolfi A, *et al.* Greater peripheral blood flow but less bleeding with propofol versus sevoflurane during spine surgery. *Spine* 2008; **33**: 2017–22.

29. Holzman A, Schmidt H, Gebhardt MM, *et al.* Propofol-induced alterations in the microcirculation of hamster striated muscle. *Br J Anaesth* 1995; **75**: 452–6.

30. Schubert A, Drummond JC, Peterson DO, Saidman LJ. The effect of high-dose fentanyl on human median somatosensory evoked responses. *Can J Anaesth* 1987; **34**: 35–40.

31. Pathak KS, Brown RH, Cascorbi HF, Nash CL. Effects of fentanyl and morphine on intraoperative somatosensory cortical-evoked potentials. *Anesth Analg* 1984; **63**: 833–7.

32. Kimball-Jones PL, Schell RM, Shook JP. The use of remifentanil infusion to allow intraoperative awakening for intentional fracturing of the anterior cervical spine. *Anesth Analg* 1999; **89**: 1059–61.

33. Imani F, Jafarian A, Hassani V, Khan ZH. Propofol-alfentanil vs. propofol-remifentanil for posterior spinal fusion including wake-up test. *Br J Anaesth* 2006; **96**: 583–6.

34. Ngwenyama NE, Knanyezi E, Anderson J, Hoernschmeyer DG, Tobias JD. Effects of

dexmedetomidine on propofol and remifentanil infusion rates during total intravenous anesthesia for spine surgery in adolescents. *Pediatr Anesth* 2008; **18**: 1190–5.

35. Bala E, Sessler DI, Nair DR, *et al.* Motor and somatosensory potentials are well maintained in patients given dexmedetomidine during spine surgery. *Anesthesiology* 2008; **109**: 417–25.

36. Anschel DJ, Aherne A, Soto RG. Successful intraoperative spinal cord monitoring during scoliosis surgery using a total intravenous anesthetic regimen including dexmedetomidine. *J Clin Neurophysiol* 2008; **25**: 56–61.

37. Tobias JD, Goble TJ, Bates G, *et al.* Effects of dexmedetomidine on intraoperative motor and somatosensory evoked potential monitoring during spinal surgery in adolescents. *Pediatr Anesth* 2008; **18**: 1082–88.

38. Mahmoud M, Sadhasivam S, Salisbury S, *et al.* Susceptibility of transcranial electric motor-evoked potentials to varying targeted blood levels of dexmedetomidine during spine surgery. *Anesthesiology* 2010; **112**: 1364–73.

39. Mahmoud M, Sadhasivam S, Sestokas AK, Samuels P, McAuliffe J. Loss of transcranial electric motor evoked potentials during pediatric spine surgery with dexmedetomidine. *Anesthesiology* 2007; **106**: 393–6.

40. Hadi BA, Al Ramadani R, Daas R, Naylor I, Zeiko R. Remifentanil in combination with ketamine versus remifentanil in spinal fusion surgery- a double blind study. *Int J Clin Pharmacol Ther* 2010; **48**: 542–8.

41. Ubags LH, Kalkman CJ, Been HD, *et al.* The use of ketamine or etomidate to supplement sufentanil/ nitrous oxide anesthesia does not disrupt the monitoring of myogenic transcranial motor evoked responses. *J Neurosurg Anesthesiol* 1997; **9**: 228–33.

42. Yang LH, Lin SM, Lee WY, *et al.* Intraoperative transcranial electrical motor evoked potential monitoring during spinal surgery under intravenous ketamine or etomidate anesthesia. *Acta Neurochir* 1994; **127**: 191–7.

43. Grundy BL, Brown RH, Greenbergh BA. Diazepam alters cortical potentials. *Anesthesiology* 1979; **51**: 538–43.

Chapter

8

Surgical techniques

8.1 Anterior cervical surgery

Iain H. Kalfas

Key points

- Anterior cervical surgery is a frequently performed spinal procedure.
- Indications for this surgery include degenerative, traumatic, neoplastic, and deformity disorders of the cervical spine.
- Surgical goals: decompression of the neural elements followed by reconstruction and stabilization of the involved spinal segments.
- Anatomic complexity of the anterior cervical region creates the potential for a variety of intraoperative and postoperative complications.
- Close collaboration between the surgical and anesthesia teams before and during anterior cervical surgery helps minimize the development of these complications and to optimize clinical outcome.

Introduction

Anterior cervical surgery is one of the more common procedures performed by neurosurgeons and orthopedic spine surgeons. It is a versatile and effective surgery that can address a wide variety of spinal disorders affecting the cervical spine.

The anterior approach to the cervical spine was first developed in the 1950s as an alternative to the more commonly performed laminectomy procedure.[1] A laminectomy is performed through a posterior approach to the cervical spine. This approach has several factors that limit its effectiveness for many patients with cervical pathology. In particular, laminectomy does not provide access to pathology lying in front of the spinal cord where a majority of cervical lesions occur. Removal of the posterior supporting elements of the cervical spine also creates the potential for the development of a postoperative spinal deformity.[2]

Over the past two decades, improvements and developments in preoperative imaging techniques, surgical microscope technology, and spinal instrumentation devices have all contributed to a rapid rise in the volume of anterior cervical surgery performed. Approximately 350 000 anterior cervical surgeries are now performed in the United States each year. It is a far more commonly performed procedure than cervical laminectomy.[3]

Indications for anterior cervical surgery

The primary indication for anterior cervical surgery is clinically correlative compression of the ventral epidural space. This is most commonly due to herniated disc material or intervertebral osteophyte (bone spur) formation (spondylosis) (Fig. 8.1). Other pathologies that can cause compression of the neural structures (spinal cord and nerve roots) include cervical trauma, deformity, neoplasms, and osteomyelitis/discitis. Anterior cervical surgery is also indicated when a disruption of the cervical bone and supporting ligamentous structures has produced an unstable spinal column that potentially places the spinal cord at risk for new or further injury.

Although less frequently performed, laminectomy remains an effective surgical option for some

Anesthesia for Spine Surgery, ed. Ehab Farag. Published by Cambridge University Press. © Cambridge University Press 2012.

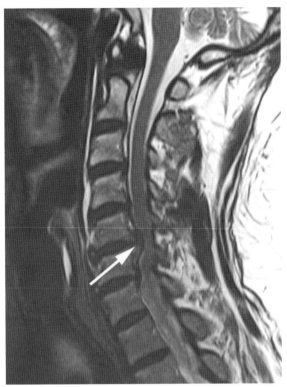

Figure 8.1 Sagittal MRI demonstrating a herniated disc (arrow) at the C5–6 level creating compression of the ventral aspect of the spinal cord.

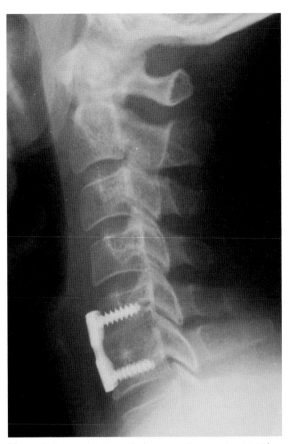

Figure 8.2 Lateral radiograph demonstrating anterior cervical fixation following a discectomy and interbody fusion.

conditions. Its primary indication is for pathology producing compression of the dorsal epidural space. It is also indicated for most intradural pathology such as spinal cord neoplasms and vascular malformations.

Rarely, both an anterior and a posterior approach may be necessary to optimally manage cervical pathology. This combined approach is typically indicated when there is a marked deformity of the cervical spine in addition to significant epidural compression. It may also be indicated for added stabilization following extensive anterior decompression requiring the removal of several vertebrae.

Surgical technique overview

The anterior cervical surgical approach can be used to access the cervical spine from the C2–3 disc space superiorly to the C7–T1 disc space inferiorly. The surgical dissection and approach follows a natural tissue plane lying between the trachea and esophagus medially and the sternocleidomastoid muscle and carotid artery laterally. These structures can be gently retracted to provide a generous exposure of the anterior surface of the cervical spine.

The most common type of anterior cervical surgery is a discectomy which involves the removal of a single or multiple intervertebral discs. This procedure is typically performed for symptoms resulting from a cervical disc herniation or from spondylosis (bone spur formation). Less frequently, one or several vertebrae as well as their adjacent intervertebral discs may need to be removed to adequately decompress the neural structures. This procedure, termed "corpectomy," is typically used for the management of cervical trauma and neoplasms that affect the structural integrity of the vertebral bodies.

Following the appropriate decompression of the neural elements through either a discectomy or a corpectomy procedure, the involved spinal column must be reconstructed. This involves placing one or several structural bone grafts into the site of the discectomy or corpectomy. Alternatively, a metal or carbon fiber cage can be used instead of a bone graft. A spinal fixation plate and screws helps secure the bone graft or cage in place and adds additional structural support to the surgical site (Fig. 8.2).

Postoperatively, patients are typically placed in a hard cervical collar for a short period. Patients requiring more extensive spinal reconstruction may require a longer period of postoperative bracing. Rarely, patients with major spinal reconstruction may need to be placed into a halo immobilization brace for several months.

A relatively recent development in anterior cervical surgery is the insertion of an artificial disc.[4] This procedure, termed cervical arthroplasty, is indicated for the treatment of single-level disc degeneration or herniation in patients with radiculopathy. It involves performing a discectomy and decompression of the epidural space followed by the insertion of an articulating device into the disc space. The theoretical advantage of arthroplasty is that it preserves segmental spinal motion and potentially reduces the incidence of degeneration of the adjacent intervertebral discs. This development of adjacent-level changes has been noted to occur at a rate of up to 3% per year following anterior cervical fusion surgery.[5]

Immediate preoperative management

Several general principles apply to all patients undergoing anterior cervical surgery. Although most patients with anterior cervical pathology can undergo gentle extension of the head and neck for endotracheal intubation, some patients will require that any extension be limited or not used at all. This is typically the case in patients with a traumatic cervical injury that has destabilized their spinal column.

Another less common contraindication to cervical extension is severe spinal canal stenosis. These patients may exhibit a finding termed Lhermitte's phenomenon. This neurologic sign occurs when affected patients extend their neck and experience a shocklike shooting down their spinal column or into their arms and legs. It indicates the presence of significant spinal cord compression with a high degree of sensitivity to motion.

Any patient with a contraindication to cervical extension should be considered for an awake intubation, preferably with fiberoptic assistance. Communication between the spinal surgeon and the anesthesiologist prior to intubation is advised to help assure the selection of the most appropriate intubation approach for each patient.

During the induction process it is critical to avoid any prolonged period of hypotension. This is particularly important in patients who present with a myelopathy due to compression of the spinal cord. Even a brief period of transient hypotension in these patients may significantly increase the potential for hypoperfusion of a spinal cord that already has its vascular supply compromised by the compressive pathology.

Following induction, the patient's head and neck are placed in a neutral to slightly extended position. The endotracheal tubing is positioned so that it extends directly over the patient's forehead. This allows for optimal access to both sides of the anterior cervical region by the surgical team. Some surgeons prefer to place their patients into gentle traction with a halter sling that fits under the chin and the back of the skull.

The administration of corticosteroids is optional. In selected patients with severe neurologic impairment due to significant neural compression, preoperative administration of corticosteroids may protect the spinal cord during surgery, although limited data exist to support this approach. Corticosteroids may also help to minimize soft tissue edema and airway issues resulting from surgical dissection and retraction. The disadvantage of the use of steroids is that they interfere with the early stages of bone healing and may compromise the long-term fusion outcome of the procedure.

The routine use of intraoperative electrophysiological monitoring (somatosensory or motor evoked potentials) during anterior cervical surgery is not conclusive. Advocates of monitoring claim that its use lowers the risk for postoperative neurologic deficits. Motor evoked potentials have been found to be far more helpful than somatosensory evoked potentials.[6]

The argument against the routine use of evoked potential monitoring is that since the risk of neurologic deterioration following anterior cervical surgery is relatively low without monitoring, the additional time and expense involved with monitoring may not justify its use for every case. The use of monitoring is best determined by each individual surgeon's personal preference and the specific surgical problem being addressed in each patient.

Surgical management

Anterior cervical surgery can be performed through either a transverse incision extending from the trachea to the sternocleidomastoid muscle or an oblique incision made along the medial border of the sternocleidomastoid muscle. Although a right-sided approach is technically easier for a right-handed surgeon, the left-sided approach to the cervical spine may offer some minimal reduction to the risk of injury to the recurrent laryngeal nerve. The recurrent laryngeal nerve on the right side lies between the trachea and esophagus but can take an aberrant course and lie more rostral than the nerve on the left side. This anatomic variance may make the nerve more prone to a retraction injury with a right-sided approach. Alternatively, a left-sided approach risks injury to the thoracic duct.

Early in the dissection process, the carotid artery is identified and retracted laterally. Injury to this vessel is very rare. Any bleeding that occurs during the approach is typically venous in origin and relatively easily controlled. The vertebral arteries are typically not visualized during the procedure unless the discectomy or corpectomy is extended too widely.

Following exposure of the spinal column, self-retaining retractor blades are positioned to retract the trachea and esophagus medially and the carotid artery and jugular vein laterally. The retractor blades are positioned under the longus colli muscles which run longitudinally on either side of the cervical spine midline. If these retractor blades are allowed to migrate from their submuscular position, they may cause a perforating injury to the esophagus or excessive retraction of the trachea. A rare complication of retractor blade migration is the development of a unilateral Horner's syndrome due to encroachment on the sympathetic chain lateral to the longus colli muscles.

Rarely, excessive pressure on the carotid artery by the lateral retractor blade may potentially compromise blood flow through the vessel. Palpation of the superficial temporal arteries may alert the anesthesia team to a possibility of reduced flow necessitating a repositioning of the retractor blades by the surgical team. Correct initial placement of the lateral retractor blade beneath the longus colli muscle minimizes the risk of reduced carotid blood flow.

Retraction of the trachea has been proposed to potentially lead to vocal cord paralysis due to endotracheal cuff pressure on the recurrent laryngeal nerve within the endolarynx. In an effort to reduce the incidence of vocal cord paralysis, one study proposed that immediately following tracheal retraction, the cuff pressure should be released and then re-inflated to the just-sealed pressure of 15 mmHg. The cuff pressure is monitored throughout the procedure and deflated with any further increases in pressure. This approach resulted in a reduction in the incidence of vocal cord paralysis from 6.4% to 1.7% in a series of 900 consecutive patients who underwent anterior cervical spine surgery.[7]

Surgical decompression proceeds with removal of the disc or bone material producing encroachment on

the neural structures. This is typically performed with the aid of a surgical microscope using a high-speed drill and a series of bone rongeurs. Although epidural venous bleeding can be encountered it is rarely excessive and relatively easy to control. It typically subsides once adequate decompression has been achieved. Leakage of cerebrospinal fluid can also occur during decompression but is relatively uncommon and can be controlled with the application of a dural sealant material.

Following adequate decompression, the structural stability of the spinal column must be reestablished. This involves placement of a suitable bone graft(s) or synthetic cage(s) into the site of the discectomy or corpectomy. In the past, bone grafts were typically harvested from the patient's iliac crest or fibula. The morbidity and pain associated with this process as well as the improvement in tissue banking practices has made the use of banked allograft bone much more common today.

The appropriately sized graft(s) or cages(s) are placed between the vertebral end plates on either side of the decompressed site. If halter traction has not been used, placement of a graft or cage into the site of reconstruction may require the anesthesia team to provide a brief period of manual inline cervical traction.

Once the bone graft(s) or cages(s) are in position, anterior cervical plate fixation is placed to further secure them (Fig. 8.2) These titanium plates are attached to the spine by screws inserted into the vertebrae on either side of the reconstructed site. In addition to enhancing the fusion rate, plate fixation also minimizes the need for postoperative bracing.[8,9]

Immediate postoperative management

Postoperatively, most patients can be extubated in the operating room. Following more extensive multilevel corpectomy procedures in which there may be excessive soft tissue edema it may be necessary to leave the patient intubated until the edema subsides. Most of these patients can be extubated 12–18 hours following surgery.

Although complications from anterior cervical surgery are relatively rare, the anatomic complexity of this region allows for the potential development of a variety of different problems. The most serious complication following this surgery is airway compromise and frank obstruction requiring urgent re-intubation or tracheostomy. This may occur in the immediate postoperative period or several days after surgery. The common causes of airway compromise following anterior cervical surgery are pharyngeal edema, wound hematoma,

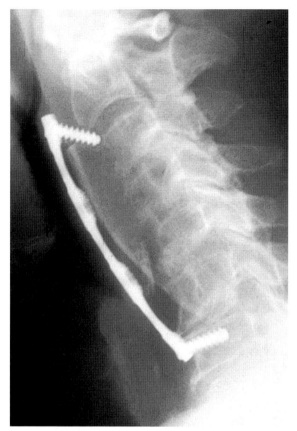

Figure 8.3 Lateral radiograph demonstrating dislodgement of an anterior fixation device and the bone graft following a three-level corpectomy procedure.

or dislodgement of the bone graft and fixation plate (Fig. 8.3).[10,11]

Sagi *et al.* reported a retrospective series of 311 patients who underwent anterior cervical surgery. Nineteen patients (6.1%) had an airway complication and six (1.9%) required re-intubation. One patient died. All airway complications except two were attributable to pharyngeal edema. Variables that were found to be statistically associated with airway complications following anterior cervical surgery were exposure of more than three vertebral bodies, blood loss >300 ml, exposure of the upper cervical spine (C2–4) and an operative time >5 hours. A history of myelopathy, spinal cord injury, pulmonary problems, smoking, anesthetic risk factors, and the absence of a wound drain did not correlate with a higher incidence of postoperative airway complications.[12]

In addition to airway obstruction other potential complications include transient sore throat, dysphagia, hoarseness, dysphonia, vocal cord paralysis, esophageal perforation, wound hematoma, and dislodgement of the fixation plate and bone graft. Injury to the spinal cord or nerve roots is relatively rare but can occur. The most common long-term complication is failure of the bone graft to fuse. A review of 4589 cases in the Cervical Spine Research Society database revealed a total complication rate of 5.3% following anterior cervical surgery.[13]

The most common neurologic complication following cervical spine surgery is C5 nerve root palsy. A meta-analysis report indicated an average incidence of C5 dermatomal weakness following anterior cervical surgery of 4.3%.[14] Most (92%) C5 palsies are unilateral and occur within the first week of surgery. Although the pathogenesis for selective C5 involvement is unclear, several theories have been promoted generally based on the root's specific anatomic location and course. Proposed mechanisms include traction of the root produced by a shifting of the spinal cord following decompression, ischemia due to involvement of the C5 radicular artery, and lack of cross-innervation of the deltoid muscles which are primarily supplied by the C5 root.[14,15] The prognosis for spontaneous recovery of a C5 motor radiculopathy is relatively good in most cases.

Postoperatively, most patients are placed into a cervical collar for a short period (1–2 weeks). They are typically discharged from the hospital 1–2 days postoperatively. The clinical outcome for patients undergoing anterior cervical surgery for radiculopathy is very good, with over 90% achieving a successful outcome.[1] Patients who undergo anterior cervical surgery for myelopathy have a clinical improvement rate of approximately 70%.[13]

Conclusion

Anterior cervical surgery is a common spinal procedure. Its use for a variety of cervical disorders has expanded with advancements in surgical microscopy, fixation devices and bone grafting technologies. The anatomic complexity of this region requires a close collaboration between the surgical and anesthesia teams in order to limit the development of complications and to optimize the clinical outcome following surgery.

References

1. Cloward RB. The anterior approach for removal of ruptured cervical discs. *J Neurosurg* 1958; **15**: 602–17.
2. Raynor RB. Anterior and posterior approaches to the cervical spinal cord, discs, and roots: a comparison of exposures and decompression. In: The Cervical Spine Research Society, Editorial Committee, ed. *The Cervical Spine*. Philadelphia: JB Lippincott; 1989: 659–69.

3. Wang MC, Kreuter W, Wolfla CE, *et al.* Trends and variations in cervical spine surgery in the United States. Medicare beneficiaries 1992–2005. *Spine* 2009; **9**: 955–61.

4. Goffin J, Van Clenbergh F, van Loon J, *et al.* Intermediate follow-up after treatment of degenerative disc disease with the Bryan cervical disc prosthesis: single and bi-level. *Spine* 2003; **28**: 2673–8.

5. Hilibrand AS, Carlson GD, Palumbo MA, *et al.* Radiculopathy and myelopathy at segments adjacent to the site of a previous anterior cervical arthrodesis. *J Bone Joint Surg* 1999; **81**: 519–28.

6. Hilibrand AS, Schwartz DM, Sethuraman V, *et al.* Comparison of transcranial electric motor and somatosensory evoked potential monitoring during cervical spine surgery. *J Bone Joint Surg* 2004; **86**: 1248–53.

7. Apfelbaum RI, Kriskovich MD, Haller JR. On the incidence, cause and prevention of recurrent laryngeal nerve palsies during anterior cervical spine surgery. *Spine* 2000; **25**: 2906–12.

8. Kalfas IH. The anterior cervical spine locking plate: a technique for surgical decompression and stabilization. In: Fessler RG, Haid RW, eds. *Techniques in Spinal Stabilization*. New York: McGraw-Hill; 1996: 25–33.

9. Kaiser MG, Haid RW, Subach BR, *et al.* Anterior cervical plating enhances arthrodesis after discectomy and fusion with cortical allograft. *Neurosurgery* 2002; **50**: 229–38.

10. Emery SE, Smith MD, Bohlman HH. Upper airway management after multi-level corpectomy for myelopathy. *J Bone Joint Surg Am* 1991; **73**: 544–50.

11. Bookvar JA, Philips MF, Telfeian AE. Results and risk factors for anterior cervicothoracic junction surgery. *J Neurosurg* 2001; **94**: 12–17.

12. Sagi HC, Beutler W, Carroll E, *et al.* Airway complications associated with surgery on the anterior cervical spine. *Spine* 2002; **9**: 949–53.

13. Zeidman SE, Ducker TB, Raycroft J. Trends and complications in cervical spine surgery: 1989–1993. *J Spinal Disord* 1997; **10**: 523–6.

14. Sakaura H, Hosono N, Mukai Y, *et al.* C5 palsy after decompression surgery for cervical myelopathy. *Spine* 2003; **28**: 2447–51.

15. Kaneko K, Hashiguchi A, Kato Y, *et al.* Investigation of motor dominant C5 paralysis after laminoplasty from the results of evoked spinal cord responses. *J Spinal Disord Tech* 2006; **19**: 358–61.

8.2   Posterior cervical surgery

Kalil G. Abdullah, Jeffrey G. Clark, Daniel Lubelski, and Thomas E. Mroz

Key points

- Posterior surgical spine surgery is a common elective procedure that is indicated for decompression and stabilization of the spinal cord and exiting nerve roots.
- It is essential to maintain vigilance in the monitoring and positioning of the cervical spine surgery patient, whether elective or traumatic due to the possibility of sudden neurologic deterioration.
- Careful positioning is paramount in this patient population to allow for appropriate surgical and airway access.
- Induction of hypotension to protect from blood loss is generally unnecessary and can result in ischemic compromise to the spinal cord.
- During traumatic intervention, mean arterial pressure should be carefully monitored and kept above 90 mmHg.

Introduction

Posterior cervical spine surgery is among the most common procedures performed by spine surgeons. A variety of indications require a posterior approach, of which several different techniques may be employed to decompress and reconstruct the spine following trauma, degeneration, neoplasm, or infection. Posterior spine surgery at any level elicits a set of considerations for the surgical team, but posterior cervical spine surgery in particular requires vigilance with regard to positioning, intubation, and intraoperative hemodynamic status. In this chapter, we briefly introduce indications for posterior spinal surgery, patient positioning, and specific considerations necessary for safe anesthesia in these patients.

Indications for posterior spine surgery

Posterior surgery is indicated when exposure of the dorsal elements of the spine or spinal cord is required. Among the most common indications for posterior surgery is cervical spondylotic myelopathy and radiculopathy. In these cases, the cervical spine is exposed through a midline incision and the bony elements including the vertebral process, lamina, and foramina are visualized and then often modified (i.e., laminoplasty) or removed (i.e., laminectomy, foraminotomy) to decompress the exiting nerve roots and/or spinal cord. In general there are two main categories of posterior surgery: decompression and fusion. Laminoforaminotomy (i.e., removing a small portion of the unilateral lamina and facet joint) addresses foraminal stenosis (i.e., *nerve root* compression) at one or more levels and does not require fusion because it does not involve removing spinous processes or interspinous ligaments, and hence, is not a destabilizing procedure. Laminectomy is typically reserved for patients with spinal cord compression at greater than three levels and is typically followed by an instrumented fusion. Laminectomy without fusion has fallen out of favor due to the known association with postlaminectomy kyphosis, and possibly late neurologic deterioration as a consequence of the structural demise. The purpose of the instrumentation is to provide provisional stability until biological fusion occurs across the surgical levels. Laminoplasty, used to treat myelopathy, is a procedure that involves making precise cuts on bilateral laminae at multiple levels, hinging the laminae open, and then fixing them in that position with small plates or sutures. This procedure does not involve fusion, and is considered as efficacious as laminectomy and fusion for the treatment of cervical myelopathy with and without radiculopathy. The majority of posterior surgery involves the subaxial spine (C3–T1); however, occipital-cervical surgery is not uncommon. Certainly, surgical approaches may vary significantly to address infection or neoplasm, but the common principles of posterior spine surgery include the need to expose, decompress, and possibly, perform an instrumented fusion.

Trauma to the cervical spine and instability due to infection or neoplasia has specific ramifications for the surgical team. Whenever destabilization occurs in the cervical spine secondary to trauma, a multitude of factors must be taken into consideration (the relevant components are discussed below). In certain situations, it may be necessary to stage surgical intervention to include anterior and posterior approaches, but that discussion is beyond the scope of this chapter. Regardless of future intervention or perioperative care, each patient with cervical trauma undergoing posterior surgery must be handled with the understanding that catastrophic neurologic deterioration is a possibility if positioning, intubation, and surgical handling are compromised. Careful collaboration with the surgical team prior to and during intubation and positioning is mandatory.

Patient positioning

Prone positioning is the standard for posterior cervical surgery. Historically, the sitting position was occasionally used but the rates of complications (e.g., air emboli, ischemia, instability) were unacceptably high. In the extremely unlikely case of morbid obesity or ventilatory restriction requiring a sitting position, then Doppler ultrasound is an option for embolism monitoring.[1]

Most patients are placed in cranial tongs for posterior cervical surgery, but some surgeons prefer a foam pillow. Advantages of the cranial tongs include intentional intraoperative positional changes, and absence of facial or ocular pressure. The decision for an awake fiberoptic intubation should be made after careful consideration of the cervical stability and the preoperative active range of motion. In patients who are deemed unstable or unable to neurologically tolerate cervical stenosis (i.e., severe stenosis) by the treating surgeon, an awake fiberoptic intubation is indicated. It is important to assess preoperative active range of motion in patients with myelopathy regardless of etiology. If active cervical extension or flexion result in subjective or objective neurologic compromise, then an awake fiberoptic intubation is indicated to avoid injury.

To prepare the prone elective patient, intubation is first accomplished and the patient is turned from supine to prone using a "log roll" technique, maintaining the neck in a neutral position. Typically, a member of the surgical team controls the head during the turn while the anesthesiologist manages the airway. To avoid elevated thoracic or abdominal pressures, cushions are placed along the margins of the upper torso. The surgeon then adjusts and negotiates the Mayfield clamp to secure the head and cervical spine in the desired position, and the bed may be placed in slight reverse Trendelenburg.[2] It is important that the endotracheal tube is secured and guided appropriately so that it is unobstructed and not in competition with any other apparatus. Unlike in surgical situations where the patient is supine, inherent difficulty will arise should the tube need to be adjusted while the surgeon is operating on the prone patient with a possibly unstable spine.

For those patients undergoing intervention following trauma, the positioning process is similar. Should these patients already have undergone halo fixation, it allows for more controlled movement of the patient from supine to prone. Patients in the emergent setting without fixation must be moved with typical stabilizing technique and can then be placed into traction by the surgeon.

Elective interventions

The most common elective procedures include laminoforaminotomy, laminectomy and fusion, and laminoplasty for spondylotic myelopathy and radiculopathy. Spinal instability is rare in cases of spondylotic myelopathy or radiculopathy involving the subaxial cervical spine. However, as mentioned, it is important to preoperatively assess the active range of motion to ensure that the patient does not neurologically decompensate in certain neck positions. Patients with rheumatoid disease, however, can have subaxial or atlantoaxial (C1–2) instability, and it is important to preoperatively discuss this particular aspect of the case with the surgeon.[3,4] Certain maneuvers can narrow the spinal canal depending on underlying pathology. Patients with subaxial spondylotic myelopathy can undergo narrowing of the spinal canal during neck extension, while those with atlantoaxial subluxation will have narrowing of the spinal canal during flexion. In these patients, a fiberoptic intubation is preferred.

The elective patient is unlikely to require additional consideration during the intubation process. The anesthetic considerations as to whether to use a fiberoptic intubation or routine direct laryngoscopy will mostly be due to the patient's other comorbidities or underlying disease process (i.e., rheumatoid arthritis, Down's syndrome) and not the specific planned surgical intervention. It should be noted that there exists a differential amount of cervical motion that occurs in the upper cervical vertebrae when using different intubation techniques. Sahin et al.[5] found, as expected, that fiberoptic laryngoscopy resulted in a significantly smaller range of motion between vertebrae when compared with direct intubation.

Patients undergoing elective procedures may require hemodynamic monitoring with a radial artery catheter, and patients with significant comorbidities may require more invasive monitoring. The patient should be carefully observed to ensure adequate perfusion of the spinal cord. States of low blood flow are often seen during spinal surgery as a result of an effect of the anesthetic drugs or the positioning of the patient.

When the patient is placed in the prone position there is often a drop in blood pressure. Dharmavaram and colleagues conducted a study comparing prone positioning systems on hemodynamic and cardiac function. They found various changes in cardiac function dependent on the manufacturer of the operating room table; some tables decreased cardiac index and stroke volume, whereas others contributed to a decrease in cardiac preload. Cardiac output was reduced in all of them.[6] The mechanism of action is thought to be poor venous return and a change in ventricular compliance.

Even moderate hypotension may exacerbate spinal cord injury that is produced from manipulation or distraction of the region during surgery. Understandably, in the hypotensive state there is limited oxygen supply and impaired clearance of metabolites. The subsequent elevated levels of carbon dioxide and lactic acid lead to lower pH and concomitant damage to the cells. These changes are irreversible, and the most successful avoidance of perioperative spinal cord injury is well-executed preventative methods and communication between the surgical and anesthetic teams.

It is important to maintain perfusion of the spinal cord in both acute injury and elective spine surgery. According to a Practice Advisory issued by a task force of the American Society of Anesthesiologists, blood pressure during induction of deliberate hypotension in healthy, nonhypotensive patients should be maintained within 24% of baseline mean arterial pressure (MAP) or with a *minimum* systolic blood pressure of 84 mmHg (range 50–120 mmHg).[7] These guidelines should absolutely be paired with clinical judgment. Specifically, the definition of "healthy" in the above report should be contextualized. Patients undergoing elective spine surgery are of a demographic that includes many comorbidities, which include obesity, peripheral vascular disease, diabetes, and other entities that negatively influence perfusion. As such, we recommend that MAP be manipulated at a higher range (80–90 mmHg MAP) to account for these factors. In a systematic review by Ahn and Fehlings, a MAP >80–85 mmHg was recommended, and it was emphasized that patients with preexisting SCI or at high risk for SCI intraoperatively should be maintained at this MAP, even if use of vasopressors is needed. Minimizing blood loss in nearly all patients undergoing elective surgery of the posterior cervical spine should not be an anesthetic priority. These surgeries typically involve minimal blood loss and in many ordinary surgeries requiring posterior intervention it is far more important to maintain perfusion to vital respiratory centers through an appropriate MAP.[8]

It is often misunderstood that hypotension is the greatest contributor to postoperative vision loss during prone position spine surgery.[9]. In the only study that has examined this phenomenon in a case–control manner, the authors found no difference in blood pressure between the group of patients with or without postoperative vision loss. Instead, length of surgery and overall blood loss were statistically significant factors.[10] Nonetheless, vigilance for postoperative vision loss is an absolutely essential component of spine surgery and has been reported in many different types of patient population, and is discussed at length elsewhere in this book.[10] Signs of hemodynamic instability should be attended to in the usual fashion, with alertness for both arterial hypo- and hypertension, and swings in blood pressure should be avoided.

Traumatic interventions

The patterns of traumatic cervical spine injuries vary, but all patients with cervical injuries (i.e., fractures, subluxations, and dislocations) should be managed the same in terms of intubation and positioning. In the emergent setting, the patient usually presents to the operating room after an appropriate traumatic workup by the surgical team. By this point, the neurologic status of the patient should have been assessed. However, there is debate as to whether or not intubation in the operating room should be performed using fiberoptic awake intubation. This provides the advantage of assessing neurologic function after intubation, and can result in minimal displacement of the neck. It is usually done under light sedation and requires a cooperative patient. The complicating aspects of awake intubation are related to risks of aspiration and a prolonged induction time. Further, this may be an understandably uncomfortable experience for the conscious patient, who may not be in a fully cooperative state. Several other methods of intubation have been proposed in case reports and small series,[11,12] and a detailed algorithm for the appropriate methods of induction following cervical trauma (including the decision as to whether or not to employ rapid-sequence induction and appropriate anesthetic regimens) can be found elsewhere.[13] Regardless of the type of intubation, immobilization of the cervical spine is paramount and must remain an urgent priority during the intubation process. It is advantageous to place the patient in a rigid cervical collar prior to positioning, as this offers additional stability. This is particularly helpful in patients with ankylosing spondylitis-related fractures in whom the cervical spines are frequently very unstable. It is imperative that the surgeon and anesthesiologist have a thorough discussion of the intubation and surgical plan prior to the intubation.

Patients with infections and tumors involving the spinal column should be considered to have unstable cervical spines unless stated otherwise by the surgeon. There a multitude of different surgeries used for these entities; however, the key tenets of decompressing the neural elements, resecting pathologic tissue, and reconstructing the spine are followed. The management of these patients from an anesthesia standpoint is similar to patients undergoing elective procedures.

Spinal cord injuries require special hemodynamic considerations. Traumatic cord injuries involve secondary mechanisms of injury, including hypoperfusion. It is extremely important to maintain proper perfusion through careful control of the blood pressure during surgery. In those patients where spinal cord injury is known or assumed, perfusion of the cord is paramount. As in elective procedures perfusion should be emphasized over blood loss. To start, MAP should be greater than 90 mmHg. The pressure should be maintained at this level, which may involve the use of vasopressors such as norepinephrine and dopamine (epinephrine should not be used as it has alpha receptor affinity, possible decreasing cord perfusion).

Vigilance to the hemodynamic state is very important during traumatic posterior cervical spine surgery. Injuries to the cervical spinal cord can result in neurogenic shock due to a loss of sympathetic tone below the site of the injury. This decreases or eliminates the ability of the cord to autoregulate perfusion. Studies suggest that the severity of abnormal cardiac control correlates well with the severity of cervical spinal cord injury[14] but is not related to the location of the injury in the upper (C1–5) or lower (C6–7) cervical spine.[15] Thus, regardless of the region of injury within the cervical spine, awareness of these phenomena should be maintained. Neurogenic shock should be immediately treated with fluids to keep central venous pressure within 4–6 mmHg. Vasopressor infusions can then be given to maintain adequate spinal cord perfusion.

Summary

The patient undergoing posterior spine surgery requires a special level of vigilance by the surgical team. Complications that may arise during intubation or preparation of the patient can be due to trauma or underlying pathology present in the cervical spine. Those patients presenting with spinal trauma must be assessed appropriately preoperatively and the intubation must proceed with minimal disruption of the spine.

References

1. Mayer HM. *Minimally Invasive Spine Surgery*. 2nd ed. New York: Springer; 2006.

2. Denaro L, D'Avella D, Denaro V. *Pitfalls in Cervical Spine Surgery*. Berlin: Springer; 2010.

3. Kim KA, Wang MY. Anesthetic considerations in the treatment of cervical myelopathy. *Spine J* 2006; **6**(6 Suppl): 207S–11S.

4. Wattenmaker I, Concepcion M, Hibberd P, Lipson S. Upper-airway obstruction and perioperative management of the airway in patients managed with posterior operations on the cervical spine for rheumatoid arthritis. *J Bone Joint Surg Am* 1994; **76**(3): 360–5.

5. Sahin A, Salman MA, Erden IA, Aypar U. Upper cervical vertebrae movement during intubating laryngeal mask, fibreoptic and direct laryngoscopy: a video-fluoroscopic study. *Eur J Anaesthesiol* 2004; **21**(10): 819–23.

6. Dharmavaram S, Jellish WS, Nockels RP, *et al.* Effect of prone positioning systems on hemodynamic and cardiac function during lumbar spine surgery: an echocardiographic study. *Spine (Phila Pa 1976)* 2006; **31**(12): 1388–93; discussion 1394.

7. American Society of Anesthesiologists Task Force on Perioperative Blindness. Practice advisory for perioperative visual loss associated with spine surgery: a report by the American Society of Anesthesiologists Task Force on Perioperative Blindness. *Anesthesiology* 2006; **104**(6): 1319–28.

8. Ahn H, Fehlings MG. Prevention, identification, and treatment of perioperative spinal cord injury. *Neurosurg Focus* 2008; **25**(5): E15.

9. Baig MN, Lubow M, Immesoete P, Bergese SD, Hamdy EA, Mendel E. Vision loss after spine surgery: review of the literature and recommendations. *Neurosurg Focus* 2007; **23**(5): E15.

10. Myers MA, Hamilton SR, Bogosian AJ, Smith CH, Wagner TA. Visual loss as a complication of spine surgery. A review of 37 cases. *Spine (Phila Pa 1976)* 1997; **22**(12): 1325–9.

11. Avitsian R, Lin J, Lotto M, Ebrahim Z. Dexmedetomidine and awake fiberoptic intubation for possible cervical spine myelopathy: a clinical series. *J Neurosurg Anesthesiol* 2005; **17**(2): 97–9.

12. Schuschnig C, Waltl B, Erlacher W, Reddy B, Stoik W, Kapral S. Intubating laryngeal mask and rapid sequence induction in patients with cervical spine injury. *Anaesthesia* 1999; **54**(8): 793–7.

13. Raw DA, Beattie JK, Hunter JM. Anaesthesia for spinal surgery in adults. *Br J Anaesth* 2003; **91**(6): 886–904.

14. Tuli S, Tuli J, Coleman WP, Geisler FH, Krassioukov A. Hemodynamic parameters and timing of surgical decompression in acute cervical spinal cord injury. *J Spinal Cord Med* 2007; **30**(5): 482–90.

15. Bilello JF, Davis JW, Cunningham MA, Groom TF, Lemaster D, Sue LP. Cervical spinal cord injury and the need for cardiovascular intervention. *Arch Surg* 2003; **138**(10): 1127–9.

8.3 Intraoperative neurophysiologic monitoring: surgeon's point of view

Manuel Saavedra and Robert F. McLain

Key points

- Spinal monitoring is provided at the surgeon's discretion – there is no standard of care.
- Motor evoked potentials (MEPs) can be obtained with partial relaxation when the patient is not paralyzed, meaning that neural responses to pressure, heat, or electroconduction are not absent. The surgeon still gets immediate feedback from surgical maneuvers that may impinge on neural tissues.

- Dorsal decompression addresses dorsal columns most directly and SEPs are often adequate. Volar compression is most common with tumors and fractures, and requires anterior column decompression. MEPs are recommended in these cases.
- When changes in latencies or amplitude are recognized during spinal cord decompression or spinal instrumentation, the first step is to check for equipment errors, then quickly

assess medication issues, patient temperature, oxygenation, and perfusion pressure. All of these should be optimized immediately at the same time the surgeon is informed of the change.

- In cases where the altered recordings appear real and directly associated with the spinal condition, surgical implants need to be assessed for direct impingement on the neural structures, spinal correction assessed for over-distraction of the cord, and margins of decompression assessed for unrecognized bone or soft tissue compression.

- Particular attention needs to paid to SCM signals that wax and wane directly with changes in blood pressure. Patients with labile systolic pressure and borderline cord perfusion are at risk for postoperative cord stroke if their postoperative blood pressure is allowed to drift downward in recovery or postoperative care. Intraoperative monitoring can identify this risk and alert the anesthesiologist to the need for tight pressure management.

Introduction

Intraoperative neurophysiologic monitoring has been used in spine surgery to minimize injury to critical neural structures from operative manipulations. Since the first recording of somatosensory evoked potentials in 1947 by Dawson,[1] the evolution of intraoperative monitoring has advanced dramatically. The advent of different types of techniques and its combinations has made possible monitoring of both motor and sensory nervous pathways according to the requirements of a variety of surgical procedures.

This chapter provides an overview of the various neurophysiologic monitoring techniques used intra-operatively, including somatosensory evoked potentials (SSEPs), motor evoked potentials (MEPs), and electromyography (EMG). Challenges of neurophysiologic monitoring include the presence of electromagnetic interference and the use of anesthetic agents that can alter recordings.

Indications for spinal monitoring

Depending on the surgery planned, the surgeon may request SSEP, MEP, EMG monitoring, or a combination of approaches in support. While these studies may be helpful in many different kinds of cases, the most common reason to request electrophysiologic monitoring is during spinal cord or nerve root manipulation. Patients who already exhibit signs of spinal cord distress or compression are particularly at risk during surgery, and monitoring of these cases is most helpful.

In cervical spine surgery, electrophysiologic monitoring is often requested simply to ensure that rare events are not missed. During cervical decompression, EMG monitoring may help avoid stress on the C5 nerve roots, one of which often experiences injury during surgery. In cases of cervical trauma, tumor, or infection, SSEPs and MEPs may detect subtle changes in cord pressure due to positioning, surgical decompression, or changes in blood pressure. SSEP and MEP monitoring are most often requested in patients with cervical myelopathy, however difficult the signals may be to obtain in patients with chronic disease. Real-time monitoring of cord function can help prevent permanent spinal cord injury.

In thoracic spine surgery, monitoring is also used in the face of spinal cord compression due to tumor, infection, or trauma, but is also useful to avoid injury when placing spinal implants such as hooks or pedicle screws. In these patient changes in cord perfusion can result in significant cord injury, and maintenance of blood pressure as well as avoidance of physical pressure on the cord may result in a much better outcome, facilitated by careful neurophysiologic monitoring.

While lumbar surgery usually avoids the spinal cord itself, the conus medullaris is at risk in upper lumbar surgery. Likewise specific nerve roots may be at risk during decompression or manipulation of the lumbar spine. Placement of pedicle screws and other spinal implants may stress the nerve roots and can potentially damage them directly. EMG monitoring as well as SEP monitoring can give important feedback during lumbar surgery.

Deformity surgery is particularly challenging in pediatric and adult patients. Congenital deformities are often associated with neurologic abnormalities, such as tethered cord or diastematomyelia, and even small changes in spinal alignment may stress the cord and cause neurologic deficit. Correction of large idiopathic curves may involve manipulation of the thoracic spinal cord or even the cervical level, and electrophysiologic monitoring may identify stress in the spinal cord long before it can be identified in any clinically helpful way. The combination of anterior surgery involving ligation of small segmental vessels with a large posterior surgery involving correction of multiple segments of the spine can put the cord at high risk for injury. Spinal monitoring during this sort of surgery can be particularly important in determining when correction is too much, and in making sure that blood pressure and other factors are optimized to maintain cord perfusion. By warning the surgeon of the need to reduce the correction, or remove specific implants, electrophysiologic monitoring can help prevent permanent and severe neurologic injuries.

Somatosensory evoked potentials (SSEPs)

Somatosensory evoked potential were initially described for monitoring the spinal cord during deformity correction for scoliosis.[2] The refinement of technology and technique has made SSEPs the mainstay in spinal cord monitoring.

SSEPs consist of monitoring neuronal integrity in the dorsal column–medial lemniscus pathway. Receptors localized in the skin, tendons, and muscles generate information on tactile discrimination, vibration and conscious proprioception. These sensory modalities relay signals to first-order neurons whose soma are located at dorsal root ganglia. They project to the spinal cord via the medial root entry zone, giving rise to the gracilis and cuneatus fasciculi, carrying sensation from the lower and upper extremities. The fibers decussate at the medullary level forming the medial lemniscus. They ascend to the thalamus and ultimately relay sensory information to the primary somatosensory cortex (Brodmann areas 3, 1, and 2).[3]

SSEPs are recorded with scalp electrodes after electric stimulation of afferent peripheral nerves. Median and ulnar nerves are used in the upper limbs while tibial and peroneal nerves are selected for monitoring the lower limbs. Figure 8.4 shows the usual location of SSEP electrodes.

Changes in amplitude greater than 50% and/or decrease in latency greater than 10% are generally accepted as a guideline for notifying the surgeon of impending spinal cord injury.[3,4] Nuwer et al., after reviewing a large multicenter survey of more than 50 000 procedures using intraoperative SSEPs, reported an overall 92% sensitivity and 98.9% specificity in the ability of SSEPs to detect new postoperative neurologic deficits.[5]

The amplitude of SSEPs can potentially be altered by the use of halogenated agents, nitrous oxide, hypothermia, hypotension, and electrical interference. Latency can be affected by temperature changes.[3]

SSEPs are generally used as a surveillance tool during spinal decompression and instrumentation. They are generally considered less sensitive to motor injuries, which may occur during anterior decompression and treatment of fractures and tumors.

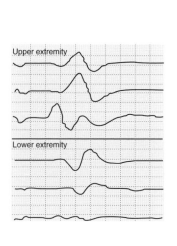

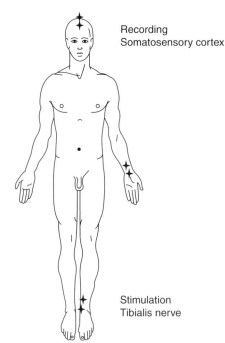

Figure 8.4 Arrangement for somatosensory evoked potential electrodes.

Recording
Somatosensory cortex

Stimulation
Tibialis nerve

Upper extremity

Lower extremity

Motor evoked potentials (MEPs)

Somatosensory evoked potentials have an excellent ability to assess the dorsal column and lateral sensory tract function. However, significant motor deficits have been seen in patients undergoing spinal surgery despite normal SSEPs.[6,7] First introduced by Levy and York in 1983,[8] motor evoked potentials were developed to assess the function of the anterior spinal columns and motor pathways.

MEP monitoring is based on transcranial stimulation (electrical) through scalp needles. The stimulus over the skull elicits a response from the underlying motor cortex at the lowest threshold. The initial voltage used is typically close to 100 V, and a train of stimuli are used to record motor evoked response from the muscles contralateral to the stimulated side. Figure 8.5 shows normal responses of different muscle groups. If no response is seen, the voltage may be increased by 50 V until MEP responses are seen.

MEP responses can be interpreted with different methods. The all-or-nothing criterion is based on complete loss of signal compared with the baseline response.[9] The amplitude criterion compares baseline responses in terms of amplitude changes.[10] The threshold criterion analyzes changes in voltage requirements compared with baseline responses.[11] Changes in waveform morphology can also be analyzed by tracking changes in the pattern and duration of MEPs.[12]

The development of multipulse stimulation has allowed monitoring with less rigorous anesthetic parameters. Total intravenous anesthesia is used for optimal acquisition of signals. Compounds such as nitrous oxide, volatile agents, and muscle relaxants are excluded, and short-acting agents such as fentanyl and propofol are relied upon to achieve anesthetic control. Although this may pose more of a challenge to the anesthesia team and possibly the surgeon, total IV anesthesia offers clear benefits in obtaining MEPs over inhaled anesthetics.[13]

Anterior spinal surgery, which often involves manipulation of structures that may be putting pressure on the spinal cord to start with, and which also may involve interruption of small blood vessels which supply the spinal cord, is often supported with MEP monitoring to determine the earliest event in which increased blood pressure support or steroids may be necessary. The MEP feedback may also alert the surgeon to the need for further decompression, or a change in the position of a graft or implant.

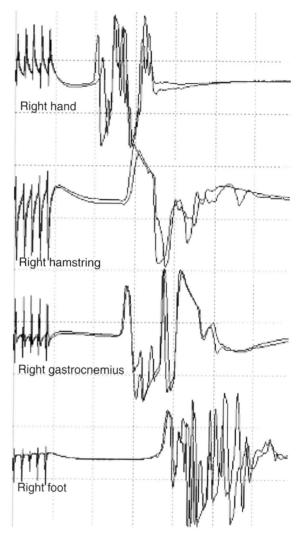

Right hand

Right hamstring

Right gastrocnemius

Right foot

Figure 8.5 Motor evoked potential – normal signal recording.

Electromyography (EMG)

Electromyography (EMG) is the recording of electrical muscle activity. In 1948, Du Bois-Reymond demonstrated the first nerve action potentials and muscle electrical activity. Changes in EMG recordings are indirect indicators of function of the innervating nerve. Intraoperative use is helpful in localization and assurance of peripheral nerve integrity and function.

Multiple EMG needles are placed into muscles of interest. Practically any muscle can be monitored, including face, tongue, and sphincter musculature. EMG is recorded continually with a low-noise amplifier. Recordings are shown on a monitor and also sent to a speaker to provide auditory feedback. Changes in electrical activity can be seen and heard. During spine surgery, EMG can be used with two techniques. The first technique captures "spontaneous EMG activity." Spontaneous muscle activity is monitored with recording electrodes placed in the muscles of interest and based on the structures at risk. Even though no stimulation is performed, surgical manipulation such as stretching, pulling, or nerve compression produces neurotonic discharges resulting in activity in the corresponding innervated muscle or muscle group. At this point the surgeon is notified in order to reassess his or her technique so as to avoid neural injury. The second technique is called "triggered EMG." This technique has been used in segmental instrumentation procedures requiring pedicle screws for fixation. The main goal is to reduce the risk of breaching walls of the vertebral pedicle in order to avoid the neural structures. Typically, a monopolar electrode is used to stimulate the top of the pedicle screw at increasing current intensities. Needle electrodes in the appropriate muscle groups will measure the muscle action potential during the stimulation. A pedicle breach would significantly reduce the stimulation threshold. A threshold response between 10 and 20 mA gives a reasonable probability that no breach of the medial wall has occurred, thresholds >15 mA indicate a 98% likelihood of accurate screw positioning on postoperative CT scan.[14] Figure 8.6 shows triggered EMG.

Sometimes, the electrodes will pick up interference from various sources that may be mistaken for spiking or training EMG activity. Potential sources of artifact responses picked up in the EMG window are cautery devices, electrocardiography leads, and high-speed drills.[3,15]

Multimodality intraoperative monitoring (MIOM)

Multimodality intraoperative monitoring (MIOM), combines SSEPs, MEPs, and EMG according to the structures at risk in surgery, taking advantage of the individual strength of each modality for accurate monitoring

Kelleher et al.,[16] after reviewing a prospective analysis of 1055 patients, showed a very low evidence supporting unimodal SSEPs or MEPs as a valid diagnostic test for measuring intraoperative neurologic injury. On the other hand, there was strong evidence suggesting that multimodality of neuromonitoring is sensitive and specific for detecting intraoperative neurologic injury during spine surgery.[3,17]

Even though there is no Class I evidence in the literature supporting the use of monitoring in spine surgery,[18] it is recommended that the use of MIOM be considered in complex spine surgery where the spinal cord or nerve roots are at risk of injury.[3,17,19]

Effects of anesthesia on recording of electrical impulses

Intraoperative neurophysiologic monitoring places certain demands on anesthesia. The main concern is to tailor the anesthetic agents in order to help maximize signal acquisition during the surgical procedure.

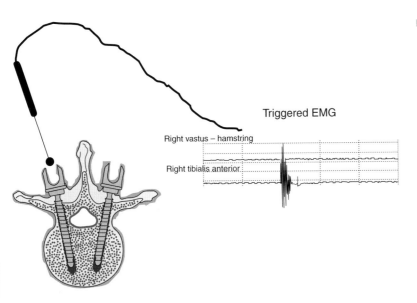

Figure 8.6 Triggered EMG.

Triggered EMG

Right vastus – hamstring

Right tibialis anterior

There are many factors that may affect evoked potential signal recording. Any physical parameter or drug that affects the axonal conduction may change the evoked potential waveform. In general, long neural tracts with more synapses are more susceptible to anesthesia. MEPs are usually more sensitive to interference by anesthesia than SSEPs. Evoked potential signals are more difficult to obtain from lower than upper extremities.[15] When the anesthetic conditions are optimized for MEPs, they are usually also acceptable for SSEPs. Another important factor is the neurologic condition of the patient. When a preexisting neurologic deficit is present, signals are more difficult to obtain.[17]

General anesthesia should be optimized to obtain useful monitoring potentials that can help guide the surgical progress. In general, most anesthetic agents depress the amplitudes and increase the latency of evoked potentials. Etomidate and ketamine are the exception to the rule, since they enhance SSEP and MEP amplitude. Either way, etomidate is limited due to the association with adrenocortical suppression.[18]

Neuromuscular blockade has a negative impact on the ability of monitoring to attain acceptable recordings.[20,21] Neuromuscular blocking agents such as succinylcholine or nondepolarizing agents such as rocuronium may be used in order to facilitate endotracheal intubation only.[20]

All halogenated inhalational agents produce a dose-related increase in latency and reduction in the amplitude of cortically recorded SSEPs.[15,19] Concentrations of 0.5 MAC of volatile anesthetics should allow acceptable acquisition of MEPs.[22] Some recommend to avoid volatile anesthetic agents and instead rely on propofol-based anesthesia.[20]

Nitrous oxide reduces SSEP cortical amplitude and increases latency when used alone or when combined with halogenated inhalational agents, opioids, or propofol.[23]

Total intravenous anesthesia (TIVA) gives the optimal conditions for intraoperative neurophysiologic monitoring.[20] Recommendations for this anesthetic approach use propofol, a synthetic narcotic such as sufentanil, an infusion of the local aesthetic lidocaine, and frequently the NMDA receptor antagonist ketamine. Propofol is used for induction and for maintenance of general anesthesia (75–150 μg/kg/min). Propofol does not affect latency but produces a dose-dependent reduction in the amplitude of MEPs.[24] Opioids have a limited impact on MEPs but there are reports suggesting a suppressive effect of alfentanil, fentanyl, remifentanil, and sufentanil.[20,25,26] Sufentanil or remifentanil are typically delivered as continuous infusion, with a loading dose of 0.5–1 μg/kg followed by an infusion of 0.2–0.5 μg/kg/h.[20] Lidocaine depresses the amplitude and prolongs the latency of SSEPs; nevertheless, the waveforms are preserved and interpretable when used as part of narcotic-based anesthesia.[27] Lidocaine infusion is used with a loading dose of 1.5 mg/kg (induction) and followed by lidocaine infusion at a rate of 40 μg/kg/h. The maximum recommended dose is 4 mg/min.[20,27]

Ketamine has the benefit of enhancing signals acquired from evoked potentials. This can be achieved with clinically relevant doses.[28] Ketamine can be used with a loading dose of 0.5–1.0 mg/kg as part of the induction, followed by an infusion of 0.3 mg/kg/h. It is administered throughout the surgical procedure and is usually terminated at least 30 minutes prior to the end of the surgery. Ketamine can be coadministered with the lidocaine infusion. The standard concentration of lidocaine is an 8% solution in dextrose-based crystalloid. Ketamine (250 mg) is added to a 250 ml IV bag of lidocaine. When the infusion pump is set for a lidocaine dose of 40 μg/kg/min, the resultant ketamine dose that will be administered is 0.3 mg/kg/h.[2]

Changes in temperature may alter intraoperative signal recording. Hypothermia increases the latency and decreases conduction velocities. Hyperthermia reduces the latency and increases the conduction velocity.[20] Hypoxemia can cause evoked potential deterioration before other clinical parameters have changed. SSEP response changes with hematocrit are consistent with this optimum range. A decrease in amplitude has been noted with mild anemia, followed by an increase in latency at hematocrits of 10–15%; further latency changes and amplitude reductions were observed at hematocrits less than 10%. These changes are partially restored by an increase in the hematocrit.[29]

An alarming change in SSEP or EMG responses can be seen when blood flow is reduced to one of the extremities. This can be expected when a tourniquet is used over the lower extremity, as in the case of harvest of a fibular graft. It may also be seen commonly during anterior approach surgery for disc replacement or interbody fusion of the lumbar spine, when pressure is placed on either the aorta or the common iliac vessels. Responses should return to normal quickly after the pressure is relieved, and after the tourniquet is removed. If this does not happen, an alarm should be sounded. This may be the first sign of a vascular thrombosis or plaque embolism that can compromise or result in loss of the lower extremity.

Table 8.1 Summary of different neuromonitoring modalities commonly used in spine surgery

	SSEPs	MEPs	EMG
Monitor	Dorsal column medial and lemniscus pathway	Function of the motor pathway. Anterolateral column	Peripheral nerve integrity and function
Abnormal recording	Decrease in amplitude (>50%) and or decrease in latency (>10%)	Complete loss of signal Changes in wave amplitude, form, threshold to stimuli response	Manipulation of peripheral nerve produces neurotonic discharges
Sensitivity/ specificity	92%/98.9%	100%/96%	46–100%/23–100%

Since it was demonstrated that temporary occlusion of segmental vessels in the thoracic spine could be reflected in SSEP changes in many patients, surgeons are more cautious about ligation of blood vessels in the thoracic region. Thoracic spine surgeons are much more likely to spare segmental vessels during anterior approaches these days, but may occasionally place a temporary clamp on a large segmental artery to determine whether vascular changes are reflected in SSEP or MEP monitoring.

Impact on surgical outcomes

Because intraoperative spinal cord injury is an uncommon event, and difficult to attribute to any single cause, very large numbers of patients are required to show significant impact of any intervention. Because of this there are few Level I data available to conclusively support the use of intraoperative monitoring in spinal surgery. Nonetheless, the devastating impact of spinal cord injury on functional outcome and survival drives surgeons to seek any opportunity to reduce risk.

Subtle changes in SSEP averaging, or in MEP signaling, can guide the surgeon to alter the surgical approach, and can alert the anesthesiologist to change the anesthetic environment. Particularly in scoliosis and deformity surgery, where the neural elements are manipulated but not seen, electrophysiologic monitoring can alert the surgical team to make changes to save the neural elements from serious irreparable injury.

If changes are seen, the surgeon can make an immediate reassessment of the implants placed and the decompression performed, and look for any evidence of pressure caused by surgical instruments, pledgets, or bone or tissue fragments. The anesthetist will immediately reassess blood pressure, raising it to an optimal level, and assess the body temperature and oxygenation. If inhaled anesthetics are being used, they should be discontinued and IV barbiturates and opioids used instead. The surgical team may choose to release the instrumentation and ease off correction, and may select specific implants to remove to see whether the changes

can be reversed. If a bone graft or cages have been placed near the spinal cord these should be removed and repositioned to ensure that there is no subtle pressure on the neural elements.

If no evident cause for the changes can be identified, a Stagnara wake-up test may be considered to verify the electrophysiologic observation. In the presence of a documented deficit, the patient will be given steroids, the implants will be locked in place without excessive correction, and the wound will be closed carefully over a drain. The patient will be transferred to an intensive care and environment where oxygenation and blood pressure can be maintained at an optimal level. Serial neurologic examinations can be carried out, and reimaging of the spine performed to identify any reversible lesion.

Summary

Surgeons will request electrophysiologic monitoring based on their anticipated needs during surgery. Combined multimodality monitoring using SSEP, MEP, and EMG (Table 8.1) modalities tends to overcome the shortcomings of each individual modality and provide the most comprehensive and sensitive test during surgery. As modalities become more reliable, surgeons will regularly depend on electrophysiologic monitoring when the spinal cord is under pressure or at risk.

References

1. Dawson GD. Cerebral responses to nerve stimulation in man. *Br Med Bull* 1950; **6**(4): 326–9.

2. Nash CL Jr, Lorig RA, Schatzinger LA, Brown RH. Spinal cord monitoring during operative treatment of the spine. *Clin Orthop Relat Res* 1977; 1977; **126**: 100–5.

3. Gonzalez A, Jeyanandarajan D, Hansen C, Zada G, Hsieh PC. Intraoperative neurophysiological monitoring during spine surgery: a review. *Neurosurg Focus* 2009; **27**(4): E6.

4. Aglio LS, Romero R, Desai S, Ramirez M, Gonzalez AA, Gugino LD. The use of transcranial magnetic stimulation

for monitoring descending spinal cord motor function. *Clin Electroencephalogr* 2002; **33**(1): 30–41.

5. Nuwer MR, Dawson EG, Carlson LG, Kanim LE, Sherman JE. Somatosensory evoked potential spinal cord monitoring reduces neurologic deficits after scoliosis surgery: results of a large multicenter survey. *Electroencephalogr Clin Neurophysiol* 1995; **96**: 6–11.

6. Hilibrand AS, Schwartz DM, Sethuraman V, Vaccaro AR, Albert TJ. Comparison of transcranial electric motor and Somatosensory evoked potential monitoring during cervical spine surgery. *J Bone Joint Surg Am* 2004; **86-A**: 1248–53.

7. Hsu B, Cree AK, Lagopoulos J, Cummine JL. Transcranial motor-evoked potentials combined with response recording through compound muscle action potential as the sole modality of spinal cord monitoring in spinal deformity surgery. *Spine* 2008; **33**: 1100–6.

8. Levy WJ Jr., York DH. Evoked potentials from the motor tracts in humans. *Neurosurgery* 1983; **12**: 422.

9. Kothbauer KF, Deletis V, Epstein FJ. Motor-evoked potential monitoring for intramedullary spinal cord tumor surgery: correlation of clinical and neurophysiological data in a series of 100 consecutive procedures. *Neurosurg Focus* 1998; **4**(5): e1.

10. Calancie B, Molano MR. Alarm criteria for motor-evoked potentials: what's wrong with the "presence-or-absence" approach? *Spine* 2008; **33**: 406–14.

11. Langeloo DD, Lelivelt A, Louis Journee H, Slappendel R, de Kleuver M. Transcranial electrical motor-evoked potential monitoring during surgery for spinal deformity: a study of 145 patients. *Spine* 2003; **28**: 1043–50.

12. Quinones-Hinojosa A, Lyon R, Zada G, *et al*. Changes in transcranial motor evoked potentials during intramedullary spinal cord tumor resection correlate with postoperative motor function. *Neurosurgery* 2005; **56**: 982–93.

13. Pechstein U, Nadstawek J, Zentner J, Schramm J. Isoflurane plus nitrous oxide versus propofol for recording of motor evoked potentials after high frequency repetitive electrical stimulation. *Electroencephalogr Clin Neurophysiol* 1998; **108**: 175–81.

14. Shi YB, Binette M, Martin WH, Pearson JM, Hart RA. Electrical stimulation for intraoperative evaluation of thoracic pedicle screw placement. *Spine* 2003; **28**: 595–601.

15. Deiner S. Highlights of anesthetic considerations for intraoperative neuromonitoring. *Semin Cardiothorac Vasc Anesth* 2010; **14**(1): 51–3.

16. Kelleher MO, Tan G, Sarjeant R, Fehlings M. Predictive value of intraoperative neurophysiological monitoring during cervical spine surgery a prospective analysis of 1055 consecutive patients. *J Neurosurg Spine* 2008; **8**: 215-221.

17. Wilson-Holden TJ, Padberg AM, *et al*. Efficacy of intraoperative monitoring for pediatric patients with spinal cord pathology undergoing spinal deformity surgery. *Spine* 1999; **24**(16): 1685–92.

18. Wagner RL, White PF, *et al*. Inhibition of adrenal steroidogenesis by the anesthetic etomidate. *N Engl J Med* 1984; **310**(22): 1415–21.

19. Zentner J, Albrecht T, *et al*. Influence of halothane, enflurane, and isoflurane on motor evoked potentials. *Neurosurgery* 1992; **31**(2): 298–305.

20. Pajewski TN, Arlet V, Phillips LH. Current approach on spinal cord monitoring: the point of view of the neurologist, the anesthesiologist and the spine surgeon. *Eur Spine J* 2007; **16** (Suppl 2): S115–29.

21. Van Dongen EP, ter Beek HT, *et al*. Within-patient variability of myogenic motor-evoked potentials to multipulse transcranial electrical stimulation during two levels of partial neuromuscular blockade in aortic surgery. *Anesth Analg* 1999; **88**(1): 22–7.

22. Sekimoto K, Nishikawa K, *et al*. The effects of volatile anesthetics on intraoperative monitoring of myogenic motor evoked potentials to transcranial electrical stimulation and on partial neuromuscular blockade during propofol/fentanyl/nitrous oxide anesthesia in humans. *J Neurosurg Anesthesiol* 2006; **18**(2): 106–11.

23. Van Dongen EP, ter Beek HT, Schepens MA, *et al*.. Effect of nitrous oxide on myogenic motor potentials evoked by a six pulse train of transcranial electrical stimuli: a possible monitor for aortic surgery. *Br J Anaesth* 1999; **82**(3): 323–8.

24. Nathan N, Tabaraud F, *et al*. Influence of propofol concentrations on multipulse transcranial motor evoked potentials. *Br J Anaesth* 2003; **91**(4): 493–7.

25. Kalkman CJ, Drummond JC, *et al*. Effects of propofol, etomidate, midazolam, and fentanyl on motor evoked responses to transcranial electrical or magnetic stimulation in humans. *Anesthesiology* 1992; **76**(4): 502–9.

26. Scheufler KM, Zentner J. Total intravenous anesthesia for intraoperative monitoring of the motor pathways: an integral view combining clinical and experimental data. *J Neurosurg* 2002; **96**(3): 571–9.

27. Schubert A, Licina MG, *et al*. Systemic lidocaine and human somatosensory-evoked potentials during sufentanil-isoflurane anaesthesia. *Can J Anaesth* 1992; **39**(6): 569–75.

28. Erb TO, Ryhult SE, *et al*. Improvement of motor-evoked potentials by ketamine and spatial facilitation during spinal surgery in a young child. *Anesth Analg* 2005; **100**(6): 1634–6.

29. Nagao S, Roccaforte P, *et al*. The effects of isovolemic hemodilution and reinfusion of packed erythrocytes on somatosensory and visual evoked potentials. *J Surg Res* 1978; **25**(6): 530–7.

8.4 An overview of minimally invasive spine surgery

R. Douglas Orr

Key points

- The minimally invasive approach allows the surgeon to perform the same operation with less collateral damage.
- Less invasive does not mean less risk.
- Initially on adoption of these techniques OR times will be longer but they should eventually become the same.
- There should be less blood loss and less postoperative pain than in open techniques.
- Each approach has subtle differences and intraoperative requirements and it is important to discuss these in advance with the surgeon.

Minimally invasive spinal surgery is a catch-all term that has been applied to a number of techniques used to treat spinal pathology. Techniques have been developed to allow decompression of the nerves and spinal cord, resection of intradural and extradural spinal tumors, correction of deformity, and stabilization of instability. The overwhelming philosophy of minimally invasive spinal surgery is to minimize the collateral damage that occurs in accessing spinal pathology through traditional open approaches. It is felt that by doing so better outcomes can be achieved. Many techniques are involved, each with their own indications, complications, and outcomes. This chapter will review many of these techniques and the rationale for their use. It will also include anesthetic considerations during these surgeries.

Traditional open approaches to the spine have been shown to cause significant muscle damage. Radiographic, histochemical, and clinical studies have shown this.[1-8] Minimally invasive approaches have been developed to lessen this injury. In general they use smaller incisions, respecting anatomic planes and separating or dilating muscles rather than cutting or detaching them. It is felt that by doing so recovery will be quicker and outcomes will be better.[9,10]

One of the earliest minimally invasive techniques was used predominantly for diagnosis, and this is epiduroscopy.[11] In this procedure a small fiberoptic endoscope is introduced into the epidural space and also potentially into the thecal sac to allow visualization of pathology. Since its development it has also been used to treat pathologies. It has been used to break down adhesions, potentially resect discs, and decompress spinal stenosis. This procedure is generally done under local anesthetic and the portal used is only a few millimeters wide. The scope is inserted through the sacral hiatus. It is advanced into the lumbar spine under radiographic guidance. Once there it can either through direct mechanical pressure or the use of lasers break down adhesions or resect compressive tissue, and corticosteroids can be directly deposited into the epidural space.[12-16] It can also be performed through an interlaminar approach.[17] There is very little blood loss and is generally done as an outpatient procedure. It has relatively limited uses and is not widely performed.

Kambin described an extraforaminal approach to the lumbar disc as a way of dealing with symptomatic lumbar disc herniations. Initially he described a two-portal technique with an arthroscope inserted from one side and a working channel to allow introduction of instruments inserted into the disc space from the opposite side.[18] This technique was later evolved through the development of working channel spinal endoscopes.[19] The scopes range in size from 5 to 8 mm in diameter. They are usually inserted under local anesthetic after tissue dilation. Through the working channel one can use a variety of graspers, drills, and lasers to remove pathology. This can be used to decompress foraminal stenosis or to resect herniated discs, and has been described for the treatment of central stenosis. This technology has been used in the cervical, lumbar, and thoracic spine.[20-26] Recent comparative studies have looked at percutaneous discectomy and compared it with open microdiscectomy in the lumbar spine. In general these studies show that patients have a shorter hospital stay and less immediate postoperative pain but equivalent long-term results.[27-31] There are no comparative studies of thoracic or cervical uses of this technique. The endoscopic transforaminal technique has not become widely accepted in North America and is done mostly in specialized outpatient centers.

The next minimally invasive technique to be developed and achieve a degree of widespread acceptance was endoscopic anterior lumbar interbody fusion.[32] This is performed through a transperitoneal approach with laparoscopic visualization. Numerous studies were published with initially good results.[33–39] As time went on further studies questioned the safety and efficacy of the technique.[40–44] It has largely been abandoned.

The modern era of more widely accepted minimally invasive spine surgery techniques began with the development of the tubular retractor by Foley. This technique was originally developed to treat far lateral and central lumbar disc herniations.[45,46] In this technique under radiographic guidance a series of dilators are used to split the muscles to allow placement of the tubular retractor. Initially the procedure used a small endoscope but now most surgeons use a microscope. Further development of the use of tubular retractors has allowed them to be used to decompress the spine for lumbar stenosis[47] and for fusion.[48]

Figure 8.7A shows the placement of the tubular retractor over a series of dilators. Figure 8.7B shows a 16 mm diameter tubular retractor being used for a microdiscectomy.

Numerous studies have looked at the use of tubular retractors for discectomies and decompressions. In general they show that in the short term patients have a faster recovery with less postoperative pain, less blood loss, and less use of narcotics.[49,50] In the longer term it does not appear as though results are any different from open techniques. These procedures do show a significant learning curve and initially operative times are longer than for the equivalent open procedure, but with experience they seem to take equivalent or less time than the open procedure.[50–52]

In order to progress from decompressive procedures to fusions it was necessary to develop the ability to place pedicle screw instrumentation through small incisions. This led to the development of a number of techniques for percutaneous pedicle screws. These screws are typically used in conjunction with some form of fusion, either an anterior lumbar interbody fusion (ALIF), a minimal access lateral fusion (LLIF), or a minimal access transforaminal lumbar interbody fusion (TLIF). The first description of this used a suprafascial implant and was not really practical.[53] The first clinical use of current types of implants was reported by Foley.[54] These screws are inserted with either fluoroscopy or image guidance. The procedure

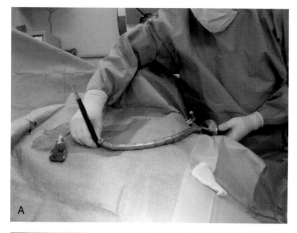

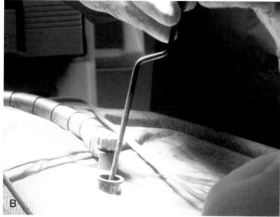

Figure 8.7 (A) Intraoperative photograph showing placement of a 16 mm tubular retractor over a series of dilators. (B) Intraoperative photograph with a Penfield probe in the 16 mm retractor during a microdiscectomy.

began by inserting a Jamshidi needle into the pedicle and then placing a guide wire over which the pedicle is prepared and the screw inserted. Figure 8.8 shows intraoperative photographs of percutaneous screw and rod placement. Technologies have been developed to allow placement of screws over multiple levels.

Percutaneous screws can be used as temporary fixation in trauma patients[55] and have occasionally been used to stabilize tumor patients in the absence of fusion. Otherwise all percutaneous instrumentation systems need to be combined with some sort of fusion. In most cases these involve placement of implants and bone graft or bone graft substitute into the intervertebral disc space. All of the current minimally invasive interbody fusion techniques developed from more standard open techniques and through the use of specialized retractors have evolved into minimally

131

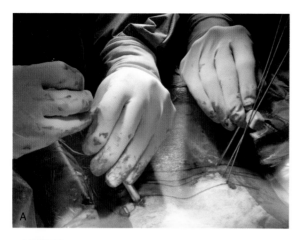

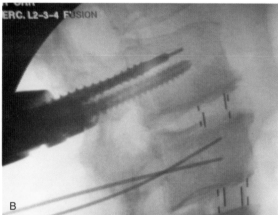

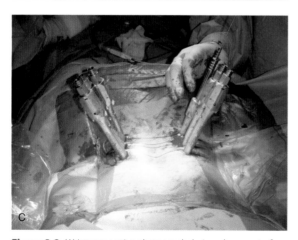

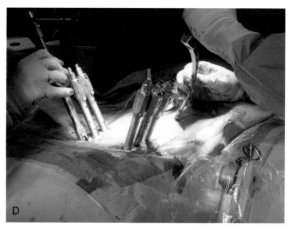

Figure 8.8 (cont.)

invasive approaches. Anterior interbody fusion (ALIF) is performed through an anterior retroperitoneal mini open approach. Typically this is done through a transverse incision overlying the rectus muscle. After the rectus sheath is divided, the remainder of the approach is done with blunt dissection and as a result is relatively atraumatic. This approach has significant intraoperative risks, particularly at the L4–5 level due to the need to mobilize the common iliac vein in order to access the disc space. Vascular injuries are uncommon but can be a significant problem.[56,57]

Posterior lumbar interbody fusion (PLIF) was initially described by Cloward[58] as an open technique. It has been adapted for use with tubular retractors.[59] In this procedure the disc is removed from a posterior approach working in the spinal canal. After removing the disc a bone graft or implant is placed. This procedure carries a risk of intraoperative nerve injury due to the necessity of retracting the thecal sac to access the disc. As a result it is often performed with intraoperative neurologic monitoring.

The transforaminal lumbar interbody fusion (TLIF) was initially described as an open technique[60] and was also converted to a minimally invasive approach.[61] The entry to the disc space is more lateral through the region of the foramen and as a result has a lower risk of neurologic injury. This is the fusion procedure that has been most widely adopted as a minimally invasive approach. Figure 8.9 shows intraoperative photographs of a TLIF being performed through a 22 mm tubular retractor.

Comparative studies looking at open versus minimally invasive TLIF fusions show that TLIF patients have a shorter postoperative stay, less blood loss, less

Figure 8.8 (A) Intraoperative photograph during placement of a percutaneous screw. On the upper right is a guide wire being placed through a Jamshidi needle. On the lower left are the dilators being placed over the wire. (B) Lateral Fluoro image showing previously placed interbody cages. A tap is being advanced over the uppermost wire and one screw has been placed. (C) After placement of 5 of 6 screws, showing the extension towers used to guide the rod into the screw heads. (D) Advancing of the rod from superior though the extension towers.

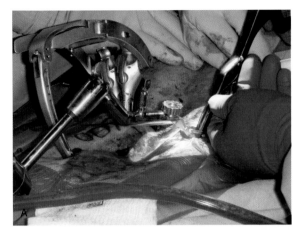

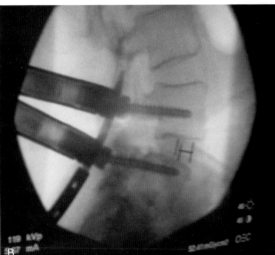

Figure 8.9 (A) Intraoperative photograph showing a Kerrison punch in a 22 mm tubular retractor during an MIS TLIF. On the left are the extension towers and rod-passing tools of a percutaneous instrumentation system. (B) Lateral Fluoro image showing interbody cage in the disc space and rod passage during MIS TLIF.

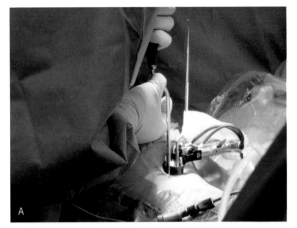

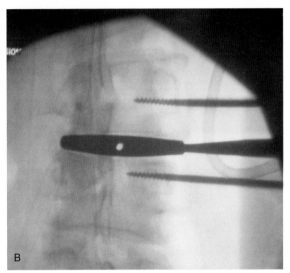

Figure 8.10 (A) Intraoperative photograph showing MIS LLIF retractor. Cables protruding from the retractor are fiberoptic light cords to assist visualization. Unlike the tubes in the previous figures the retractor is expandable. (B) AP Fluoro image showing placement of an implant trial in the disc space. Screws are temporary retaining pins to hold the retractor in position.

postoperative narcotic use, and a faster recovery. At 1 year and 2 years there is no difference in outcome compared with open procedures.[62–66] Early in the learning experience operative times tend to be longer than seen in open techniques, but with experience the operation can be done in equal or shorter time.[65,67,68]

Minimally invasive lateral fusion (LLIF) is done through a retroperitoneal and trans-psoas approach. In this procedure the patient is placed in a lateral position. Under a combination of direct palpation and radiographic guidance a probe is placed down onto the spine through the psoas muscle. Because of the presence of the lumbar nervous plexus this approach is done with stimulated EMG monitoring to lessen the risk of

nerve injury. After placement of a probe into the disc space, serial dilators are used to enlarge the approach until a retractor can be placed.[69] Figure 8.10 shows the retractor in place and a trial implant in position. This technique can be used over multiple levels and has now been used in the minimally invasive treatment of scoliosis.[70] This procedure does not require mobilization of the great vessels and so has a low risk of vascular complication.[71] There is a relatively high risk of injury to the lumbosacral plexus and this necessitates EMG monitoring.[72] In general, high fusion rates can be obtained with good clinical success. These procedures are often backed up with posterior instrumentation.[71] They can be done stand-alone and are sometimes augmented with an anterior plate.[73]

The trans-sacral lumbar interbody fusion is a technique for fusion of L5–S1, and now L4–5 and L5–S1. It utilizes the presacral interval as an approach and is done through a paracoccygeal incision.[74] It has been reported to have good clinical success and low complication rates,[75] though rectal injury has been reported.[76]

Minimally invasive treatment of idiopathic scoliosis and kyphosis

Thoracoscopy has been used extensively for anterior release and instrumentation in idiopathic scoliosis and kyphosis and is used as an alternative to open thoracotomy. It is associated with shorter operative times, faster recovery, and better cosmesis.[77] Thorascopic instrumentation for correction of scoliosis has been done, but many have abandoned it to due to higher complication rates – particularly late hardware failure.[78–81] This can be done with the patient either in the lateral position or as a simultaneous prone procedure accompanied by posterior instrumentation.[82] In either case double-lumen intubation is used and the lung collapses on the upper side. Scoliosis can be treated either from the convexity or the concavity. It is important for the anesthesiologist to be aware of which side the approach will be done from when it comes time to deflate the lung.

Conditions treated with minimally invasive spine surgery

Initial reports of minimally invasive surgery in the spine looked at common degenerative conditions such as herniated disc, lumbar spinal stenosis, degenerative disc disease, and spondylolisthesis. As techniques have evolved many more conditions are able to be treated through minimally invasive techniques. Trauma,[83] deformity,[84–86] and tumors[87–89] have all been reported to have been treated to minimally invasively. As these techniques evolve it is likely that there will be a minimally invasive option for most spinal surgeries.

Anesthetic considerations in minimally invasive spine surgery

In general minimally invasive techniques allow spine surgeons to do the same procedures with less collateral damage. It is important to remember that smaller incision does not mean smaller risk to the patient. As a result it is important to be prepared for the potential

complications of the procedure just as one would for a traditional open operation. In the case of any anterior surgery there is the risk of catastrophic bleeding if the great vessels are injured. This can occur with all of the interbody techniques and, in the case of vascular injury during a posterior interbody technique, may not be readily apparent. In patients with sudden loss of blood pressure this should be considered.

If a surgeon is just beginning to use minimally invasive techniques, operative times will typically be longer than with the equivalent open procedure. With time and experience this should decrease to similar operative times and sometimes even shorter as there is less time needed to open and close the incision. For the anesthesiologist it is important to know where the surgeon is on the learning curve and to plan accordingly. Long procedure duration early in the experience can increase problems with core body temperature and pressure over bony prominences.

In general minimally invasive surgery (MIS) techniques have lower intraoperative blood loss. As a result there should be lower demand for fluids intraoperatively. At the author's institution one of our early MIS patients had a postoperative myocardial infarct attributed to volume overload after receiving a 2 l fluid bolus before a kyphoplasty that had 15 ml blood losses.

Most studies have shown less immediate postoperative pain and lower postoperative narcotic demands. In the author's practice most open spinal fusion patients require PCA IV narcotics for the first 24–48 h where most MIS patients can be managed with PO pain medication.

Depending on the technique used, neuromuscular blockade may be required or contraindicated. In the ALIF approach it is vital to have blockade to allow retraction. Loss of blockade during the procedure can lead to loss of retraction and risk of vessel injury. In contrast, the need for stimulated EMG monitoring during LLIF surgery means that neuromuscular blockade is contraindicated. In some case both procedures are done and as a result blockade is required for part of the procedure and contraindicated later. In these cases short-acting blockade agents must be used. It is important to confirm with the surgeon before the start of the procedure what the requirement for blockade is.

Conclusion

Minimally invasive techniques are rapidly evolving and are changing the way that spine surgery is done. In the future it will be a larger part of most practices. It has been shown to lead to less postoperative pain, lower blood loss, shorter hospital stays, and shorter recovery. In many cases patients are preferentially seeking out minimally invasive options as they perceive these techniques are superior. Long-term studies have yet to show benefits in the long term over traditional open techniques, but if these techniques have equivalent success and equivalent complication rates then the improved short-term outcome would justify the more widespread adoption of these techniques. Those that do not have equivalent outcomes should fall out of favor over time, as has been seen with laparoscopic ALIF and thorascopic instrumentation for scoliosis.

These techniques still carry the same risks as the open procedures and in some cases the smaller incision makes complications harder to deal with. Anesthesiologists must remember this and be prepared for the possibility.

References

1. Gejo R, *et al.* Serial changes in trunk muscle performance after posterior lumbar surgery. *Spine* 1999; **24**(10): 1023–8.

2. Kawaguchi Y, Matsui H, Tsuji H. Changes in serum creatine phosphokinase MM isoenzyme after lumbar spine surgery. *Spine* 1997; **22**(9): 1018–23.

3. Kawaguchi Y, *et al.* Back muscle injury after posterior lumbar spine surgery. Topographic evaluation of intramuscular pressure and blood flow in the porcine back muscle during surgery. *Spine* 1996; **21**(22): 2683–8.

4. Kawaguchi Y, Matsui H, Tsuji H. Back muscle injury after posterior lumbar spine surgery. A histologic and enzymatic analysis. *Spine* 1996; **21**(8): 941–4.

5. Kawaguchi Y, Matsui H, Tsuji H. Back muscle injury after posterior lumbar spine surgery. Part 2: Histologic and histochemical analyses in humans. *Spine* 1994; **19**(22): 2598–602.

6. Styf JR, Willen J. The effects of external compression by three different retractors on pressure in the erector spine muscles during and after posterior lumbar spine surgery in humans. *Spine* 1998; **23**(3): 354–8.

7. Weber BR, *et al.* Posterior surgical approach to the lumbar spine and its effect on the multifidus muscle. *Spine* 1997; **22**(15): 1765–72.

8. Motosuneya T, *et al.* Severe scoliosis associated with Costello syndrome: a case report. *J Orthop Surg* 2006; **14**(3): 346–9.

9. Fessler R, *et al.*, The development of minimally invasive spine surgery. *Neurosurg Clin N Am* 2006; **17**(4): 401–9.

10. German JW, Foley KT. Minimal access surgical techniques in the management of the painful lumbar motion segment. *Spine* 2005; **30**(16 Suppl): S52–9.

11. Blomberg R. A method for epiduroscopy and spinaloscopy. Presentation of preliminary results. *Acta Anaesthesiol Scand* 1985; **29**(1): 113–16.

12. Ruetten S, Meyer O, Godolias G. Endoscopic surgery of the lumbar epidural space (epiduroscopy): results of therapeutic intervention in 93 patients. *Minim Invasive Neurosurg* 2003; **46**(1): 1–4.

13. Kitahata LM. Recent advances in epiduroscopy. *J Anesth* 2002; **16**(3): 222–8.

14. Ruetten S, Meyer O, Godolias G. Application of holmium: YAG laser in epiduroscopy: extended practicabilities in the treatment of chronic back pain syndrome. *J Clin Laser Med Surg* 2002; **20**(4): 203–6.

15. Gillespie G, MacKenzie P. Epiduroscopy – a review. *Scott Med J* 2004; **49**(3): 79–81.

16. Igarashi T, *et al.* Lysis of adhesions and epidural injection of steroid/local anaesthetic during epiduroscopy potentially alleviate low back and leg pain in elderly patients with lumbar spinal stenosis. *Br J Anaesth* 2004; **93**(2): 181–7.

17. Avellanal M, Diaz-Reganon G. Interlaminar approach for epiduroscopy in patients with failed back surgery syndrome. *Br J Anaesth* 2008; **101**(2): 244–9.

18. Kambin P. Diagnostic and therapeutic spinal arthroscopy. *Neurosurg Clin N Am* 1996; **7**(1): 65–76.

19. Kambin P, Savitz MH. Arthroscopic microdiscectomy: an alternative to open disc surgery. *Mt Sinai J Med* 2000; **67**(4): 283–7.

20. Mathews HH. Transforaminal endoscopic microdiscectomy. *Neurosurg Clin N Am* 1996; **7**(1): 59–63.

21. Ditsworth DA. Endoscopic transforaminal lumbar discectomy and reconfiguration: a postero-lateral approach into the spinal canal. *Surg Neurol* 1998; **49**(6): 588–97; discussion 597–8.

22. Jho HD. Endoscopic transpedicular thoracic discectomy. *Neurosurg Focus* 2000; **9**(4): e4.

23. Yeung AT, Yeung CA. Advances in endoscopic disc and spine surgery: foraminal approach. *Surg Technol Int* 2003; **11**: 255–63.

24. Choi G, *et al.* Percutaneous endoscopic interlaminar discectomy for intracanalicular disc herniations at L5-S1 using a rigid working channel endoscope. *Neurosurgery* 2006; **58**(1 Suppl): ONS59–68; discussion ONS59–68.

25. Ruetten S, *et al.* Use of newly developed instruments and endoscopes: full-endoscopic resection of lumbar disc herniations via the interlaminar and lateral transforaminal approach. *J Neurosurg Spine* 2007; **6**(6): 521–30.

26. Nellensteijn J, *et al*. Transforaminal endoscopic surgery for symptomatic lumbar disc herniations: a systematic review of the literature. *Eur Spine J* 2010; **19**(2): 181–204.

27. Peng CW, Yeo W, Tan SB. Percutaneous endoscopic discectomy: clinical results and how it affects the quality of life. *J Spinal Disord Tech* 2010; **23**(6): 425–30.

28. Peng ZW, *et al*. A case-control study comparing percutaneous radiofrequency ablation alone or combined with transcatheter arterial chemoembolization for hepatocellular carcinoma. *Eur J Surg Oncol* 2010; **36**(3): 257–63.

29. Peng CW, YeoW, Tan SB. Percutaneous endoscopic lumbar discectomy: clinical and quality of life outcomes with a minimum 2 year follow-up. *J Orthop Surg Res* 2009; **4**: 20.

30. Lee DY, *et al*. Comparison of percutaneous endoscopic lumbar discectomy and open lumbar microdiscectomy for recurrent disc herniation. *J Korean Neurosurg Soc* 2009; **46**(6): 515–21.

31. Kim MJ, *et al*. Targeted percutaneous transforaminal endoscopic diskectomy in 295 patients: comparison with results of microscopic diskectomy. *Surg Neurol* 2007; **68**(6): 623–31.

32. Zucherman JF, *et al.*, Instrumented laparoscopic spinal fusion. Preliminary results. *Spine* 1995; **20**(18): 2029–34; discussion 2034–5.

33. Olsen D, McCord D, Law M. Laparoscopic discectomy with anterior interbody fusion of L5–S1. *Surg Endosc* 1996; **10**(12): 1158–63.

34. Regan JJ, *et al*. Laparoscopic fusion of the lumbar spine in a multicenter series of the first 34 consecutive patients. *Surg Laparosc Endosc* 1996; **6**(6): 459–68.

35. Zdeblick TA. Laparoscopic spinal fusion. *Orthop Clin North Am* 1998; **29**(4): 635–45.

36. Burkus JK, *et al*. Six-year outcomes of anterior lumbar interbody arthrodesis with use of interbody fusion cages and recombinant human bone morphogenetic protein-2. *J Bone Joint Surg Am* 2009; **91**(5): 1181–9.

37. DeBerard MS, *et al.*, Outcomes of posterolateral versus BAK titanium cage interbody lumbar fusion in injured workers: a retrospective cohort study. *J South Orthop Assoc* 2002; **11**(3): 157–66.

38. Regan JJ, *et al*. Laparoscopic approach to L4-L5 for interbody fusion using BAK cages: experience in the first 58 cases. *Spine* 1999; **24**(20): 2171–4.

39. Kleeman TJ, *et al*. Laparoscopic anterior lumbar interbody fusion at L4-L5: an anatomic evaluation and approach classification. *Spine* 2002; **27**(13): 1390–5.

40. Pellise F, *et al*. Low fusion rate after L5-S1 laparoscopic anterior lumbar interbody fusion using twin stand-alone carbon fiber cages. *Spine* 2002; **27**(15): 1665–9.

41. Zdeblick TA, David SM. A prospective comparison of surgical approach for anterior L4-L5 fusion: laparoscopic versus mini anterior lumbar interbody fusion. *Spine* 2000; **25**(20): 2682–7.

42. Liu JC, *et al*. Is laparoscopic anterior lumbar interbody fusion a useful minimally invasive procedure? *Neurosurgery* 2002; **51**(5 Suppl): S155–8.

43. Kaiser MG, *et al*. Comparison of the mini-open versus laparoscopic approach for anterior lumbar interbody fusion: a retrospective review. *Neurosurgery* 2002; **51**(1): 97–103; discussion 103–5.

44. Button G, *et al*. Three- to six-year follow-up of stand-alone BAK cages implanted by a single surgeon. *Spine J* 2005; **5**(2): 155–60.

45. Perez-Cruet MJ, *et al*. Microendoscopic lumbar discectomy: technical note. *Neurosurgery* 2002; **51**(5 Suppl): S129–36.

46. Foley KT, Smith MM, Rampersaud YR. Microendoscopic approach to far-lateral lumbar disc herniation. *Neurosurg Focus* 1999; **7**(5): e5.

47. Khoo LT, Fessler RG. Microendoscopic decompressive laminotomy for the treatment of lumbar stenosis. *Neurosurgery* 2002; **51**(5 Suppl): S146–54.

48. Foley KT, Holly LT, Schwender JD. Minimally invasive lumbar fusion. *Spine* 2003; **28**(15 Suppl): S26–35.

49. Rahman M, *et al*. Comparison of techniques for decompressive lumbar laminectomy: the minimally invasive versus the "classic" open approach. *Minim Invasive Neurosurg* 2008; **51**(2): 100–5.

50. Yagi M, *et al*. Postoperative outcome after modified unilateral-approach microendoscopic midline decompression for degenerative spinal stenosis. *J Neurosurg Spine* 2009; **10**(4): 293–9.

51. Fourney DR, *et al*. Does minimal access tubular assisted spine surgery increase or decrease complications in spinal decompression or fusion? *Spine* 2010; **35**(9 Suppl): S57–65.

52. Parikh K, *et al*. Operative results and learning curve: microscope-assisted tubular microsurgery for 1- and 2-level discectomies and laminectomies. *Neurosurg Focus* 2008; **25**(2): E14.

53. Lowery GL, Kulkarni SS. Posterior percutaneous spine instrumentation. *Eur Spine J* 2000; **9** (Suppl 1): S126–30.

54. Foley KT, Gupta SK. Percutaneous pedicle screw fixation of the lumbar spine: preliminary clinical results. *J Neurosurg* 2002; **97**(1 Suppl): 7–12.

55. Beringer W, *et al.*, Percutaneous pedicle screw instrumentation for temporary internal bracing of nondisplaced bony Chance fractures. *J Spinal Disord Tech* 2007; **20**(3): 242–7.

56. Brau SA, *et al*. Vascular injury during anterior lumbar surgery. *Spine J* 2004; **4**(4): 409–12.

57. Brau SA. Mini-open approach to the spine for anterior lumbar interbody fusion: description of the procedure, results and complications. *Spine J* 2002; **2**(3): 216–23.

58. Cloward RB. The treatment of ruptured lumbar intervertebral disc by vertebral body fusion. III. Method of use of banked bone. *Ann Surg* 1952; **136**(6): 987–92.

59. Khoo LT, *et al*. Minimally invasive percutaneous posterior lumbar interbody fusion. *Neurosurgery* 2002; **51**(5 Suppl): S166–71.

60. Blume HG. Unilateral posterior lumbar interbody fusion: simplified dowel technique. *Clin Orthop Relat Res* 1985; (193): 75–84.

61. Schwender JD, et al. Minimally invasive transforaminal lumbar interbody fusion (TLIF): technical feasibility and initial results. *J Spinal Disord Tech* 2005; **18** (Suppl): S1–6.

62. Adogwa O, *et al*. Comparative effectiveness of minimally invasive versus open transforaminal lumbar interbody fusion: 2-year assessment of narcotic use, return to work, disability, and quality of life. *J Spinal Disord Tech* 2011 Dec; **24**(8): 479–84.

63. Karikari IO, Isaacs RE. Minimally invasive transforaminal lumbar interbody fusion: a review of techniques and outcomes. *Spine* 2010; **35**(26 Suppl): S294–301.

64. Wang J, *et al*. Minimally invasive or open transforaminal lumbar interbody fusion as revision surgery for patients previously treated by open discectomy and decompression of the lumbar spine. *Eur Spine J* 2011; **20**(4): 632–8.

65. Villavicencio AT, *et al*. Minimally invasive versus open transforaminal lumbar interbody fusion. *Surg Neurol Int* 2010; **1**: 12.

66. Wu RH, Fraser JF, Hartl R. Minimal access versus open transforaminal lumbar interbody fusion: meta-analysis of fusion rates. *Spine* 2010; **35**(26): 2273–81.

67. Wang J, *et al*. Comparison of one-level minimally invasive and open transforaminal lumbar interbody fusion in degenerative and isthmic spondylolisthesis grades 1 and 2. *Eur Spine J* 2010; **19**(10): 1780–4.

68. Peng CW, *et al*. Clinical and radiological outcomes of minimally invasive versus open transforaminal lumbar interbody fusion. *Spine* 2009; **34**(13): 1385–9.

69. Ozgur BM, *et al*. Extreme Lateral Interbody Fusion (XLIF): a novel surgical technique for anterior lumbar interbody fusion. *Spine J* 2006; **6**(4): 435–43.

70. Anand N, *et al*. Minimally invasive multilevel percutaneous correction and fusion for adult lumbar degenerative scoliosis: a technique and feasibility study. *J Spinal Disord Tech* 2008; **21**(7): 459–67.

71. Rodgers WB, Gerber EJ, Patterson J. Intraoperative and early postoperative complications in extreme lateral interbody fusion: an analysis of 600 cases. *Spine* 2011; **36**(1): 26–32.

72. Tohmeh AG, Rodgers WB, Peterson MD. Dynamically evoked, discrete-threshold electromyography in the extreme lateral interbody fusion approach. *J Neurosurg Spine*, 2011; **14**(1): 31–7.

73. Sharma AK, *et al*. Lateral lumbar interbody fusion: clinical and radiographic outcomes at 1 year: a preliminary report. *J Spinal Disord Tech* 2011 Jun; **24**(4): 242–50.

74. Marotta N, *et al*. A novel minimally invasive presacral approach and instrumentation technique for anterior L5-S1 intervertebral discectomy and fusion: technical description and case presentations. *Neurosurg Focus* 2006; **20**(1): E9.

75. Patil SS, *et al*. Clinical and radiological outcomes of axial lumbar interbody fusion. *Orthopedics* 2010; **33**(12): 883.

76. Botolin S, *et al*. High rectal injury during trans-1 axial lumbar interbody fusion L5-S1 fixation: a case report. *Spine* 2010; **35**(4): E144–8.

77. Newton PO, *et al*. Anterior release and fusion in pediatric spinal deformity. A comparison of early outcome and cost of thoracoscopic and open thoracotomy approaches. *Spine* 1997; **22**(12): 1398–406.

78. Wong HK, *et al*. Results of thoracoscopic instrumented fusion versus conventional posterior instrumented fusion in adolescent idiopathic scoliosis undergoing selective thoracic fusion. *Spine* 2004; **29**(18): 2031–8; discussion 2039.

79. Newton PO, *et al*. Thoracoscopic multilevel anterior instrumented fusion in a goat model. *Spine* 2003; **28**(14): 1614–19; discussion 1620.

80. Kim DH, Jaikumar S, Kam AC. Minimally invasive spine instrumentation. *Neurosurgery* 2002; **51**(5 Suppl): S15–25.

81. Newton PO, *et al*. Surgical treatment of main thoracic scoliosis with thoracoscopic anterior instrumentation. Surgical technique. *J Bone Joint Surg Am* 2009; **91** (2 Suppl): 233–48.

82. Lieberman IH, *et al*. Prone position endoscopic transthoracic release with simultaneous posterior instrumentation for spinal deformity: a description of the technique. *Spine* 2000; **25**(17): 2251–7.

83. Rampersaud YR, Annand N. Dekutoski MB. Use of minimally invasive surgical techniques in the management of thoracolumbar trauma: current concepts. *Spine* 2006; **31**(11 Suppl): S96–102; discussion S104.

84. Wang MY, Mummaneni PV. Minimally invasive surgery for thoracolumbar spinal deformity: initial clinical experience with clinical and radiographic outcomes. *Neurosurg Focus* 2010; **28**(3): E9.

85. Dakwar E, *et al*. Early outcomes and safety of the minimally invasive, lateral retroperitoneal transpsoas approach for adult degenerative scoliosis. *Neurosurg Focus* 2010; **28**(3): E8.

137

86. Anand N, *et al*. Mid-term to long-term clinical and functional outcomes of minimally invasive correction and fusion for adults with scoliosis. *Neurosurg Focus* 2010; **28**(3): E6.

87. Haji FA, *et al*. Minimally invasive approach for the resection of spinal neoplasm. *Spine* 2011; **36**(15): E1018–26.

88. Mannion RJ, *et al*. Safety and efficacy of intradural extramedullary spinal tumor removal using a minimally invasive approach. *Neurosurgery* 2011; **68**(1 Suppl Operative): 208–16; discussion 216.

89. Uribe JS, *et al*., Minimally invasive surgery treatment for thoracic spine tumor removal: a mini-open, lateral approach. *Spine* 2010; **35**(26 Suppl): S347–54.

8.5   Posterior lumbar interbody fusion

Virgilio Matheus and William Bingaman

Key points

This chapter will:
- Review the indications for performing a posterior lumbar interbody fusion.
- Explain the critical portions of the surgical procedure from an anesthesia point of view.
- Discuss possible complications related to the procedure.
- Review some critical steps the anesthesiologist can follow to minimize complications
- Summarize the postprocedural care.

Introduction

Posterior lumbar interbody fusion (PLIF) is a surgical intervention to restore and stabilize the sagittal alignment of the spine and distract the neuroforaminal space. Cloward first introduced it in 1945 with the intention to treat disc herniations.[1] The operation is performed via a posterior approach with wide laminectomy, which allows excellent neural decompression and access to the anterior vertebral column (disc space) for distraction and stabilization.

Indications

Lumbar spondylolisthesis is the condition most commonly treated by lumbar fusion (Fig. 8.11). Spondylolisthesis results most commonly from degenerative disease but also may occur due to trauma, infection, or iatrogenic causes following lumbar decompression surgery. The pathophysiology of lumbar spondylolisthesis involves anterior translation of the spine at the involved level due to instability in the supporting spinal structures including the disc and facet joints. This leads to mechanical back pain and eventually radicular lower

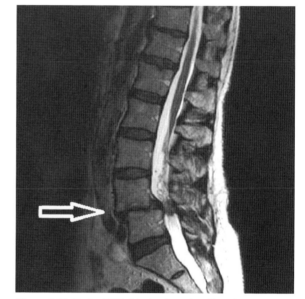

Figure 8.11 Sagittal MRI of the lumbar spine. Note the anterior displacement of L4 on L5 (arrow) representing a grade II spondylolisthesis.

extremity pain as the nerve root exiting at the involved level becomes chronically compressed. Other less common indications for PLIF include recurrent lumbar disc herniation, chronic medically intractable degenerative disc disease, and pseudoarthrosis after attempted lumbar posterolateral transverse process fusions (Table 8.2). Relative contraindications include previous interbody fusion attempts, upper level spinal pathology (places the spinal cord at risk from retraction), and multiple levels of spinal instability where PLIF may lead to excessive blood loss. General contraindications to any lumbar fusion procedure include advanced osteoporosis and significant preexisting medical conditions that place the patient at risk.

Table 8.2 Common indications for PLIF

Indications	Contraindications	Complications
Spondylolisthesis	Pathology above L2 where retraction may cause cord injury.	Hardware failure or misplacement
Recurrent disc herniation	Severe osteoporosis precluding safe hardware implantation	General surgical complications (e.g., infection, bleeding)
Failure of intertransverse process fusion	Previous lumbar decompression with severe epidural scaring	Radiculopathy from manipulation of the nerve roots
Degenerative disc disease	Arachnoiditis	Vascular injury (iliac vessels)

Procedure

Positioning and patient preparation

Given the prone positioning, the potential for long operative times, and the potential for blood loss requiring transfusion, general anesthesia with endotracheal intubation is usually the recommended technique. It is worth mentioning that since most of these patients have degenerative disease of the spine, the anesthesiologist and spine surgeon should discuss the safety and feasibility of maneuvering the cervical spine for intubation purposes. Once the airway is secured, the endotracheal tube is securely fastened to avoid dislodgement in the prone position. Traditional intraoperative monitoring should include intra-arterial monitoring of blood pressure, bladder catheterization, and adequate intravenous access. Central venous pressure monitoring is also sometimes recommended depending on the underlying medical condition of the patient. Prior to final positioning, the surgical team should discuss whether the patient's head will be placed on a face cushion or head clamp system to decrease the incidence of postoperative vision loss (Fig. 8.12). Careful attention should be paid to the patient's eyes to avoid corneal abrasions, which have a much higher incidence in the prone position. The blood loss expected for posterior lumbar fusion differs depending on several variables including single vs. multiple operative levels, abdominal decompression (positioning and surgical table), surgeon's experience, and open vs. minimally invasive technique (Fig. 8.13). Recent studies have quoted an average blood loss of 900 ml without iliac crest bone graft harvesting and 1400 ml when bone graft is harvested.[2] More recent studies quote lower blood losses ranging between 200 and 300 ml.[3] Careful attention to patient positioning can help to reduce blood loss by relaxing the abdominal musculature and decreasing the amount of blood present in the epidural venous plexus.[4,5] Finally, intraoperative cell salvage can be utilized to minimize the risks associated with blood transfusion.

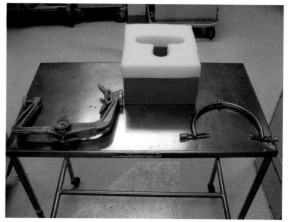

Figure 8.12 Variety of available head-holding systems. On the left is the rigid head holder allowing clamp fixation of the head; in the center is the foam pillow; and on the right are cranial tongs allowing the head to move freely when attached to a pulley system.

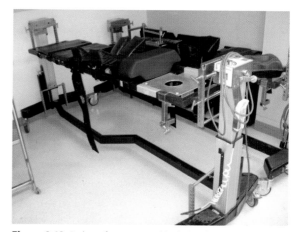

Figure 8.13 Jackson frame surgical bed. The abdomen is allowed to freely hang through the center opening, relieving pressure and decreasing venous congestion in the epidural plexus.

Attention to other intraoperative concerns includes the avoidance of hypothermia through the use of body warmers and the possible need for electrophysiologic monitoring to avoid nerve root injury. While not a "standard of care," intraoperative nerve root monitoring is sometimes performed and may necessitate a change in anesthetic management.

Surgical technique

A midline incision is made at the desired level of the lumbar spine. The subcutaneous tissue is dissected using electrocautery down to the level of the dorsal fascia. A subperiosteal exposure of the lumbar spine is performed. Careful attention to hemostasis during exposure is critical to avoid excessive blood loss over the course of the procedure. Intraoperative radiographic verification of the correct level is made. A bilateral laminectomy is performed exposing the thecal sac. Careful mobilization of the dural sac as well as the exiting root is performed medially in order to expose the vertebral disc. The aim of laminectomy is to allow for relief of the spinal stenosis and allow exposure of the pedicles for safe insertion of the titanium pedicle screws for stabilization. For this part of the procedure fluoroscopy or stereotactic navigation may be used to accomplish adequate placement of the intervertebral hardware.[6] Once the pedicle screws are placed, the annulus of the affected disc space is divided and the disc space is sequentially opened with mechanical disc space distractors. This is made safer by removal of the inferior facet joint of the superior vertebral level allowing for wider exposure and easier preparation of the interbody space. Once the disc space height is restored to the desired value, titanium plates or rods are placed across the pedicle screws to hold the disc space in the correct position. At this point, the disc material is removed with a combination of disc shavers and curettes to allow for placement of

intervertebral spacers and bone graft. This intervertebral bone graft will be compressed when the patient stands up and will serve as the ultimate strength of the surgical fusion. After the spacers are placed, the remainder of the disc space is packed with morselized bone taken from the iliac crest or from the bone removed during the surgical decompression. After this is completed, the nerve root foramina are checked to make sure the roots are adequately decompressed. Thorough inspection of the hardware, decompression site, and hemostasis is performed one last time, after which adequate closure by layers is performed. A final intraoperative radiograph may be obtained to verify adequate positioning of the hardware prior to emergence from anesthesia (Fig. 8.14). A subfascial drain will be inserted prior to skin closure based on the surgeon's preference. In some instances the surgeon will place an epidural catheter prior to closure for postoperative pain control.

Postprocedural care

Normal postoperative care will include avoiding hypertension, adequate analgesia, and safe mobilization of the patient in the hospital environment. Antibiotics are given from just prior to the induction of anesthesia and stopped within 24 hours afterwards. Corticosteroid therapy may be utilized to help reduce inflammation and improve patient comfort. Assessment by physical and occupational therapy allows for safe mobilization and discharge planning. Orthotics is generally consulted to fit the patient for a rigid or semi-rigid lumbar orthosis. Attention to hospital risk management includes prevention of deep venous thrombosis through the use of a variety of antithrombotic devices/drugs

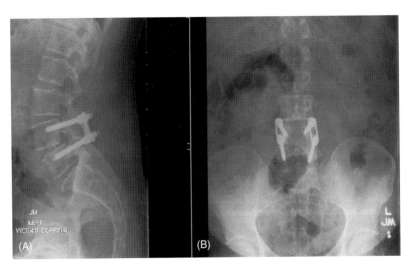

Figure 8.14 AP (A) and lateral (B) weight-bearing radiographs of the lumbar spine following surgery. Note the construct composed by the pedicle screws and ramps interconnecting both vertebral bodies. Small radiopaque dots in the disc space represent the interbody graft in place.

and the prevention of urine and wound infection by aggressive control of blood sugar and aseptic technique.

Complications

Complications can be divided into those specific to the operation and those common to spinal surgery. The general complications include risk of blood loss, infection, deep venous thrombosis, urinary tract infection, ileus, and cardiopulmonary complications related to general anesthesia.[7–9] Complications specific to the procedure are centered on nerve root or thecal sac injury due to manipulation/retraction of the neural elements during surgery and those related to implantation of the hardware. Postoperative neuralgia occurs in approximately 7% of patients, likely related to surgical manipulation of the involved nerve root.[10] Hardware complications include improper placement and/or migration. The hardware consists of titanium pedicle screws, rods/plates, and the interbody spacers. As with any implanted device, improper placement can result in neural or vascular injury. A potentially devastating complication is violation of the anterior longitudinal ligament and iliac vessel injury leading to catastrophic hemorrhage. Long-term complications include pseudoarthrosis (failure of the bony fusion) and adjacent segment failure and may lead to ongoing back pain requiring further surgery. The overall complication rate associated with PLIF varies widely in the literature with rates ranging from 6.7% to 68%.[8,9] It is important to note that most of these are transient with no resulting permanent neurologic deficits.

Conclusion

Posterior lumbar interbody fusion is a safe and effective technique to treat disorders of the intervertebral disc, especially lumbar spondylolisthesis.

References

1. Cloward RB. The treatment of ruptured intervertebral discs by vertebral body fusion. I. Indications, operative techniques, after care. *J Neurosurg* 1953; **10**: 154–68.

2. Yasuhisa A, Masaki T, Hisashi K. Comparative study of iliac bone graft and carbon cage with local bone graft in posterior lumbar interbody fusion. *J Orthop Surg* 2002; **10**(1): 1–7.

3. Freudenberger C, Lindley E, Beard E, *et al.* Posterior vs. anterior lumbar interbody fusion with anterior tension band plating: retrospective analysis. *Orthopedics* 2009; **32**(7): 492.

4. Singh A, Ramappa M, Bhatia C, Krishna M. Less invasive posterior lumbar interbody fusion and obesity: clinical outcomes and return to work. *Spine* 2010; **35**(24): 2116–20.

5. Frymoyer J, Wiesel S. Thoracolumbar spine-Interbody fusion. In: *The Adult and Pediatric Spine: Principles, Practice and Surgery*. 3rd ed. Philadelphia, PA: Lippincott Williams & Wilkins; 2003: 1141–6.

6. A. Vaccaro, T. Albert. Posterior lumbar interbody fusion. In: *Spine Surgery: Tricks of the Trade*. 2nd ed. New York: Thieme; 2008: 1154–5.

7. Hosono N, Namekata M, Makino T, *et al.* Perioperative complications of primary posterior lumbar interbody fusion for nonisthmic spondylolisthesis: analysis of risk factors. *J Neurosurg Spine* 2008; **9**: 403–7.

8. Cho KJ, Park SR, Kim JH, *et al.* Complications in posterior fusion and instrumentation for degenerative lumbar scoliosis. *Spine* 2007; **32**: 2232–7.

9. Krishna M, Pollock RD, Bhatia C. Incidence, etiology, classification, and management of neuralgia after posterior lumbar interbody fusion surgery in 226 patients. *Spine* 2008; **8**: 374–9.

10. Kasis AG, Marshman LA, Krishna M, *et al.* Significantly improved outcomes with a less invasive posterior lumbar interbody fusion incorporating total facetectomy. *Spine* 2009; **34**: 572–7.

8.6 Minimally invasive procedures for vertebral compression fractures

Jason E. Pope and Nagy Mekhail

Key points

- Vertebral compression fractures are common in the aged population and carry significant morbidity and mortality consequences.

- The sites of vertebral compression fracture are commonly in the thoracolumbar junction (T12/L1), followed by T7/T8,

- Risk factors for vertebral compression fractures are most commonly a consequence of osteoporosis, and are less commonly associated with primary or secondary cancers.

- Management of vertebral compression fractures follows the principles of orthopedic fracture management
- Vertebral augmentation procedures are very effective in eliminating pain and disability in the appropriately selected patient.
- There are multiple flaws in the literature discounting its benefit for selected patients.

Introduction

Vertebral compression fractures (VCFs) are most commonly a consequence of osteoporosis and less frequently of primary or metastatic cancers. Osteoporosis is a systemic skeletal disease that is characterized by reduced bone strength, caused by a deficiency in peak bone mass during growth and development, inadequate bone formation, and excessive bone resorption, resulting in disruption in architecture and mass.[1] Secondary osteoporosis can be a consequence of medications (steroids, chemotherapy, anticonvulsants), endocrinopathies (hyperthyroidism, Cushing's syndrome, hyperparathyroidism, and hypogonadism), toxins (alcohol, tobacco), cancers, and malnutrition. The National Osteoporosis Foundation estimates that 100 million people worldwide and 44 million people in the United States are at risk for developing osteoporosis. Over 2 million fragility fractures in the United States can be attributed to osteoporosis, of which 26% are vertebral body fractures.[2]. Moreover, two-thirds are left undiagnosed and even fewer are appropriately treated.[2] Not surprisingly, VCF prevalence increases with age, as 1 in 2 women and 1 in 4 men over the age of 50 years will have an osteoporosis-related fracture.[2,3]

Vertebral compression fractures are the most common osteoporotic fracture and an estimated 700 000 occur annually.[4] Over 150 000 people are hospitalized for pain and management of spinal fractures each year.[5] Approximately 260 000 patients are diagnosed with their first painful fracture each year,[5] and after the first, the risk of a subsequent VCF increases 5-fold, 12-fold after two or more, and 75-fold after two or more and low bone mass below the 33rd percentile.[6] VCFs commonly occur spontaneously and can result from minimal or no trauma. Minor activities, such as bending, lifting, and coughing have been implicated with developing vertebral compression fractures.[7] The sites of fracture are commonly in the thoracolumbar

junction (T12/L1), followed by (T7/T8), whereas the morphology of vertebral compression fractures can vary through crush, biconcave, and wedge (most common).[8] A high degree of clinical suspicion for cancer needs to be maintained in fractures outside of these locations and in patients without the commonly associated risks factors (see below).

Dreadfully, an estimated 75 000–100 000 cancer-related fractures occur annually. Metastatic disease, including all stages of multiple myeloma, stage III prostate cancer, and stage IV breast and lung cancer are commonly implicated in VCFs;[9-13] 30–70% of those who die from cancer annually have bone metastasis.[14] Distribution of tumor types causing VCF includes: lung (20%); breast (6%); myeloma (22%); prostate (32%); and others, including bladder, thyroid, and survival of pediatric solid tumors (20%).[15] Metastatic bone lesions are either osteoblastic or osteolytic, where the latter predispose to a higher risk of fracture.[16] Osteoblastic lesions are characterized by increased bone density, maintained bone strength, but decreased bone integrity (stiffness), and are common in prostate cancer. Osteolytic lesions are characterized by decreased bone density and decreased strength and integrity, and are common in patients with multiple myeloma. Not only does cancer cause VCF, so does its treatment.[17] The long-term use of oral glucocorticoids increases the risk of fracture 2.6-fold.[18]

The consequences of vertebral compression fractures are far reaching. Patient-associated consequences are both physical and psychological. Physical consequences include bone pain, disability, radiculopathy, spinal cord compression, kyphosis, and related reduction on lung volume, abdominal content compression, impaired physical function, impaired gait, sleep disorders, decreased adult activities of daily living (ADL), and hypercalcemia. Patients with VCF are 2–3 times more likely to die of pulmonary causes, i.e., pneumonia because of increased work of breathing, decreased functional residual capacity, and the associated kyphosis causing reduced lung capacity. Psychological consequences include depression, reduced self-esteem, anxiety, reduced autonomy, and reduction in the quality of life.[19] Van Schoor looked at 334 people aged 65 or older with VCF assessed by radiography and SF-12 (quality of life measure) and reported that patients with three or more vertebral compression fractures had a loss of quality of life compared with patients with stroke.[19] VCFs increase the risk of mortality.[5] Johnell reported a mortality of near 80% for patients 5 years after vertebral compression fracture (mean age of patients at the time of fracture was 78.6 years).[20]

The economic burden is as telling as the consequences of VCF for the patient. Annual costs of osteoporotic fractures continue to rise; estimates were as high as $13.8 billion in 1995 with an increase to $16.7 billion in 2003.[21,22] Two minimally invasive options for vertebral body augmentation are vertebroplasty and kyphoplasty. Both entail injecting polymethylmethacrylate into the fractured vertebrae to fix the fracture and relieve the pain. A detailed discussion of these techniques follows.

Patient selection

An appropriate history, physical examination, and radiographic testing are a necessity and cannot be understated. As alluded to previously, historical indicators for suspicion of VCF include age greater than 50 years, exposure to known medications with known bone strength and architecture detriment (including glucocorticoid therapy), endocrinopathies, known cancers with either primary or metastatic vertebral body sites, a diagnosis of osteoporosis, and female sex. Furthermore, relatively minor or no traumatic history is often reported, and includes cough, sneeze, bending, and twisting maneuvers. Often, patients report awakening with pain. The pain is typically localized and axial in nature, with or without a bandlike radiation, and can be elicited longitudinally up to 10 cm (4 inches) (one to two levels) from the VCF (caudal presentation is more common than rostral, anecdotally). The pain is typically exacerbated by movement. Spinal percussion may be helpful to delineate the symptomatic vertebral compression fracture level, but this sign is not sensitive or specific.[23] Indications, as well as relative and absolute contraindications are listed in Tables 8.3–8.5.[24]

Radiologic correlation is paramount. Modalities employed include plain films, magnetic resonance imaging, bone scan, and computed tomography. Axial and sagittal MRI are generally recommended currently, as it provides anatomic detail and suggests fracture age. Uniformly, acute fractures typically have a low T1 and high T2 signal and T2 STIR signal on MRI, secondary to edema and increased water content.

Computed tomography (CT) with a bone scan is an excellent imaging modality when MRI cannot be used, either secondary to inability to tolerate MRI positioning or if the patient has preexisting implanted metal devices (ferromagnetic). Bone scans with increased tracer uptake are suggestive of recent fracture. CT scans differentiate fat from other soft tissue and accurately describe bony architecture. Importantly, CT exposes the patient to ionizing radiation, whereas MRI does not.

Table 8.3 Indications for vertebral augmentation

- Symptomatic VCF
- Osteoporotic/osteolytic/malignant/benign fractures refractory to conservative medical therapy
- Multiple compression fractures where further spinal deformity would result in depressed respiratory function
- Painful fracture secondary to osteonecrosis (Kummels disease)[a]
- Unstable fracture with movement of wedge deformity
- Chronic nonunion traumatic fracture
- Pain localization and presentation suggestive of VCF (bandlike, localized, axial)
- Ideally acute/subacute fractures (<1 year old) although symptomatic chronic fractures suitable candidates
- Older patient age > younger patient age

[a] Vascular necrosis of the vertebral body after a vertebral compression fracture.

Table 8.4 Absolute contraindications for vertebral augmentation

- Asymptomatic stable fracture
- Effective conservative medical measurement
- Systemic or localized infection
- Osteomyelitis of target vertebra
- Uncorrected coagulopathy
- Allergy to bone cement or contrast agents
- Acute traumatic fracture of nonosteoporotic vertebra
- Prophylaxis in osteoporotic patients
- Fractured pedicles
- Burst fracture (traumatic injury resulting in pieces of vertebral body shattering into surrounding tissues)[a]
- Retropulsed fragment causing significant canal compromise[b]

[a] Although some authors advocate using vertebroplasty for burst fracture management.[25]
[b] Some authors consider retropulsed fragments relative contraindications.
[a,b] Both conditions may require open fixation rather than minimally invasive techniques.

Table 8.5 Relative contraindications for vertebral compression fractures

- Radicular pain (caused by a compressive syndrome unrelated to vertebral body collapse
- Younger age
- Tumor extension into the epidural space
- Severe vertebral body collapse >70% (vertebra plana)

143

Management

Management of vertebral compression fractures is largely medical or surgical. Medical management includes symptom reduction by conservative management: analgesics, bracing, and institution of preventative measures (supplementation of calcium and vitamin D; calcitonin; antireabsorption agents (bisphosphonates); chemotherapy/radiation therapy for cancer; and hormonal therapy (estrogen, PTH). There are questions regarding conservative management with analgesics: How long should they be trialed while attempting to mitigate the aforementioned VCF sequelae? Innately, orthopedic principles of fracture management include anatomy restoration, rigid fixation, minimal tissue disruption, and safe and early mobilization.[26] In can be argued that conservative management for symptomatic VCF does not fulfill these well-established principles.

Techniques

Vertebroplasty

Deramond and Gilbert introduced vertebroplasty in France in 1984 for treatment of hemangiomas. The procedure was then employed in the United States in 1993. The procedure is typically performed in an outpatient setting under monitored anesthesia care and local anesthesia. Routinely, perioperative antibiotics are given within 30 minutes prior to the procedure. The procedure itself takes between 30 and 60 minutes, with the majority of the time dedicated to patient positioning and fluoroscopic C-arm alignment, and biplanar fluoroscopy is advocated. The patient is self-positioned prone to ensure reduce joint stress and minimize risk of intraoperative compressive neuropathy. True AP and true lateral fluoroscopic views are required for successful and safe needle placement. In the AP projection, the pedicle outline is the waist of the pedicle, not the base. A true AP projection is where the pedicles are in the upper half of the vertebral body, the spinous process is equidistant between the pedicles, and the end plates are parallel. True lateral projection assurance is confirmed by parallel end plates and superimposed pedicles. Two common approaches are described: extrapedicular or transpedicular, and both are intended to be bilateral. Transpedicular approaches, where appropriate (low thoracic and lumbar) have been advocated to reduce the chance of cement extravasations. It is vitally important to consider fracture orientation and trajectory before needle positioning. For the transpedicular approach,

after true AP and lateral images are confirmed, a mark is placed approximately 5 cm (2 inches) lateral and parallel to the superior end plate of the target vertebral body, with the projected trajectory to the upper posterior portion of the pedicle waist (10–11:00 on LEFT and 2–3:00 on the RIGHT). After local infiltration with local anesthetic (50:50 mixture of 0.75% bupivacaine and 2% lidocaine with epinephrine 1:400 000), the tip of the trochar is advanced to the pedicle. Precise correction of trajectory is paramount and should be checked with sequential AP and lateral images. For the extrapedicular approach, the trajectory is similar to the transpedicular approach, although entry is outside the pedicles, either lateral to the junction of the transverse process and superior articular process or between the rib and transverse process at the superior lateral pedicle wall, depending on the level of the thoracic vertebra. An en-face, coaxial approach may aid in tool placement, but is usually not advocated.

There are some authors who advocate venography prior to cement injection to evaluate for potential routes of cement extravasation. The physical properties of cement are different from those of the contrast medium (i.e., viscosity), and injectate radiographic spread correlation is not guaranteed.[27] Venography is therefore not routinely performed, exclusive of vascular lesions. In patients with osteoporosis or hemangiomas, 2.5–4 cm^3 of cement can provide optimal filling of the vertebra; in tumor smaller volumes of 1.5–2.5 cm^3 are sufficient.[28] The cement is mixed and the viscosity is checked, as it is recommended that it should have "toothpaste" consistency. The injection should be monitored under live fluoroscopy with care in emptying the trocar before removing it to avoid extravasation. The patient is instructed to remain prone until the cement hardens (8–15 minutes). Some advocate a postprocedure CT scan, while others do not.[29] The patient is to stay recumbent for 3–5 h and neurologic evaluation is performed. Refer to Fig. 8.15.

Kyphoplasty

Kyphoplasty is a variation of percutaneous vertebroplasty, where the difference lies in mechanical fracture reduction and cavity creation through the percutaneous introduction of an inflatable balloon tamp (IBT). Typically, this procedure is performed under general anesthesia. Patient positioning, imaging, and trocar placement are the same as for vertebroplasty. Biopsy is usually taken to determine or confirm the cause of the vertebral body compression fracture. The IBT has

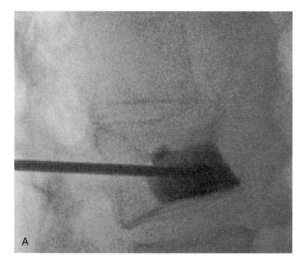

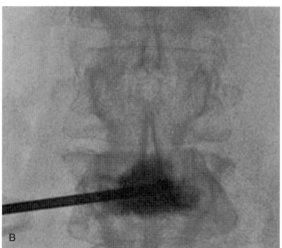

Figure 8.15 Lateral (A) and AP (B) images of vertebroplasty.

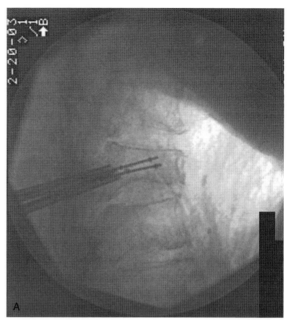

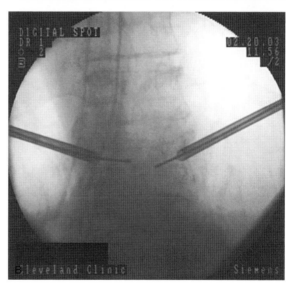

Figure 8.16 Lateral (A) and AP (B) fluoroscopic views of trocar placement for kyphoplasty.

bidirectional and unidirectional inflating properties, and can range from 10 to 20 mm in length. It is crucial to understand that the operator controls the volume of IBT inflation, as it is recommended to increase the volume in 0.25 cm³ increments (180° turn of plunger). The maximum pressure recommended is 400 psi (2.76 Mpa) without decay and the maximum volume is 4 cm³ for the 10 and 15 mm IBT and 6 cm³ for the 20 mm IBT. The goal is IBT introduction into the anterior one-third of the vertebral body. The IBT is then removed and the bone filler device (BFD) is introduced approximately 3–5 mm into anterior cortex. Cement mixing is similar to that for vertebroplasty, although the consistency is usually much more viscous, and the cement appears "doughy"; it usually takes 8 minutes, depending on ambient temperature, rigor in mixing, and handling.

The more viscous cement is recommended for kyphoplasty because the injection occurs under lower pressure and fills an iatrogenic void, in contrast to vertebroplasty where injection is under high pressure without cavity creation. It is recommended not to add additives to the cement, e.g., antibiotics. It is recommended to inject the cement via the BFD to 5 mm of posterior wall, starting anteriorly, under live fluoroscopy to completely fill the void created and to reduce occurrence of extravasation.[30] Refer to Figs. 8.16 through 8.18.

145

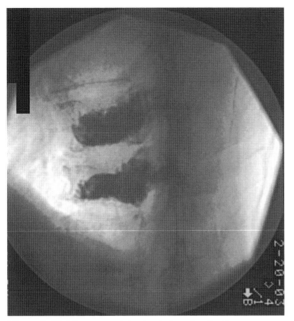

Figure 8.17 After cement injection in lateral projection.

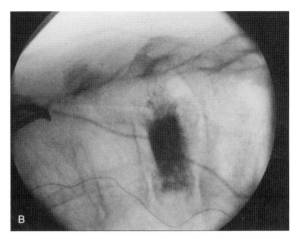

Figure 8.18 (*cont.*)

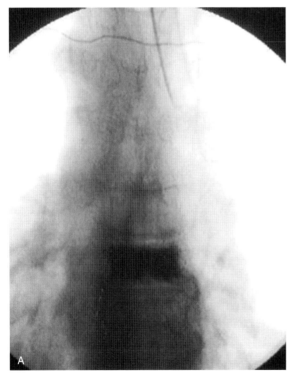

Figure 8.18 Anteroposterior (A) and lateral (B) images of kyphoplasty.

Table 8.6 Technical considerations

Kyphoplasty	Vertebroplasty
In-patient procedure, increasingly outpatient	Outpatient
General anesthesia, monitored anesthesia care	Monitored anesthesia care
Single or bi trans/extrapedicular	Single or bi trans/extrapedicular
8 G trochar	11–13 G trochar
Procedure time slower than vertebroplasty	Procedure time faster than kyphoplasty
Cost $$$$	Cost $
VCF anatomy restoration ++++	++
Cement viscosity higher	Cement viscosity lower
Injection under lower pressure	Injection with higher pressure

Central cavity creation

As described briefly earlier, kyphoplasty utilizes curettes to create a space to accommodate the IBT and cement deposition. A variation of vertebroplasty involving similar mechanisms with IBT deployment has also been described.[31] Important technical considerations regarding the decision to perform either procedure are listed in Table 8.6.

Complications

Complications associated with vertebral body augmentation are procedure specific and are traditionally either procedural or extravasations of cement in nature. Collectively, the clinically meaningful complication rate of vertebroplasty is reported to be approximately

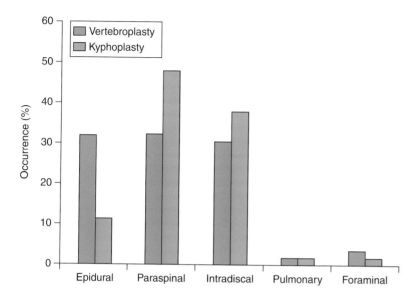

Figure 8.19 Percentage of occurrence and distribution of cement leakage by location in vertebroplasty and kyphoplasty. (From Hulme P, Kebs J, Ferguson S, Berlemann U, Vertebroplasty and kyphoplasty: a systematic review of 69 clinical studies. *Spine* 2006;31:1983–2001. Reproduced with permission.)

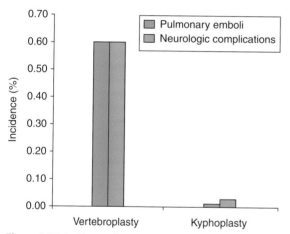

Figure 8.20 Incidence of severe clinical complications following vertebroplasty and kyphoplasty. (Created from data presented in Moreland DB, Landi MK, Grand W, Vertebroplasty: Techniques to avoid complications. *Spine J* 2001;1:66–71.)

suspected of increasing adjacent vertebral body compression fractures, with rates of 12–52%.[35] Severe clinical complications for vertebroplasty and kyphoplasty, including pulmonary emboli and neurologic seque-lae occurred at rates of 0.6% and 0.1%, and 0.6% and 0.03%, respectively.[33] Pulmonary emboli likely resulted from venous uptake via paravertebral veins. Other pulmonary reactions to cement, as for long bone fracture repair, can induce a pulmonary hypertension.

Extravasation management is dependent on symptomatology and includes observation or surgical decompression. Perivertebral leakage of cement has been reported to occur in up to 65% of treated osteoporotic VCFs.[36] Nevertheless, the majority of patients are asymptomatic.[37,38] Some may experience transient neurologic findings, from mechanical compression or chemical irritation, but these rarely persist for more than 4 weeks.

Outcomes and efficacy

Relief observed after vertebral body augmentation has consistently been reported to occur almost immediately after the procedure to 1–2 days postoperatively.[39,40] The hypothesized mechanisms of pain relief from vertebral body augmentation include immobilization of the fracture, and/or intraosseous neural destruction from the exothermic PMMA (polymethylmethacrylate) reaction, and/or a direct neural cytotoxic effect of the PMMA. However, recent studies suggest that mechanical stabilization is the most likely mode of pain relief.[41,42]

1–3%, and complications include infection, bleeding, increased pain, numbness, tingling, extravasation of cement, paralysis, and death. The overall complication rate of vertebroplasty, as reported by Murphy and Deramond in 2000, was 1.3% for osteoporosis, 10% for cancer, and 2.5% for hemangiomas.[32] In comparison, Hulme reviewed the distribution of cement leakage and percentage of occurrence for kyphoplasty and vertebroplasty and reported, respectively, 11% and 32% epidural, 48% and 32.5% paraspinal, 38% and 30.5% intradiscal, 1.5% and 1.7% pulmonary, and 1.5% and 1.7% foraminal. Refer to Figs. 8.19 and 8.20.[33,34] Both vertebral body restoration procedures have been

The biomechanics of the spine following vertebral body augmentation have been investigated as there have been some suggestions of an increased risk of adjacent vertebral body fracture, and that the risk may be different after vertebral body augmentation with cavity creation (kyphoplasty). Under normal physiologic conditions, load is shared between the discs, the vertebral bodies, the ligaments, and the facets. Anterior load shift, increased vertebral body stiffness, and load transfer through the intervertebral disc are suggested reasons for potential increased potential for VCF at adjacent levels. See Fig. 8.21. The response of a FSU (functional stiff component) to a load is governed by the less stiff component, i.e., the intervertebral disc, which is not severely disrupted. In a prospective study of 25 patients with 34 fractures who were treated with vertebroplasty and followed for 2 years, 52% had developed at least one VCF, where the odds ratio of developing an adjacent VCF to a treated, augmented vertebra was 2.27 versus 1.44 for a new fracture unrelated to the treated vertebra and was not statistically significant.[43] Although static compression tests demonstrate continued slight redistribution of stress and stiffness following augmentation that may contribute to adjacent vertebral body fracture,[44] it is clear that subsequent VCF development is multifactorial and may be a consequence of progression of disease rather than slightly altered biomechanics of a slightly increased load and geometric misalignment.

Luo et al. demonstrated that vertebral augmentation could restore normal spine mechanics.[45] Numerous studies have reported incidence rates of VCF after augmentation with PMMA for kyphoplasty and vertebroplasty but are inconsistent in fracture definitions and time spans, with interpretation confounded by age, sex, bone density, and disease progression, to name a few factors. Furthermore, when comparing the biomechanics of the spine following fusion with the alteration following vertebral body augmentation, it is clear that vertebral body augmentation is more physiologic. Compared with anatomy restoration by postural reduction (commonly lordotic positioning), kyphoplasty doubled the final height achieved by the former and was maintained throughout follow-up of 1 year.

The clinical benefits of vertebral body augmentation are seemingly impressive. As demonstrated by Ledlie and Renfro, in 77 patients followed for 2 years after kyphoplasty, 90% had complete pain relief; use of analgesic medications decreased 87%; there were no procedure-related complications; and vertebral body

Mean normal stress
Augmented

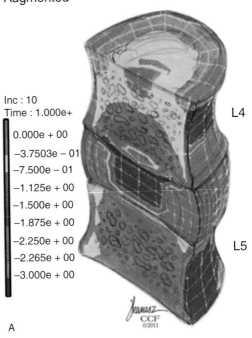

Inc : 10
Time : 1.000e+

0.000e + 00
−3.7503e − 01
−7.500e − 01
−1.125e + 00
−1.500e + 00
−1.875e + 00
−2.250e + 00
−2.265e + 00
−3.000e + 00

A

L4

L5

Mean normal stress
Non-augmented

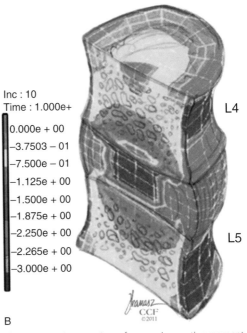

Inc : 10
Time : 1.000e+

0.000e + 00
−3.7503 − 01
−7.500e − 01
−1.125e + 00
−1.500e + 00
−1.875e + 00
−2.250e + 00
−2.265e + 00
−3.000e + 00

B

L4

L5

Figure 8.21 A comparison of stresses in a motion segment, showing the load shift that results from rigid cement augmentation. (Adapted from Hadley C. Abdulreham A, Zoarski GH, Biomechanics of vertebral bone augmentation. *Neuroimag Clin N Am* 2010 159–67.)

augmentation was maintained.[46] Comparing augmentation with medical management at 6 months, Komp *et al.* demonstrated progressive vertebral body height loss in 94% of patients and subsequent fracture rate of 65% with nonsurgical treatment, against 0% vertebral body height loss and 37% subsequent fracture rate following kyphoplasty.[47] Komp *et al.* also demonstrated that kyphoplasty improved pain and function by VAS (visual analogue scale) reduction and Oswestry Back Disability Index reduction in patients compared with nonsurgical management in fractures with mean age of 1 month that were followed to 6 months.[47] Furthermore, in comparing chronic fracture management greater than 1 year old, kyphoplasty improved pain and function by VAS and EVOS Functional Scale at 6 months.[48]

Controversy persists between kyphoplasty and vertebroplasty.[49–52] Regarding anatomy restoration, both vertebroplasty[46] and kyphoplasty improve height and angular deformity; however, most agree that kyphoplasty is more effective. Kyphoplasty, on average, improved angular deformity by 53% in one study and 47% in another.[53,54] Hiwatashi *et al*, however, concluded that the statistical significance of height restoration was not significant.[55] Furthermore, Ledlie and Renfro reported maintained height of 88% prefracture height at 2 years.[46] Kumar *et al.* prospectively analyzed 52 patients randomized to either kyphoplasty or vertebroplasty with mean follow-up of approximately 42 weeks, recording outcomes pre- and post-procedure using VAS, Oswestry Disability Index, the EuroQol-5D questionnaire, and the Short-Form 36 Health Survey. Both vertebroplasty and kyphoplasty were effective at improving pain on VAS (8.0–5.5 cm vs. 7.5–2.5 cm), functional disability (57.6–38.4 vs. 50.7–28.8), and quality of life. However, kyphoplasty provides better results, which are maintained over long-term follow-up.[52]

Interestingly, Liu *et al.* randomly assigned 100 patients with thoracolumbar compression fractures to either kyphoplasty or vertebroplasty using PMMA and assessed VAS scores and vertebral body height an kyphotic wedge angle from reconstructed CT images with follow-up to 6 months and concluded that degree of pain reduction, wedge angle improvement, and vertebral body height improvement did not differ significantly and, secondarily to expense, suggested vertebroplasty for osteoporotic VCFs.[52]

Literature support, as shown, can seemingly substantiate both sides of the debate on kyphoplasty vs vertebroplasty. Reported advantages of either procedure need to be weighed against their risks. Table 8.6

lists some of the differences and similarities between kyphoplasty and vertebroplasty. After factoring in operating room time, general anesthesia, and overnight admission, kyphoplasty costs 10–20 times more than vertebroplasty.[49] Ignoring the extrapolated costs, the vertebroplasty kit without cement costs approximately $400, whereas the kyphoplasty kit costs $3400.[49]

Despite the kyphoplasty vs. vertebroplasty debate, a mountain of evidence exists suggesting their appropriate use in the management of vertebral compression fractures to reduce both morbidity and mortality. In stark contradiction, the *New England Journal of Medicine* published two articles regarding the routine use of vertebroplasty in fracture management in 2009 and concluded that there was no beneficial effect of vertebroplasty as compared with a sham procedure in patients with painful osteoporotic vertebral fractures up to 3 months of follow-up, and that there was no statistically significant difference in pain improvement in the sham procedure vs. vertebroplasty in pain and pain-related disability.[56,57] In a later reply, Buchbinder *et al.* state that[58]

> Vertebroplasty appears to confer no benefit over sham procedure or usual care, and it poses risk…it would be neither appropriate nor moral to offer this treatment in routine care.

Let us look a bit closer. Buchbinder *et al.* performed a multicenter, randomized double-blind, placebo-controlled trial in which participants with one or two painful osteoporotic vertebral fractures that were of less than 12 months' duration and unhealed, as confirmed by magnetic resonance imaging, were randomly assigned to undergo vertebroplasty or a sham procedure. The sham procedure was introduction of the trocar to the posterolateral portion of the facet, with the sharp stylet being replaced with a blunt one to mimic tapping and entry into the vertebral body after local infiltration of osteum with local anesthetics.

Participants were stratified according to treatment center, sex, and duration of symptoms (<6 weeks or ≥6 weeks). Outcomes were assessed at 1 week and at 1, 3, and 6 months and included the primary outcome of pain assessment by NRS at 3 months, and secondary outcomes of quality of life (QUALEFFO), a VCF-specific questionnaire, AQoL (Assessment of Quality of Life) questionnaire, sensitive to the elderly, and the EQ-5D (European Quality of Life-5 Dimensions scale).

The Kallmes study involved the random assignment of 131 patients who had one to three painful osteoporotic vertebral compression fractures to undergo either vertebroplasty or simulated procedure (as described previously) following 4 weeks of medical management, and patients were followed at 3, 14, and 90 days with the primary outcome of pain relief with the modified Roland–Morris Disability Questionnaire (RDQ) and numerical rating scale (NRS), where secondary measures were EQ-5D and the Study of Osteoporosis Fracture–Activities of Daily Living (SOF-ADL).

There were multiple flaws. No physical examination was performed and therefore pain could not be attributed specifically to the VCF discovered on MRI. Furthermore, other sources of back pain were not controlled, as the aged population commonly has symptomatic facet arthropathy. This could explain the description of pain relief following the procedure (i.e., blocking of the medial branches with local infiltration in the sham group). Furthermore, because "pain generators" rarely occur in an isolated presentation, the specificity and sensitivity of the outcomes for VCF and vertebroplasty versus sham is uncertain, as no follow-up examination was performed. Interestingly, both studies only treated only two levels (some patients had three levels of evidence VCF). One hundred and forty-one patients declined to participate in the Buchbinder study, while 300 declined to participate in the Kallmes study without an exclusion explanation. One explanation could be that they feared randomization into the sham group because of severe pain.

In the natural course osteoporotic fractures typically heal at 6–8 weeks, although MRI evidence of fracture lingers. Furthermore, in-patients were excluded in the study and medical management was required for 4 weeks, removing the subacute VCF patient population and resulting in intervention on healed VCF. Only 32% and 44% of subjects enrolled in these studies were within this time frame, for Buchbinder and Kallmes, respectively.[59] These articles were overwhelmingly accepted as unequivocal evidence and incorrectly deride vertebroplasty as ineffective.

Conclusions

Comparative effectiveness research and evidence-based medicine are paramount to ensuring appropriate and accessible patient-centered pain care. Vertebroplasty and kyphoplasty are techniques that can reduce morbidity and mortality associated with vertebral compression fracture. Most contend that kyphoplasty, although more expensive and often requiring general anesthesia and 23-hour observation, is better at restoring vertebral body height, with equivocal evidence of reduction in cement extravasations secondary to central cavity creation.

References

1. Raisz LG. Pathogenesis of osteoporosis: concepts, conflicts, and prospects. *J Clin Invest* 2005; **115**(2): 3318–25.

2. National Osteoporosis Foundation. http://www.nof.org (accessed December 1, 2011).

3. Oneil TW, Felsenberg D, Varlow J, *et al.* Prevalence of vertebral deformity in European men and women: the European vertebral osteoporosis study. *J Bone Miner Res* 1996; **11**: 1010–18.

4. Riggs BL, Melton LJ. The worldwide problem of osteoporosis: insights afforded by epidemiology. *Bone* 1995; **17**: 505–11.

5. Cooper C, Atkinson EJ, O'Fallon WM, *et al.* Incidence of clinically diagnosed vertebral fractures: a population-based study in Rochester, Minnesota, 1985–1989. *J Bone Miner Res* 1992; **7**: 221–7.

6. Ross PD, Davis JW, Epstein RS, Wasnich RD. Pre-existing fractures and bone mass predict vertebral fracture incidence in woman. *Ann Intern Med* 1991; **114**(11): 919–23.

7. Aslan S, Karicioglu O, Katirici Y, *et al.* Speed-bump induced spinal cord injury. *Am J Emerg Med* 2005; **23**: 563.

8. Nevit MC, Ross PD, Palermo L, *et al.* Association of prevalent vertebral fractures, bone density, and alendronate treatment with incident vertebral fractures: effect of number and spinal location of fractures. *Bone* 1999; **25**: 613–19.

9. Berenson JR, Lichtenstein A, Porter L, *et al.* Efficacy of pamidronate in reducing skeletal event in patients with advanced multiple myeloma. *NEJM* **334**(8): 488–93.

10. Brinker H, Westin J, Abildgaard N, *et al.* Failure of oral pamidronate to reduce skeletal morbidity in multiple myeloma: a double blind placebo controlled trial. *Br J Haematol* 1998; **101**: 280–6.

11. Melton LJ, Kyle RA, Achenbach SJ, Oberg AL, Rajkumar SV. Fracture risk with multiple myeloma: a population-based study. *J Bone Miner Res* 2005; **20**: 487–93.

12. Berruti A, Dogliotti L, Bitossi R, *et al.* Incidence of skeletal complications in patients with bone metastatic prostate cancer and hormone refractory disease. *J Urol* 2000; **164**: 1248–53.

13. Diamond TH, Bucci J, Kersley JH, *et al.* Osteoporosis and spinal fractures in men with prostate cancer: risk factors and effects of androgen deprivation therapy. *J Urol* 2004. **172**: 529–32.

14. Coleman RE. Metastatic bone disease: clinical features, pathophysiology and treatment strategies. *Cancer Treat Rev* 2001; **27**: 165–76.

15. Bilariki K, Anagnostou E, Masse V, *et al.* Low bone mineral density and high incidences of fractures and

vitamin d deficiency in 52 pediatric cancer survivors. *Horm Res Paediatr* 2010; **74**(5): 319–27.

16. Patel B, DeGroot H. Evaluation of the risk of pathologic fractures secondary to metastatic bone disease. *Orthop J* 2001; **24**: 612–17.

17. Una Cidón E. Steroids, cancer and vertebral fractures: a dreaded complication. *J Oncol Pharm Pract* 2011; **17**(3): 279–281.

18. Van Staa TP, Leufkens HG, Abenhaim L, Zhang B, Cooper C. Use of oral corticosteroids and risk of fractures. *J Bone Miner Res* 2000; **15**(6): 993–1000.

19. Silverman SL, Minshall ME, Shen W, Harper KD, Xiw S. The relationship of health-related quality of life to prevalent and incident vertebral fractures in postmenopausal women with osteoporosis: results from the Multiple Outcomes of Raloxifene Evaluation Study. *Arthritis Rheum* 2001; **44**(11): 2611–19.

20. Johnell O. Mortality after osteoporotic fractures. *Osteoporosis Int* 2004; **15**: 38–42.

21. Truumees E. Osteoporosis [Editorial]. *Spine* 2001; **26**: 930–2.

22. Silverman SL. The clinical consequences of vertebral compression fractures. *Bone* 1992; **13**(suppl 2): 27–31.

23. Gaughen JR, Jensen ME, Schweickert PA, *et al.* Lack of preoperative spinous process tenderness does not affect clinical success of percutaneous vertebroplasty. *J Vasc Interv Radiol* 2002; **13**: 1135–8.

24. Soin A, Mekhail N. Minimally invasive procedures for vertebral compression fractures. *Raj's Practical Management of Pain*. 4th ed. Chapter 61. New York: Elsevier Mosby; 2008: 1119–26.

25. Shin JJ, Chin DK, Yoon YS. Percutaneous vertebroplasty for the treatment of osteoporotic burst fractures. *Acta Neurochir (Wien)* 2009 Feb; **151** (2): 141–8.

26. Helfet DL, Kloen P, Anand N, Rosen H. Open reduction and internal fixation of delayed unions and nonunions of fractures of the distal part of the humerus. *J Bone Joint Surg Am* 2003; **85**: 33–40.

27. Gaughen JR, Jensen ME, Schweickert PP, *et al.* Relevance of antecedent venography in percutaneous vertebroplasty for the treatment of osteoporotic compression fractures. *AJNR* 2002; **23**: 594–6.

28. Gangi A, Wong LLS, Guth S, *et al.* Percutaneous vertebroplasty: indications, techniques and results. *Semin Intervent Radiol* 2002; **19**: 265–70.

29. Venmans A, Klazen CA, Lohle PN, *et al.* Percutaneous vertebroplasty and pulmonary cement embolism: results from VERTOS II. *AJNR Am J Neuroradiol* 2010 Sep; **31**(8): 1451–3.

30. Miller JC. *Radiology Grand Rounds Massachusetts General Hospital Department of Radiology* 2009 July; **7**(7).

31. Vallejo R, Benyamin R, Floyd B, *et al.* Percutaneous cement injection into a created cavity for the treatment of vertebral body fracture: preliminary results of a new vertebroplasty technique. *Clin J Pain* 2006; **22**: 182–9.

32. Murphy KJ, Deramond H. Percutaneous vertebroplasty in benign and malignant disease. *Neuroimaging Clin N Am* 2000; **10**: 535–45.

33. Moreland DB, Landi MK, Grand W. Vertebroplasty: techniques to avoid complications. *Spine J* 2001; **1**: 66–71.

34. Hulme P, Kebs J, Ferguson S, Berlemann U. Vertebroplasty and kyphoplasty: a systematic review of 69 clinical studies. *Spine* 2006; **31**: 1983–2001.

35. Fribourg D, Tang C, Sra P, Delamerter R, Bae H. Incidence of subsequent vertebral body fracture after kyphoplasty. *Spine* 2004; **29**(20): 2270–6.

36. Cortet B, Cotton A, Boutry N. Percutaneous vertebroplasty in the treatment of osteoporotic vertebral compression fractures: an open prospective study. *J Rheumatol* 1999; **26**: 2222–8.

37. Schmidt R, Cakir B, Mattes T. Cement leakage during vertebroplasty: an underestimated problem? *Eur Spine J* 2005; **14**: 466–73.

38. Nassbaum DA, Gailloud P, Murphy K. A review of complications associated with vertebroplasty and kyphoplasty as reported to the food and drug administration medical device related website. *J Vasc Interv Radiol* 2004; **15**: 1185–92.

39. Deramond H, Depriester C, Galibert P, *et al.* Percutaneous vertebroplasty with polymethylmethacrylate. Technique, indications, and results. *Radiol Clin North Am* 1998; **36**: 533–46.

40. Truumees E, Hilirand A, Vaccaro AR. Percutaneous vertebral augmentation. *Spine J* 2004; **4**: 218–29.

41. Urrutia J, Bono CM, Mery P, Rojas C. Early histologic changes following polymethylmethacrylate injection (vertebroplasty) in rabbit lumbar vertebrae. *Spine* 2008; **33**(8): 877–82.

42. Hadley C. Abdulreham A, Zoarski GH. Biomechanics of vertebral bone augmentation. *Neuroimaging Clin N Am* 2010; **20**(2): 159–67.

43. Grados F, Depriester C, Cayrolle G, *et al.* Long-term observations of vertebral osteoporotic fractures treated by percutaneous vertebroplasty. *Rheumatology* 2000; **39**(12): 1410–14.

44. Baroud G, Nemes J, Heini P, *et al.* Load shift of the intervertebral disc after a vertebroplasty: a finite-element study. *Eur Spine J* 2003; **12**: 423.

45. Luo J, Adams MA, Dolan P. Vertebroplasty and kyphoplasty can restore normal spine mechanics following osteoporotic vertebral fracture. *J Osteoporos* 2010. doi:10.4061/2010/729257.

46. Ledlie JT, Renfro MB. Kyphoplasty treatment of vertebral fractures: 2 year outcomes show sustained benefits. *Spine* 2006; **31**: 2213–20.

47. Komp M, Ruetten S, Godolias G. Minimally-invasive therapy for functionally unstable osteoporotic vertebral fractures by means of kyphoplasty: prospective comparative study of 19 surgically and 17 conservatively treated patients. *J Miner Stoffwechs* 2004; **11**(Suppl 1): 13–15.

48. Kasperk C, Hillmeier J, Noldge G, et al. Treatment of painful vertebral fractures by kyphoplasty in patients with primary osteoporosis: a prospective nonrandomized controlled study. *J Bone Miner Res* 2005; **20**: 604–12.

49. Mathis JM, Ortiz O, Zoarski GH. Vertebroplasty versus kyphoplasty: a comparison and contrast. *Am J Neuroradiol* 2004; **25**: 840–5.

50. Kumar K, Nguyen R, Bishop S. A comparative analysis of the results of vertebroplasty and kyphoplasty in osteoporotic vertebral compression fractures. *Neurosurgery* 2010 Sep; **67**(3 Suppl Operative): 171–88; discussion 188.

51. Anselmetti GC, Muto M, Guglielmi G, Masala S. Percutaneous vertebroplasty or kyphoplasty. *Radiol Clin North Am.* 2010 May; **48**(3): 641–9.

52. Liu JT, Liao WJ, Tan WC, et al. Balloon kyphoplasty versus vertebroplasty for treatment of osteoporotic vertebral compression fracture: a prospective, comparative, and randomized clinical study. *Osteoporos Int* 2010 Feb; **21**(2): 359–64.

53. Gaitanis IN, Carandang G, Phillips FM, et al. Restoring geometric and loading alignment of the thoracic spine with a vertebral compression fracture: effects of balloon (bone tamp) inflation and spinal extension. *Spine J* 2005; **5**: 45–54.

54. Crandall D, Slaughter D, Hankins PJ, Moore C, Jerman J. Acute vs. chronic vertebral compression fractures with kyphoplasty: early results. *Spine J* 2004; **4**(4): 418–24.

55. Hiwatashi A, Westesson A, Ypshiura T, et al. Kyphoplasty and vertebroplasty produce the same degree of height restoration. *Am J Neuroradiol* Apr 2009; **30**: 669–73.

56. Buchbinder R, Osborne RH, Ebeling PR, et al. Randomized trial of vertebroplasty for painful osteoporotic vertebral fractures. *N Engl J Med* 2009; **361**: 557–68.

57. Kallmes DF, Comstock BA, Heagerty PJ, et al. A randomized trial of vertebroplasty for osteoporotic spinal fractures. *N Engl J Med* 2009; **361**: 569–79.

58. Buchbinder R, Osborne R, Staples M. Correspondence Reply. *N Engl J Med* **361**; 21.

59. Lotz JC. Trials of vertebroplasty for vertebral fractures. *N Engl J Med.* 2009; **361**(21):2098; author reply 2099–100.

8.7 Endoscopic surgery for Chiari malformation type I

Rodolfo Hakim and Xiao Di

Key points

- The symptoms and signs of Chiari I malformation patients can be diverse.
- Patients with Chiari I tend to have a crowded posterior fossa.
- The current surgical techniques proposed for the treatment of symptomatic Chiari I malformation are very diverse among different authors.
- A purely endoscopic decompressive surgery is a novel technique in a minimally invasive modality.

Introduction

The management of Chiari malformation type I (CM I) with less postoperative complications and recurrence continues to pose great challenges to surgeons, especially when associated with syringomyelia.[1,2] Although the complete pathogenic mechanisms are yet to be elucidated, it is widely accepted that either an inborn or an acquired descent of the cerebellar tonsils creates a craniospinal pressure dissociation and an impaired cerebrospinal fluid (CSF) flow due to crowding at the level of the craniovertebral junction (CVJ).[3,4] Consequently, the first line of surgical therapy offered at many institutions is a craniovertebral decompression, usually including suboccipital craniectomy with removal of the posterior arch of the atlas. Sometimes a laminectomy of the axis with or without intradural exploration, reduction of the tonsils, duraplasty, and even a shunt implantation for syringomyelia may be included as part of the surgical treatment. The specific surgical steps in this operation continue to undergo modifications as surgeons attempt to identify the optimum procedure. In addition, postoperative complications including pseudomeningocele, meningitis, CSF leak, intradural adhesions, cerebellar ptosis, and cervical instability have brought about not only failures of the operation but also potentially severe consequences for some of the patients.

In order to simplify and make the surgical decompression less invasive, a novel and entirely endoscopic procedure has been employed for the decompression of Chiari malformation type I.

We describe here a new, minimally invasive technique for removing the subocciput as well as the posterior elements of the cervical vertebrae under direct endoscopic visualization. The aim of this procedure is to ameliorate as much as possible the clinical symptoms. This is done by enlarging the foramen magnum and vicinity and thereby facilitating the flow of CSF at the CVJ.

Clinical manifestations of Chiari I

The symptoms and the clinical presentation of Chiari I malformation are diverse. Although headache is the most common symptom, ocular, otoneurologic, brainstem, lower cranial nerve, cerebellar, and spinal cord disorders may occur as well. The headache is more common in the suboccipital region; its description can range from a light pressure to intense pounding that can radiate upward to the vertex or all the way to the retroorbital region as well as downward to the neck and shoulders. It usually intensifies when lowering the head's position and with Valsalva maneuvers.

The ocular symptoms that can occur in Chiari I patients are phosphenes, photophobia, blurred vision, diplopia, visual field cuts, and visual blackouts. Funduscopic examination may reveal bilateral papilledema as well as decreased or absent venous pulsations. Among the otoneurologic symptoms, one may find dizziness, vertigo, loss of equilibrium, oscillopsia, tinnitus, nausea and vomiting, and hypo- or hyperacusia. On examination, rotary, lateral, and/or downbeat nystagmus may be found.[2,5–26]

The symptoms correlated with the brainstem, lower cranial nerves, and the cerebellum that can be described by the patient are sleep apnea, syncope, shortness of breath, dysphagia, dysarthria, facial pain or numbness, throat pain, palpitations, hoarseness, incoordination, tremor, and decreased fine motor function. On examination, one may find facial hypoesthesia, trigeminal and/or glossopharyngeal neuralgia, glossal atrophy,

an impaired gag reflex, vocal cord paralysis, decreased trapezius muscle strength, dysmetria, and truncal and apendicular ataxia.

With regard to the spinal cord, the symptoms occurring from anterior cord compression, posterior cord compression, or a cord syrinx are motor (atrophy, spasticity, and muscle weakness) or sensory (anesthesia, hypoalgesia, hyperesthesia, burning dysesthesia, decreased temperature sensation, and decreased positional sense). Also, urinary and/or fecal incontinence as well as impotence are described. On examination, scoliosis, muscle weakness, muscle atrophy, decreased fine-motor ability, trophic phenomena, hyper- or hyporeflexia, Babinski sign, and dissociated sensory loss may be found.

Pathophysiology

Although it is difficult to assess, patients with Chiari I malformation seem to share a common denominator which is a tight or crowded posterior fossa. It has been suggested that this is a disorder of the para-axial mesoderm in which the posterior fossa is underdeveloped and therefore its normally developed contents are tight or overcrowded.[10] With time, the result can be a "downward squeeze" of the normally developed hindbrain through the foramen magnum establishing as an anatomical cerebellar tonsillar herniation. The clinical manifestations may be due to direct compression of the nearby nervous structures and probably from a caudal and cephalad restricted CSF flow through the foramen magnum. A genetic component with autosomal dominant or recessive inheritance has been documented in those families where more than one member has a Chiari I.

Interestingly, a "secondary" or "acquired" form of Chiari I is sometimes found in patients with pseudotumor cerebri, posterior fossa lesions with mass effect, hydrocephalus, central nervous system infections, multiple lumbar punctures, spinal CSF fistulas, and/or lumboperitoneal shunts.[27–29]

Surgical technique

General anesthesia is induced in the patient using endotracheal intubation. The neck should be kept in neutral position during intubation and positioning especially in those patients with a tight craniocervical junction, brainstem or spinal cord compression, or with a syrinx. Venous and arterial lines are placed. It is very important to have a constant arterial pressure as well as heart rate monitoring throughout the head pinning and patient positioning as well as during surgery; inadvertent pressure, trauma, or ischemia over the brainstem and spinal cord can usually be suspected by sudden bradycardia and hypotension. Also, it must be kept in mind that besides the neural structures involved and exposed during the procedure, the vertebral arteries are near or within the surgical field and therefore can be inadvertently injured as well. Electrophysiological monitoring such as somatosensory and/or motor evoked potentials are utilized throughout the case, more so in those patients with any of the following: articular instability/ligamentous laxity, tight craniocervical junction, the presence of a syrinx, progressive neurologic deficit, or any signs of brainstem involvement. Broad-spectrum antibiotics are given for 24 hours after surgery; the first dose is given ideally at least 30 minutes (but not more than 60 minutes) prior to skin incision. Cefazolin is our first choice antibiotic although, if the patient is allergic, we usually use vancomycin as an option. All patients will have a Foley catheter placed. Diuretics are not used routinely. We try to stay away from the use of steroids to avoid their side effects. Since most of our patients are healthy individuals except for their Chiari malformation, we try to keep their perioperative management as physiological as possible.

A Mayfield frame is pinned to the patient's head while the patient is supine. The frame with pediatric-size pins is used on patients younger than 10 years of age; other adult-size pins are used on patients. The single-pin arm of the frame is preferably positioned on the right side of the head (nondominant hemisphere) and the double-pin arm is positioned on the left (dominant side). From the physics point of view there is less likelihood of penetrating the inner cranial bone table on the side with the two pins. This is because the pressure exerted by the two-pin side is distributed between the two pins, while on the one-pin side the same but opposite pressure will be distributed to only one pin. Therefore, the probability of injury occuring (such as a dural tear, epidural and/or subdural hematoma, brain contusion, cortical vascular injury, etc.) from a perforating pin on the dominant side would be less. One pin from each side of the frame is positioned slightly below the cephalic equator (toward the frontal direction instead of the occipital), thereby providing support for the weight of the head and the pressure exerted over it during the surgery. The patient is then placed in the prone position over two chest rolls, one on each side of the chest; these are placed underneath the patient

and longitudinally to the body's axis to secure good expansion of the chest and therefore facilitate adequate ventilation. Emphasis on making sure that the shoulders are being supported by the chest rolls is important; this provides more stability and therefore decreases unnecessary torque and pull on the neck. Also, it is not uncommon for patients to complain of shoulder, lower neck, and interscapular postoperative pain when the unsupported shoulders have been pulling forward by gravity. In female patients, the breasts should be positioned within the space between the chest rolls so that they are free from pressure points.

Although a moderate neck flexion definitely facilitates surgical exposure in most cases, a slightly anteflexed or even neutral head position provides us with an approach to the CVJ, especially when the patient's condition does not allow the neck adequate flexion. As a general rule a minimum distance of about two finger widths should exist between the jaw and the sternum when flexing the head. One must keep in mind that overflexion poses risks for vascular, spinal cord, and brainstem injuries in an already tight craniocervical space, as well as decreased venous jugular blood flow and compromise of the airway or endotracheal tube obstruction.

The last checkpoint in the patient positioning phase is to observe the inclination of the head in relation to the heart on the horizontal axis: we usually tilt the head of the bed upward to a point where the head is at or slightly above the level of the heart and the operative field is nearly parallel to the floor. This will facilitate venous drainage and therefore keep facial edema to a minimum, as well as decreasing intraoperative bone and venous bleeding.

Once the patient is prepped and draped, a 2 cm longitudinal midline skin incision is made from the superior portion of the spinous process of the axis to the CVJ. This is an important strategic position, allowing a surgical trajectory to cover the C1 laminae and the subocciput. The subcutaneous tissue is divided along the incision line. Muscle splitting and dissection are performed along the midline in a cranial direction, exposing first the lower edge of the foramen magnum. Afterwards, the posterior arch of the atlas is exposed once the inferior capitis rectus minor muscles are resected bilaterally from the posterior tubercle of C1. These are the only muscles resected in this procedure. The next step consists in performing a small craniectomy (2 cm in the rostrocaudal diameter and 3–4 cm in the lateralateral diameter) on the occiput at

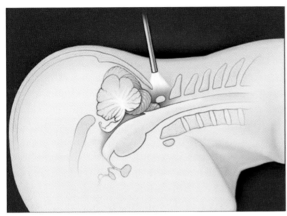

Figure 8.22 The endoscopic panoramic field of view fits well in the craniovertebral junction angle.

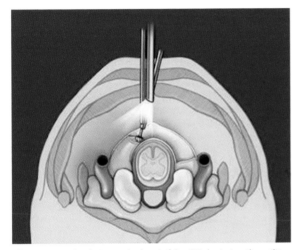

Figure 8.23 Axial view at the level of the CVJ depicting the utility of the 30° endoscope in bilateral corner trimming of the foramen magnum and the C1 laminae.

the level of the foramen magnum. This step is visually accomplished with the 0-degree endoscope (Fig. 8.22). Afterwards, a C1 laminectomy is performed; its width is approximately the same as the width of the occipital craniectomy.

A high-speed drill (Midas-Rex drill; Medtronic, USA) and Kerrison punch are used to remove the bone and to maximally widen the craniectomy on the foramen rim as well as to extend laterally the laminectomy on C1 to the condyles and the lateral masses on each side. This latter step is done under direct visualization using a 30° endoscope (Fig. 8.23). Once there is a sufficient bony decompression at the CVJ, then the atlantooccipital membrane is resected thus exposing the dura mater. Afterwards, the external layer of the CVJ dura is incised (dural splitting). Intraoperative ultrasound is applied to assess CSF flow at the CVJ and from the foramen of Magendie, thereby determining whether any further adjunctive procedure such as dural opening is needed. For those patients who require an intradural procedure such as a cerebellar tonsillectomy for further decompression, the dura is left open. Although procedures such as duroplasty and plugging of the obex are sometimes performed in conventional Chiari surgery, they are not used in endoscopic Chiari surgery.

The entire surgical procedure is performed under the assistance of video monitoring. After adequate decompression has been achieved, the muscle fascia and the skin are suture-closed and small Steristrips are applied. Patients who undergo this procedure stay in the hospital between 1 and 3 days, although the majority leave on postoperative day 2.

Advantages of the endoscopic technique

The treatment of symptomatic Chiari malformation with surgery has been widely recommended, although the surgical techniques proposed are extremely diverse.[30–32] Some authors favor cervical decompression only, without any decompression of the posterior fossa.[33] Others support suboccipital and cervical bone decompression with durotomy,[34] limited occipital decompression with durotomy and C1 laminectomy,[35] dissection of arachnoidal adhesions when present, exploration of the fourth ventricle,[36] and plugging of the obex if hydromyelia is present.[37] Yet others have advocated that in addition to occipital craniectomy, C1 laminectomy, durotomy, and duroplasty should also be performed.[34] Other authors include in the surgical treatment durotomy but without duroplasty.[38] Yet others suggest that coagulation of the cerebellar tonsils should also be performed.[39] To date, no optimal standard treatment procedure for Chiari malformation has been commonly accepted except for a consensus that bony decompression is essential for any of the adjunct procedures such as a duroplasty, shrinkage or resection of the cerebellar tonsils, obex plugging, syringostomy, or shunting for syringomyelia. There has been a marked trend in recent years among several surgeons to attempt to simplify the procedure with bony decompression only, with dural splitting instead of dural opening, or with simple dural opening without duraplasty and without manipulation of the cerebellar tonsils or syrinx.[35,40] The endoscopic Chiari decompressive procedure, as described in this

155

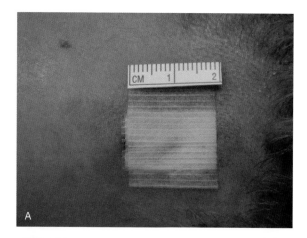

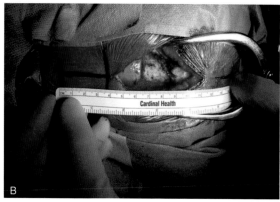

Figure 8.24 An advantage of the endoscopic technique over conventional open surgery is the fact that less superficial and deep tissue dissection and trauma is necessary in order to achieve adequate surgical exposure. The patient in (A) had an endoscopic Chiari decompression. After the wound is closed, the sutured skin is covered with Steristrips. The patient in (B) had previous open surgery for Chiari decompression. Three years later the symptoms (headache and neck pain) persisted. CT and MRI studies showed that further bilateral bone removal was necessary in the foramen magnum and in C1. The photograph was taken at the time of the second surgery. The black marking line, which extends above and below the surgical wound, shows the extent of the scar from the first surgery.

chapter, was introduced on the basis of the principles of simplicity and minimal invasiveness.

The natural angle of the CVJ is optimal since the panoramic view of the endoscope can easily cover an area extending from the occiput to the C1 lamina (Fig. 8.22). With this wide-angle field of view, bony decompression can readily be performed from the lower third of the occiput and the C1 laminae to the upper portion of the C2 laminae, under direct 0-degree endoscopic visualization. The 30° endoscope is especially useful for looking in more detail bilaterally at the corners of the posterior rim of the foramen magnum and C1 laminae,

and therefore enabling one to maximally drill and safely widen them. This is an advantage that the endoscopic technique has over both conventional and microscopic surgeries since, in order to achieve this in the latter two types of surgeries, a sufficiently lengthy incision and a traumatically wide tissue dissection and exposure need to be obtained in the first place (Fig. 8.24).

Another intraoperative tool that has been useful in the endoscopic technique is ultrasonography. The use of ultrasound was previously described by Milhorat and is useful in some of the conventional surgeries as well. It was adopted to detect the motion of the cerebellar tonsils (using monochrome video imaging) as well as the biphasic CSF flow around the CMJ (using color video imaging).[41]

Conclusion

We have briefly described a new endoscopic technique for decompressing the CMJ. This technique is minimally invasive and is associated with an excellent clinical outcome.

Compared with conventional open surgery, endoscopic decompressive surgery is considered to be less invasive because of the following. (1) Patient neck flexion is not as critical as it is in conventional Chiari surgery. This is important especially in patients who have difficulty flexing their neck. (2) The skin incision is as small as 2 cm in length. (3) There is minimal injury of the CMJ muscles and ligaments, thereby minimizing the instability of the CMJ.

References

1. Holly LT, Batzdorf U. Management of cerebellar ptosis following craniovertebral decompression for Chiari I malformation. *J Neurosurg* 2001 Jan; **94**(1): 21–6.

2. Milhorat TH, Chou MW, Trinidad EM, *et al.* Chiari I malformation redefined: clinical and radiographic findings for 364 symptomatic patients. *Neurosurgery* 1999; **44**(5): 1005–17.

3. Schijman E. History, anatomic forms, and pathogenesis of Chiari I malformations. *Childs Nerv Syst* 2004; **20**(5): 323–8.

4. Sgouros S, Kountouri M, Natarajan K. Posterior fossa volume in children with Chiari malformation Type I. *J Neurosurg* 2006 **105** (2 Suppl Pediatrics): 101–6.

5. Cockerhamn K, Bejjani G, Monya D. The role of spontaneous venous pulsations in the diagnosis of adult Chiari malformation. *Internet J Neurol* 2009; **10**(2).

6. Aboulezz AO, Sartor K, Geyer CA, Gado MH. Position of cerebellar tonsils in the normal population and

in patients with Chiari malformation: a quantitative approach to MR imaging. *J Comput Assist Tomogr* 1985; **9**: 1033–6.

7. Barkovich AJ, Wippold FJ, Sherman JL, Citrin CM. Significance of cerebellar tonsillar position on MR. *AJNR* 1986: **7**: 795–9.

8. Meadow J, Kraut M, Guarnieri M, Haroun RI, Carson BS. Asymptomatic Chiari type I malformations identified on magnetic resonance imaging. *J Neurosurg* 2000; **92**: 920–6.

9. Mikulis DJ, Diaz O, Egglin TK, Sanchez R. Variance of the position of the cerebellar tonsils with age: preliminary report. *Radiology* 1992; **183**: 725–8.

10. Saez RJ, Onofrio BM, Yanagihara T. Experience with Arnold-Chiari malformation: 1960–1970. *J Neurosurg* 1976; **45**:416–422.

11. Pillay PK, Awad IA, Little JR, Hahn JF. Symptomatic Chiari malformation in adults: a new classification based on magnetic resonance imaging with clinical and prognostic significance. *Neurosurgery* 1991: **28**: 639–45.

12. Giuseffi V, Wall M. Siegel PZ, Rojas PB. Symptoms and disease associations in idiopathic intracranial hypertension (pseudotumor cerebri): a case–control study. *Neurology* 1991; **41**: 239–43.

13. Round R, Keane JR. The minor symptoms of increased intracranial pressure: 101 patients with benign intracranial hypertension. *Neurology* 1988; **38**: 1461–4.

14. Bortoluzzi M, Dilauro L, Marini G. Benign intracranial hypertension with spinal and radicular pain. *J Neurosurg* 1982; **57**: 833–6.

15. Groves MD, McCutcheon IE, Ginsberg LE, Athanassios P. Radicular pain can be a symptom of elevated intracranial pressure. *Neurology* 1999; **52**: 1093–5.

16. Mueller DM, Oro JJ. Prospective analysis of presenting symptoms among 265 patients with radiographic evidence of Chiari malformation type I with or without syringomyelia. *Am Acad Nurse Pract* 2004; **16**(3): 134–8.

17. Levin BE: The clinical definition of spontaneous pulsations of the retinal veins. *Arch Neurol* 1978; **35**: 37–40.

18. Marcellis J, Silberstein SD. Idiopathic intracranial hypertension without papilledema. *Arch Neurol* 1991; **48**: 392–9.

19. Radhakrishnan K, Ahlskog JE, Garrity JA, Kurland LT. Subject Review – Idiopathic intracranial hypertension. *Mayo Clin Proc* 1994; **69**: 169–80.

20. Sullivan HC. Fatal tonsillar herniation in pseudotumor cerebri. *Neurology* 1991; **41**: 1142–4.

21. Wang SJ, Silberstein SD, Patterson S, Young WB. Idiopathic intracranial hypertension without papilledema. A case control study in a headache center. *Neurology* 1998; **51**: 245–9.

22. Aguiar PH, Tella OI, Pereira CU, Godinho, F, Simm R. Chiari type I presenting as left glossopharyngeal neuralgia with cardiac syncope. *Neurosurg Rev* 2002; **25**(1–2): 99–102.

23. Inoue M, *et al.* Idiopathic scoliosis as a presenting sign of familial neurologic abnormalities. *Spine* 2003; **28**: 40–45.

24. Bunc G, Vorsic M. Presentation of a previously asymptomatic Chiari I Malformation by a flexion injury to the neck. *J Neurotrauma* 2001; **18**(6): 645–8.

25. Vaphiades MS, Eggenberger ER, Miller NR, Frohman L, Krisht A. Resolution of papilledema after neurosurgical decompression for primary Chiari I malformation. *Am J Ophthalmol* 2002; **133**: 673–8.

26. Kumar A, Patni AH, Charbel F. The Chiari I malformation and the neurotologist. *Otol Neurotol* 2002; **23**: 727–35.

27. Sathi S, Stieg PE. "Acquired" Chiari I malformation after multiple lumbar punctures: case report. *Neurosurgery* 1993; **32**: 306–9.

28. Welch K, Shillito J, Strand R, Fischer EG, Winston KR. Chiari I malformations – an acquired disorder? *J Neurosurg* 1981; **55**: 604–9.

29. Huang PP, Constantini S. "Acquired" Chiari I malformation. Case report. *J Neurosurg* 1994; **80**: 1099–102.

30. Dyste GN, Menezes AH, Van Gilder JC. Symptomatic Chiari malformations: an analysis of presentation, management, and long-term outcome. *J Neurosurg* 1989; **71**: 159–68.

31. Fischer EG. Posterior fossa decompression for Chiari I deformity, including resection of the cerebellar tonsils. *Childs Nerv Syst* 1995: **11**: 625–9.

32. Gardner WJ, Angel J. The mechanism of syringomyelia and its surgical correction. *Clin Neurosurg* 1959; **6**: 131–40.

33. Parks TS, Hoffman HJ, Cail WS. Arnold–Chiari malformation: manifestations and management. *Neurosurgery: State of the Art Reviews* 1986; **1**: 81–99.

34. Park JK, Gleason PL, Madsen JR, Goumnerova LC, Scott RM. Presentation and management of Chiari I malformation in children. *Pediatr Neurosurg* 1997; **26**: 190–6.

35. Krieger MD, McComb JG, Levy ML. Toward a simpler surgical management of Chiari I malformation in a pediatric population. *Pediatr Neurosurg* 1999; **30**: 113–21.

36. Piatt JH Jr, D'Agostino A. The Chiari malformation: lesions discovered within the fourth ventricle. *Pediatr Neurosurg* 1999; **30**: 79–85.

37. Hoffman HJ, Hendrick EB, Humphreys RP. Manifestations and management of Arnold–Chiari malformation in patients with myelomeningocele. *Childs Brain* 1975; **1**: 255–9.

38. Munshi I, Frim D, Stine-Reyes R, *et al.* Effects of posterior fossa decompression with and without duraplasty on Chiari malformation-associated hydromyelia. *Neurosurgery* 2000; **46**(6): 1384–90.

39. Williams B: Syringomyelia. *Neurosurg Clin N Am* 1990; **13**: 653–85.

40. Yeh DD, Koch B, Crone KR: Intraoperative ultrasonography used to determine the extent of surgery necessary during posterior fossa decompression in children with Chiari malformation Type I. *J Neurosurg* (1 Suppl Pediatrics) 2006; **105**: 26–32.

41. Milhorat TH: Tailored operative technique for Chiari Type I malformation using intraoperative color Doppler ultrasonography. *Neurosurgery* 2003; **53**: 899–906.

8.8 Posterior and anterior thoracic surgery

Matthew Grosso and Michael Steinmetz

Key points

- Surgical teams have a variety of options when approaching the thoracic spine. These options should be considered on the basis of spinal cord pathology, risk of complications, and necessary degree of exposure.
- In general, anterior approaches allow for enhanced exposure but may carry a higher morbidity burden because of manipulation of the abdominal and thoracic cavities.
- The T4 to T8 spinal cord is at particular risk for ischemia because of relatively reduced perfusion.
- Posterior approaches are often indicated for fractures or spondylosis of the posterior spinal elements, and/or spinal cord compression with minimal anterior column involvement.
- The costotransversectomy and lateral extracavitary approaches are posterolateral approaches that allow exposure of both anterior and posterior aspects of the thoracic spine, but require longer operating time and surgical expertise.

Introduction

The thoracic spine is susceptible to trauma fractures, spinal metastases, primary bone and meningeal tumors, bacterial infection, disc herniations, and a variety of rheumatic diseases, all which can lead to neurologic symptoms as a result of radiculopathy or myelopathy. A variety of surgical techniques have been developed for exposure of the thoracic spine. These approaches provide the surgeon with a diversity of options so that optimal exposure and flexibility can be achieved for each patient's specific pathology. In addition, each technique has its own risks and associated complications that an experienced surgical team must be familiar with.

Critical vasculature to the thoracic spine

The spinal cord is supplied by one anterior and two posterior spinal arteries. In the thoracic region, the radicular arteries contribute to the spinal arteries. These arteries are originally derived from the segmental vessels originating from the aorta. Each segmental artery divides into an intercostal and a dorsal branch. The dorsal branch passes lateral to the intervertebral foramen to give off the spinal branch, which further divides into the anterior and posterior radicular arteries. The majority of these smaller radicular arteries supply the meninges, and only a small portion reaches the spinal cord itself. However, at various vertebral levels, the segmental arteries also give rise to longitudinally oriented radicular arteries called segmental medullary arteries. These vessels reinforce the longitudinal blood supply of the spinal cord. The largest of these segmental medullary arteries is the artery of Adamkiewicz, which arises in the lower thoracic or upper lumbar area. Two other segmental medullary vessels, usually around the T1 and T7 vertebral areas, provide the major blood supply for the thoracic cord. It is important to note that there is considerable variation in the presence and location of these arteries, and that the region from

T4 to T8 is a particularly vulnerable zone because of relatively decreased perfusion. This watershed zone is thus vulnerable to ischemic complications. Spinal cord ischemia and resulting paraplegia following unilateral interruption of the blood supply to the thoracic cord, including for the artery of Adamkiewicz, are very rare. However, bilateral disruption can lead to neurologic deficits including paraplegia and paraparesis. Causes of bilateral disruption include aortic aneurism rupture or repair, aortic dissection, and decreased aortic perfusion. Methods to reduce ischemic complications caused by bilateral segmental vessel disruption include steps to avoid hypotension and/or anemia, limit the sacrifice of segmental vessels especially the artery of Adamkiewicz, and increase spinal cord perfusion pressure by the diversion of cerebrospinal fluid drainage.[1] There is lower risk for ischemia associated with posterior spinal approaches compared with the anterior spine. For the more invasive costotransversectomy and lateral extracavitary approaches, it may be appropriate to obtain a spinal angiogram to avoid sacrificing critical segmental vessels.

Anterior approaches

Anterior approaches to the thoracic spine can allow optimal visualization and access to the anterior spinal structures. However, these approaches present a challenge because of the significant obstacles to exposure as a result of a crowded thoracic cavity. Anterior approaches are most often indicated for trauma fractures of the vertebral bodies, osteomyelitis, vertebral body tumors, midline disc herniations, and fixed kyphoscoliotic deformities.[2–4]

There are three general categories for anterior approaches to the thoracic spine. Choosing the appropriate strategy depends upon the spinal level, as well as the underlying pathology.

For anterior pathologies at the cervicothoracic junction, a transmanubrial approach is most often indicated. This technique allows for exposure of C5–T3 vertebrae. Below T3 (or T2 depending upon the patient), the great vessels of the mediastinum prevent further access. The anterior cervical exposure aspect of the approach is usually performed from the left side because of a lower incidence of laryngeal nerve nonrecurrence, and thus reduced potential for injury, compared with the right. The patient is placed in a supine position with the head turned away from the side of the approach, and the neck slightly extended. The operative approach to this strategy begins with a skin incision 1–2 cm above the left clavicle that extends from the lateral border of the sternocleidomastoid to the midline of the jugular notch. The incision is then extended vertically and caudally half way down the sternum. The platysma muscle is mobilized and divided in the direction of the incision. Dissection of the superficial and middle layers of the cervical fascia allows mobilization of the strap muscles and sternocleidomastoid. The sternocleidomastoid and jugular vein are mobilized laterally, and the sternohyoid and sternothyroid medially. Prior to resection of the manubrium, the sternohyoid muscle is detached from its sternal and clavicular insertion sites. The manubrium is then cut using a power saw or drill, and brought down to the level of the sternal angle. Following opening of the manubrium, the pleura is carefully dissected on both sides and retracted. Blunt dissection medial to the carotid sheath is recommended to move inferiorly to the prevertebral fascia. Sharp division of this fascia allows for placement of retractors to move the carotid sheath laterally and the tracheoesophageal structures medially, providing optimal exposure of anterior spinal elements. Significant concerns with the transmanubrial approach involve potential damage to the carotid sheath, esophagus, and trachea. Proper precautions must also be taken to avoid damage to the external jugular vein, recurrent laryngeal nerve, and medial branches of the supraclavicular nerves. From a left-sided approach, a thoracic duct injury is also possible. Depending on the degree of exposure achieved following the supraclavicular incision, a median sternotomy may not be necessary.[5]

Exposure of the anterior T2–T12 vertebral levels may be safely achieved through a standard thoracotomy approach. The entire vertebral body may be isolated. Decompression of the spinal cord and anterior instrumentation may be applied from this approach. The first step when choosing a thoracotomy is determining the rib levels. This decision is made based on the pathologic process. It is recommended that for pathologies that require direct anterior exposure, the incision is made one or two levels above the vertebral level of pathology to give adequate exposure while working down the lesion.[6] Alternatively, fluoroscopy may be used to place the incision optimally over the pathology. The primary advantages of this approach include a direct ventral multilevel exposure and bilateral ventral access for decompression.

Thoracotomy requires placement of the patient in the lateral decubitus position, with special care taken to

159

Table 8.7 Indications, advantages, and disadvantages of approaches to thoracic spine surgery

Approach	Type	Indications	Advantages	Disadvantages
Anterior	Transmanubrial	Exposure of C5–T3 vertebral bodies Anterior compression of the spinal cord Anterior instrumentation	Allows access to the lower cervical and upper thoracic vertebra	Possible damage to the carotid sheath, esophagus, trachea, and recurrent laryngeal nerve
	Thoracotomy	Exposure of T2–L2 vertebral bodies and pedicles Anterior compression of the spinal cord or anterior release for scoliosis Anterior instrumentation	Multilevel ventrolateral exposure An alternative **retropleural approach** avoids pulmonary compromise but limits exposure levels	Pulmonary compromise, and spinal cord ischemia
	Thoracoabdominal	Exposure of T10–L4 vertebral bodies and pedicles Anterior compression of the spinal cord Anterior instrumentation	Multilevel ventrolateral exposure at the thoracolumbar junction	Pulmonary compromise, diaphragmatic detachment, manipulation of two body cavities
Posterior	Dorsal midline	Exposure of posterior elements of T1–L5 Laminectomy or fusion of posterior elements Posterior instrumentation	Safe and simple procedure with low morbidity	Limited to exposure of posterior elements and posterior spinal cord
	Transpedicular	Exposure of posterior elements of T1–L5, and access to the posterolateral vertebral disc and a portion of the vertebral body Herniated disc removal and vertebral body biopsy	Safe and simple procedure with low morbidity Alternative **transfacet approach** removes the facet but preserves the pedicle to maintain spinal stability	Limited to exposure of posterolateral disc space
Posterolateral	Costotransversectomy	Exposure of posterior elements of T1–L5, and large portion of vertebral disc and body Vertebral body resection, spinal fusions, and certain types of anterior and posterior decompression Posterior instrumentation	Simultaneous access of anterior and posterior spine without complication of anterior approaches	Anterior instrumentation is not possible Limited exposure of anterior elements as compared with anterior approaches Large soft tissue exposure Possible intrusion of pleural sac
	Lateral extracavitary	Exposure of posterior elements of T1–L5, and access to large portion of vertebral disc and body Corpectomies, and posterior decompression Posterior instrumentation	Simultaneous access of anterior and posterior spine without complication of anterior approaches More lateral exposure compared with costotransversectomy allows superior visualization of thecal sac	Significant operating time and technically demanding Possible intrusion of pleural sac

support the axilla and other areas susceptible to pressure damage. A right or left thoracotomy may be used. The decision is based largely upon the location of the pathology and the surgeon's experience. Above T9 a right-sided approach is often utilized to avoid manipulating the aorta, while below T9 the spine is usually approached from the left to avoid the liver. In general a left-sided thoracotomy may be easier due to the ease of manipulation of the aorta. An incision is made along the predetermined intercostal level from the lateral border of the paraspinous musculature to the costochondral junction. Rib exposure is achieved by sectioning of the appropriate thoracic musculature according to the rib level. The periosteum of the rib is exposed, scored with cautery, and elevated off the rib surface; then a portion of the rib, as far posteriorly as necessary, is removed using a rib cutter. Entry into the chest is achieved by cutting through the parietal pleura. Once entry into the pleural cavity has been achieved, a retractor is placed to spread the ribs, and the lung is manually deflated. A double-lumen endotracheal tube is recommended to facilitate lung retraction in unilateral ventilation. This achieves exposure of the ventrolateral aspect of the vertebral column for decompression via corpectomy and discectomy, and placement of instrumentation (Table 8.7). During closure, the parietal pleura is reconnected with sutures, and the lung is reinflated. Disadvantages associated with this approach include a higher morbidity accompanying pulmonary compromise, the need for thoracostomy drainage tubes, and the possibility of spinal cord ischemia when approaching from the left side caused by damage to the major radiculomedullary artery of Adamkiewics.[7] There is also a moderate risk for pain syndrome to develop such as intercostal neuralgia, and a possibility for shoulder pathology. An alternative retropleural approach to the T2–T10 vertebrae avoids the morbidity associated with pleural cavity entry, but provides limited exposure to multiple levels.

For pathologies at the thoracolumbar junction, a variety of thoracoabdominal approaches may be used. Approaches to this junction are complicated by the presence of the diaphragm. This dome-shaped muscle originates on the lower six ribs and inserts onto a variety of structures caudally that include the tip of the T12 rib, the L1 transverse process, the medial arcuate ligaments, and the anterior vertebral lumbar column via the diaphragmatic crus. Once again, patients are placed in the lateral decubitus position. Rib incisions for this approach vary depending on the level of pathology, but T10–T12 is most common. These incisions are brought more ventrally than their thoracotomy counterparts. For an incision at the 10th rib, removal of the rib and splitting of the costal cartilage exposes the retroperitoneal space. Blunt dissection of the peritoneum off the inferior aspect of the diaphragm allows for direct exposure of the abdominal musculature (Fig. 8.25A). The diaphragm can then be opened with cuts at its peripheral attachment of the costal margin, lateral arcuate ligament, and medial arcuate ligament at the L1 transverse process (Fig. 8.25B). Once the medial posterior diaphragm is free from its attachments, exposure of anterolateral thoracolumbar elements is achieved. This approach has similar complications as the thoracotomy approach related to pulmonary compromise and

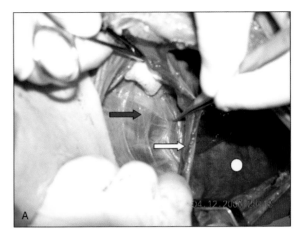

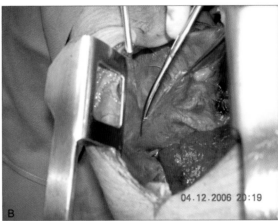

Figure 8.25 Diaphragmatic exposure for the thoracoabdominal approach. (A) After removal of the 10th rib, the internal oblique and transverse abdominis muscles are split to identify the peritoneum (blue arrow). The peritoneum is being dissected from the undersurface of the diaphragm (white arrow). The pleural cavity is indicated by a white dot. (B) The diaphragm is being split with an approximately 1 cm lateral margin.

the need for a thoracostomy drainage tube. In addition, this approach carries risks associated with diaphragm detachment and the manipulation of two major body cavities. A more medial cutting of the diaphragm may compromise the innervation of this muscle thus leading to hemidiaphragm paralysis.

Posterior approaches

Posterior approaches to the spine can be divided into the posterolateral and true posterior approaches. The posterolateral approaches include the extracavitary and costotransversectomy techniques. The standard posterior strategies consist of the midline (laminectomy) and transpedicular approaches. In general, posterior strategies carry a lower mortality burden than anterior strategies because they do not normally involve disruption of the thoracic and abdominal cavities. They are most often indicated for fractures or spondylosis of the posterior spinal elements, and spinal cord compression with minimal anterior components due to a variety of pathologies.[8]

Choosing the appropriate approach depends on the lateral angle desired for anterior vertebral access. The midline approach is a common technique used most often used for a laminectomy or fusion of the posterior spine elements, with or without instrumentation. Decompressive laminectomies are only useful for pathology that causes posterior compression of the spinal cord. If simultaneous anterior compression exists, another strategy or multiple approaches must be utilized. Patients are placed in the prone position and an incision is made along the midline of the back, using the spinous processes as guidance. The incision is made to the deep thoracic fascia, so that the transverse processes are visible. The paraspinous muscles are stripped bilaterally to expose the posterior spine. Precautions should be taken to preserve the facet capsules unless fusion is warranted. After proper exposure is achieved, laminectomy can be performed. The more lateral the laminectomy, the greater the concern for disruption of the epidural venous plexus, which can lead to excessive bleeding.[1] Moreover, excessive removal of the facet joints may lead to iatrogenic instability. The midline approach is a relatively safe and simple procedure, but is limited in its exposure of anything but the most posterior spinal elements and posterior cord.[8]

The transpedicular approach was first described by Patterson and Arbit as an alternative method to remove a herniated thoracic disc from the spinal canal.[9] In this approach, a midline incision is made at the level of interest, followed by mobilization of the paraspinal musculature on the side of interest. Once one-sided exposure of the facet joint is achieved, a high-speed drill may be used to remove the entire facet joint and associated pedicle. This provides access to the intervertebral space for disc removal. The exiting nerve root may be sacrificed to improve access. Care must be taken to prevent spinal fluid leakage following sacrifice. The authors prefer to place a titanium clip proximal to the dorsal root ganglion prior to severing the nerve. In addition, a portion of the anterolateral vertebral body can be removed if warranted. The transpedicular approach is a simple, relatively safe procedure, but is limited in its exposure of the anterior vertebral elements. The transfacet approach is a variation of this strategy that

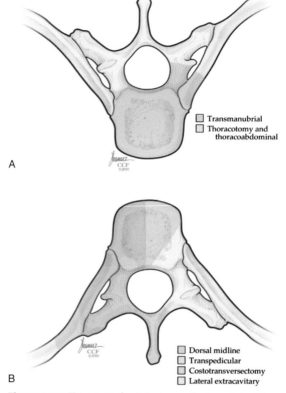

Figure 8.26 The extent of vertebral access for the anterior (A) and posterior (B) thoracic spine approaches. Each approach color highlights the *additional* area covered and includes the shaded area in transpedicular (green) and dorsal midline approach (red), but not the lateral extracavitary (purple).

removes the facet but preserves the pedicle to maintain spinal stability.

Posterolateral approaches allow exposure of the lateral aspects of the thoracic vertebrae, including the vertebral body, without invading the pleural cavity (Fig. 8.26B). The costotransversectomy was originally developed to drain spine abscesses in tuberculosis patients. The approach allows this dorsolateral exposure, but is much more limited compared to the thoracotomy. Today, the approach may also be used for a partial vertebral body resection, a variety of spinal fusions, and certain types of anterior and posterior decompression. For anterior pathologies, a thoracotomy may be preferred, but the costotransversectomy approach is often used for high-risk patients because of its lower morbidity or when anterior decompression is to be combined with posterior fixation. The patient is usually placed in the prone position, although the lateral decubitus position is used as well. A paramedian or curvilinear incision is made 5–8 cm from the midline, with the rib to be exposed centered along the line. Subcutaneous fat and muscle is dissected to expose the appropriate rib. The trapezius, latissimus dorsi, and paraspinous muscles all must be dissected for exposure of the thoracic spine. An incision in the rib is performed using a rib cutter 6 to 8 cm from the costovertebral articulation, and disarticulation is achieved by removing the appropriate costotransverse ligaments. Care should be taken to avoid cutting the neurovascular bundle at the inferior aspect of the rib. Following disarticulation, the transverse process is removed. Once the sympathetic trunk and parietal pleura are elevated, pedicle, facet, and vertebral body dissection can be performed. A disadvantage to this procedure is possible complications related to the large soft tissue exposure such as secondary blood loss and postoperative pain. In addition, the surgical team must also be ready for accidental intrusion into the pleural cavity.

The lateral extracavitary approach is considered a modification of the costotransversectomy. It differs primarily in its route past the paraspinal muscles. This approach provides appropriate exposure to perform corpectomies, posterior decompression, and posterior instrumentation in one procedure. The patient is placed in the prone position. A midline incision is made three spinous processes above to three spinous processes below the desired vertebral level, and then the incision is curved to form a "hockey stick" cut. A standard subperiosteal dissection to the transverse processes is performed. The trapezius and rhomboid muscles are dissected off the spinous processes to form a musculocutaneous flap, and the paraspinal muscles are retracted medially, exposing the posterior spine and rib cage. For vertebral body exposure, the corresponding rib and the rib immediately below are removed in a similar fashion to that described in the costotransversectomy. The intercostal nerves and arteries should be followed to the vertebral foramen, which will allow for identification of the pedicle. The pedicle can be removed using a high-speed drill, allowing exposure of the spinal canal, dural sac, and lateral aspect of the vertebral body. The primary advantages of this approach are superior visualization of the thecal sac and combined anterior and posterior exposure. However, the approach requires significant operating time and is technically demanding, leading to increased morbidities when compared with other approaches.[10] As in the costotransversectomy, the surgical team must also be prepared for minor and major pleural injuries.

Conclusion

Today's surgeon has a diversity of procedures to choose from when confronted with thoracic spine pathology. Location of pathology, degree of decompression, desired fusion location, risk of complications, and need for instrumentation are all important factors when deciding on a surgical approach. The unique anatomy of the thoracic spine and its proximity to the vital structures of the thoracic cavity make a thorough understanding of the anatomy and a cohesive surgical team essential to a safe and successful surgery.

References

1. Stambough JL. Thoracic spine: anterior. In: Herkowitz H, ed. *Rothman-Simeone. The Spine.* Philadelphia: Elsevier; 2006: 1459–85.

2. Cook WA. Transthoracic vertebral surgery. *Ann Thorac Surg* 1971; **12**(1): 54–68.

3. Hodgson AR, Stock FE. Anterior spinal fusion. A preliminary communication on the radical treatment of Pott's disease and Pott's paraplegia. 1956. *Clin Orthop Relat Res* 1994 (300): 16–23.

4. Woodard E. Surgical exposures of the thoracic and thoracolumbar spine. In: Benzel E, Stillerman C, eds. *The Thoracic Spine.* St. Louis, MO: Quality Medical Publishing; 1999: 208–26.

5. Papdopoulos SM, Fessler R. Thoracic spine. In: *Spine Surgery: Techniques, Complication Avoidance, and Management.* Philadelphia: Churchill Livingston; 2004: 281–93.

6. Watkins R. Thoracic spine: anterior. In: Herkowitz H, ed. *Rothman-Simeone. The Spine.* Philadelphia: Elsevier; 2006: 290–307.

7. Ikard RW. Methods and complications of anterior exposure of the thoracic and lumbar spine. *Arch Surg* 2006; **141**(10): 1025–34.

8. Lee D, Lemma M, Kostuik J. Surgical approaches to the thoracic and thoracolumbar spine. In: Frymoyer J, Wiesel S, eds. *Adult and Pediatric Spine.* Philadelphia: Lippincott Williams & Wilkins; 2004: 1011–41.

9. Patterson RH, Arbit E. A surgical approach through the pedicle to protruded thoracic discs. *J Neurosurg* 1978; **48**(5): 768–72.

10. Resnick DK, Benzel EC. Lateral extracavitary approach for thoracic and thoracolumbar spine trauma: operative complications. *Neurosurgery* 1998; **43**(4): 796–802; discussion 802–3.

8.9   Surgery for intramedullary spinal cord tumors

John H. Shin and Edward C. Benzel

Key points

- Ependymoma is the most common intramedullary spinal cord tumor in adults.
- If evoked potential monitoring is employed, baseline testing prior to positioning, adds significant value.
- Usually, a midline myelotomy is performed for the resection of intramedullary tumors. Distortion of the normal anatomy due to tumor mass effect, may make identification of the true midline difficult.
- Once the tumor is reached, a biopsy is performed and a frozen section is obtained.
- When changes in SSEPs and MEPs occur, an expeditious and systematic review of surgical and anesthetic factors should be performed.

Introduction

Intramedullary spinal cord tumors are rare, with an incidence of approximately 1.1 cases per 100 000.[1] They account for 2–4% of central nervous system tumors and represent 15% of adult and 35% of pediatric primary intradural tumors.[2–4] Without treatment, they may cause significant neurologic dysfunction, morbidity, and mortality.

By definition, these tumors are intradural and located within the spinal cord parenchyma, as opposed to metastatic spine tumors, which are more common and are usually extradural. Ependymoma is the most common intramedullary tumor in adults, followed by astrocytoma and hemangioblastoma, while astrocytomas are most common in children. When possible, the goal of surgery is complete resection. In the absence of compete resection, control rates using adjuvant therapies such as chemotherapy and radiation therapy for residual, recurrent, or malignant disease have not been consistently reported, with a wide variance of treatment protocols among centers.[5–9] Though complete resection is desirable, this is limited mainly by tumor histology and the presence of an adequate plane of dissection between the tumor and spinal cord.[10] Numerous series have observed the significance of these factors towards long-term outcomes.[11–13] Though this plane is often easily identified with ependymomas and hemangioblastomas, it is less so with astrocytomas, hence limiting the potential for complete resection and progression-free survival.

Due to the rarity of these lesions, there have been no prospective randomized studies to guide clinical decision making.[14] There is, however, a significant body of retrospective data detailing the observations of experienced surgeons since the first case of intramedullary tumor resection was reported in 1911.[15] In general, it is recommended that surgery be performed early in patients with progressive neurologic symptoms as the preoperative neurologic examination is regarded as the main predictor of long-term outcome.[14]

In the last decade, advances in microsurgical techniques, general anesthesia, and intraoperative electrophysiological monitoring have allowed surgeons to operate with greater certainty as real-time feedback from intraoperative monitoring has provided surgeons with indicators of potentially reversible neurologic events. Strategies to reverse these changes may then be performed by both surgeon and anesthesiologist. Despite these advances, surgical morbidity remains high and communication among surgeon, anesthesiologist, and monitoring technician is critical.

In this chapter, we describe the surgical technique of intramedullary tumor resection and highlight the significance of anesthesia strategies in the intraoperative management of these patients.

Surgical technique

After the induction of general anesthesia and placement of electrodes required for intraoperative electrophysiological monitoring, the patient is carefully positioned prone on the operating table as these tumors are almost always approached dorsally. Short-acting muscle relaxants may be used for induction and intubation, but are otherwise discontinued as they interfere with monitoring of muscle motor evoked potentials (MEPs).[16] The use of halogenated anesthetics is also discouraged as they elevate muscle MEP stimulus thresholds and block these signals in a dose-dependent fashion. A constant infusion of propofol and fentanyl is typically recommended as both have minimal effects on somatosensory evoked (SSEP) and MEP monitoring.[16]

Baseline electrophysiological recordings are obtained prior to positioning so that changes occurring during positioning can be addressed. Patients with preexisting severe sensory or motor deficits will have diminished responses at baseline. A bite block is also placed in the mouth as tongue lacerations have been reported during stimulation for MEP.[17] For patients with cervical or upper thoracic tumors, head and neck immobilization using the Mayfield head holder is critical to minimize movement during surgery, particularly during microdissection; a foam pillow may otherwise be used. Perioperative administration of steroids is at the discretion of the surgeon.

After a localizing radiograph over the intended spinal level is obtained, the skin is incised and exposure of the dorsal spinal elements is performed using electrocautery and subperiosteal elevation. Tissue retractors are placed and laminectomies are performed over the appropriate levels, exposing the dura mater. Once hemostasis is achieved, the dura is incised and the edges are tacked up to the surrounding tissue. (Fig. 8.27) There is often an egress of cerebrospinal fluid with the dural opening which relaxes the spinal cord and infrequently causes hemodynamic changes. Depending on the morphology of the tumor, the spinal cord may appear swollen or asymmetrically enlarged due to the

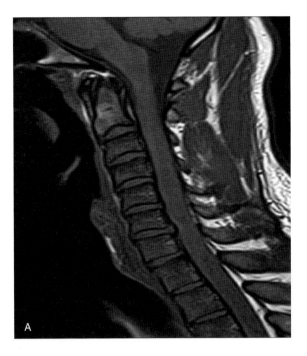

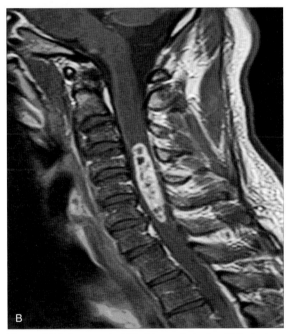

Figure 8.28 Preoperative MRI of the cervical spine. (A) Sagittal T1-weighted image. (B) Sagittal T1-weighted image with contrast. Note the heterogeneous signal intensity within the spinal cord. This represents cystic or hemorrhagic cavities within the tumor. (C) Sagittal T2-weighted image. Edema within the spinal cord spreads rostrally to the brainstem and caudally to the thoracic spinal cord. (D) Axial T1-weighted image with contrast. The spinal cord is thinned out and wraps around the tumor ventrally.

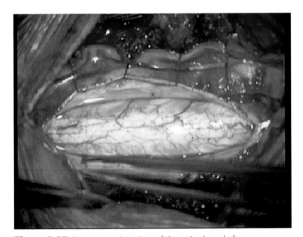

Figure 8.27 Intraoperative view of the spinal cord after laminectomy and dural opening. The dural edges are tacked up to the surrounding muscle in order to enhance the visualization of the spinal cord.

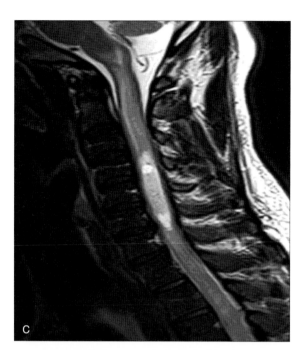

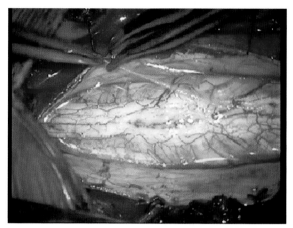

Figure 8.29 The arachnoid is dissected away from the surface of the spinal cord. A midline myelotomy is performed after dissection and cauterization of dorsal vessels.

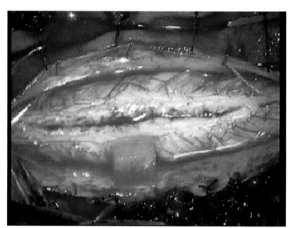

Figure 8.30 A midline myelotomy is performed along the full length of the underlying tumor. This minimizes retraction and pulling of the spinal cord during microdissection of the tumor.

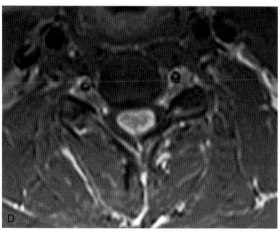

Figure 8.28 (*cont.*)

expansive nature of the underlying tumor. There may also be a slight discoloration that represents either a cystic or hemorrhagic component within the tumor. Preoperative MRI is reviewed to verify the rostral and caudal extent of the tumor (Fig. 8.28). Intraoperative ultrasound may also be used to identify its location once the dura is open. The operating microscope is then brought into the field and under high power magnification, the arachnoid is sharply dissected, further exposing the spinal cord (Fig. 8.29).

A midline myelotomy is performed, but distortion of the normal anatomy due to tumor may make identification of the true midline difficult. With intramedullary tumors, the spinal cord is frequently rotated and enlarged with loss of the posterior median sulcus as an identifiable anatomic landmark. Small blood vessels on the dorsal surface are dissected and cauterized as needed. The pial surface is then incised and the dorsal columns are separated over the length of the tumor to avoid unnecessary traction of the spinal cord (Fig. 8.30). Sharp dissection is performed until the tumor is reached (Fig. 8.31). Drainage of a cystic or hemorrhagic component may result in further relaxation of the spinal cord.

Once the tumor is reached, a biopsy is performed and a frozen section is obtained. The identification of tissue histology as well as a plane of dissection between the tumor and spinal cord will determine the potential for complete resection. Although the surgical strategy

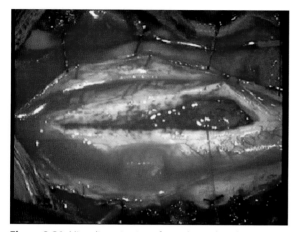

Figure 8.31 Microdissection is performed, revealing the tumor (ependymoma).

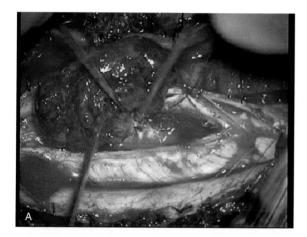

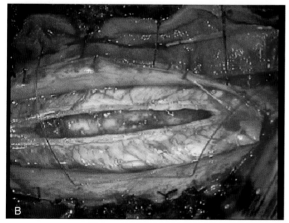

Figure 8.32 Tumor dissection and resection. (A) A plane of dissection is identified between the spinal cord and ependymoma, facilitating resection of the tumor. Ventral arterial feeders to the tumor are identified, dissected, cauterized, and cut. (B) Cavity within the spinal cord as seen after resection of the tumor.

may vary technically depending on whether the tumor is an ependymoma or astrocytoma, the general concept is to first debulk large tumors to minimize trauma to the spinal cord. If a plane is identified, dissection is performed circumferentially to the ventral surface, where most tumors receive their vascular supply. These vessels are subsequently dissected, cauterized, and cut until the tumor is dissected free from the spinal cord. (Fig. 8.32) As tumor resection proceeds, intraoperative monitoring is checked frequently to guide the extent of resection. Should there be any changes, a number of maneuvers may be implemented to attempt to reverse them. Strategies to address changes in these evoked potentials are discussed later in this chapter. Though the significance of these findings is often debated, the sensitivity and specificity of MEP in particular have been shown to correlate with long-term neurologic deficits. Following tumor resection, the surgical cavity is irrigated with warm saline prior to closure.

Role of electrophysiological monitoring

Intraoperative electrophysiological monitoring is a critical component to spinal cord tumor surgery. The rationale for using monitoring is to maximize tumor resection and minimize neurologic morbidity. Because intramedullary tumors are within the substance of the spinal cord, manipulation of the spinal cord is anticipated. If these changes are identified early, corrective surgical and anesthetic maneuvers can be performed to minimize permanent neurologic damage. The point at which these deficits become permanent or the degree to which recovery of evoked responses is required to reverse a potential neurologic insult, however, is not clear and is subject to debate.

Evoked potentials represent an assessment of the electrical potentials produced in response to stimulating the nervous system by sensory or electrical stimulation. Somatosensory evoked potentials are produced by stimulation of the sensory system. These responses arise from the action potentials or graded polysynaptic potentials during propagation of an electrical impulse from the periphery to the brain and can be recorded over the scalp, as well as at various sites along the anatomic pathway using surface or subdermal needle electrodes.[16]

SSEPs have been used for decades in spine surgery and were initially thought to be predictive of postoperative motor deficits. However, as experience grew, it became clear that the maintenance of SSEPs during surgery did not guarantee preservation of motor function.[18] Changes in latency and amplitude in SSEPs have typically been considered indicators of surgically induced injuries. Several investigators have shown that a 50% decrease of amplitude and simultaneous 10% increase in latencies are sensitive indicators for the possibility of new postoperative motor deficits.[16,19] According to Jones et al.,[20] a decrease of 60% in amplitude of an SSEP is associated with a 50% risk of a postoperative motor deficit.

Because SSEP and MEP pathways are served by different vascular distributions, namely the posterior and anterior spinal arteries respectively, it is possible that injury to the motor tract can occur without changes in SSEPs when monitoring with SSEPs alone.[18,21] For this reason, both SSEPs and MEPs are now typically used in spine tumor surgery.

Motor evoked potentials assess the function of the motor cortex and the descending motor pathways through the corticospinal tracts. In this technique, muscle activity is recorded after stimulation of the motor pathway through transcranial electrical motor cortex stimulation. In general, evoked potentials are described in terms of the poststimulation latency in milliseconds and peak-to-peak amplitude in millivolts. These correspond to the time between the application of a stimulus and the occurrence of a peak in the waveform. These MEPs can be recorded from the spinal cord, either in the form of D waves or from the peripheral muscles. It is the combination of these recordings that provides useful feedback to the surgeon. D waves are recorded by an electrode placed in the epidural space caudal to the area of resection. These recordings represent a pool of high-conduction velocity fibers within the corticospinal tracts that support locomotion.[19,22,23] Muscle MEP responses are optimally recorded from muscles known to have strong pyramidal innervation, namely the thenar, hypothenar, tibialis anterior, and flexor hallucis brevis muscles.

Interpretation of both of these responses may help identify a window of reversibility should a change in recordings be found. According to some investigators, as long as the D wave is preserved with an amplitude of at least 50% of the baseline value, a loss of muscle MEPs during surgery correlates with a transient paraparesis or paraplegia.[24] A decrease of more than 50% of the baseline D wave amplitude is associated with a long-term postoperative motor deficit.[19] The exact mechanism for this is unclear, however it is postulated that since the D wave is generated exclusively by fast neurons of the

corticospinal tracts and muscle MEPs are generated by corticospinal as well as other descending pathways, an injury to the other pathways can be compensated by the corticospinal tracts but not vice versa.[24,25]

Sala et al.[17] recently reviewed their experience of intramedullary spinal cord tumor surgery with and without the use of monitoring. In this series, 50 operations performed before the introduction of MEP monitoring were compared with 50 consecutive operations performed with monitoring. Preoperative neurologic status, histological findings, tumor location, and extent of removal were found to be independent of outcome. At the time of surgery, the disappearance of muscle MEP led to modification of surgical technique and surgery was not discontinued as long as D wave amplitude remained greater than 50% of baseline. A decrement of more than 50% in D wave amplitude without recovery was the major indication to stop surgery. At 1 year, patients in the monitoring group had significantly better outcomes, though the rates of early motor dysfunction at discharge were similar between groups.

Kothbauer et al.[25] also performed a retrospective analysis of the pre- and postoperative motor status of 100 consecutive patients who underwent surgery for intramedullary tumors using intraoperative monitoring with D waves and MEPs. The authors report that the sensitivity of muscle MEPs to detect postoperative motor deficits was 100% and its specificity was 91%. In this series, no motor deficits were detected postoperatively in patients with stable MEP. Patients with preserved D wave amplitude up to 50% of the baseline amplitude with a complete loss of muscle MEPs suffered only transient paraplegia. Despite the transient weakness, all recovered within a few hours to a few weeks.

Intraoperative strategies for recovery of potentials

In addition to surgical manipulation of the spinal cord, various physiologic factors can affect evoked responses. These include hypotension, hypoxemia, hypothermia, acidosis, low circulating blood volume, and electrolyte imbalance.[26] When a change in responses occurs, it is important to systematically assess for each of these.

Likewise, several surgical strategies may help recover lost or diminished potentials. Signals may recover spontaneously if surgery is stopped immediately after muscle MEPs have disappeared or after D wave amplitude has decreased significantly. Sala *et al.*[16,24] describe a "stop and go" strategy during which surgery is stopped for half an hour or more to allow muscle MEPs and/or D waves to recover on their own before proceeding with surgery.

Irrigation of the surgical field with warm saline irrigation has also been shown to recover both SSEPs and MEPs.[16] Whether this is due to the effect of temperature, of irrigation, or a combination of the two is not clear. It is theorized that irrigation dilutes potassium that accumulates in the extracellular space and blocks conduction. This is based on experimental spinal cord injury models in which traumatic injury to the spinal cord induces a disruption of cell membranes with subsequent accumulation of potassium in the extracellular space.

Another mechanism of spinal cord injury during surgery is related to ischemia secondary to decreased perfusion pressure or vasospasm. The extent to which the spinal cord can tolerate a decrease in perfusion pressure is unknown. Applying papaverine locally to the spinal cord and increasing the mean arterial pressure may improve perfusion to the spinal cord and counteract any ongoing ischemia due to vasospasm or hypoperfusion.

Considerations for anesthesia

With the use of SSEP and MEP monitoring during spine tumor surgery, special consideration must be given to the agents used for induction and maintenance of anesthesia. A coordinated effort involving the monitoring technician, anesthesiologist, and surgeon is critical to developing an effective management strategy as changes in the physiologic milieu and anesthesia may affect the quality of electrophysiological recordings and impact surgical decision making.

Many inhalational anesthetics substantially affect cortical function and suppress both SSEPs and MEPs.[26] It is essential to moderate the amount of inhalational or intravenous anesthesia. Halogenated inhalational anesthetics such as desflurane, enflurane, halothane, isoflurane, and sevoflurane produce dose-related reduction in SSEP amplitude and increase in latency. This effect varies from isoflurane (most potent) to halothane (least potent).[26] They also elevate muscle MEP stimulus thresholds and block these potentials in a dose-dependent fashion at cortical and spinal levels. Nitrous oxide, a nonhalogenated inhalational anesthetic, reduces SSEP amplitude and increases latency when used alone or when combined with halogenated inhalational agents or opioid agents. When compared with other inhalational anesthetic agents, nitrous oxide produces more profound changes in SSEP and muscle recordings from transcranial motor stimulation than any other agent.

Intravenous analgesic agents, such as opioids and ketamine are less likely to affect SSEPs.[27] The effects of opioids appears to be related to drug concentration, as maximal changes occur after bolus delivery. One study of fentanyl suggested that the effect on evoked responses may be minimized by using a drug infusion to avoid transient bolus effects.[28] Intravenous sedative-hypnotic drugs such as droperidol, barbiturates, benzodiazepines, etomidate, and propofol produce dose-related depression of evoked responses to a lesser degree than do inhalational agents. For this reason, a constant infusion of propofol and fentanyl has typically been used in intramedullary tumor surgery as these allow for minimal interference with intraoperative monitoring.[16]

The use of muscle relaxants has been shown to have no direct deleterious effects on SSEP but can significantly alter or completely block intraoperative MEP.[16] Other than their use during induction, muscle relaxants should otherwise be avoided during surgery, particularly during the intradural portion of surgery where monitoring is critical.

Conclusion

Intramedullary spinal cord tumors are rare lesions for which the mainstay of treatment is surgery. Despite advances in neurosurgical technique, the overall morbidity rates remain high with approximately 20% of patients sustaining permanent neurologic injury as a result of surgery.[14] Many factors have been associated with functional outcomes following surgery including tumor histology, extent of resection, and the use of intraoperative monitoring. When changes in SSEPs and MEPs occur, an expeditious and systematic review of surgical and anesthetic factors should be performed in concert among surgeon, anesthesiologist, and monitoring technician to prevent permanent neurologic damage.

References

1. Benes V 3rd, Barsa P, Benes V Jr., Suchomel P. Prognostic factors in intramedullary astrocytomas: a literature review. *Eur Spine J* 2009; **18**: 1397–422.

2. Constantini S, Houten J, Miller DC, *et al.* Intramedullary spinal cord tumors in children under the age of 3 years. *J Neurosurg* 1996; **85**: 1036–43.

3. Constantini S, Miller DC, Allen JC, *et al.* Radical excision of intramedullary spinal cord tumors: surgical morbidity and long-term follow-up evaluation in 164 children and young adults. *J Neurosurg* 2000; **93**: 183–93.

4. Cooper PR. Outcome after operative treatment of intramedullary spinal cord tumors in adults: intermediate and long-term results in 51 patients. *Neurosurgery* 1989; **25**: 855–9.

5. Bouffet E, Amat D, Devaux Y, Desuzinges C. Chemotherapy for spinal cord astrocytoma. *Med Pediatr Oncol* 1997; **29**: 560–2.

6. Chamberlain MC. Salvage chemotherapy for recurrent spinal cord ependymoma. *Cancer* 2002; **95**: 997–1002.

7. Chamberlain MC. Temozolomide for recurrent low-grade spinal cord gliomas in adults. *Cancer* 2008; **113**: 1019–24.

8. Cohen AR, Wisoff JH, Allen JC, Epstein F. Malignant astrocytomas of the spinal cord. *J Neurosurg* 1989; **70**: 50–4.

9. Garcia DM. Primary spinal cord tumors treated with surgery and postoperative irradiation. *Int J Radiat Oncol Biol Phys* 1985; **11**: 1933–9.

10. Karikari IO, Nimjee SM, Hodges TR, *et al.* Impact of tumor histology on resectability and neurological outcome in primary intramedullary spinal cord tumors: a single-center experience with 102 patients. *Neurosurgery* 2011; **68**: 188–97.

11. Garces-Ambrossi GL, McGirt MJ, Mehta VA, *et al.* Factors associated with progression-free survival and long-term neurological outcome after resection of intramedullary spinal cord tumors: analysis of 101 consecutive cases. *J Neurosurg Spine* 2009; **11**: 591–9.

12. McCormick PC, Torres R, Post KD, Stein BM. Intramedullary ependymoma of the spinal cord. *J Neurosurg* 1990; **72**: 523–2.

13. McGirt MJ, Goldstein IM, Chaichana KL, *et al.* Extent of surgical resection of malignant astrocytomas of the spinal cord: outcome analysis of 35 patients. *Neurosurgery* 2008; **63**: 55–60; discussion 60–61.

14. Harrop JS, Ganju A, Groff M, Bilsky M. Primary intramedullary tumors of the spinal cord. *Spine (Phila Pa 1976)* 2009; **34**: S69–77.

15. Sciubba DM, Liang D, Kothbauer KF, Noggle JC, Jallo GI. The evolution of intramedullary spinal cord tumor surgery. *Neurosurgery* 2009; **65**: 84–91; discussion 91–92.

16. Deletis V, Sala F. Intraoperative neurophysiological monitoring of the spinal cord during spinal cord and spine surgery: a review focus on the corticospinal tracts. *Clin Neurophysiol* 2008; **119**: 248–64.

17. Sala F, Palandri G, Basso E, *et al.* Motor evoked potential monitoring improves outcome after surgery for intramedullary spinal cord tumors: a historical control study. *Neurosurgery* 2006; **58**: 1129–43; discussion 1129–43.

18. Lesser RP, Raudzens P, Luders H, *et al.* Postoperative neurological deficits may occur despite unchanged intraoperative somatosensory evoked potentials. *Ann Neurol* 1986; **19**: 22–5.

19. Morota N, Deletis V, Constantini S, *et al.* The role of motor evoked potentials during surgery for intramedullary spinal cord tumors. *Neurosurgery* 1997; **41**: 1327–36.

20. Jones SJ, Harrison R, Koh KF, Mendoza N, Crockard HA. Motor evoked potential monitoring during spinal surgery: responses of distal limb muscles to transcranial cortical stimulation with pulse trains. *Electroencephalogr Clin Neurophysiol* 1996; **100**: 375–83.

21. Ginsburg HH, Shetter AG, Raudzens PA. Postoperative paraplegia with preserved intraoperative somatosensory evoked potentials. Case report. *J Neurosurg* 1985; **63**: 296–300.

22. Levy WJ, York DH, McCaffrey M, Tanzer F. Motor evoked potentials from transcranial stimulation of the motor cortex in humans. *Neurosurgery* 1984; **15**: 287–302.

23. Patton HD, Amassian VE. Single and multiple-unit analysis of cortical stage of pyramidal tract activation. *J Neurophysiol* 1954; **17**: 345–63.

24. Sala F, Bricolo A, Faccioli F, Lanteri P, Gerosa M. Surgery for intramedullary spinal cord tumors: the role of intraoperative (neurophysiological) monitoring. *Eur Spine J* 2007; **16 Suppl 2**: S130–9.

25. Kothbauer KF, Deletis V, Epstein FJ. Motor-evoked potential monitoring for intramedullary spinal cord tumor surgery: correlation of clinical and neurophysiological data in a series of 100 consecutive procedures. *Neurosurg Focus* 1998; **4**: e1.

26. Sloan TB, Heyer EJ. Anesthesia for intraoperative neurophysiologic monitoring of the spinal cord. *J Clin Neurophysiol* 2002; **19**: 430–43.

27. Scheufler KM, Zentner J. Total intravenous anesthesia for intraoperative monitoring of the motor pathways: an integral view combining clinical and experimental data. *J Neurosurg* 2002; **96**: 571–9.

28. Pathak KS, Brown RH, Nash CL Jr., Cascorbi HF. Continuous opioid infusion for scoliosis fusion surgery. *Anesth Analg* 1983; **62**: 841–5.

8.10 Avoiding complications: surgeon's point of view

Michael Kelly and Richard Schlenk

Key points

- It is critical to the safety of spine surgical patients that anesthetic risk assessment must take into consideration cervical instability.
- Preoperative antibiotics should always be considered except for cases of primary spinal infections when administration is often recommended after surgical cultures are obtained.
- The use of steroids for any indication should be discussed with the surgeon prior to the operation and utilized with caution and on a case-to-case basis.
- Understanding spinal surgical positioning and the impact of variations is crucial to avoiding injury to the spine and avoidance of peripheral nerve neuropraxia.
- The anesthesia team should harbor knowledge of nuances of spine approaches specific to intraoperative complication avoidance and management.

Introduction

The words complication and spine surgery often find themselves in close association with one another. Spine surgery is typically elective, so tolerance for complications is often low. However, spine surgery is also complex and generally of higher risk, which creates a challenging situation when weighing risks and benefits of surgical intervention. This chapter will discuss the risks associated with spine surgery and how such risks might be avoided or at least reduced. Above all, close collaboration among spine surgeons, anesthesiologists, and medical doctors is essential to reducing complications in these patients.

Preoperative risk assessment

Avoiding complications in spine surgery begins, when possible, with careful patient selection and preoperative evaluation. A complete medical evaluation includes basic historical information such as medical problems, surgeries, current medications, allergies, substance use, and prior issues with anesthesia or surgery. Of particular importance is identifying preoperative medical conditions that increase the risk of surgery and anesthesia for the patient. These conditions include heart disease, diabetes, chronic obstructive pulmonary disease, and bleeding dyscrasias. Preoperative optimization of cardiac, pulmonary, renal, and nutritional status has been correlated with improved outcomes in surgical patients overall.[1]

Some authors have argued for a protocol-based approach to patient selection for high-risk spine surgery.[2] Systematic preoperative evaluation of patients by medical, surgical, and anesthesia teams can identify high-risk medical conditions and assess the safety and timing of surgery from a multidisciplinary perspective. These medical risks can then be weighed against the type and duration of surgery including number of levels, estimated blood loss, and expected postoperative course.

Careful physical examination can also yield important information regarding positioning during surgery and airway issues. In particular, surgical approaches to the cervical spine often require meticulous attention to positioning and can make intubation more challenging particularly in the setting of instability. Flexion and extension maneuvers can be performed while the patient is awake to assess for evidence of neurologic symptoms.[3] In particular, patients with severe arthritis or complex trauma with instability may have limited neck and jaw mobility necessitating fiberoptic intubation.[4] Knowledge of these circumstances before surgery promotes safety and efficiency in the operating room.

Antibiotics

The rate of infection from spine surgery has been reported between 0.3% and 9% in some studies.[5,6] These rates are relatively high in comparison with quoted rates from the orthopedic literature as well as other clean, noncontaminated procedures. The higher risk associated with spine surgery is attributed to many factors. For example, blood glucose control in patients with known history of diabetes has been described as one of the leading risk factors for postoperative wound infection.[7] Other medical conditions including age >60 years, obesity, smoking, and malnutrition have all been associated with increased rates of postoperative wound infection. Intraoperative factors including operative time, estimated blood loss, and staging of spinal procedures can also raise the risk of postoperative wound infection nearly threefold.[8,9]

Some controversy exists around the use of perioperative antibiotics in spine surgery. Most surgeons give some form of antibiotic therapy perioperatively. However, choice of antibiotic, duration of therapy, and timing of administration are not uniform. Studies have shown a preponderance of Gram-positive organisms in postoperative spine infections. These findings suggest that a single perioperative dose of first-generation cephalosporin is often adequate in reducing postoperative infection. Multiple-dose regimens have not demonstrated clear benefit but are a common practice among some surgeons. In 2007, guidelines published by the North American Spine Society (NASS) cite level B evidence supporting the use of perioperative antibiotics in spine surgery.[10] The only instance in which antibiotics would be held preoperatively would be in a case of primary spinal infection, where broad-spectrum antimicrobial medications should be administered after cultures are obtained surgically.

Studies have also shown that the volume of irrigation used during surgery is associated with a lower risk of postoperative infections. A minimum of 2 liters of saline irrigation in the surgical wound prior to closure was associated with lower rates of infection in the study by Watanabe *et al.* mentioned above.[7] This saline is often infused with antibiotic such as bacitracin. Of course, intraoperative sterile technique, judicious use of antibiotics, and wound irrigation are only the first efforts in preventing postoperative infections. Proper blood glucose control, early mobilization after surgery, and adequate wound care are all essential factors in preventing operative site infections.

Steroids

Controversy exists regarding steroid use in traumatic spinal cord injury. Initial data suggested that high-dose (30 mg/kg) administration of methylprednisolone in the setting of an acute injury is associated with improved outcome in animal models.[11,12] However, subsequent studies failed to demonstrate a clear benefit and point to the comorbidities associated with use of high-dose steroids. The National Acute Spinal Cord Injury Studies (NASCIS) II and III suggest that high-dose therapy administered within 8 h of initial injury does confer a benefit in the setting of incomplete or complete spinal cord injury.[13]

However, these findings have been criticized by many who cite the known side effects of high-dose steroids therapy including infection and avascular necrosis.[14] The American College of Surgeons (ACS) no longer mandates its use. A recent survey indicates that 90% of spine surgeons polled use the therapy even though only 24% believe that it provides a clinical benefit.[15]

In the setting of routine, elective spine surgery, steroids are used in smaller doses, more frequently, and with less controversy. Low doses (5–10 mg) of Decadron (dexamethasone) are typically given before cases involving large disc herniations, spinal cord tumors, and severe canal stenosis. Such perioperative treatment is thought to preserve neural structures from inflammation and swelling postoperatively.

Steroids are usually given for no longer than 24–48 hours to avoid known complications associated with long-term steroid therapy. In patients who have undergone spinal fusion, steroids are used sparingly due to their inhibition of bone growth and remodeling. For patients taking chronic steroids, stress-dose steroids are also commonly given to prevent adrenal crisis.

Positioning

Positioning in spine surgery can pose unique challenges to both the anesthesia and surgical teams. A wide variety of positions are used in spine surgery including supine, prone, lateral, sitting, and kneeling positions, each of which demands close attention to detail before the operation can begin.

Special consideration should be made for patients demonstrating significant spinal stenosis and/or instability of the cervical spine. Cervical stenosis is defined as narrowing of the spinal canal that causes compression of the spinal cord and/or nerve roots. Severe stenosis can often place patients at significant risk for iatrogenic injury of the spinal cord and/or nerve roots during positioning.[16] Special care must be taken during intubation in these patients as well. Excessive extension in the setting of severe stenosis has been associated with the development of central cord syndrome.[17]

In patients with instability or malalignment of the spinal column, traction is often employed to reestablish proper alignment and to decompress neural elements prior to surgical decompression.[18] Preoperatively, patients are placed in a traction system using standard counterweight techniques and a head fixation device such as Gardner–Wells tongs. Initially, a 4.5 kg (10 lb) weight is added to the traction device to account for the head. Additional weights of this value are added for each additional level requiring traction in the cervical spine.[19] Weight is typically added every 30 to 60 minutes with interval radiographs to confirm alignment and to avoid injury due to overdistraction.

Supine

This position is frequently used for procedures designed for ventral pathology involving either the disc, the vertebral body, or both. Arms are typically tucked or remain wrapped on an arm board, with careful attention to padding of pressure points, particularly the ulnar, radial, and peroneal nerves. Failure to adequately pad these areas can lead to nerve palsies including grip weakness, wrist drop, and foot drop, respectively.

In the cervical spine, the neck is often placed in the neutral position usually with slight extension, unless contraindicated, for better surgical exposure. These patients often require fiberoptic intubation due to limitations in neck mobility. Occasionally patients can undergo awake intubation and positioning to ensure that neural structures are not compromised before the surgery begins. If concern arises during the procedure and neuromonitoring is not available, an intraoperative "wake-up test" can be performed to check for neurologic function.[20]

Prone

This position is the standard for most pathology involving the dorsal elements of the spine including the spinous processes, lamina, facet joints, pedicles, and even spinal cord. For cases involving the cervical spine, the head is usually placed in a fixation device such as a Mayfield Head Holder or Gardner–Wells tongs. The fixation device stabilizes the cervical spine during surgery and allows manipulation of the cervical spine after decompression to correct kyphosis, promote lordosis, or reestablish normal alignment of the spinal column.

During positioning, the spine surgeon controls the head and neck as the patient is rolled over into a prone position ensuring that the spine remains in neutral position. Special care must be taken to maintain neutral position during transition from the bed to the operating table, particularly when there is instability or severe canal stenosis. In some cases, neurophysiologic monitoring such as somatosensory evoked potentials (SSEPs) can be used to ensure preservation of neurologic function during prone positioning and throughout the surgery. While in prone position, careful attention must be given to padding pressure points including the chest, anterior superior iliac spine, and thighs.

Perioperative visual loss or ischemic optic neuropathy (ION) has been reported for patients placed in the prone position, particularly during lengthy spine operations. The incidence of visual loss after spine surgery is reported between 0.002% and 0.2%.[21] Although the pathophysiology remains unknown, ischemia is presumed to be the mechanism.[22] Risk factors include more than 5 hours duration in the prone position, blood loss greater than 1 liter, hypotension, elevated venous pressure, use of vasoconstricting agents, and head positioning.[23] Studies suggest that MAPs below 65 mmHg and head positioning devices such as the horseshoe may exacerbate ischemic. Current studies are now focused on monitoring intraocular pressure as a metric for preventing ION.

Lateral

Lateral position can be used for procedures that involve the need for access to the lateral thoracic or lumbar spine. The approach is typical for anterior exposures that require corpectomy in these regions for traumatic, infectious, or neoplastic pathologies. These procedures are usually lengthy and require that all pressure points are meticulously addressed. Less commonly the lateral position is used for the placement of catheter systems into the abdomen, including intrathecal baclofen pumps and lumbar peritoneal shunts. Typically, patients undergo intubation and are then turned on their side using a conformational "bean bag" to preserve the position for the duration of the case. Adequate padding of the hip and shoulder as well as an axillary role is important for avoiding postoperative joint pain, nerve injury, and skin breakdown.

Sitting

The sitting position is perhaps the most challenging position for the anesthesiologist and surgeon alike. Major risks include cardiac instability, venous air embolism (VAE), and quadriplegia. Venous pooling is often encountered in this position which must be countered by adequate intravenous fluid administration and compression stockings to avoid hypotension particularly when cord ischemia is a concern.

Venous air embolism occurs when approximately 5 ml/kg of air enters the circulation and travels to the heart causing severe right heart strain and cardiorespiratory collapse.[24] In the setting of a patent foramen oval or right to left cardiac shunt, VAE can lead to stroke. Although the incidence of VAE during spine surgery is much lower than in cranial surgery (7% vs. 43%), the complication carries significant morbidity when it occurs.[25] Contraindications for the sitting position include: patent foramen oval or right to left cardiac shunt, evidence of cerebral ischemia in the upright position while awake, and cardiac instability.[20]

In the sitting position, patients are often monitored with precordial Doppler and careful attention is given to the end-tidal CO_2 and the central venous pressure. Treatment of a VAE includes stopping the source of venous bleeding, flooding the field with irrigation, packing the wound, aspirating the central venous line, discontinuing nitrous oxide if in use, and sometimes turning the patient on his/her left side. Continuous supportive treatment with intravenous fluids and pressors should be included when necessary.[26]

Kneeling

The kneeling position shares much in common with the prone position. Careful attention must be given to padding the chest and iliac crests as well as in ensuring that the arms are positioned at less than ninety degrees from the body to reduce stretch on the brachial plexus and peripheral nerves. The abdomen must also be decompressed as much as possible to promote venous return and thereby reduce epidural venous bleeding during surgery. This position is not recommended in those patients with recent knee replacement surgery and/or severe cervical spine stenosis/instability as the position can place unsafe strain at these locations.

Surgical approaches

The wide variety of surgical approaches used in spine surgery creates many challenges to safe and effective intraoperative care. Each approach contains unique risks and benefits depending upon the pathology in question and the goals of surgery. Knowledge of the risks inherent in each approach can prove useful in anticipating and preventing complications during surgery. Listed below are several common approaches used in the cervical, thoracic, and lumbar spine and the major complications associated with each.

Transoral/lateral transcondylar approach

This approach is often used for ventral pathology in the upper cervical spine. Major complications include hemorrhage, infection, and tongue swelling. Hemorrhage most frequently results from injury to the vertebral artery or smaller perforating vessels. Meticulous operative hemostasis and monitoring of coagulation parameters reduces the risk of bleeding and hematoma

formation. Infections are typically reduced with preoperative oral antibiotics and betadyne mouth lavage. Tongue swelling is treated with perioperative steroids and periodic massage. A small risk of intraoperative CSF leak also exists which is treated with primary closure using suture and fibrin glue as well as lumbar drain placement if the leak persists.[27]

Dorsal/ventral subaxial cervical approach

Complications in this region include vascular injury, nerve root injury, mediastinal injury, and thoracic duct injury. The carotid artery, vertebral artery, jugular vein, and brachiocephalic vein are all at risk using this approach. If encountered, the injury is typically primarily repaired, but blood loss can be substantial and maintenance of normal blood pressure is important particularly when spinal cord perfusion is concerned.

Nerve root injury is most common at the C5 level and usually results from overly aggressive decompression.[28] The recurrent laryngeal nerve is injured in 3–11% of cases and leads to postoperative hoarseness that usually improves over time. A study by Apfelbaum et al. showed that monitoring endotracheal cuff pressure and releasing the pressure after retractor placement reduces paralysis rates from 6.4% to 1.7%.[29] The sympathetic chain is also susceptible to injury in the lower thoracic spine that can cause a Horner's syndrome postoperatively. Such nerve injury can be avoided by proper retractor placement and careful, midline surgical exposure. In rare cases, injury to the hypoglossal nerve occurs resulting in dysphagia of varying degrees.[30]

Although rare, serious esophagus and trachea injuries have been reported to occur in approximately 0.01% of cervical spine surgeries. More commonly, postoperative dysphagia and esophageal dysmotility has been observed in approximately 10% of postoperative patients.[31] Intermittently relieving traction of tissues during surgery is helpful in reducing this complication. Rare reports of injury to the thoracic duct have also been reported, although such complications are unusual since the duct is typically lateral to most surgical approaches.

Cervicothoracic junction approach

Ventral approaches at this level are technically challenging and carry a higher complication rate due to the natural kyphosis of the spinal column at this level and the presence of the mediastinum. Complications are consistent with those present in the subaxial spine but carry a higher risk as surgical repair at such levels is often difficult. Perhaps the only additional consideration at this level is the risk of damage to the lung apex, particularly in more lateral approaches to the brachial plexus, first rib, and/or clavicle. Dorsal approaches at this level often carry less risk and are primarily associated with nerve root injury.

Thoracic, lumbar, and sacral approaches

Approaches to the thoracic and lumbosacral spine share many of the same types of risks described for the cervical spine but also present their own unique challenges. Ventral approaches to the thoracic spine require, by design, thoracotomy and chest tube placement. Postoperatively these patients often suffer from increased pain, decreased mobility, and increased rates of pneumonia and atelectasis. At the thoracolumbar junction, takedown of the diaphragm for ventral exposure often carries the highest morbidity.[32,33]

Dorsal and dorsolateral approaches including the transpedicular, costotransversectomy, and lateral extracavitary approaches all spare the need for direct thoracotomy and thus avoid the postoperative morbidity inherent in direct ventral approaches. Overall, the morbidity rates for these approaches remain low at approximately 1–4% and include pneumonia, pleural tear, infection, bowel obstruction, and neurologic dysfunction. Risk of injury to the thoracic spinal cord remains low at approximately 1% according to some studies.[34] Such risk can be reduced by maintaining adequate spinal cord perfusion, both intraoperatively and postoperatively. Mean arterial blood pressure (MAP) goals are usually kept in the 80–90 mmHg range in such settings.

Ventral and dorsal approaches to the lumbar and sacral spine carry less risk to neural structures as the canal widens and the spinal cord ends typically about the level of L2. Large-vessel injury remains the most common serious injury from ventral approaches with incidence rates reported between 8% and 12%. Such injury is most often secondary to venous laceration usually resulting from retraction injury. The use of an "approach surgeon" has been associated with a reduced complication rate in some studies but remains controversial to date.[35] Although rare, vascular injuries have been reported from dorsal approaches and carry a mortality rate as high as 10–40% depending on the type and location of the injury.[36] The artery of Adamkiewicz is a large artery supplying the thoracolumbar spinal cord. It typically exits the aorta on the left side at lower thoracic or upper lumbar levels. Injury to this vessel can result in an extensive spinal cord infarction. Preoperative angiography is often used to identify the anatomic location of this vessel in order to avoid injury during surgery.

Visceral injury is rare in ventral approaches since the exposure is carried out in a retroperitoneal fashion although post-operative ileus is present frequently. Injury to the lumbar sympathetic plexus occurs in about 6% of all ventral approaches to the lumbosacral spine and usually results from retraction injury. Patients typically report an ipsilateral warm leg after surgery that often resolves spontaneously. Injury to the superior hypogastric plexus is often a troubling complication after surgery and can result in bladder dysfunction in female patients and retrograde ejaculation/sterility in male patients.[37] Careful surgical technique and avoidance of electrocautery in the region of the prevertebral fascia is the best way to avoid such complications.

Durotomy

Unintended durotomy is a common complication from spinal surgery at any level. Recent data suggest that the rate of unintended durotomy is about 1.6%. Risk increases with age, revision surgery, kyphosis, spondylolisthesis, and degenerative disease of the spine. It is also less common in the cervical spine than in the thoracic or lumbar spine.[38]

Management includes primary repair of the defect occasionally with fibrin glue or muscle patching. When primary repair is either incomplete or unsuccessful, a lumbar drain is typically inserted and left in place for 2–3 days postoperatively. Most patients recover well after durotomy and studies indicate that incidental durotomy does not seem to impact long-term outcomes including pain, physical function, infection, and mortality.[39] Occasionally, a CSF leak can persist requiring additional surgery due to risk of infection and or wound breakdown.

Summary

Avoiding complications in spine surgery is a complex endeavor for the spine surgeon and anesthesiologist alike. The process begins with a thorough, multidisciplinary selection of patients suitable for surgery, which includes preoperative optimization of cardiac, pulmonary, renal, and nutritional status. Additional measures such as a perioperative antibiotic regimen and steroid therapy can also improve outcomes when used appropriately. Special care must be given to patients with severe stenosis and/or instability. Knowledge of proper positioning technique and awareness of the risks inherent in each surgical procedure allows both the anesthesia and surgical teams to anticipate potential complications and improve outcomes in patients undergoing spine surgery.

References

1. Hu SS, Berven SH. Preparing the adult deformity patient for spinal surgery. *Spine* 2006; **31**(19 Suppl): S126–31.

2. Halpin RJ, Sugrue PA, Gould RW, *et al.* Standardizing care for high-risk patients in spine surgery: the northwestern high-risk spine protocol. *Spine* 2010; **35**(25): 2232–8.

3. Kim KA, Wang MY. Anesthetic considerations in the treatment of cervical myelopathy. *Spine J* 2006; **6**(6 Suppl): 207S–11S.

4. Bonhomme V, Hans P. Management of the unstable cervical spine: elective versus emergent cases. *Curr Opin Anaesthesiol* 2009; **22**(5): 579–85.

5. Dempsey R, Rapp RP, Young B, Johnston S, Tibbs P. Prophylactic parenteral antibiotics in clean neurosurgical procedures: A review. *J Neurosurg.* 1988; **69**(1): 52–7.

6. Dobzyniak MA, Fischgrund JS, Hankins S, Herkowitz HN. Single versus multiple dose antibiotic prophylaxis in lumbar disc surgery. *Spine* 2003; **28**(21): E453–5.

7. Watanabe M, Sakai D, Matsuyama D, *et al.* Risk factors for surgical site infection following spine surgery: Efficacy of intraoperative saline irrigation. *J Neurosurg Spine* 2010; **12**(5): 540–6.

8. Schuster JM, Rechtine G, Norvell DC, Dettori JR. The influence of perioperative risk factors and therapeutic interventions on infection rates after spine surgery: A systematic review. *Spine* 2010; **35**(9 Suppl): S125–37.

9. Fang A, Hu SS, Endres N, Bradford DS. Risk factors for infection after spinal surgery. *Spine* 2005; **30**(12): 1460–5.

10. Watters WC,3rd, Baisden J, Bono CM, *et al.* Antibiotic prophylaxis in spine surgery: an evidence-based clinical guideline for the use of prophylactic antibiotics in spine surgery. *Spine J* 2009; **9**(2): 142–6.

11. Braughler JM, Hall ED. Current application of "high-dose" steroid therapy for CNS injury. A pharmacological perspective. *J Neurosurg* 1985; **62**(6): 806–10.

12. Hall ED, Wolf DL, Braughler JM. Effects of a single large dose of methylprednisolone sodium succinate on experimental posttraumatic spinal cord ischemia: dose-response and time-action analysis. *J Neurosurg* 1984; **61**(1): 124–30.

13. Bracken MB, Shepard MJ, Holford TR, *et al.* Administration of methylprednisolone for 24 or 48 h or tirilazad mesylate for 48 h in the treatment of acute spinal cord injury. Results of the third national acute spinal cord injury randomized controlled trial. National acute spinal cord injury study. *JAMA* 1997; **277**(20): 1597–604.

14. Short DJ, El Masry WS, Jones PW. High dose methylprednisolone in the management of acute spinal cord injury – a systematic review from a clinical perspective. *Spinal Cord* 2000; **38**(5): 273–86.

15. Eck JC, Nachtigall D, Humphreys SC, Hodges SD. Questionnaire survey of spine surgeons on the use of methylprednisolone for acute spinal cord injury. *Spine* 2006; **31**(9): E250–3.

16. Ghafoor AU, Martin TW, Gopalakrishnan S, Viswamitra S. Caring for the patients with cervical spine injuries: What have we learned? *J Clin Anesth* 2005; **17**(8): 640–9.

17. Aarabi B, Koltz M, Ibrahimi D. Hyperextension cervical spine injuries and traumatic central cord syndrome. *Neurosurg Focus* 2008; **25**(5): E9.

18. Kim CW, Perry A, Garfin SR. Spinal instability: The orthopedic approach. *Semin Musculoskelet Radiol* 2005; **9**(1): 77–87.

19. Morone MA, Ball PA. Spinal traction. In: Benzel EC, ed. *Spine Surgery: Techniques, Complication Avoidance, and Management.* 2nd ed. Philadelphia, PA: Elsevier; 2005: 1905–13.

20. Bertrand ML, Beerle BJ. Anesthesia. In: Benzel EC, ed. *Spine Surgery: Techniques, Complication Avoidance, and Management.* 2nd ed. Philadelphia, PA: Elsevier; 2005: 1823–36.

21. Newman NJ. Perioperative visual loss after nonocular surgeries. *Am J Ophthalmol* 2008; **145**(4): 604–10.

22. Ho VT, Newman NJ, Song S, Ksiazek S, Roth S. Ischemic optic neuropathy following spine surgery. *J Neurosurg Anesthesiol* 2005; **17**(1): 38–44.

23. Lee LA, Newman NJ, Wagner TA, Dettori JR, Dettori NJ. Postoperative ischemic optic neuropathy. *Spine* 2010; **35**(9 Suppl): S105–16.

24. Mirski MA, Lele AV, Fitzsimmons L, Toung TJ. Diagnosis and treatment of vascular air embolism. *Anesthesiology* 2007; **106**(1): 164–77.

25. Losasso TJ, Muzzi DA, Dietz NM, Cucchiara RF. Fifty percent nitrous oxide does not increase the risk of venous air embolism in neurosurgical patients operated upon in the sitting position. *Anesthesiology* 1992; **77**(1): 21–30.

26. Shaikh N, Ummunisa F. Acute management of vascular air embolism. *J Emerg Trauma Shock* 2009; **2**(3): 180–5.

27. Zileli M, Naderi S, Benzel EC. Preoperative and surgical planning for avoiding complications. In: Benzel EC, ed. *Spine Surgery: Techniques, Complication Avoidance, and*

Management. 2nd ed. Philadelphia, PA: Elsevier; 2005: 233–41.

28. Saunders RL. On the pathogenesis of the radiculopathy complicating multilevel corpectomy. *Neurosurgery* 1995; **37**(3): 408–12; discussion 412–13.

29. Apfelbaum RI, Kriskovich MD, Haller JR. On the incidence, cause, and prevention of recurrent laryngeal nerve palsies during anterior cervical spine surgery. *Spine* 2000; **25**(22): 2906–12.

30. Park SH, Sung JK, Lee SH, Park J, Hwang JH, Hwang SK. High anterior cervical approach to the upper cervical spine. *Surg Neurol* 2007; **68**(5): 519–24; discussion 524.

31. Patel NP, Wolcott WP, Johnson JP, *et al.* Esophageal injury associated with anterior cervical spine surgery. *Surg Neurol* 2008; **69**(1): 20–4; discussion 24.

32. McCormick WE, Will SF, Benzel EC. Surgery for thoracic disc disease: complication avoidance: Overview and management. *Neurosurg Focus* 2000; **9**(4): e13.

33. Stillerman CB, Chen TC, Couldwell WT, Zhang W, Weiss MH. Experience in the surgical management of 82 symptomatic herniated thoracic discs and review of the literature. *J Neurosurg* 1998; **88**(4): 623–33.

34. Fessler RG, Sturgill M. Review: Complications of surgery for thoracic disc disease. *Surg Neurol* 1998; **49**(6): 609–18.

35. Jarrett CD, Heller JG, Tsai L. Anterior exposure of the lumbar spine with and without an "access surgeon": Morbidity analysis of 265 consecutive cases. *J Spinal Disord Tech* 2009; **22**(8): 559–64.

36. Papadoulas S, Konstantinou D, Kourea HP, *et al.* Vascular injury complicating lumbar disc surgery. A systematic review. *Eur J Vasc Endovasc Surg* 2002; **24**(3): 189–95.

37. Kang BU, Choi WC, Lee SH, *et al.* An analysis of general surgery-related complications in a series of 412 minilaparotomic anterior lumbosacral procedures. *J Neurosurg Spine* 2009; **10**(1): 60–5.

38. Williams BJ, Sansur CA, Smith JS, *et al.* Incidence of unintended durotomy in spine surgery based on 108,478 cases. *Neurosurgery* 2011; **68**(1): 117–23; discussion 123–4.

39. Desai A, Ball PA, Bekelis K, *et al.* SPORT: Does incidental durotomy affect long-term outcomes in cases of spinal stenosis? *Neurosurgery* 2011; **69**(1): 38–44; discussion 44.

Chapter

9

Anesthesia for cervical spine surgery

Alaa A. Abd-Elsayed and Ehab Farag

Key points

- Surgery on the cervical spine is one of the most commonly performed surgical procedures. Anesthesiologists should be aware of the anatomy of the cervical spine and syndromes associated with cervical spine abnormalities.
- Fiberoptic intubation is least likely to cause cervical spine movement during endotracheal intubation.
- It is very important to maintain a normal or a slightly higher blood pressure during cervical spine surgery to avoid spinal cord hypoperfusion.
- Direct laryngoscopy can cause central cord syndrome in patients with cervical spondylosis.
- The incidence of quadriplegia during cervical spine surgery is between 0.1% and 0.4%.

Introduction

Cervical spine surgery is one of the most frequently performed spine procedures. In the United States between 1990 and 2000, surgery to treat degenerative cervical spine disease increased twofold, from 29 to 55 cases per 100 000 people (100 000 hospitalizations per year).

Anesthetic management for cervical spine surgery requires understanding the anatomy of the cervical spine, the pathophysiology of cervical degenerative disease, and proper upper airway management during cervical spine surgery. The aim of this chapter is to present the most recent evidence-based findings pertinent to anesthesia for cervical spine surgery.

Anatomy of the cervical spine

The general characteristics of the 3rd through 6th cervical vertebrae are as follows:

- The **body** of these four vertebrae is small, and broader from side to side than from front to back.

- The anterior and posterior surfaces are flat and equally deep. The anterior surface is lower than the posterior. Its inferior border extends downward, overlapping the upper and forepart of the vertebra below.
- The upper surface is concave transversely, with a projecting lip on either side.
- The lower surface is concave from front to back, convex from side to side, and has laterally shallow concavities that receive the corresponding projecting lips of the underlying vertebra.

- The **pedicles** are directed laterally and backward, and are attached midway between the upper and lower borders of the body, making the superior vertebral notch as deep as that of the inferior, but also narrower.
- The **laminae** are narrow, and thinner at the top than at the bottom; the vertebral foramen is large and triangular.
- The **spinous process** is short and bifid; the two divisions are often unequal in size.
- The superior and inferior **articular processes** of cervical vertebrae are fused on one or both sides, forming articular pillars, columns of bone that project laterally from the juncture of the pedicle and lamina.
  - The articular facets are flat and oval.
  - The superior facet is positioned backward, upward, and slightly medially.
  - The inferior facet is positioned forward, downward, and slightly laterally.
- The **foramen transversarium** pierces each of the transverse processes, which, in the upper six vertebrae, gives passage to the **vertebral artery** and **vein,** and to a plexus of **sympathetic**

Anesthesia for Spine Surgery, ed. Ehab Farag. Published by Cambridge University Press. © Cambridge University Press 2012.

nerves. Each process consists of an anterior and a posterior part, both of which are joined outside the foramen by a bar of bone that exhibits a deep sulcus on its upper surface for the passage of the corresponding **spinal nerve.**

- The anterior part of each process, named the costal process or costal element, is the homologue of the **rib** in the **thoracic** region. It arises from the side of the body, is directed laterally in front of the foramen, and ends in the **anterior tubercle.**

- The posterior part, the true transverse process, springs from the vertebral arch behind the foramen, and is directed forward and laterally; it ends in a flattened vertical tubercle, the **posterior tubercle.**

Special cervical vertebrae (C1, C2, and C7)

C1 (**atlas**): The topmost vertebra, along with C2, forms the joint connecting the **skull and spine.** The major characteristic of this vertebra is that it lacks a distinctive body (Fig. 9.1).

C2 (**axis**): This forms the pivot upon which C1 rotates. The most distinctive characteristic of this vertebra is its strong **odontoid process** (dens), which rises perpendicularly from the upper surface of the body. The body is deeper in front than behind, and prolonged downward anteriorly so as to overlap the upper and front part of the third vertebra (Fig. 9.2). The interval between the posterior aspect of the odontoid process and the anterior aspect of the posterior ring of the atlas is termed the posterior atlas–dens interval and is the space available for the cord. The space available for the cord at C1 may be divided into cord and half space; the space allows for some encroachment of the spinal lumen without compromising the cord. At lower cervical levels (between C4 and C7), the spinal cord normally fills approximately 75% of the cross-sectional area of the canal.

C7 (**vertebra prominens**): The most distinctive characteristic of this vertebra is its long and prominent spinous process, hence the name vertebra prominens. In some subjects, this vertebra is associated with an abnormal pair of ribs, as the **cervical ribs**. Although usually small, they occasionally compress blood vessels

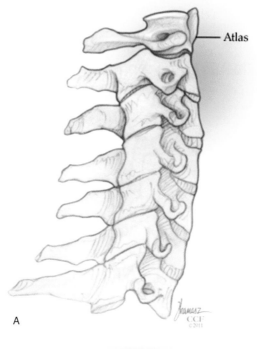

A

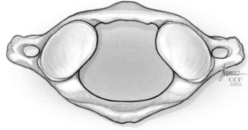

B

Figure 9.1 The atlas.

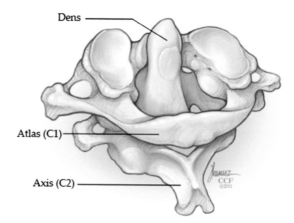

Figure 9.2 Relationship between the axis and the atlas.

179

(such as the **subclavian artery**) or nerves in the **brachial plexus,** causing ischemic muscle pain, numbness, tingling, and weakness in the upper limb.

Movements of the cervical spine

Nodding of the head originates predominantly through **flexion** and **extension** at the joint between the atlas and the occipital bone, the **atlantooccipital joint**. However, the cervical spine is comparatively mobile, and some component of this movement is due to flexion and extension of the vertebral column itself.

Shaking or rotating the head left and right originates almost entirely at the **atlantoaxial joint.** A small amount of rotation of the vertebral column itself contributes to the movement.

Landmarks

- Base of nose and the hard palate correspond to C1.
- Teeth (when mouth remains closed) correspond to C2.
- Mandible and hyoid bone correspond to C3.
- The thyroid cartilage lies from C4 to C5.
- The cricoid cartilage lies from C6 to C7.

Movement of the cervical spine with intubation

The anesthesiologist must align the pharyngeal and laryngeal axis during intubation. In addition, to place a tube via direct laryngoscopy, the anesthesiologist must be able to obtain a line-of-sight view between the eye and enough of the glottis to allow placement of the endotracheal (ET) tube through the trachea. Placement of the tube requires a complex series of movements. The primary force applied by the laryngoscope is upward lift, which results in extension of the occiput and the O–C1 interspace. The lift also results in flexion at lower vertebrae. There is evidence that laryngoscopy results in maximal extension at O and C1, with flexion below C2. Any intervention that requires this combination of extension and flexion movements will make it more difficult for the glottis to be visualized. External stabilization methods may reduce movement during direct laryngoscopy (DL) but they will also make glottic visualization more difficult.

Atlantoaxial instability, observed in patients with rheumatoid arthritis (RA) and Down's syndrome, holds important clinical significance for anesthesiologists. In atlantoaxial instability, the odontoid process is no longer firmly held against the back of the anterior arch of C1, due either to disruption of the transverse ligament or to damage of the odontoid process itself.

In patients with severe or longstanding RA, the transverse ligament as well as several joints in the neck are destroyed. Roughly 30% of patients with severe disease will exhibit some instability at C1–C2, although few patients require surgical correction. It is advisable for all patients with severe RA to have periodic flexion and extension radiographs, certainly prior to undergoing any surgical procedure. Similarly, roughly 15% of patients with Down's syndrome exhibit laxity in the transverse ligament. It is advisable that all Down's patients have radiography at ages 3, 12, and 18 years, before any surgical procedure that requires DL or extensive neck manipulation, or before they engage in vigorous sports.

Atlantoaxial instability arises from the fact that C1 is a rigid ring affixed firmly to the base of the skull. If the transverse ligament is damaged, lifting the skull and C1 will result in an increase in the anterior atlantodental interval and hence a decrease in the posterior atlantodental interval. In other words, C2 remains fixed while C1 slides anteriorly, with the cord becoming compressed or trapped in the space behind the odontoid.[1]

Five other conditions which may affect the cervical spine and which are significant during intubation are as follows:

1. **Achondroplasia**
   Radiologic images show a large skull with a narrow foramen magnum and relatively small skull base and short flattened vertebral bodies with relatively large intervertebral disc heights.[2] Up to 85% of infants born with achondroplasia may exhibit neurologic findings, including respiratory irregularity.[3,4] The rate of sudden infant death syndrome is significantly higher in children with achondroplasia.

2. **Klippel–Feil syndrome** and **Klippel–Feil variant**
   These are conventionally recognized as a triad of low-lying hairline, short neck, and cervical fusion abnormalities. Patients with cervical fusion abnormalities alone are said to exhibit the Klippel–Feil variant. Associated abnormalities include scoliosis, rib abnormalities, Sprengel deformity, synkinesis, and genitourinary and cardiovascular disorders.[5,6] Patients have limited neck motion and are usually difficult to intubate.

3. **Neurofibromatosis type 1 (NF1)**
   This is characterized by progressive cervical kyphosis, which may occur because of intrinsic ligamentous abnormality and abnormal bony architecture. Cervical kyphosis also may occur

following resection of soft tissue or extradural neurofibromas.

4. **Chiari malformation**

   This congenital anomaly is characterized by crowding of the posterior fossa by the neural elements and hindbrain herniation through the foramen magnum. There are four types of Chiari malformation. Type I, most common in adults, occurs in up to 0.5% of the population. Type II is more severe and associated with a myelomeningocele. Types III and IV are associated with high early mortality. Anomalies of the base of the skull and upper cervical spine are seen in many patients with type I and may include occipitalization of C1, fusion of C1 to C2, Klippel–Feil deformity, or cervical spina bifida occulta.[7]

5. **Common skeletal dysplasias**

   These are all characterized by the presence of a hypoplastic or aplastic dens with varying degrees of atlantoaxial subluxation.

   - Morquio's syndrome (mucopolysaccharidosis IV): autosomal recessive. Type A (severe) and type B (mild) are recognized by the enzymes involved.
   - Spondyloepiphyseal dysplasia: autosomal dominant.
   - Diastrophic dwarfism: autosomal recessive.
   - Osteogenesis imperfecta.

Preoperative assessment

As in other situations, preoperative assessment should routinely include the patient's past medical history and most importantly the patient's baseline blood pressure. Maintaining tight control of blood within 10% of basal mean arterial pressure (MAP) is crucial to maintaining perfusion to a myelopathic spinal cord during surgery. Examination of the patient's ability to flex and extend the neck without symptoms while awake is a very important step in assessing upper airway management during surgery. The anesthesiologist should examine the patient for the presence or absence of Lhermitte's sign, sometimes called the "barber chair" phenomenon. Lhermitte's sign is an electrical sensation that runs down the back and into the limbs from involvement of the posterior columns, and is produced by flexion or by extending the neck. This sign suggests compression of the spinal cord in the neck from any cause such as cervical spondylosis, disc herniation, tumor, or Arnold–Chiari malformation. The presence of Lhermitte's should alert the

anesthesiologist to use extra caution in maintaining a neutral head position during intubation and throughout the whole procedure. It is advisable to use awake fiberoptic intubation in these patients. The indication for surgery is important in predicting the degree of difficult intubation.

Cervical spondylosis, the commonest indication for cervical spine surgery, suggests difficult laryngoscopy. It has been suggested that anterior osteophytes can make direct laryngoscopy difficult in patients with cervical spondylosis.

Another important pathology is RA. Patients with RA can be classified into two groups, those who require surgery for atlantoaxial subluxation and those who require surgery for vertical subluxation of the axis. Vertical subluxation of the axis occurs when an intervertebral joint is lost, resulting in a short, stiff neck in such patients. The high prevalence of difficult laryngoscopy in RA patients is a consequence of the combination of occipito-atlanto-axial disease and temporomandibular joint disease. RA patients have impaired mandibular protrusion due to an impaired temporomandibular joint. Mandibular protrusion is essential for mouth opening: 30% of mouth opening ability depends on it.[8] The co-occurrence of occipito-atlanto-axial disease and poor protrusion in RA patients carries serious implications for laryngoscopy. Failure of extension at the craniocervical junction during laryngoscopy was found to result in anterior bowing of the cervical spine, which pushed the larynx forward.[9] Extension at the craniocervical junction is also necessary for full mouth opening. Deviation of the glottis from the midline has been reported in cervical RA. Finally, direct laryngoscopy in patients with undiagnosed atlantoaxial subluxation was reported to cause quadriplegia.[10]

Cervical radiculopathy and myelopathy

The presence of cervical radiculopathy or myelopathy represents an important symptom that should be examined in the preoperative setting. Neurologic symptoms in cervical spondylosis result from a cascade of degenerative changes that most likely begin at the cervical disc. Age-related changes result in a progressive loss of disc viscoelastic properties. The disc loses height and bulges posteriorly into the canal. With loss of height the vertebral bodies drift toward one another. Posteriorly, infolding occurs in the ligamentum flavum and facet joint capsule, causing a decrease in canal and foraminal dimensions. Osteophytes form around the disc margins and at the facet joints. The posteriorly protruded disc material, osteophytes, or thickened soft tissue within the canal or foramen results in extrinsic pressure on the nerve root or spinal cord. Mechanical distortion of the nerve root may lead to motor weakness or sensory deficits. Within the compressed nerve root, intrinsic blood vessels show increased permeability and nerve root edema. Chronic edema and fibrosis within the nerve root will result in nerve root pain or radiculopathy. Cervical spondylotic myelopathy is the manifestation of cumulative signs that result from a decrease in the space available for the cervical spinal cord.

A congenital decrease in the anterior–posterior diameter of the spinal canal can play a role in the development of cervical myelopathy. Individuals with an anterior–posterior diameter of the spinal canal of <13 mm (normal 17–18 mm) are considered to have congenital cervical stenosis. There is a strong association between flattening of the cord within the narrowed spinal canal and the development of cervical myelopathy. Ono and colleagues described an anterior–posterior cord compression ratio that was calculated by dividing the anterior–posterior diameter of the cord by the cord's transverse diameter.[11] Patients with substantial flattening of the cord (banana-shaped spinal cord) suggested by an anterior–posterior ratio of <0.40 tended to have worse neurologic function. The increase in this ratio to ≥0.40 or an increase in transverse area to >40 mm was a strong predictor of recovery following surgery.

Dynamic factors in the cervical spinal column affect the degree of cord compression. Hyperextension narrows the spinal canal by shingling the laminae and buckling the ligamentum flavum. Translation or angulation between vertebral bodies in flexion or extension can result in narrowing of the space available for the cord. Patients who lack cord compression statically may compress the cord dynamically, leading to the development of myelopathic symptoms. Retrolisthesis of the vertebral body can result in pinching of the spinal cord between the inferior–posterior margin of a vertebral body and the superior edge of the lamina caudad to it (Fig. 9.3). This compression may be aggravated in extension, and it may be relieved in flexion as the retrolisthesis tends to reduce. Hypermobility cephalad to a degenerated and stiffened segment is commonly seen at the third and fourth cervical levels in elderly patients and it may result in myelopathy. Breig and colleagues[12] showed that the spinal cord stretches with flexion of the cervical spine and shortens and thickens with extension: the "Poisson effect." Thickening of the cord in extension makes it more

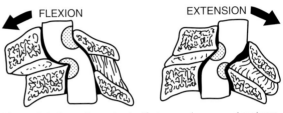

Figure 9.3 Dynamic mechanical factors, such as normal or abnormal motion, can create the so-called pioneer phenomenon, which may be associated with different patterns of encroachment of the cord. (From Bernhardt M, Hynes RA, Blume HW, White AA, Current concepts review: cervical spondylitic myelopathy. *Journal of Bone and Joint Surgery American* 1993;75:119–28. Used with permission.)

susceptible to pressure from the infolded ligamentum flavum or lamina. In flexion, the stretched cord may be prone to higher intrinsic pressure if it is abutting against a disc or vertebral body anteriorly.[13] Prone positioning is often associated with modest degrees of extension and therefore the cord might sustain excessive pressure induced by soft encroachment on the spinal canal with extension and aggravated by the preexisting canal compromise. The clinical relevance of these findings is that a persistent malposition of an abnormal neck may result in cord ischemia and neurologic injury. Prone positioning is also associated with increases in vena caval pressures, which may further reduce cord blood flow, already compromised by cord compression, by increasing resistance in the venous outflow channels.[7]

In sum, the best way to reduce neurologic complications during anesthetic management for cervical spine is to keep the head in neutral position as much as possible during surgery.

Mechanism of myelopathy

Severe compression results in direct injury to neurons and a secondary cascade of events including ischemia, excitotoxicity, and apoptosis in the spinal cord.[14] The central gray matter and the lateral columns manifest the most changes, with cystic cavitation, gliosis, and demyelination most prominent caudad to the site of compression. The posterior columns and poster lateral tracts show wallerian degeneration cephalad to the site of compression. These irreversible changes may explain why some patients do not recover following decompressive surgery.[13]

Nurick classification of cervical myelopathy

The severity of cervical spondylotic myelopathy can be graded according to the Nurick grading system. The

Table 9.1 Nurick classification of cervical myelopathy

Grade 1: Spinal cord disease with no problem walking
Grade 2: Slight difficulty walking but can work
Grade 3: Difficulty walking and cannot work full-time
Grade 4: Can only walk with help of a frame walker
Grade 5: Chair-bound or bedridden

Nurick system grades disability in cervical spondylotic myelopathy on the basis of gait abnormality (Table 9.1). Patients with grade 1 have no difficulty in walking, whereas grade 5 patients are chair-bound or bedridden.[15]

Atypical presentations of cervical spondylosis

Cervical angina is a symptom mimicking ischemic heart disease but produced by cervical radiculopathy. Chronic breast pain in women may be due to cervical radiculopathy. Marked spurring along the anterior aspects of the vertebral bodies due to proliferative degenerative changes may manifest as dysphagia, dyspnea, or dysphonia as a result of pressure on the esophagus, larynx, or trachea. Similar hypertrophic spurs resulting from the uncovertebral joints and facet joints can occlude the vertebral artery in its foramen and result in thrombosis of the vertebral artery. If thrombosis spreads to the posterior inferior cerebellar artery, it may lead to palsy of the ipsilateral cranial nerves V, IX, X, and XI. Horner's syndrome, cerebellar ataxia, and possibly death – a constellation known as Wallenberg's syndrome – occurs.[13]

Airway management for cervical spine surgery

Patients with disorders of the cervical spine have a higher incidence of difficult intubation than do matched controls, and the incidence increases with the severity of the disease.[16] A patient with atlantoaxial instability is in supine position; passive movement of the head with either flexion or extension may cause the atlas and the axis to separate, and this may result in increased subluxation. In addition, sniffing may significantly increase subluxation.[7] If a small, flat pillow, with a doughnut-shaped pillow on top, is placed beneath the patient's head, it will provide support to the upper cervical spine by moving the odontoid process forward, closing the anterior atlas–dens interval, and increasing the posterior atlas–dens interval.[7]

The primary force applied during DL is upward lift with a little angular force. This force can be as high as 50–70 N (45 N is sufficient to lift 4.5 kg or 10 lbs). The more difficult the exposure, as in cervical spondylosis, the greater is the force that is usually applied and thus the greater likelihood of cervical injury during intubation. DL with the MAC 3 blade results in near maximal extension at the occiput and C1.[17,18] Fiberoptic intubation is accordingly an ideal method, for it entails the least degree of upper cervical spine motion when cervical spine movement is not feasible.[19] Surveys indicate that the majority of anesthesiologists in theUnited States prefer to use a fiberoptic bronchoscope to intubate at-risk patients and to do so with the patient awake.[20]

The use of the laryngeal mask airway (LMA) or intubating laryngeal mask airway (ILMA) is not recommended for upper airway management in unstable cervical spine, as these exert high pressure against the upper cervical vertebrae during insertion, during inflation and while in situ.[21]

Manual in-line stabilization (MILS) and cricoid pressure

The goal in MILS is to apply force to the head and neck equal in magnitude and opposite in direction to those generated by DL so as to limit the movement that might result during airway management; traction forces should be avoided. However, MILS not only failed to reduce movement at the site of instability in cadaver models but also limited the anesthesiologists' ability to visualize the vocal cords.[22,23] However, cricoid pressure, as long as it was not excessive, did not result in movement in a cadaver model of an injured upper cervical spine.[24]

Central cord syndrome and direct laryngoscopy

Central cord syndrome (CCS) was first described by Schneider in 1954. Classic CCS presents as underlying cervical spondylosis in the older patient above 60 years old who sustains a hyperextension injury without any evidence of damage to the bony spine. The pathologic mechanism involves compression of the cord, by osteophytes anteriorly and by infolded ligamentum flavum posteriorly, impinging on the central cord spinal cord and leading to ischemia, edema, or hematomyelia. Cumulatively, this mechanism results in subsequent injury to the lateral corticospinal tracts.

Hyperextension often seems mild, as in direct intubation, but in the setting of cervical spondylosis it can result in marked neurologic injury. Younger patients with congenital cervical stenosis also are at increased risk of sustaining CCS as a result of hyperextension injury.

Finally, it is noteworthy that patients with chronic renal failure are prone to spinal degenerative disease. The term destructive spondyloarthropathy (DSA) is used to describe a process occurring in hemodialysis patients which affects the cervical spine. Therefore, the head of a patient with chronic renal failure should be kept in neutral position during endotracheal intubation and during surgery.[25]

CCS presents on a spectrum, from weakness confined to the hands and forearms, with sensory preservation, to complete quadriparesis. The upper extremities, particularly the hands and forearms are more severely affected than the lower extremities.[26–28]

Chin lift, jaw thrust, and DL can cumulatively cause movement in the cervical spine, and thereby induce spinal cord injury. Lee and Andree[29] have shown the difficulty of intubating patients with spondylosis. In addition, case reports have addressed cervical traumatic injury after intubation using DL in patients without preexisting cervical spine fracture.[25,27,29,30] During cervical spine surgery it is advisable to use either awake or asleep fiberoptic intubation, while keeping the patient's neck in neutral position to avoid cervical spine injury.

Induction and maintenance of anesthesia

Induction of anesthesia is unusually challenging during cervical spine surgery. During this period the spinal cord has not yet been mechanically decompressed, the neck musculature is unable to provide protective stabilization, and the patient cannot be assessed neurologically. Neck motion during this phase can be considerable, producing dynamic spinal cord compression that could result in cervical spine injury. It should be remembered that neck extension in patients with cervical spondylosis can narrow the diameter of the spinal canal, whereas in those with rheumatoid disease or Down's syndrome, neck flexion will widen the atlantodental interval, narrowing the spinal canal.

Anterior cervical surgery is straightforward, as the patient remains in the supine position. However, for posterior cervical procedures, the patient will be placed in prone position. Special care should be exercised during prone positioning to avoid injury to the spinal cord. The head is usually positioned in a Mayfield skull clamp, and turning must be accomplished without excessive neck motion. The neck is typically placed in a slightly flexed or neutral position for patients with spondylotic myelopathy or slightly extended for patients with atlantoaxial subluxation so as to maximize the diameter of the spinal cord.[31] If the patient has severe cervical myelopathy or a severely unstable neck, perform awake fiberoptic intubation. While the patient is wake and under light sedation, the surgeon applies a Mayfield skull clamp to the patient's head after applying local anesthetics to the clamp sites and then the patient is turned prone. Only after positioning the patient and performing neurologic examination while the patient is still awake, do we induce anesthesia.

During maintenance of anesthesia, close attention must be paid to maintaining adequate blood pressure during surgery. The chronically compressed cervical cord appears to have limited perfusion reserves and as a result may be more susceptible to ischemic injury. Dogs with chronic cervical cord compression exhibited signs of cord dysfunction at systemic arterial blood pressures 20–30 mmHg greater than dogs without cord compression.[32] These findings indicate that patients with severe cervical stenosis may be susceptible to cervical cord ischemic injury by neck movement and/or hypotension that would not otherwise cause injury in the absence of this condition.[33] Therefore, blood pressure should be maintained at or slightly above the patient's baseline. During surgery, blood pressure is preferably monitored using an arterial line so that even transient reductions in perfusion can be identified. Furthermore, hypotension strategies to control blood loss should be avoided as they can threaten spinal cord function and are ineffective, as most bleeding is of venous or bony origin.[34]

During anterior cervical discectomy (ACD) with fusion (ACDF) or without, some degree of pressure on the carotid artery is an inescapable element of this procedure. In order to expose the anterior surface of the cervical vertebral column, the surgeon should displace the carotid sheath and the strap muscles laterally and achieve medial displacement of the trachea and the esophagus. The surgeon should palpate the carotid pulse superior to the retractor. This maneuver is non-quantitative and raises the possibility of false-positive confirmation of adequate flow because of arterial pulsation transmitted through soft tissue. Therefore maintaining adequate blood pressure during this procedure is crucial for maintaining cerebral perfusion and avoiding ischemic stroke if the circle of Willis fails to maintain compensatory collateral flow.[35,36]

Complications associated with cervical spine surgery

The immediate postoperative period after extensive cervical spine surgery is crucial as emergency re-intubation or tracheostomy can lead to graft-related neurologic complications, hypoxia, and death. Risk factors contribute to delays in extubation or necessitate tracheostomy following complex cervical spine procedures. Risk factors include obesity, operative time greater than 10 hours, ACDF including C2 level, and asthma. Additional rare risk factors include recurrent laryngeal nerve (RLN) palsy (<1% with left-sided approaches), esophageal perforation, and new postoperative spinal cord deficits.[36] When these risk factors are present, it is preferable to postpone immediate postoperative extubation and instead to extubate over a tube exchanger with fiberoptic examination in order to identify residual postoperative tracheal and/or vocal cord swelling.[36]

- The development of postoperative wound hematoma is a potentially catastrophic complication. It usually presents mainly as a neck mass associated with dysphagia and occasionally as respiratory distress. Its incidence varies between 1% and 11%. The management of this complication requires immediate awake fiberoptic intubation and reoperation to evacuate the neck hematoma.

- RLN palsy is one of the most commonly reported ACDF-related complications. RLN injury could be caused by direct nerve injury at the time of neck dissection, surgical retractor placement, or endotracheal balloon insufflation pressure.[37] Releasing the air from the endotracheal cuff and reinflating after the retractor blade placement decreased the rate of temporary vocal cord paralysis from 6.4% to 1.69% in one study.[38] Interestingly, clinically silent RLN palsy was found in 16% of patients in ACDF surgery in a study by Jung and colleagues.[39] RLN injury is clinically expressed as postoperative airway obstruction, hoarseness, vocal fatigue, persistent cough, aspiration, and dysphagia.[40] The incidence of this complication during ACDF has been reported to range from 0.2% to 16.7%. RLN injury

is more common with the right-sided approach than the left-sided one, for the right RLN has a shorter, more oblique course than the left RLN.[41] Patients that are at higher risk for developing RLN palsy, such as those who have previously undergone neck surgery, patients with an enlarged thyroid gland, and patients with preexisting hoarseness might be candidates for preoperative laryngoscopic examination before they undergo ACD surgery.[39,40]

- Esophageal or pharyngeal perforation during ACDF is a rare but potentially serious complication. After surgery, the presence of subcutaneous emphysema or widening and haziness of the mediastinum on radiographs or CT scan might be indicative of esophageal injury, and the patient should be further evaluated and appropriately treated.

- Vascular injury during ACDF, mainly to the vertebral artery (VA), has been reported as high as 0.3%.[41,42] An anomalous and tortuous course of the VA, the presence of an aberrant artery, previous irradiation, and the presence of dense scar tissue all constitute risk factors for intraoperative VA injury.[39]

- The incidence of severe intraoperative cervical cord injury (quadriplegia) during cervical spine surgery is between 0.1% and 0.4% (1–4 per 1000).

The ASA closed claims analysis for spinal cord injury shows that the main nonsurgical factors for spinal cord injury during cervical spine surgery include head or neck position during surgery or intubation and/or arterial blood pressure; patients with preexisting cord injury from either trauma or myelopathy are the most susceptible.[34]

Conclusion

Appropriate anesthetic management for cervical spine surgery demands proper understanding of the anatomy of the cervical spine, the pathophysiology of cervical stenosis or instability, and associated complications.

References

1. Todd M. Cervical spine anatomy and function for the anesthesiologist. *Can J Anaesth* 2001; **48**: R1–5.

2. Hecht JT, Nelson FW, Butler IJ, *et al.* Computerized tomography of the foramen magnum: achondroplastic values compared to normal standards. *Am J Med Genet* 1985; **20**: 355–60.

3. Reid CS, Pyeritz RE, Kopits SE, *et al.* Cervicomedullary cord compression in young children with achondroplasia: value of comprehensive neurologic and respiratory evaluation. *Basic Life Sci* 1988; **48**: 199–206.

4. Reid CS, Pyeritz RE, Kopits SE, *et al.* Cervicomedullary cord compression in young children with achondroplasia: value of comprehensive neurologic and respiratory evaluation. *J Pediatr* 1987; **110**: 522–30.

5. Hensinger RN, Lang JE, MacEwen GD. Klippel–Feil syndrome: a constellation of associated anomalies. *J Bone Joint Surg Am* 1974; **56**: 1246–53.

6. Herman MJ, Pizzutillo PD. Cervical spine disorders in children. *Orthop Clin North Am* 1999; **30**: 457–66.

7. Crosby ET. Considerations for airway management for cervical spine surgery in adults. *Anesthesiol Clin* 2007; **25**: 511–33.

8. Calder I, Calder J, Crockard HA. Difficult direct laryngoscopy in patients with cervical spine disease. *Anaesthesia* 1995; **50**: 756–63.

9. Nichol HC, Zuck D. Difficult laryngoscopy – the "anterior" larynx and the atlanto-occipital gap. *Br J Anaesth* 1983; **55**: 141–4.

10. Bollensen E, Schönle PW, Braun U, *et al.* [An unnoticed dislocation of the dens axis in a patient with primary chronic polyarthritis undergoing intensive therapy]. *Anesthetist* 1991; **40**: 294–97. [In German].

11. Ono K, Ota H, Tada K, *et al.* Cervical myelopathy secondary to multiple spondylotic protrusions. A clinico-pathologic study. *Spine* 1977; **2**: 109–25.

12. Breig A, Turnbull I, Hassler O. Effects of mechanical stresses on the spinal cord in cervical spondylosis. A study on fresh cadaver material. *J Neurosurg* 1966; **25**: 45–56.

13. Raj Rao. Neck pain, cervical radiculopathy, and cervical myelopathy. *J Bone Joint Surg Am* 2002; **84**: 1872–81.

14. Baptiste DC, Fehlings MG. Pathophysiology of cervical myelopathy. *Spine J* 2006; **6**(6 Suppl): 190S–7S.

15. Nurick S. The pathogenesis of the spinal cord disorder associated with cervical spondylosis. *Brain* 1972; **95**: 87–100.

16. Lee TC, Yang LC, Chen HJ. Effect of patient position and hypotensive anesthesia on inferior vena caval pressure. *Spine* 1998; **23**: 941–7.

17. Sawin PD, Todd MM, Traynelis VC, *et al.* Cervical spine motion with direct laryngoscopy and orotracheal intubation. An in vivo cinefluoroscopic study of subjects without cervical abnormality. *Anesthesiology* 1996; **85**: 26–36.

18. Watts AD, Gelb AW, Bach DB, *et al.* Comparison of the Bullard and Macintosh laryngoscopes for endotracheal intubation of patients with a potential cervical spine injury. *Anesthesiology* 1997; **87**: 1335–42.

19. Sahin A, Salman MA, Erden IA, *et al.* Upper cervical vertebrae movement during intubating laryngeal mask, fibreoptic and direct laryngoscopy: a video-fluoroscopic study. *Eur J Anaesthesiol* 2004; **21**: 819–23.

20. Crosby ET. Airway management in adults after cervical spine trauma. *Anesthesiology* 2006; **104**: 1293–318.

21. Keller C, Brimacombe J, Keller K. Pressures exerted against the cervical vertebrae by the standard and intubating laryngeal mask airways: a randomized, controlled, cross-over study in fresh cadavers. *Anesth Analg* 1999; **89**: 1296–300.

22. Santoni BG, Hindman BJ, Puttlitz CM, *et al.* Manual in-line stabilization increases pressures applied by the laryngoscope blade during direct laryngoscopy and orotracheal intubation. *Anesthesiology* 2009; **110**: 24–31.

23. Lennarson PJ, Smith D, Todd MM, *et al.* Segmental cervical spine motion during orotracheal intubation of the intact and injured spine with and without external stabilization. *J Neurosurg* 2000; **92**: 201–6.

24. Donaldson WF 3rd, Heil BV, Donaldson VP, *et al.* The effect of airway maneuvers on the unstable C1-C2 segment. A cadaver study. *Spine* 1997; **22**: 1215–18.

25. Schneir RC, Cherry G, Pantek H The syndrome of acute central spinal cord injury: with special reference to the mechanisms involved in hyperextension injuries of cervical spine. *J Neurosurg* 1954; **11**: 546–77.

26. Mercieri M, Paolini S, Mercieri A, *et al.* Tetraplegia following parathyroidectomy in two long-term haemodialysis patients. *Anaesthesia* 2009; **64**: 1010–13.

27. Nowak DD, Lee JK, Gelb DE, *et al.* Central cord syndrome. *J Am Acad Orthop Surg* 2009; **17**: 756–65.

28. Buchowski JM, Kebaish KM, Suk KS, *et al.* Central cord syndrome after total hip arthroplasty: a patient report. *Spine* 2005; **30**: E103–5.

29. Lee HC, Andree RA. Cervical spondylosis and difficult intubation. *Anesth Analg* 1979; **58**: 434–5.

30. Clinchot DM, Colachis SC 3rd. An unusual case of traumatic spinal cord injury: case report. *Spinal Cord* 1997; **35**: 181–2.

31. Yan K, Diggan MF. A case of central cord syndrome caused by intubation: a case report. *J Spinal Cord Med* 1997; **20**: 230–2.

32. Kim KA, Wang MY. Anesthetic considerations in the treatment of cervical myelopathy. *Spine J* 2006; **6**(Suppl): 207S–11S.

33. Hukuda S, Wilson CB. Experimental cervical myelopathy: effects of compression and ischemia on the canine cervical cord. *J Neurosurg* 1972; **37**: 631–52.

34. Hindman BJ, Palecek JP, Posner KL, *et al.* Cervical spinal cord, root, and bony spine injuries: A closed claims analysis. *Anesthesiology* 2011; **114**: 782–95.

35. Tsuji T, Matsuyama Y, Sato K, *et al*. Evaluation of spinal cord blood flow during prostaglandin E1-induced hypotension with power Doppler ultrasonography. *Spinal Cord* 2001; **39**: 31–6.

36. Drummond JC, Englander RN, Gallo CJ. Cerebral ischemia as an apparent complication of anterior cervical discectomy in a patient with an incomplete circle of Willis. *Anesth Analg* 2006; **102**: 896–9.

37. Epstein NF, Hollingsworth R, Nardi D, *et al*. Can airway complications following multilevel anterior cervical surgery be avoided? *J Neurosurg* 2001; **94**(2 Suppl): 185–8.

38. Sperry RJ, Johnson JO, Apfelbaum RI. Endotracheal tube cuff pressure increases significantly during anterior cervical fusion with the Caspar instrumentation system. *Anesth Analg* 1993; **76**: 1318–21.

39. Jung A, Schramm J, Lehnerdt K, *et al*. Recurrent laryngeal nerve palsy during anterior cervical spine surgery: a prospective study. *J Neurosurg Spine* 2005; **2**: 123–7.

40. Fountas KN, Kapsalaki EZ, Nikolakakos LG, *et al*. Anterior cervical discectomy and fusion associated complications. *Spine* 2007; **32**: 2310–17.

41. Apfelbaum RI, Kriskovich MD, Haller JR. On the incidence, cause, and prevention of recurrent laryngeal nerve palsies during anterior cervical spine surgery. *Spine* 2000; **25**: 2906–12.

42. Taylor BA, VaccaroAR, Albert TJ Complications of anterior and posterior surgical approaches in the treatment of cervical disc disease. *Semin Spine Surg* 1999; **11**: 337–46.

Chapter

10

Anesthesia for thoracic spine surgery

Rafi Avitsian

Key points

- Surgical procedures on the thoracic spine are performed for a variety of disorders with different levels of invasiveness and patients are diverse in their preoperative condition.
- In anterior thoracic spine procedures as well as video-assisted thoracoscopic procedures there may be a need for one-lung ventilation.
- Vertebroplasty and kyphoplasty have been used to decrease pain and correct spine deformities after traumatic or pathologic fractures.
- Emergent and urgent thoracic spine procedures may be indicated when acute enlargement of a space-occupying lesion compresses against the spinal cord.
- Hemodynamic changes after spinal cord injury may be as a result of spinal shock or autonomic dysreflexia, depending on timing after the injury.

Introduction

Surgical procedures on the thoracic spine have specific and unique characteristics. The adult spinal cord ends at the T12 or L1 level, causing more disability with each higher level of injury. Apart from anatomic differences in the vertebrae, the close proximity to vital organs such as heart, lungs, and kidneys makes surgical procedures on the thoracic spine more challenging and the morbidity of surgical complications graver. Compared with the rest of spine, the thoracic spine has unique drawbacks regarding surgical access. Although relatively superficial in the posterior approach in surgical procedures, the close proximity of the lungs and pleura can increase likelihood of injury to these vital organs. In anterior approach, however, the deep location in relation to vital organs such as heart, major vessels and lungs makes the surgical procedure challenging. The

level of injury in thoracic spine is also important and can affect the autonomic reflexes and cause dysreflexia. Thoracic spine procedures are also performed for correction of scoliosis; patients with scoliosis may have respiratory problems making perioperative management more demanding. This chapter will discuss the anatomic characteristics of the thoracic spine; outline the surgical procedures and anesthetic considerations; and describe possible complications and their management specific for open surgical procedures, thoracoscopic procedures, vertebroplasty, and kyphoplasty. Etiologies leading to emergent and urgent thoracic spinal cord procedures as well as spinal shock and autonomic dysreflexia will also be discussed at the end of this chapter.

Anatomy

The thoracic vertebral column is formed by the 12 thoracic vertebrae, which have their specific distinctive characteristics. The body part in the thoracic vertebrae is larger than in the cervical vertebrae, but the vertebral foramen is smaller (Fig. 10.1). The main distinctive feature of the thoracic vertebrae is the costal facet on each side, which provides an articular surface to join to its corresponding rib. The spinous processes, especially in the mid thoracic region, are long and face downward, making access to the intervertebral foramen more difficult. The anterior and posterior longitudinal ligaments connect the vertebral bodies to create the vertebral column, which has a natural posterior convexity compared with that of the cervical and lumbar regions. The vascular supply of the thoracic vertebral column is of utmost importance. The spinal cord is supplied by two posterior, but only a single anterior one. These longitudinal arteries are fed by radiculomedullary arteries, branches of the intercostal arteries originating from the aorta. The number and position of radiculomedullary arteries vary between individuals, but one major

Anesthesia for Spine Surgery, ed. Ehab Farag. Published by Cambridge University Press. © Cambridge University Press 2012.

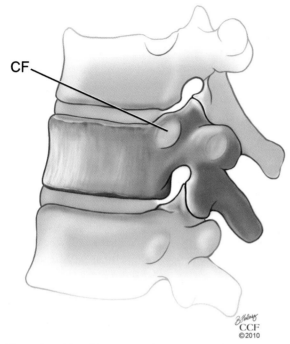

CF

Figure 10.1 Typical thoracic vertebrae., CF = costal facet.

radiculomedullary artery (Adamkiewicz) originates between T8 and L2. During surgical procedure, aortic stent placement or as a result of thrombosis, this artery, which is a major supplier of blood to the spinal cord, may be damaged or obstructed, causing spinal cord ischemia. The anterior longitudinal artery supplies the major part of the spinal cord including the anterior horn motor portion.

Open thoracic spine procedures

Surgical procedures on the thoracic spine are performed for a variety of diseases and disorders; thus patients undergoing these procedures have a wide range of preoperative medical conditions. The invasiveness of the surgical procedures together with the preoperative medical condition of the patient are important determinants of the outcome[1] and are essential in determining the anesthetic plan and postoperative care. A young athletic patient undergoing thoracic sympathetic ablation for hyperhidrosis is different from an elderly diabetic with chronic renal problems undergoing thoracic vertebral corpectomy for excision of metastatic renal cell carcinoma. Thoracic procedures may be performed for correction of deformities, trauma, excision of tumors, degenerative diseases, and infections. A detailed description of surgical procedures in adolescents for correction of scoliosis will be discussed

elsewhere in this book; in this chapter the general perioperative anesthetic considerations of patients undergoing open thoracic spine procedures are reviewed.

Preoperative evaluation

A detailed history and physical examination followed by appropriate laboratory studies is important for anesthetic planning. Patients undergoing thoracic spine surgery may have pulmonary involvement which could be from the restrictive effect of spinal deformity on the lung causing a restrictive lung disease, pulmonary hypertension secondary to severe scoliosis,[2] chronic obstructive pulmonary disease (COPD), and lobectomies for primary or metastatic lung cancers. Patient history and activity level is an important determinant for deciding on preoperative pulmonary function testing; however, for some procedures including severe spinal deformities such as scoliosis, a pulmonary function test is decisive of indication for surgery. Cardiac involvement, including ischemic heart disease is also seen in some patients. In patients with known coronary disease or those with multiple risk factors, further testing and cardiology consultation may be indicated to identify the baseline cardiac function and further medical or interventional optimization, although in urgent or emergent cases there may not be adequate time for any intervention. Congenital cardiac disorders may also be seen in patients undergoing scoliosis correction.[3] Other congenital abnormalities, especially skeletal involvement, should also be considered in patients undergoing spine procedures.[4] Thorough airway examination is indicated to identify patients with difficult intubations; a detailed intubation plan is necessary in patients with cervical spine instability to minimize cervical motion during intubation. A complete review of systems will identify other organ involvement and facilitate the outlining of an effective anesthetic plan. Most centers include a standardized laboratory testing in the preoperative assessment of patients, but a goal-directed laboratory evaluation according to findings in history and physical examination is more appropriate. In most centers a complete blood count and a basic metabolic panel including electrolytes and renal function testing is routine. Evaluation of coagulation profile is also helpful in identifying patients with subclinical coagulation problems and determining whether coagulation has returned to a normal state after discontinuation of anticoagulants. It will also provide a baseline for intraoperative decision making for a cut-off point for blood product replacement.[5] Chest radiography has most likely been ordered by the surgeon to evaluate the surgical site and can give information about pulmonary involvement as well as cardiac condition. Patients presenting with malignancies are prone to development of deep venous thrombosis (DVT) and preoperative evaluation with lower extremity ultrasound should be considered in suspected patients. A review of medication history is also necessary; anticoagulants and antiplatelet drugs are usually discontinued, but in patients who may have an increased tendency for thrombotic complications if off these medications for even a short period of time (e.g., after cardiac stenting,[6] hypercoagulable states, etc.) there may be a need for early hospitalization to "bridge" with short-acting anticoagulants until return to baseline medication is possible postoperatively.[7]. Continuation of beta blockers in the perioperative period may reduce mortality,[8] but increased risk of hypotension, bradycardia, and stroke should be taken into consideration.[9]

Intraoperative considerations

In patients with comorbidities that can affect the surgical outcome, a more invasive monitoring plan is necessary. As mentioned before, the invasiveness of the procedure is also an important determinant of outcome and hence the monitoring plan. Usually posterior approach thoracic spine surgery is technically easier than anterior approach since it does not necessitate surgical exposure of the thoracic cage. Any type of instrumentation and fixation does have a higher chance of intraoperative hemorrhage and surgical complications including injury to the adjacent organs. Simple posterior procedures such as laminectomies in patients with American Society of Anesthesiologists (ASA) physical status classification P1 and P2 can usually be done with ASA standard monitoring. As the procedure becomes more invasive and/or in patients with higher preoperative risks, addition of invasive monitoring is indicated. An arterial line will provide means of a more continuous hemodynamic monitoring in patients with a narrower margin of safety for keeping adequate spinal blood perfusion pressure as a result of the pathologic state. It also provides a route for accessing blood for arterial blood gas and other laboratory evaluations. In some patients with large body habitus, monitoring blood pressure with a traditional blood pressure cuff may be inaccurate; positioning these patients in the prone position may also cause major hemodynamic changes because of increased abdominal pressure causing a decreased preload. The author recommends using

invasive arterial pressure monitoring in surgical procedures where the dura is opened, where a multilevel procedure is involved, when instrumentation is a part of procedure, when there is a high chance of fluid shift or blood loss, when induced hypotension is planned, and when the medical history necessitates keeping the blood pressure in a narrow range. Also in patients who will undergo intraoperative neurophysiologic monitoring, since having an adequate perfusion pressure in the spine is essential in interpretation of evoked potential changes and since anesthetic methods should be altered to allow these monitoring a more close hemodynamic monitoring is indicated. A central line access may be indicated in major surgical procedures where there is a possibility of large fluid shifts, a need for a large-bore access for rapid transfusion, as well as a reliable route for infusion of inotropic agents. In anterior approach surgeries that require a thoracotomy, if central access is attempted through the jugular or subclavian veins, it is preferable to access on the nondependent side, the side which the lung is deflated. Thus if there is an inadvertent pneumothorax during the central access it will be on the same side as lung deflation rather than causing a bilateral pneumothorax. Although monitoring the central venous pressure in the prone position may not be an accurate indicator of a true preload, the trend of changes during the surgical procedure may help in altering the anesthetic management. Monitoring of the temperature is also necessary since a decrease in body temperature can affect intraoperative blood loss,[10] and also neurophysiologic monitoring.[11] Hypothermia may also increase perioperative infection rate.[12] Measuring urine output could also be a good guide for renal perfusion and estimation of fluid status in procedures where surgical bleeding or fluid shifts are expected. A "wake-up test," once common for monitoring the integrity of the spinal cord,[13] is now done more infrequently and is replaced by neuromonitoring of the evoked potentials. The wake-up test involves decreasing the anesthetic to a level at which the patient can follow commands. Although it may show the integrity of the motor function usually in the lower extremity, this is only at a certain point of time during the procedure and cannot give any information about incidents other than that point of time; sensory changes may not be monitored effectively in a wake-up test either. It is also very uncomfortable for the patient, thus it has lost its popularity. Electrophysiological monitoring is discussed in a separate chapter in detail; however, it is worth mentioning that somatosensory and motor evoked potentials are useful tools in monitoring spinal cord perfusion and physiologic status in procedures where surgical injury or hemodynamic changes can cause neuronal injury.

Current recommendation regarding prophylactic antibiotic administration is to administer the antibiotic within one hour before surgical incision.[14] In prolonged cases there may be a need to repeat the antibiotic dose. In patients who are on continuous antibiotic management the need for additional doses and/or additional antibiotic coverage is based on antibiotic type, timing, and discussion with the surgeon. When there is an infectious source for the vertebral pathology, the surgeon may request administration of the antibiotic to be delayed in order to get a sample for culture from the infected tissue. Currently there is stress on timing of antibiotic administration to a level that the financial reimbursement is being linked to this health care improvement initiative.[15]

Apart from a few exceptions where surgical procedure may necessitate having a patient awake for monitoring (e.g., implantation of spinal cord stimulators), all thoracic spine procedures are performed under general anesthesia. Anesthesia is usually induced with intravenous anesthetic agents and maintenance is accomplished with a balanced anesthesia technique including volatile or intravenous infusion of anesthetics, opioids, and muscle relaxants. Formulation will depend on procedure, patient medical history, and postoperative plan. If neuromonitoring is part of the surgical plan, a lower level of volatile anesthetics and nitrous oxide is recommended to decrease the chance of suppression of monitoring waveforms. In some cases a total intravenous anesthetic is advocated during neuromonitoring. Total muscle relaxation is avoided where motor evoked potentials or electromyography is part of the monitoring plan. Patients with long-standing history of opioid use may have a higher tolerance to these medications and a higher dose may be necessary for titration. Inclusion of a continuous infusion of opioids in the anesthetic plan will decrease the need for higher anesthetic doses; the choice, however, should also take into consideration the postoperative pain management plan. Use of a short-acting agent such as remifentanil can provide a more awake patient immediately postoperatively for an early neurologic examination, but it can cause severe, postoperative pain if additional longer-acting opioids are not administered in a timely manner. A discussion with the surgical team for postoperative pain management is also helpful since if possible, intraoperative placement of an epidural catheter may provide more effective pain control and decrease the need for higher doses of intravenous opioids.

Acute hemodynamic changes are common in thoracic spine trauma. In acute stages there may be spinal shock as well as hemorrhage from other organs causing hypoperfusion of the spinal cord. In chronic situations after thoracic spinal cord trauma, dysautonomia can cause sudden hemodynamic changes necessitating acute intervention. Autonomic dysreflexia is discussed in a separate part of this chapter.

During the procedure, especially when there is increasing blood loss, the surgeon may ask for a decrease in the blood pressure to be able to control the bleeding. Recently there has been an increased stress on maintaining adequate blood pressure to avoid postoperative ischemic optic neuropathy.[16] In one analysis of 93 spine cases with postoperative visual loss, Lee et al. showed that 27% of patients who had postoperative visual loss had undergone a period of deliberate hypotension.[17] However, more studies are needed to reflect the independent or multifactorial causes of this complication.[17]

Patient positioning is important and should be planned after a discussion with the surgeon. If an anterior approach is a part of the surgery, the anesthetic plan should include the ability for one-lung ventilation to allow surgical exposure. This is usually achieved using a double-lumen endotracheal tube or a bronchial blocker. The reader is encouraged to read the section on "Thoracoscopic procedures" in this chapter and Chapter 11 on "Lung isolation during thoracic spine surgery." In some instances the anterior approach is followed by a posterior spine fusion; oxygenation and ventilation after re-expansion of the lung as well as hemodynamic stability should be evaluated before deciding on proceeding to the posterior approach, or delaying it and performing the procedure in a staged manner. The anterior approach is usually performed in left lateral decubitus position with the arms on a double arm board and knees in semi-flexed position to decrease pressure. For posterior approach a Jackson frame table with or without a Wilson frame is an option for thoracolumbar procedures. The Jackson frame can result in decreased pressure on the abdomen, which translates into less inferior vena cava pressure and less epidural venous engorgement and can cause a decrease in intraoperative bleeding but it has the downside of exposing a larger area of the body surface and increasing the risk of hypothermia. A regular operating room table with parallel chest rolls is also common for posterior thoracic spine procedures. In both cases, pressure on the thoracic cage may cause restriction in ventilation and increase peak inspiratory pressures on the ventilator to reach an adequate tidal volume. Ensuring adequacy of oxygenation and ventilation is essential after positioning and before surgical incision. A regular stretcher should always be available if there is a need for emergency positioning of the patient in supine position (e.g., for resuscitation or endotracheal tube repositioning). Careful padding of pressure points is important to avoid nerve injuries regardless of the surgery bed used. During prone position the upper extremities may be placed on arm boards with attention to avoiding extension of shoulders and elbows beyond a 90° angle if the surgery is on the lower part of the thoracic spine. In higher thoracic or cervicothoracic procedures the arms should be tucked in neutral position at the sides. After positioning of the arms, adequate flow and function of the intravenous lines and arterial line should be confirmed. Positioning of the head is also an essential element of patient preparation. Many types of head positioning have been suggested, including three-pronged Mayfield head clamp, two-pronged Gardner traction head holder, horseshoe head holder, or foam padding. The intraocular pressure increases in an anesthetized patient in prone position.[18] Appropriate positioning on the horseshoe holder or foam pad should ensure no pressure on the orbit since it may cause increased intraocular pressure, ischemia, and blindness;[19] the positioning should be checked at the start of the case and periodically. The sitting position has also been used for sympathectomy for hyperhidrosis, although currently thoracoscopy is the method of choice for this procedure.[20] All necessary precautions regarding sitting positions including those relating to nerve injury following positioning, possibility of air embolism, and hemodynamic instability should be taken into consideration if this position is chosen for the procedure.[21]

Postoperative considerations

The decision on extubation at the end of the surgical procedure depends on the invasiveness of the procedure, the amount of blood loss and fluid shifts, ventilatory status after re-inflation of the deflated lung, and other criteria of extubation including muscle strength and body temperature. After prolonged prone positioning, especially following large amount of fluids or blood product transfusion, there may be a significant amount of facial and upper airway edema. Detection of a leak around the endotracheal tube after deflation of the cuff may be used as an indicator that the patient can maintain

an open airway after extubation despite the edema. To complete this test the patient should have spontaneous respiration; after suctioning the oral contents the circuit is disconnected and the proximal end of the endotracheal tube is obstructed with the thumb, and after deflating the cuff the patient should be able to continue respiration around the deflated cuff of the endotracheal tube, confirmed by auscultation over the larynx. Even if extubation criteria are met, a plan for re-intubation should always be available if the patient cannot maintain adequate oxygenation or ventilation. As discussed for thoracoscopic procedures for lung isolation, after re-inflation of the lung and wound closure, a chest tube is placed. If a double-lumen tube is used and the patient is to remain intubated the bronchial cuff should be deflated and the double-lumen tube positioned in a tracheal position, or the double-lumen exchanged to a single-lumen endotracheal tube. This can be done over a tube-exchanger catheter to avoid loss of airway since the operative edema may cause difficult intubation. If the patient is to be transferred intubated to an intensive care setting, a complete report to the intensive care personnel is necessary. The patient should be transported under continuous monitoring and rescue medications and airway management devices should accompany the sedated patient. Sedation can be provided by midazolam, propofol infusion, or dexmedetomidine infusion. It is better to use a short-acting sedative since early neurologic examination is desired after admission to the ICU.

Not all open surgical procedures on the thoracic spine, even in anterior approach cases, need postoperative intensive care or an intubation period. Routine postoperative care in the postoperative care unit (PACU) should include treatment of nausea and vomiting, pain management and hemodynamic issues. Pain control is important especially in patients with a history of chronic opioid use. In cases where the surgeon has placed an epidural catheter, epidural patient-controlled analgesia (PCA) could be used in the early postoperative period. In patients who do not have an epidural catheter, intravenous boluses or intravenous PCA can be used. Although epidural analgesia can have fewer complications, including nausea and pruritus,[22] the possibility of motor blockade and interference with postoperative neurologic examination should be realized, especially if local anesthetics are the main components of the analgesic mixture.[23] After thoracotomy, use of intrapleural opioids and/or analgesics have also been described;[24] the possibility of local anesthetic toxicity should also be kept in mind.[25]

Table 10.1 Comparison between posterior spinal fusion with thoracic pedicle screws and video-assisted thoracoscopic surgery in terms of operative time, estimated blood loss, transfusion, and length of stay

	Posterior spinal fusion with thoracic pedicle screws	Video-assisted thoracoscopic surgery	p value[a]
Operative time[b] (min)	245.9±120.4	325.6±85.9	0.03[c]
Estimated blood loss[b] (ml)	1018±731	371±216	0.001[c]
Rate of transfusion[d] (%)	29	18	0.69
Patients who received Cell Saver transfusion[d] (%)	65	0	<0.001[c]
Cell Saver amount† (ml)	382±267	0	<0.001[c]
Length of stay[b] (days)	4.8 ±1.0	4.8 ±1.4	0.89

Reprinted with permission from: Lonner BS *et al.*, Video-assisted thoracoscopic spinal fusion compared with posterior spinal fusion with thoracic pedicle screws for thoracic adolescent idiopathic scoliosis. *J Bone Joint Surg Am* 2009; **91**(2): 398–408.
[a] *p* values were calculated with one-way analysis of variance unless otherwise noted.
[b] The values are given as the mean and the standard deviation.
[c] Statistically significant.
[d] *p* value was calculated with the chi-square test.

Complications

Complications from positioning include nerve injuries from inadequate pressure point padding, skin abrasions, facial swelling and sliding of the head when positioned in the head holder. Skin abrasions are usually seen in heavy patients positioned in beds with smaller points of contact (e.g., Jackson frame table). Chemosis and conjunctival swelling may be seen after prone spine surgery. Duration of surgery, amount of fluids given and position of the head are important determinants of amount of swelling.[26] Atelectasis, pneumonia, and pulmonary failure after one-lung ventilation are discussed elsewhere. If the head is not held in the Mayfield head holder pins appropriately, it may slide, causing cervical spine injury and laceration of the scalp or face. Surgical complications include hemorrhage and nerve injury. Thoracic surgical procedures, in particular those performed for tumors and trauma may encounter a large amount of blood loss. Blood transfusion especially in large quantities can put the patient at risk of infection, coagulopathy, immunosuppression, transfusion reaction, and transfusion-related acute lung injury.[5] Surgical instrumentation can cause entry in vessels or other organs or nerve injury. As mentioned previously, neuromonitoring can be helpful in decreasing the latter.

Thoracoscopic procedures

In an effort to decrease the invasiveness of procedures performed on the thoracic spine, in recent years thoracoscopic approach has been an important topic of discussion. Lately indications for thoracoscopy have evolved, ranging from simple procedures including anterior discectomy and biopsy to anterior release, instrumentation, and fusions.[27] Video-assisted thoracoscopy (VATS) has also been used in sympathectomy for hyperhidrosis[28] and as a part of an anterior–posterior approach to correct spine deformities.[29] The main aim of VATS is to improve outcome in terms of shorter operating time, better postoperative pain control, less pain, and faster recovery. In a study Rosenthal and Dickman published their experience in anterior discectomy using VATS, comparing this procedure with an open thoracotomy, and showed a mean improvement of 1 hour in operating time and less than half the blood loss in VATS procedures. They also showed reduced hospital stay, chest tube drainage, and pain medication requirement.[30] In another study on adolescent patients with thoracic idiopathic scoliosis, Lonner *et al.* compared VATS-assisted fusion with posterior spinal fusion with thoracic pedicle screws. They observed that VATS significantly increased the operative time but reduced blood loss, although the amount of transfusion and length of stay were the same in the two groups (Table 10.1). They also showed that in the VATS group on average the number of levels fused was significantly smaller than in the posterior spinal fusion group (5.9 compared with 8.9). Although both groups had similar improvement from baseline in terms of pulmonary function at 2 years, the posterior spinal fusion group had significantly improved peak flow measurement compared with the VATS group.[31] Patient selection is an important step for this procedure since there are surgical contraindications (e.g., excessive kyphosis >40°) that can worsen the outcome.[27]

193

Preoperative evaluation

Although the aim of VATS is to minimize invasiveness, the anesthetic management should not be thought easier than that of a "major open" spine procedure. Preoperative evaluation should include a careful history and physical examination. Although most patients undergoing procedures to correct scoliosis are young and in the adolescent age group, VATS may also be performed in patients with advanced age. There may be other anomalies with scoliosis even in younger age groups (e.g., progressive scoliosis in central core disease with susceptibility to malignant hyperthermia[32]). The extent of physiologic changes during VATS surgery depends on preoperative condition as well as the extent of surgical invasiveness. Patients undergoing multilevel fusion or corpectomy are considered to have higher-risk procedures than discectomy or sympathectomy. Procedures under VATS require one-lung ventilation to allow visualization of the thoracic spine. Spinal deformity or pain could be severe enough to cause a restrictive pulmonary pattern; thus preoperative pulmonary function testing can give important information regarding the feasibility of anesthesia, one-lung ventilation, and the need for postoperative controlled ventilation. A detailed history to uncover pulmonary involvement including pulmonary hypertension, COPD, smoking, and obstructive sleep apnea can also help in decision making for postoperative management. A detailed discussion with the patient regarding the possibility of blood loss and transfusion and a postoperative intubated period is crucial. A thorough airway examination is important since some of these patients may have cervical spine involvement. Preoperative ECG and need for further cardiac evaluation will depend on patient history and functional capacity. In patients with connective tissue disorders, renal and hematologic involvement as well as coagulation problems should also be investigated. Preoperative laboratory studies are helpful in diagnosing the asymptomatic conditions. A current blood type and screen – and in cases where the possibility of blood loss is high, the starting hematocrit is low, or there is an antibody in type and screening process – available, cross-matched blood is also essential before the procedure starts.

Intraoperative considerations

The anesthetic plan consists of a balanced general anesthesia with endotracheal intubation. Intubation should be planned to provide the ability for one-lung ventilation. This is usually accomplished by using a double-lumen tube or a bronchial blocker. In addition to ASA standard monitoring, invasive arterial pressure monitoring can provide accurate and timely information about hemodynamic changes that can occur during thoracoscopy. During the procedure, especially with one-lung ventilation the major vessels and heart can be displaced, causing major hemodynamic changes. An arterial line can also give access to intermittent arterial blood gas evaluation to assess adequacy of oxygenation and ventilation during one-lung ventilation. The decision on placement of a central venous access line is similar to that in open thoracic vertebral surgical procedures and is dependent on preoperative patient status, invasiveness of the procedure, expected fluid shifts and blood loss, and also the need for inotropic infusion. It should be noted that during thoracoscopy, shifting of intrathoracic vessels and positioning of the patient would give an inaccurate measurement of central venous pressure. Also attempts at central line positioning, if the internal jugular or subclavian vein is chosen, should be on the side that will have the lung deflated to decrease the chance of bilateral pneumothorax. An arterial line is also usually placed on the dependent side to have a better correlation with the level of the heart as well as a more accurate reading if the nondependent subclavian artery becomes narrower under pressure. Bleeding depends on the invasiveness of the procedure and could range from minimal in less-invasive procedures such as sympathectomy to more than 2000 ml in a spinal metastasis or corpectomy.[33] Large-bore intravenous access is essential for rapid blood transfusion if it becomes necessary.

The majority of VATS procedures are done in a left lateral decubitus position (Fig. 10.2) with hips and knees flexed, since a larger area of the spine is visible beside the azygous veins on the right side than on the left side where the aorta is present, however, below the T9 level left-sided thoracoscopy is also possible. Thus in the majority of cases the right lung is deflated. Although lung isolation is discussed in Chapter 11, we should mention that a left-sided, double-lumen endotracheal tube is preferred since the branching of the superior lobe of the right lung from the right main bronchus is more proximal, causing a higher chance of obstruction of its opening by the bronchial cuff if a right-sided double-lumen tube is used. Use of bronchial blockers is also described for one-lung ventilation.

After induction of general anesthesia, the trachea is intubated with a double-lumen tube and positioning is confirmed with bronchoscopic examination. This confirmation should be repeated after positioning the

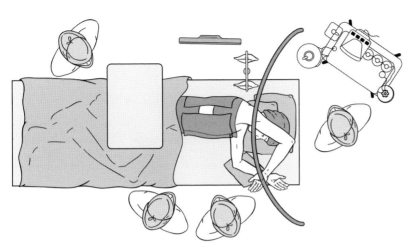

Figure 10.2 Patient positioning during thoracoscopy.

patient. Special attention should be directed to careful padding of pressure points during positioning. After each repositioning and intermittently, monitoring devices as well as intravenous and arterial lines should be checked for proper functioning (Fig. 10.2). Placement of a warming forced-air blanket is recommended to decrease patient heat loss during prolonged procedure. Anesthesia is maintained using volatile agents in conjunction with opioids. If neuromonitoring is part of the surgical plan, other recommendations for anesthesia during neuromonitoring are implemented including using a lower concentration of volatile agent with infusion of an opioid.[33] Alternatively total intravenous anesthesia (TIVA) can be used to avoid significant suppression of neuromonitoring waveforms. If motor evoked potentials are also monitored, muscle relaxation should be avoided. An opioid infusion such as remifentanil or sufentanil can help in patient immobility during the procedure but can not replace muscle relaxants. Nitrous oxide is usually avoided during one-lung ventilation to decrease the chance of hypoxia. The lung is usually deflated after initiation of one-lung ventilation; an arterial blood gas evaluation at this point can help in deciding the ventilator settings (see Chapter 11). High airway pressures after lung deflation may cause barotrauma or pneumothorax on the dependent lung. In some instances, one-lung ventilation cannot be achieved following technical difficulties in lung isolation or inadequate oxygenation and/or ventilation; these cases may need to be converted to an open procedure or a posterior approach. After the procedure the deflated lung is re-inflated and two-lung ventilation is restarted. In prolonged cases the absorption of alveolar air in the deflated lung can cause atelectasis

and accumulation of secretions, called "Down lung" syndrome. In some cases, after the thoracoscopy the patient should be turned to a prone position for continuation of the procedure with posterior approach. In such cases it is recommended that the double-lumen endotracheal tube be changed to a single-lumen tube. Since there is a risk of inability of re-intubation following airway edema, use of a tube exchanger is recommended. The same method should be used if a combined anterior–posterior approach is not planned but the patient is to remain intubated postoperatively. In some cases the risk of losing the airway is high and if the anesthesiologist is unwilling to exchange the tube until airway edema is subsided, the bronchial cuff of the double-lumen tube should be deflated and the tube pulled back so the two lumens are in the tracheal position. A chest tube is placed by the surgical team at the time of closure.

Postoperative considerations

Similarly to open thoracic vertebral procedures, the decision to emerge and extubate the patient should be reached at the end of the procedure according to length of sugery and amount of fluid shifts, hemodynamic stability, ventilatory status, and preoperative condition of the patient. If patients are to be left intubated in the immediate postoperative period, they should be transported to an intensive care unit capable of continuous hemodynamic monitoring and familiar with the management of thoracic surgical procedures. A detailed report of the anesthetic course and complications should be provided to the intensive care unit physician and nursing staff in order to achieve efficient postoperative care. Continuous monitoring en route is advised in these cases. In patients who would be extubated immediately or shortly after the end of the procedure, treatment of pain is an important concern. If not treated adequately, the pain may decrease the ventilatory effort, which could contribute to further atelectasis. In their study, Lonner *et al.* showed that at first postoperative visit (3–5 weeks) the decrease in vital capacity and peak flow in the thoracoscopic group was significantly larger than in posterior fusion in patients who underwent spinal fusion for adolescent idiopathic scoliosis, but at the time of final follow-up this difference was not significant.[34] Acute lung injury can be seen in patients undergoing sequential anterior then posterior correction of spinal deformities in up to 15% of cases. Transfusion, direct trauma to the lung, systemic inflammatory response, and fat and bone marrow embolization have all been suggested as etiologic factors.[35]

Complications

Anesthetic-related complications include the Down lung syndrome with excess secretion and atelectasis noted on the chest radiograph after re-inflation. Mucus plugs can also be a cause of atelectasis and bronchoscopy should be used for treatment of these cases. Nerve injuries may also occur as a result of improper positioning. Surgical complications include vessel injury causing hemorrhage, lymphatic injury causing chylothorax, nerve injury, and inadvertent entry into viscera. Cardiac complications include hypotension following decreased preload, hypoxia causing myocardial infarction, and arrhythmia.[36] The surgical and anesthetic teams should be ready to convert the procedure to an open one to treat possible complications. Horner's syndrome has also been described following transthoracic endoscopic sympathectomy.[37] In cases where instrumentation is used, inadvertent entry into the opposite lung during instrumentation can cause a bilateral pneumothorax. Postoperative intercostal neuralgia has also been described. In Rosenthal and Dickman's study comparing thoracoscopy with thoracotomy for excision of herniated thoracic discs, neuralgia was more severe and prolonged in the thoracotomy group.[30] Complications from thoracoscopic sympathectomy include gustatory sweating (facial sweating associated with eating), pneumothorax, nasal obstruction, Horner's syndrome, and intercostal neuralgia.[37]

Vertebroplasty and kyphoplasty

With increasing age, the bone mass within the vertebral body decreases, making it more fragile and

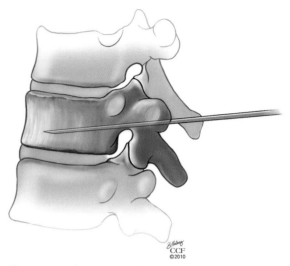

Figure 10.3 Schematic view of trocar insertion for vertebroplasty in thoracic vertebra.

susceptible to fracture. Osteoporosis is a major cause of vertebral compression fractures affecting more than 700 000 people annually in the USA and results in significant health care cost.[38] Decreased height of the vertebral body causes pressure on the sensory nerves and can also pressurize the spinal cord. Injection of supportive material within the vertebral body can increase its stability and prevent further compression fractures (Fig. 10.3). This is the basis of percutaneous vertebroplasty, during which synthetic bone material such as polymethylmethacrylate is injected within the vertebral body (Fig. 10.4). In contrast, during kyphoplasty the deformity of the vertebral body is corrected (Fig. 10.5). This procedure is usually performed to treat destructive pathologic conditions, for example, lesions from multiple myeloma or metastatic lesions. During kyphoplasty the height of the vertebral body should be corrected before injection of cement material. This is done by inserting a balloon within the vertebral body which upon inflation can relatively correct the deformed vertebra. After this correction, which is performed under fluoroscopic guidance, the cement material is infused. A study performed by Schofer *et al.* showed that kyphoplasty and vertebroplasty both caused significant pain relief and quality of life was similar within the two therapy groups; however, kyphoplasty led to an ongoing reduction of freshly fractured vertebrae and lower rate of cement leakage.[39] Contraindications to these procedures are uncontrolled coagulopathy, presence of local or systemic infection, and epidural or foraminal extension of the lesion causing neurologic deficit.

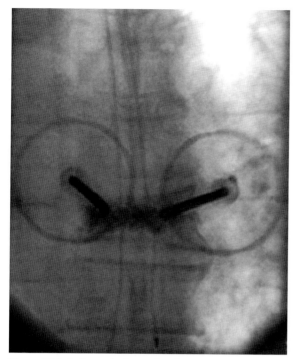

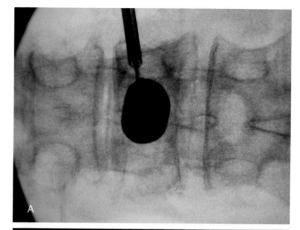

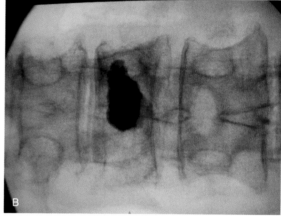

Figure 10.4 Radiograph of a vertebroplasty procedure.

Preoperative evaluation

Most patients undergoing kyphoplasty or vertebroplasty are either advanced in age or have significant comorbidities resulting from their primary disease (e.g., metastatic tumor). Thus, even though surgically these procedures may not seem as complicated as some of the major open spine surgeries, the anesthetic care may be complicated. A complete preoperative evaluation is essential for a good anesthetic plan and favorable outcome. Special attention should be directed to concomitant cardiac disorders. These patients may have undiagnosed ischemic cardiac conditions and may not tolerate adequate mobilization to determine the true functional class. Most of these patients are in dire pain from the fracture and may not tolerate any cardiac stress test. In many metastatic patients also the procedure is being performed as a palliative measure to decrease pain, thus even if ischemic cardiac pathology is detected, they may not be candidates for revascularization or stenting. Although the importance of cardiac evaluation in patients suspected of having ischemic heart disease in elective cases should not be underestimated, any perioperative study should be done with consideration of the patient's health status, prognosis, and indication of any cardiac intervention. The pulmonary system is also affected in these patients. These patients may have

Figure 10.5 The two stages of kyphoplasty with (A) correction of deformity by inflation of a balloon and (B) injection of synthetic bone material.

chronic obstructive pulmonary disease (COPD) or have a decreased vital capacity if the decrease in the height of the thoracic vertebral column is significant. They may also have primary or metastatic pulmonary malignancies or have undergone a pneumonectomy. Attention to the primary malignancy is also very important. In multiple myeloma, patients may present with anemia, neutropenia, or thrombocytopenia, elevated creatinine, and hypercalcemia. About 60% of patients with plasma cell malignancy have vertebral involvement mostly at T6–L4.[38]. Patients undergoing these procedures may also have opioid dependency following chronic use of pain medications. Pain may also inhibit these patients from movement, making them prone to deep venous thrombosis especially if the underlying disease is a malignancy.

Intraoperative considerations

As mentioned, patients undergoing kyphoplasty or vertebroplasty may have severe pain during movement.

197

There may be a need for opioid boluses before transporting these patients from the stretcher; however, respiratory suppression of these agents should be kept in mind and continuous monitoring of oxygenation and ventilation should be applied when large amounts of opioids are given to these patients. These procedures are performed in the prone position and in many instances on a fluoroscopic bed or a Jackson frame with the assistance of portable fluoroscopy. Since there may be other parts of the skeletal system involved in bony disruption, transport from one bed to another should be done with extra care. Although these procedures have been done successfully under sedation,[40] in many cases discomfort from lying in the prone position may necessitate deeper sedation and use of narcotics that may suppress respiratory effort. Monitored anesthesia care with midazolam and fentanyl, propofol infusion with or without an opioid (e.g., alfentanil or remifentanil), as well as dexmedetomidine infusion have all been described. Although use of supraglottic airway devices has been reported, many anesthesiologists are hesitant to use these devices in patients in prone position, and in any case they should be readily available in all cases under sedation.[38] Spinal anesthesia under fluoroscopic guidance has also been described for this procedure.[41] The already compromised respiratory function following thoracic vertebral fracture may be worsened in prone position when the thoracic cage is placed on the operating table, increasing its restrictive pattern. For reasons mentioned above, most cases need a general anesthetic for this procedure. In patients on chronic steroid therapy, a stress dose of steroids should be considered. Information regarding involvement of the cervical spine and physical examination of the airway including cervical range of motion is essential in planning the intubation method. Although induction and positioning of these patients may be stimulating, the rest of the procedure may be less painful, with the exception of the time when the kyphoplasty balloon is inflated or cement is injected. Titration of the anesthetic agent and opioids accordingly will decrease the chance of large hemodynamic changes. Monitoring is usually possible with ASA standard monitoring. Use of invasive monitoring (e.g., arterial line) is usually reserved only for cases where the severity of medical problems and comorbidities calls for a closer hemodynamic monitoring.

Postoperative considerations

In many instances, patients experience improvement of symptoms postoperatively. However, pain control in the postoperative area is essential. These procedures are mostly done on an outpatient basis. The postanesthesia care unit personnel should evaluate patients for pain and nausea before discharge.

Complications

Most complications are due to incorrect positioning of the needle or working cannula in the vertebral body. In the thoracic region a costotransversal approach, where the needle is positioned between the transverse process and the origin of the rib, should be performed with care and continuous fluoroscopic monitoring. Incorrect placement can cause vascular or cardiac dissection or neural injury; however, the main complication is cement leakage. The posterior wall of the vertebral body is an important landmark for evaluating leakage. Cement may leak to the disc area, pressurize nerve roots, and even cause paraplegia.[42] Another devastating complication is intravascular injection of the cement, which can cause hemodynamic changes, pulmonary emboli, anaphylactic reaction to contrast or cement, and cardiovascular collapse.[43] In these situations a rapid termination of the procedure, supine placement of the patient, and resuscitative measures should be taken.

Other minimally invasive procedures are also described for thoracic vertebrae including disc or vertebral body biopsy, epidural injections, and radiofrequency ablation of the upper thoracic sympathetic chain for hyperhidrosis.[44] Anesthesia is usually not required for these procedures, which are routinely preformed under sedation. However, in some patients underlying medical conditions or severe pain may necessitate involvement of an anesthesiologist. As mentioned for vertebroplasty and kyphoplasty, a careful preoperative history and physical examination are essential for a proper anesthetic plan.

Thoracic spine emergencies, spinal shock and autonomic dysreflexia

Emergent and urgent procedures on the thoracic spine are indicated for a multitude of etiologies (Table 10.2). A good understanding of the clinical picture, laboratory findings, and imaging characteristics is important in determining a suitable anesthetic plan.

Epidural hematoma can have a compressive effect on the spinal cord, causing progressive clinical signs and symptoms. In many cases it is spontaneous, but a relative cause can also be found including surgical complication after a recent surgical procedure, coagulopathy,

Table 10.2 Etiologies that can lead to emergent thoracic spinal procedure

Spinal epidural hematoma
Epidural abscess
Spinal arterial thrombosis
Aortic dissection
Vascular procedures decreasing spinal blood flow
Trauma
Pathologic fractures
Disc herniations
Spondylitis
Metastatic tumors
Spinal cord tumors

Table 10.3 Mechanism of spinal cord injury

Immediate neural injury from tissue disruption after shearing or compression forces
Compression from disrupted adjacent tissue (e.g., bony fragments)
Ischemia from compression of adjacent tissue
Local vascular alterations and ischemia
Loss of autoregulation
Ischemia following global hypotension (hypovolemic shock, spinal shock)
Reperfusion injury with oxygen-derived free radicals
Release of free radicals and lipid peroxidases
Inflammatory response and cytokine release
Excitotoxicity by glutamate release increasing intracellular calcium
Airway compromise resulting in hypoxemia and hypoventilation

trauma, or vascular malformation. Symptoms begin with back pain radiating to the extremities and progress to sensory and motor deficit as well as urinary retention. Postoperative epidural hematoma can occur following rupture of the internal vertebral venous plexus during surgery. Although the presentation may be delayed, an early postoperative neurologic examination can help in diagnosing the early-onset ones. Epidural hematoma after spinal anesthesia can present with a more rapid progression of pain to sensorimotor deficit and loss of sphincter tone.[45] Hematoma as a result of epidural anesthesia has a low incidence of about 1:150 000–1:190 000[46–47] and is often seen as a result of traumatic insertion or after removal of the catheter. Anticoagulation after a spinal or epidural anesthesia is a matter of much debate; currently it is recommended to wait 2 hours after spinal anesthesia needle placement or epidural catheter removal unless there was a bloody aspirate, after which the anticoagulation should be further delayed or avoided.[48] The risks of being off anticoagulation and postoperative bleeding should be weighed before starting the anticoagulation.

Epidural abscess can have a similarly progressive course, although there is a more subtle form with additional signs and symptoms including back pain, fever, elevated white count, and neurologic deficit. Epidural abscesses can be a complication of epidural anesthesia and are usually seen after poor aseptic technique, prolonged catheterization, or traumatic insertion.[49] However, in a meta-analysis by Reihsaus *et al.* only 5.5% of patients with spinal epidural abscess had a history of epidural anesthesia.[50]. In this meta-analysis the main risk factors included diabetes mellitus, trauma, intravenous drug abuse, and alcoholism. The thoracic spine was involved in 35%, cervicothoracic in 7%, and thoracolumbar in 7%.

Vascular catastrophes including aortic aneurysm or anterior spinal artery syndrome may also be part of the differential diagnosis of progressive neurologic deficiencies. Improvement in spinal cord perfusion is the main goal in treatment in these situations. Although trauma to the spine will not be discussed in detail in this chapter, it should be noted that it is an important etiology for thoracic spine emergencies. Many pathophysiologic mechanisms are involved in spinal injury following trauma (Table 10.3). Pathologic fractures as well as acute disc herniations may also present similarly to trauma.

Although in modern medicine availability of rapid radiologic diagnostic measures can give a timely and accurate diagnosis of the pathologic segment, an understanding of clinical signs and symptoms relative to the level of involvement is important in the initial evaluation and monitoring of the progression. Table 10.4 shows the motor sensory and reflex examinations in relation to the segment involved. Supplementary examination and history of the presentation can also help in determining the diagnosis.

Spinal shock: After spinal cord injury initially there is a loss of spinal reflexes below the level of injury. The muscles innervated by the spinal root nerves bellow the injury are paralyzed and flaccid. Some reflexes start to recover earlier and there may be a difference in neurologic examination as time progresses.[51] Not only the reflexes below the injured cord are inhibited, there may also be cephalad effects of spinal cord injury known as Schiff–Sherrington phenomenon.[52] This could be seen as a transient loss of upper extremity reflexes in higher thoracic spinal cord injuries. One of

199

Table 10.4 Examinations for determining level of spinal cord injury.

A: Distribution of the involved spinal levels according to sensory examination

Corresponding level	Feeling at
C2	Occiput
C3	Thyroid cartilage
C4	Suprasternal notch
C5	Below clavicle
C6	Thumb
C7	Index finger
C8	Small finger
T4	Nipple line
T10	Umbilicus
L1	Femoral artery region
L2–L3	Medial thigh
L4	Knee
L5	Lateral calf
S1	Lateral foot
S2–S4	Perianal area

B: Motor examination

Testing level	Can you
C4	spontaneous breathing
C5	Shrug your shoulders
C6	Flex your elbow
C7	Extend your elbow
C8–T1	Flex your fingers
T1–T12	Take a deep breath (intercostals)
L1–L2	Flex your hip
L3	Adduct your hip
L4	Abduct your hip
L5	Bring up your foot
S1–S2	Push down your foot

C: Diminished reflexes and involved roots

Level involved	Diminished reflex
C6	Biceps
C7	Triceps
L4	Knee
S1	Achilles

labia minus lateral to the clitoris is touched in females. This is also one of the first normal reflexes to recover. A pathologic reflex to appear early is the Delayed Plantar Response in which there is a delay in flexion and then relaxation of the great and other toes after moving a blunt object from heel to the toes on the lateral side and then continuing on the volar aspect of the metatarsal heads. This reflex needs an unusually stronger stimulus than what is used during Babinski. Loss or blunting of sympathetic reflexes with intact vagal cranial nerve may cause bradyarrhythmias, hypotension and atrioventricular conduction blocks. In spinal cord injuries hypotension is seen following the pooling of blood in lower extremities because of the loss of sympathetic tone. Temperature control is also affected, and there may be a transient small bowel ileus. During the next hours to days after spinal cord injury the reflexes return. The Babinski reflex is also performed by touching the lateral side of the plantar surface and moving up towards the toes by a blunt object. The normal (negative Babinski) sign is when the toes flex and the foot everts. This also returns with the other deep tendon reflexes.

Autonomic dysreflexia

After the acute and subacute phase of spinal cord injury is passed, the cutaneous as well as deep tendon reflexes and Babinski sign become hyperactive. This is usually seen after the first month of injury. The vagally mediated hypotension and bradyarrhythmias that peaked at the fourth day after injury decrease and are usually resolved by 2–6 weeks.[53] At this time the exaggerated sympathetic response to stimuli below the injury will appear and will persist indefinitely. This phenomenon, also known as autonomic dysreflexia can also be seen during the first month of spinal cord injury. In one report it was seen as early as 4 days after spinal cord injury.[54] Since the bulbospinal inputs to the sympathetic preganglionic neurons are lost, the regulation of sympathetic reflexes in the spine is by dorsal root afferent and spinal interneurons.[55] The pathophysiology of autonomic dysreflexia has been described by Vaidyanathan et al. as changes in sympathetic preganglionic neurons, neurobiochemical changes in the spinal cord distal to the injury, remodeling of the spinal cord circuits, hypersensitivity of vascular alpha-adrenoreceptors in tetraplegic patients, and spillover of norepinephrine below the lesion with peripheral stimulation.[55] Recently sympathetic nonadrenergic transmission has also been shown to be involved in the pathophysiology of hypertension.[56] Any stimulation,

the important reflexes that can determine spinal cord injury is the disappearance of bulbocavernosus reflex. In this reflex the anal sphincter is contracted if the glans penis is squeezed or the Foley catheter tugged in men or especially in the perineal region, or distension of the bladder or rectum can result in overactivity of the sympathetic nervous system. The cluster of sympathetic hyperactivity symptoms includes excessive increase in blood pressure as a result of preganglionic sympathetic activation in the distal spinal cord. The elevated blood pressure can stimulate the baroreceptors and cause a supraspinal baroreceptor reflex resulting in bradycardia, although tachycardia and other arrhythmias have also been reported. The pathophysiology is explained by disruption of regulatory and inhibitory pathways from the brain to the spinal reflexes at the level of spine injury. In patients with spinal cord injury there is no regulatory effect of the brain and the spinal reflex arc can trigger a massive activation of sympathetic and sacral parasympathetic outflow. Vasoconstriction below the lesion can cause pallor, while above the lesion there may be flushing and sweating. Other symptoms in an awake patient include shivering, anxiety, headache, and chest tightness. In addition to hypertension, bradycardia, and arrhythmias, other signs include dilated pupils, visual disturbances, piloerection, or aphasia. Severe or untreated cases can result in cerebral hemorrhage, cardiac dysrhythmias, seizures, and death. The anesthesiologist should be aware of possible complications and sudden hemodynamic changes in these patients. Deeper states of anesthesia and complete inhibition of reflexes during painful procedures below the spinal cord injury site, even though the patient is unable to feel the pain, are advised. In treatment of hypertension alpha-1 adrenergic blockers (e.g., prazocin), alpha-2 adrenergic agonists (e.g., clonidine), calcium channel blockers (e.g., nifedipine), as well as monoamine oxidase inhibitors and diuretics have been used. Another important anesthetic issue is monitoring of body temperature. Impairment of a sweating mechanism may even cause hyperthermia. On the other hand, inability to shiver and cutaneous vasodilation can cause hypothermia.

References

1. Schuster JM, Rechtine G, Norvell DC, Dettori JR. The influence of perioperative risk factors and therapeutic interventions on infection rates after spine surgery: a systematic review. *Spine* 2010; **35**(9 Suppl): S125–37.

2. Koumbourlis AC. Scoliosis and the respiratory system. *Paediatr Respir Rev* 2006; **7**(2): 152–60.

3. Campbell RM, Jr. Spine deformities in rare congenital syndromes: clinical issues. *Spine* 2009; **34**(17): 1815–27.

4. Takaso M, Nakazawa T, Imura T, *et al.* Surgical correction of spinal deformity in patients with congenital muscular dystrophy. *J Orthop Sci* 2010; **15**(4): 493–501.

5. Ornstein E, Berko R. Anesthesia techniques in complex spine surgery. *Neurosurg Clin N Am* 2006; **17**(3): 191–203.

6. Brilakis ES, Banerjee S, Berger PB. Perioperative management of patients with coronary stents. *J Am Coll Cardiol* 2007; **49**(22): 2145–50.

7. Faltas B, Kouides PA. Update on perioperative bridging in patients on chronic oral anticoagulation. *Expert Rev Cardiovasc Ther* 2009; **7**(12): 1533–9.

8. Angeli F, Verdecchia P, Karthikeyan G, *et al.* ss-Blockers reduce mortality in patients undergoing high-risk noncardiac surgery. *Am J Cardiovasc Drugs* 2010; **10**(4): 247–59.

9. White CM, Talati R, Phung OJ, *et al.* Benefits and risks associated with beta-blocker prophylaxis in noncardiac surgery. *Am J Health Syst Pharm* 2010; **67**(7): 523–30.

10. Rajagopalan S, Mascha E, Na J, Sessler DI. The effects of mild perioperative hypothermia on blood loss and transfusion requirement. *Anesthesiology* 2008; **108**(1): 71–7.

11. Seyal M, Mull B. Mechanisms of signal change during intraoperative somatosensory evoked potential monitoring of the spinal cord. *J Clin Neurophysiol* 2002; **19**(5): 409–15.

12. Hranjec T, Swenson BR, Sawyer RG. Surgical site infection prevention: how we do it. *Surg Infect (Larchmt)* 2010; **11**(3): 289–94.

13. Vauzelle C, Stagnara P, Jouvinroux P. Functional monitoring of spinal cord activity during spinal surgery. *Clin Orthop Relat Res* 1973; (93): 173–8.

14. Bratzler DW, Houck PM. Antimicrobial prophylaxis for surgery: an advisory statement from the National Surgical Infection Prevention Project. *Am J Surg* 2005; **189**(4): 395–404.

15. Fahy BG, Bowe EA, Conigliaro J. Perioperative antibiotic process improvement reaps rewards. *Am J Med Qual* 2011 May-Jun; **26**(3): 185–92.

16. Patil CG, Lad EM, Lad SP, Ho C, Boakye M. Visual loss after spine surgery: a population-based study. *Spine* 2008; **33**(13): 1491–6.

17. Lee LA, Roth S, Posner KL, *et al.* The American Society of Anesthesiologists Postoperative Visual Loss Registry: analysis of 93 spine surgery cases with postoperative visual loss. *Anesthesiology* 2006; **105**(4): 652–9.

18. Hunt K, Bajekal R, Calder I, *et al.* Changes in intraocular pressure in anesthetized prone patients. *J Neurosurg Anesthesiol* 2004; **16**(4): 287–90.

19. Leibovitch I, Casson R, Laforest C, Selva D. Ischemic orbital compartment syndrome as a complication of spinal surgery in the prone position. *Ophthalmology* 2006; **113**(1): 105–8.

20. Hashmonai M, Kopelman D, Assalia A. The treatment of primary palmar hyperhidrosis: a review. *Surg Today* 2000; **30**(3): 211–18.

21. Gale T, Leslie K. Anaesthesia for neurosurgery in the sitting position. *J Clin Neurosci* 2004; **11**(7): 693–6.

22. Blumenthal S, Borgeat A, Nadig M, Min K. Postoperative analgesia after anterior correction of thoracic scoliosis: a prospective randomized study comparing continuous double epidural catheter technique with intravenous morphine. *Spine* 2006; **31**(15): 1646–51.

23. Raw DA, Beattie JK, Hunter JM. Anaesthesia for spinal surgery in adults. *Br J Anaesth* 2003; **91**(6): 886–904.

24. Inderbitzi R, Flueckiger K, Ris HB. Pain relief and respiratory mechanics during continuous intrapleural bupivacaine administration after thoracotomy. *Thorac Cardiovasc Surg* 1992; **40**(2): 87–9.

25. Raffin L, Fletcher D, Sperandio M, *et al.* Interpleural infusion of 2% lidocaine with 1: 200,000 epinephrine for postthoracotomy analgesia. *Anesth Analg* 1994; **79**(2): 328–34.

26. Jeon YT, Park YO, won HJ, *et al.* Effect of head position on postoperative chemosis after prone spinal surgery. *J Neurosurg Anesthesiol* 2007; **19**(1): 1–4.

27. Sucato DJ. Thoracoscopic anterior instrumentation and fusion for idiopathic scoliosis. *J Am Acad Orthop Surg* 2003; **11**(4): 221–7.

28. Krasna MJ. Thoracoscopic sympathectomy. *Thorac Surg Clin* 2010; **20**(2): 323–30.

29. Schubert A, Deogaonkar A, Lotto M, Niezgoda J, Luciano M. Anesthesia for minimally invasive cranial and spinal surgery. *J Neurosurg Anesthesiol* 2006; **18**(1): 47–56.

30. Rosenthal D, Dickman CA. Thoracoscopic microsurgical excision of herniated thoracic discs. *J Neurosurg* 1998; **89**(2): 224–35.

31. Lonner BS, Auerbach JD, Estreicher M, Milby AH, Kean KE. Video-assisted thoracoscopic spinal fusion compared with posterior spinal fusion with thoracic pedicle screws for thoracic adolescent idiopathic scoliosis. *J Bone Joint Surg Am* 2009; **91**(2): 398–408.

32. Miyamoto K, Shimizu K, Matsumoto S, *et al.* Surgical treatment of scoliosis associated with central core disease: minimizing the effects of malignant hyperthermia with provocation tests. *J Pediatr Orthop B* 2007; **16**(3): 239–42.

33. Lotto ML, Banoub M, Schubert A. Effects of anesthetic agents and physiologic changes on intraoperative motor evoked potentials. *J Neurosurg Anesthesiol* 2004; **16**(1): 32–42.

34. Lonner BS, Kondrachov D, Siddiqi F, Hayes V, Scharf C. Thoracoscopic spinal fusion compared with posterior spinal fusion for the treatment of thoracic adolescent idiopathic scoliosis. *J Bone Joint Surg Am* 2006; **88**(5): 1022–34.

35. Urban MK, Jules-Elysee KM, Beckman JB, *et al.* Pulmonary injury in patients undergoing complex spine surgery. *Spine J* 2005; **5**(3): 269–76.

36. Dieter RA, Jr., Kuzycz GB. Complications and contraindications of thoracoscopy. *Int Surg* 1997; **82**(3): 232–9.

37. Lai YT, Yang LH, Chio CC, Chen HH. Complications in patients with palmar hyperhidrosis treated with transthoracic endoscopic sympathectomy. *Neurosurgery* 1997; **41**(1): 110–13.

38. Frost EA, Johnson DM. Anesthetic considerations during vertebroplasty, kyphoplasty, and intradiscal electrothermal therapy. *Int Anesthesiol Clin* 2009; **47**(2): 45–55.

39. Schofer MD, Efe T, Timmesfeld N, Kortmann HR, Quante M. Comparison of kyphoplasty and vertebroplasty in the treatment of fresh vertebral compression fractures. *Arch Orthop Trauma Surg* 2009; **129**(10): 1391–9.

40. Della PA, Andreula C, Frass M. Assisted sedation: a safe and easy method for pain-free percutaneous vertebroplasty. *Minerva Anestesiol* 2008; **74**(3): 57–62.

41. Hannallah M, Gibby E, Watson V. Fluoroscopy-guided, small-dose spinal anesthesia for kyphoplasty: a collaborative effort between the anesthesiologist and interventional radiologist. *Anesth Analg* 2008; **106**(4): 1329–30.

42. Anselmetti GC, Muto M, Guglielmi G, Masala S. Percutaneous vertebroplasty or kyphoplasty. *Radiol Clin North Am* 2010; **48**(3): 641–9.

43. Childers JC, Jr. Cardiovascular collapse and death during vertebroplasty. *Radiology* 2003; **228**(3): 902–3.

44. Kelekis AD, Somon T, Yilmaz H, *et al.* Interventional spine procedures. *Eur J Radiol* 2005; **55**(3): 362–83.

45. Vandermeulen EP, Van Aken H, Vermylen J. Anticoagulants and spinal-epidural anesthesia. *Anesth Analg* 1994; **79**(6): 1165–77.

46. Al Mutair A, Bednar DA. Spinal epidural hematoma. *J Am Acad Orthop Surg* 2010; **18**(8): 494–502.

47. Wulf H. Epidural anaesthesia and spinal haematoma. *Can J Anaesth* 1996; **43**(12): 1260–71.

48. Spector LR, Madigan L, Rhyne A, Darden B, Kim D. Cauda equina syndrome. *J Am Acad Orthop Surg* 2008; **16**(8): 471–9.

49. Reynolds F. Neurological infections after neuraxial anesthesia. *Anesthesiol Clin* 2008; **26**(1): 23–52, v.

50. Reihsaus E, Waldbaur H, Seeling W. Spinal epidural abscess: a meta-analysis of 915 patients. *Neurosurg Rev* 2000; **23**(4): 175–204.

51. Ditunno JF, Little JW, Tessler A, Burns AS. Spinal shock revisited: a four-phase model. *Spinal Cord* 2004; **42**(7): 383–95.

52. Atkinson PP, Atkinson JL. Spinal shock. *Mayo Clin Proc* 1996; **71**(4): 384–9.

53. Lehmann KG, Lane JG, Piepmeier JM, Batsford WP. Cardiovascular abnormalities accompanying acute spinal cord injury in humans: incidence, time course and severity. *J Am Coll Cardiol* 1987; **10**(1): 46–52.

54. Krassioukov AV, Furlan JC, Fehlings MG. Autonomic dysreflexia in acute spinal cord injury: an under-recognized clinical entity. *J Neurotrauma* 2003; **20**(8): 707–16.

55. Vaidyanathan S, Soni BM, Sett P, *et al.* Pathophysiology of autonomic dysreflexia: long-term treatment with terazosin in adult and paediatric spinal cord injury patients manifesting recurrent dysreflexic episodes. *Spinal Cord* 1998; **36**(11): 761–70.

56. Groothuis JT, Rongen GA, Deinum J, *et al.* Sympathetic nonadrenergic transmission contributes to autonomic dysreflexia in spinal cord-injured individuals. *Hypertension* 2010; **55**(3): 636–43.

Chapter

11

Lung isolation during thoracic spine surgery

Gordon Finlayson and Jay B. Brodsky

Key points

- In order to provide lung isolation and selective lung collapse for a thoracic spinal procedure the anesthesiologist must be familiar with the different equipment and techniques available. Complications, both minor and major, can result from device malposition, traumatic placement, and/or poor management of single-lung ventilation.

- The presence of cervicothoracic spinal deformities or major trauma may make tracheal intubation more difficult in patients requiring single-lung ventilation for corrective spine surgery.

- For many thoracic spine surgery patients, postoperative mechanical ventilation may be required. Ventilatory support may be due to extensive intraoperative surgical manipulation, large-volume fluid resuscitation, prolonged single-lung ventilation, prone positioning, or the presence of spinal cord injuries.

- Lung isolation for thoracic spine surgery is most safely achieved using a bronchial blocker, particularly when faced with a difficult tracheal intubation. Bronchial blockade may be the only safe means of providing single-lung ventilation in children too small for the smallest double-lumen tube. If postoperative ventilation is needed, the blocker can simply be withdrawn from the tracheal tube, thus avoiding a tube exchange if a double-lumen tube is used.

- Strategies for single-lung ventilation are adopted from techniques in patients undergoing lung resection surgery and are aimed at establishing adequate gas exchange while minimizing ventilator induced lung injury.

Introduction

The ability to perform complex surgical procedures inside the chest is a relatively recent innovation only made possible by the development of anesthetic techniques that allow for safe lung isolation and selective lung collapse.[1] The first means for providing one-lung ventilation, described 80 years ago, was by endobronchial intubation with a cuffed endotracheal tube. Shortly thereafter, a variety of different bronchial blockers were designed to be advanced alongside a tracheal tube into a bronchus. Obstruction of ventilation to that lung by the bronchial blocker facilitated lung collapse while protecting the contralateral, ventilated lung from contamination. In 1949 the Swedish physiologist Eric Carlens described the first double-cuffed, double-lumen endobronchial tube. Carlens intended to use his tube for differential spirometry, but the surgeon V.O. Bjork recognized the advantages of using a Carlens tube for thoracic operations. The introduction of double-lumen tubes into clinical anesthetic practice permitted further major advances in intrathoracic surgery.

The general indications for providing lung isolation are either to facilitate surgical exposure and/or to provide anatomic or physiologic separation of the lungs. The list of surgical procedures benefiting from lung isolation is expansive. Basically, any operation requiring an intrathoracic approach can be helped by collapsing the lung on the operative side. In addition, anatomic separation can protect the healthy lung when it is threatened by contamination from secretions, pus, blood, or even tumor material. Physiologic separation is necessary when the adequacy of alveolar gas exchange is threatened because of heterogeneous compliance between the two lungs, resulting in a mismatch of ventilation and perfusion. Using a double-lumen tube to achieve lung separation can also allow independent, differential ventilation to each lung as might

Anesthesia for Spine Surgery, ed. Ehab Farag. Published by Cambridge University Press. © Cambridge University Press 2012.

be necessary in a trauma patient with a lung contusion or a flail chest.

For the majority of thoracic spine operations, the objective of lung isolation is to provide easy access to the thoracic spine through the thoracic cavity. This chapter will review the equipment and techniques currently used in clinical practice to provide lung separation and will highlight the potential complications of these techniques in patients undergoing spine procedures.

Equipment and techniques

There are three general techniques for providing routine lung isolation. Lung separation can be achieved (a) by selective endobronchial intubation with a tracheal tube, (b) with some form of bronchial blockade, or (c) by placement of a double-lumen tube (Fig. 11.1).

Endobronchial tubes

Endobronchial tubes are seldom used for elective lung isolation in contemporary thoracic surgical practice. Under emergency circumstances, a conventional single-lumen tracheal tube can be guided into a main-stem bronchus (either blindly or aided by bronchoscopy or fluoroscopy) to provide selective ventilation or to prevent aspiration of debris or blood from the contralateral, nonventilated lung. Conventional tracheal tubes are not designed for endobronchial placement. Tracheal tubes have a very long cuff and a long distal extension of their lumen past the cuff. When positioned entirely within the bronchus, the long cuff and luminal extension of a standard tracheal tube will obstruct the upper-lobe bronchus on that side. In this situation both the contralateral diseased lung and the upper lobe of the intubated lung will not be ventilated, and this will usually result in severe hypoxemia.[2] This is especially true if the right bronchus is intubated since the right main bronchus is so short. Modern tubes specifically designed for endobronchial placement incorporating a very narrow cuff and short distal lumen are available but are not widely used.[3]

Bronchial blockade

Although various devices have been employed since the inception of this technique, the general principle and design of all bronchial blockers are conceptually straightforward. Today's bronchial blockers are all basically thin plastic tubes with a distal inflatable balloon. When positioned correctly the inflated balloon is meant to occlude a main-stem or lobar bronchus to facilitate lung collapse and lung isolation.

In the past any balloon-tipped catheter, like a Fogarty occlusion embolectomy catheter (Edwards Lifesciences, Irvine, CA, USA) or a pulmonary artery wedge catheter, was typically placed alongside or through a single-lumen endotracheal tube and guided by bronchoscopy into position.[4] The major disadvantage of using these devices as blockers is that they are designed and intended for other purposes. Their balloons have low-volume, high-pressure properties that are a potential cause of bronchial injury. Contemporary bronchial blockers are specifically designed for safe airway blockade and incorporate high-volume, low-pressure balloons to minimize mucosal trauma. Many modern blockers have a patent inner channel in the catheter to hasten lung deflation and allow for the application of continuous positive airway pressure (CPAP) if needed.

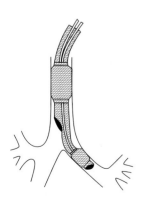
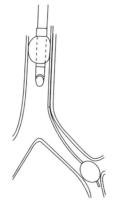
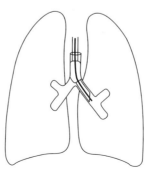

Figure 11.1 Lung separation can be achieved (A) by a double-lumen tube which allows inflation or collapse of either lung, (B) by a bronchial blocker catheter placed in the lung or bronchus that is intended to be deflated, or (C) by selective endobronchial intubation with a tracheal tube into the lung intended to be ventilated.

A   Double-lumen tube   B   Bronchial blocker   C   Endobronchial tube

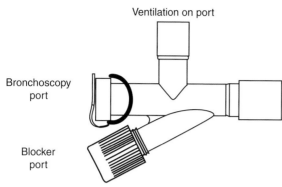

Ventilation on port

Bronchoscopy port

Blocker port

Figure 11.2 Bronchial blockers are placed either alongside or within the lumen of a standard tracheal tube. A special 3-port connector (Arndt® Multi-Port Airway Adaptor) allows advancement of a blocker under direct vision by a bronchoscope without interfering with ventilation during blocker placement.

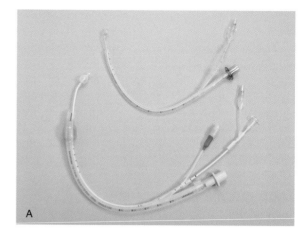

A

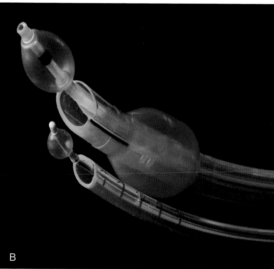

B

Figure 11.3 (A) The Univent® Tube incorporates a dedicated blocker channel within the wall of a tracheal tube. The tracheal tubes come in a variety of sizes including un-cuffed tubes for pediatric patients. (B) The balloon-tipped blocker catheter is advanced down the narrow channel of the main body of the Univent® Tube into the bronchus of the lung to be collapsed.

Blockers are usually placed either alongside or within the lumen of a standard tracheal tube. When placed within the lumen of a tracheal tube, a special connector is used that allows advancement of the blocker under direct vision by a bronchoscope without interfering with ventilation during blocker placement (Fig. 11.2). Proper blocker position within the airway normally requires the use of a bronchoscope. Another approach is the Univent® Tube (Vitaid, Lewinston, NY, USA), which incorporates a dedicated blocker channel within the wall of a tracheal tube (Fig. 11.3). The blocker is advanced down this narrow channel into a bronchus. Additional rotation of the main body of the tracheal tube improves the success of catheter placement.

All blockers have special features to help direct the catheter to its desired position, where, once inflated, the balloon at the tip of the blocker then serves to obstruct ventilation to that lung (Fig. 11.4). The simplest solution is the placement of an angle at the distal tip of the blocker catheter so that rotation at the proximal end of the catheter deflects the distal end in the same direction (Uniblocker®, Vitaid).

A recent novel method to achieve bronchial blockade is with the Papworth BiVent Endotracheal Tube® (P3 Medical Limited, Bristol, UK).[5] This is a unique double-lumen tube, which unlike other double-lumen tubes, has two lumens of equal length that end in a forked tongue that seats on the carina. Any blocker device can be advanced down either the right or the left lumen of the BiVent tube allowing rapid and reliable lung isolation without the need for fiberoptic endoscopic guidance.

The Cohen® Flexitip Endobronchial Blocker (Cook Critical Care, Bloomington, IN, USA) uses a rotational

wheel at the operator's end to mechanically maneuver the distal end of the blocker into position (Fig. 11.5). The wire-guided Arndt® Endobronchial Blocker (Cook Critical Care) has a removable wire lasso placed in the central channel of the blocker that is snared to the end of a fiberoptic bronchoscope. The bronchoscope is advanced into the appropriate bronchus and the blocker's snare slides over the bronchoscope moving the blocker into position. The bronchoscope is then removed and the snare is withdrawn into the lumen of the blocker (Fig. 11.6).

The latest entry for bronchial blockade is the EZ-Blocker® (AnaesthetIQ BV, Rotterdam, The Netherlands)[6] (Fig. 11.7A). Its distal end is a Y shape,

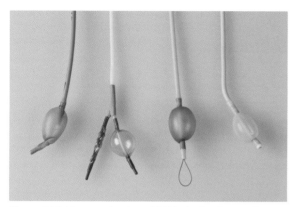

Figure 11.4 Every modern bronchial blocker has features that help direct it into the desired position. Once inflated, the balloon at the distal tip of the blocker catheter serves to prevent ventilation beyond the balloon obstruction causing collapse of the lung. Shown are the distal portions of the Cohen® Flexitip Endobronchial Blocker, the E-Z-blocker®, the Arndt® Endobronchial Blocker and the Uniblocker®.

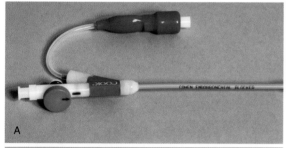

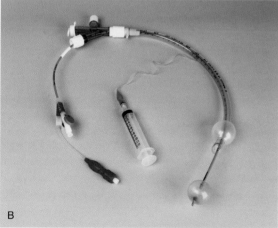

Figure 11.5 (A) The Cohen® Flexitip Endobronchial Blocker uses a rotational wheel at the operator's end to mechanically maneuver the distal end of the blocker into position. (B) This photograph shows the Cohen® Flexitip Endobronchial Blocker in the 3-port Arndt® Multi-port Airway Adaptor. Any blocker can be advanced through one port, a fiberoptic bronchoscope in a second port allows direct visual observation of catheter placement, while ventilation can continue through the third port.

consisting of two 4 cm-long distal extensions, each with a polyurethane spherically shaped cuff. The extensions are fully symmetrical and colored differently (blue and yellow) for identification purposes. The symmetrical design facilitates introduction and positioning of the device with each of the extensions in a main-stem bronchus. Like all other blockers it is introduced and positioned under direct vision using a bronchoscope, but it has the potential for placement under emergency situations "blindly" without direct visualization. When the proper position is reached, the cuff in the extension of the main-stem bronchus of the lung to be collapsed can be inflated and lung isolation achieved. Owing to its Y shape, the blocker remains in position (Fig. 11.7B)

Detailed reviews of techniques for proper bronchial blocker placement are readily available for the interested reader. It is fundamental that basic tracheobronchial anatomy and bronchoscopic skills are achieved before attempting blocker placement.[7] Although lung collapse may be slightly delayed with a blocker compared with a double-lumen tube, in adult patients surgical conditions are usually more than adequate.[8] Since all double-lumen tubes currently commercially available are too large for many children, bronchial blockade remains the technique of choice for one-lung separation in the pediatric patient population (Table 11.1).

The two most commonly encountered problems with blockers are the failure to intubate the intended bronchus and proximal herniation of the balloon towards the tracheal carina (particularly during patient positioning). When difficulty is encountered in directing a blocker to its intended location the following strategies should be considered. In the absence of contraindications (e.g., unstable cervical injury) the patient's head and neck are rotated and flexed with the ear directed toward the shoulder contralateral to the bronchus that needs to be blocked. This movement helps with tracheal and bronchial alignment so that the blocker can be passed along a straighter course under bronchoscopic visualization. Should this maneuver fail, the bronchoscope can be inserted distally into the bronchus, serving as a stylet to guide endobronchial intubation of an uncut tracheal tube. Once the single-lumen tube is advanced into the bronchus, the blocker can be passed distally through it, then the blocker catheter is held firmly in place until the breathing tube is withdrawn and repositioned in the trachea.

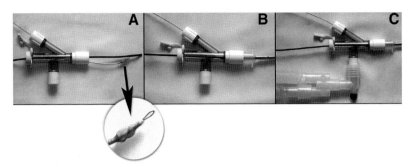

Figure 11.6 The wire-guided Arndt® Endobronchial Blocker has a removable wire lasso placed in the central channel of the blocker that is snared to the end of a fiberoptic bronchoscope. The bronchoscope is advanced into the bronchus and the blocker's snare slides over the bronchoscope, moving the blocker into position. The bronchoscope is then removed and the snare is withdrawn into the lumen of the blocker.

Table 11.1 Tube selection for single-lung ventilation in children. For pediatric patients, bronchial blockade or placement of a single-lumen tube in a main-stem bronchus are the only practical means of achieving selective lung collapse. The smallest double-lumen tubes commercially available are size 26 Fr which is too large for most children younger than 8–10 years of age

Age (years)	ETT (ID)	BB (Fr)	Univent®	DLT (Fr)
0.5–1	3.5–4.0	5		
1–2	4.0–4.5	5		
2–4	4.5–5.0	5		
4–6	5.0–5.5	5		
6–8	5.5–6.0	6	3.5	
8–10	6.0 cuffed	6	3.5	26
10–12	6.5 cuffed	6	4.5	26–28
12–14	6.5–7 cuffed	6	4.5	32
14–16	7.0 cuffed	7	6.0	35
16–18	7.0–8.0 cuffed	7	7.0	35

Double-lumen tubes

Double-lumen tubes are regarded as the gold standard technique for achieving lung separation. The basic design of all double-lumen tubes is similar to the tube introduced by Carlens. A typical double-lumen tube consists of two single-lumen tubes of unequal length molded together (Fig. 11.8A). The lumen of the shorter tube ends within the trachea and the longer tube is positioned within a main-stem bronchus. There is a proximal cuff on the tracheal portion and a distal cuff on the longer, bronchial lumen. Inflating the tracheal cuff allows positive-pressure ventilation to both lungs. When both the bronchial and tracheal cuffs are inflated, the lungs can be ventilated together or separately. Selectively clamping the lumen to either lung at a connector at the proximal limb end of the tube enables separation and collapse of that lung while ventilation continues through the other, unclamped lumen to the ventilated lung (Fig. 11.8B).

Modern double-lumen tubes are manufactured from clear polyvinyl plastic material which allows for inspection of condensation, blood, or purulent secretions in either lumen. Suction catheters or a small fiberoptic bronchoscope can be passed down either lumen to inspect the airway and also to enable pulmonary toilette.

Tracheal intubation and correct positioning of a double-lumen tube can be more challenging than placement of a standard tracheal tube. This is an important consideration when providing lung isolation for a patient with an anticipated difficult airway. Their larger tube diameter is the primary contributing factor; this obscures visualization of the vocal cords and resists advancement beyond the glottic inlet. Individual double-lumen tubes are designed for placement in either the left or right bronchus. Either a left or a right double-lumen tube can be utilized to isolate either lung. Airway anatomy in humans is asymmetric; the left main bronchus in an adult is usually 4–5 cm long while the right main bronchus is <2 cm and is often even shorter. Because of the longer left bronchus, a left-sided double-lumen tube offers a wider "margin of safety" for placement and greater range of movement within the airway without jeopardizing herniation into the trachea or obstruction of a distal bronchial orifice. Therefore, left-sided double-lumen tubes are usually preferred unless safe placement is precluded by left bronchial obstruction or prior surgical intervention. A variety of right-sided double-lumen tubes are manufactured by different companies. Each is individually designed in different ways to minimize obstruction of the right upper lobe bronchial orifice, but the "margin of safety" for any right-sided double-lumen tube is never as great as with a left-sided tube.

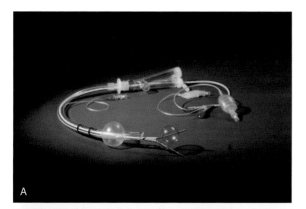

A

Figure 11.7 (A) The EZ-Blocker® has a Y-shaped distal end which consists of two 4 cm-long extensions, each with a polyurethane spherically shaped balloon cuff. The symmetrical extensions are each positioned in one or the other main-stem bronchi under direct visual guidance with a fiberoptic bronchoscope. (B) The EZ-Blocker® is advanced until it engages the tracheal carina. In this position each balloon-tipped extension will be in one of the two main bronchi. The balloon in the main-stem bronchus of the lung to be collapsed is then inflated for bronchial blockade. Owing to its Y shape, the blocker remains in position and there is little chance of balloon displacement into the trachea.

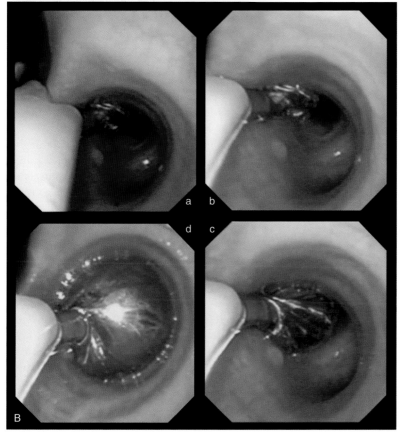

B

In selecting the optimal size of double-lumen tube there remains another concern, particularly between sex and ethnic groups. The patient's preoperative chest radiograph or chest computed tomography scan should always be reviewed before selecting any lung isolation device. This will help to identify distorted airway anatomy that could complicate tube placement, and can also aid in the selection of an appropriately sized device.[9] Although patient sex and height have been used to choose a double-lumen tube, the direct measurement of bronchial width, or the measurement of tracheal width to predict bronchial width (left bronchial width = 0.68 × [tracheal width]) is a more accurate predictor of actual airway size and should be used to select an appropriate double-lumen tube size. Using sex and height alone will frequently under- or overestimate correct size. Selecting a double-lumen tube that is too large, or one that is too small, can lead to injury and other complications.

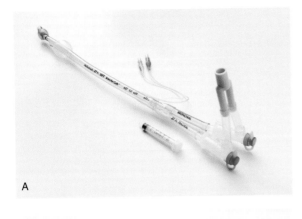

A

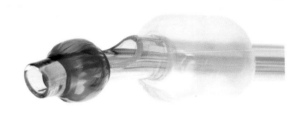

B

Figure 11.8 (A) The basic design of all double-lumen tubes consists of two single-lumen tubes of unequal length molded together. The lumen of the shorter tube ends within the trachea and the longer tube is positioned within a main-stem bronchus. (B) A double-lumen tube has two cuffs. There is a proximal cuff on the tracheal portion and a distal cuff on the bronchial lumen. Inflating the tracheal cuff allows positive-pressure ventilation to both lungs. When both the bronchial and tracheal cuffs are inflated, the lungs can be ventilated together or separately. Selectively clamping the lumen to either lung at a connector at the proximal limb end of the tube enables separation and collapse of that lung while ventilation continues through the other, unclamped lumen to the ventilated lung.

Usually, a larger double-lumen tube, one whose bronchial lumen just fits the intended bronchus, is preferred. There is less resistance to air flow during one-lung ventilation through the wider lumen of a larger tube, and less chance for development of auto-PEEP in patients with chronic obstructive pulmonary disease. A larger lumen more easily accommodates a fiberoptic bronchoscope or suction catheter. In experienced hands a left-sided double-lumen tube can be placed by clinical examination and auscultation[10], but most clinicians use a fiberoptic bronchoscope for visual guidance and/or to confirm correct placement. Unless one is familiar with airway anatomy, use of a bronchoscope does not always guarantee accurate placement of a double-lumen tube or bronchial blocker.[11]

Table 11.2 Advantages of double-lumen tubes

- Same tube can be used to isolate either right or left- lung
- Easy to position; does not always require fiberoptic bronchoscopy
- Less likely to be displaced than the balloon of bronchial blocker
- Each lung is protected from contamination
- Either lung can be collapsed and reexpanded at will during surgery
- Allows suction for pulmonary toilette of operated lung
- Allows bronchoscopic inspection of either lung
- Continuous positive airway pressure (CPAP) can be applied to operated lung to treat hypoxemia
- Allows split-lung, simultaneous, independent ventilation to both lungs

Advantages of a double-lumen tube include the ability to provide rapid lung collapse and reliable lung isolation (Table 11.2). It is the only device that allows either lung to be collapsed and re-expanded at will as many times as necessary during surgery. Only with a double-lumen tube can one alternate between single-lung and two-lung ventilation during the procedure. This feature is desirable for assessing air leaks during lung resection surgery but is seldom needed during spine procedures. The application of CPAP to the collapsed lung through the large lumen of a double-lumen tube improves oxygenation during one-lung ventilation in the event of intraoperative hypoxemia. Suctioning of fluid, secretions, or blood in the airway of the collapsed lung is easily performed while still maintaining isolation and lung collapse. Prolonged postoperative ventilation, although not ideal, is possible with a double-lumen tube in situ.[12] Usually if postoperative ventilation is needed, an airway exchange catheter (AEC) can be used to change from a double-lumen to a single-lumen tube at the completion of surgery.

Lung isolation in the difficult airway

Factors contributing to difficult airway management or lung separation in spine surgery patients can include distorted tracheobronchial anatomy and restricted cervical spine mobility from associated comorbidities (e.g., rheumatoid arthritis, ankylosing spondylitis). Further, the spine surgery patient may be susceptible to failed extubation owing to airway edema (prolonged prone position, massive fluid resuscitation, or surgical manipulation) and/or ventilatory insufficiency from spinal cord injury.

Table 11.3 Guidelines for using an airway exchange catheter (AEC)

1. Select an AEC >70 cm length when using with a double-lumen tube

2. Choose an AEC with a large outer diameter in preference to a tube with a relatively small inner diameter

3. Always lubricate the AEC

4. Test the fit between the AEC and the tube before attempting tube exchange

5. Never advance the AEC against resistance

6. Use a laryngoscope to lift supraglottic tissue to facilitate tube passage at the glottis

7. If passage is obstructed, rotate the tube 90° counterclockwise to avoid arytenoid or vocal cord impingement

8. Note the depth markings on both the AEC and in situ tube; never insert the AEC deeper than 25 cm into the airway

9. Have a system for jet ventilation available if the tube cannot be advanced

Table 11.4 Suggested ventilation strategies during one-lung ventilation

- Minimize absolute duration of one-lung ventilation
- Unless patient is hypoxemic, reduce fraction inspired O_2 (F_iO_2) <60%
- Target tidal volume (V_T) = 4–6 ml/kg (ideal body weight, IBW)
- Avoid ventilator plateau pressure (P_{plat}) >30 cmH_2O
- Use positive end-expiratory pressure (PEEP) 5–10 cmH_2O
- Allow permissive hypercapnea if patient predisposed to air trapping

Intubation with a double-lumen tube can be more challenging than with a standard single-lumen tube. When difficult tracheal intubation is anticipated or encountered, lung isolation is most easily accomplished using a bronchial blocker via a single-lumen tube. If both laryngoscopy and mask ventilation are anticipated to be difficult, maintenance of spontaneous ventilation is key to avoiding a "can't intubate, can't ventilate" scenario. The best technique for accomplishing tracheal intubation is a matter of practitioner preference, patient anatomy, and patient cooperation. Most anesthesiologists rely upon fiberoptic bronchoscopy or video-laryngoscopy to access the airway under these circumstances. Once the airway is secure with a single-lumen tube, lung isolation can be achieved with a blocker. Alternatively, an AEC may be placed as a stylet to advance a double-lumen tube or exchange a single-lumen tube for a double-lumen tube.

Some important points are worth highlighting when using an AEC to assist the difficult placement of a double-lumen tube[13] (Table 11.3). First, ensure that the exchange catheter is of sufficient length (>70 cm) and passes easily through the bronchial lumen of a double-lumen tube. Avoid placement of the catheter beyond 25 cm (at the teeth) to minimize the risk of distal airway perforation. Close approximation of the AEC width and inner diameter of the bronchial lumen will help to reduce resistance when passing through the glottis. Performing laryngoscopy to lift

the supraglottic structures and counterclockwise rotation of the tube may also help prevent this. Should difficulties persist, two exchange catheters may need to be inserted (in each lumen) to lessen impingement on the glottis.

Management of one-lung ventilation

The traditional ventilator strategies for one-lung ventilation have recently been challenged. Previously, management of one-lung ventilation focused primarily upon avoiding hypoxemic events. Although controversial,[14,15] contemporary ventilator management now focuses upon maintaining low tidal volumes (~6 ml/kg ideal body weight) and minimizing plateau pressures (<30 cmH_2O) to avoid lung injury (Table 11.4). The primary impetus to reduce intraoperative lung volumes has been extrapolated from critical care literature in patients with acute respiratory distress syndrome (ARDS). With emerging awareness of the morbidity associated with acute lung injury complicating lung resection surgery, these same principles have been recommended for all one-lung ventilation scenarios. Although incompletely understood and still unproven, it is hypothesized that ventilator-induced lung injury from large tidal volume single-lung ventilation may predispose to ARDS. Despite an absence of convincing, supportive evidence, many experts advocate adopting a low-tidal volume, pressure-limited ventilation strategy.

If a low-tidal volume strategy is used, PEEP (5–10 cmH_2O) should be applied to the dependent lung to improve oxygenation by minimizing the compressive atelectasis that occurs from displacement of the mediastinum and cephalad migration of the diaphragm. Permissive hypercapnea is usually associated with this technique. In the trauma patient with multiple injuries, hypovolemia, and shock, the addition of a respiratory acidosis combined with an already present metabolic acidosis may not be well tolerated. In addition, low tidal ventilation in the patient with severe COPD when combined with an increased respiratory rate to maintain normocapnea may predispose to air trapping and dynamic hyperinflation.

Placement of any device for lung isolation is most easily performed with the patient supine. Final operative positioning of the patient often results in proximal movement of the double-lumen tube or bronchial blocker.[16] This may occur more often when a patient is placed in the prone position for a posterior approach during spine operations, but there are no studies that confirm this. However, it seems reasonable to recommend that tubes and blockers be initially intentionally placed more distal than normal, and then re-advanced if necessary into optimal position under direct fiberoptic visualization after the patient is moved.

Complications of lung separation

The actual incidence of complications related to the provision of lung isolation is not known. Complications are generally due to traumatic tube placement, unrecognized malposition of the tube or blocker, or result from the management of single-lung ventilation.

Minor tracheobronchial trauma following one-lung ventilation is relatively common, particularly with the use of double-lumen tubes,[17] but these complications are usually not clinically significant.[18] Sore throat and hoarseness are the most frequent clinical manifestations and are generally self-limited. Traumatic glottic edema is rarely of consequence in otherwise normal patients, but ultimately may lead to respiratory insufficiency or obstruction in susceptible patients. Prolonged surgery in the prone or supine positions with massive fluid resuscitation can contribute to airway edema making exchange to a single-lumen tube from a double-lumen tube hazardous.

Fortunately, catastrophic traumatic airway injuries are rare and primary literature on this subject is limited to case reports. Tracheal laceration and bronchial rupture are potentially lethal complications of lung isolation. Although it seems counterintuitive, in a comprehensive review of airway rupture from double-lumen tubes a major risk factor identified was selection of an undersized tube.[19] The authors felt that smaller double-lumen tubes are more likely to be advanced too deeply into the airway, causing injury, and their bronchial cuff required inflation with larger volumes of air in order to seal the airway. Deep penetration into the airway with associated trauma and pressure injury

from cuff over-inflation are the usual causes of airway injury. Bronchoscopically guided tube placement, limiting the volume of air used to inflate the bronchial cuff, and avoiding the use of nitrous oxide may help to limit these injuries.

Depending on the operative site and lung isolation device used, malposition of a double-lumen tube or bronchial blocker may result in a variety of clinical problems. Typically a poorly positioned lung isolation device will manifest either as failure of lung isolation or by obstruction to ventilation. These difficulties can present immediately following tube placement, after patient repositioning for surgery, or at any time during the procedure due to surgical manipulation.

When ventilation is obstructed it is often due to the bronchial cuff or blocker balloon being displaced outward into the trachea. It is imperative to deflate the balloon or cuff to reestablish ventilation to both lungs. If the lung on the operated side fails to collapse, troubleshooting begins with fiberoptic examination of the airway to remedy double-lumen tube or blocker position. Commonly this also occurs because the device has herniated proximally and the lungs are no longer isolated from each other. A useful trick is to palpate the pilot balloon to the bronchial cuff of the double-lumen tube. A reduction in tension of that pilot balloon usually means the bronchial cuff has pulled out into the larger trachea.

Hypoxemia during one-lung ventilation (defined as an S_pO_2 <90% with F_1O_2 >0.5) occurs in approximately 5% of patients.[20] Multiple factors influence the development of hypoxemia. Matching of ventilation and perfusion is paramount to maintaining adequate gas exchange (Table 11.5). During operative lung collapse, an obligatory shunt is created. During one-lung ventilation with the patient in the lateral position, pulmonary blood flow is preferentially distributed to the dependent, nonoperative lung due to gravity and hypoxic pulmonary vasoconstriction. Improper tube placement with obstruction of the upper lobe in the ventilated lung combined with intentional collapse of the lung on the operated side is a common cause of hypoxemia. This is always associated with a very high peak inspiratory pressure, even when low tidal volumes are used. The differential diagnosis, which must always be considered, is tension pneumothorax in the dependent, ventilated hemithorax.[21]

Dependent lung compressive atelectasis occurs from downward movement of mediastinal structures

Table 11.5 Management of hypoxemia during one-lung ventilation

- Increase F_iO_2
- Confirm correct position of the double-lumen tube or bronchial blocker by inspection with a fiberoptic bronchoscope; re-adjust position if indicated
- Optimize ventilation of nonoperative lung (suction secretions; consider increasing PEEP; perform lung recruitment maneuver)
- Consider causes other than the obligatory intrapulmonary shunt from operative collapse
  - Ventilated lung atelectasis
  - Low cardiac output
  - Pneumothorax
- Inform surgical team, provide CPAP or intermittent ventilation to operative (collapsed) lung

and encroachment by abdominal contents on the diaphragm. Judicious use of PEEP and selective lung recruitment maneuvers can ameliorate oxygenation, especially when a low tidal volume strategy is implemented. Reabsorption atelectasis may be associated with 100% F_iO_2 or bronchial obstruction from secretions. In this event, fiberoptic inspection may be both diagnostic and therapeutic. Cardiac arrhythmias or hypotension are other major causes of hypoxemia during one-lung ventilation. Reduced perfusion to the dependent lung leads to an increase in dead-space in the ventilated lung.

Should hypoxemia persist despite proper double-lumen tube or blocker position after optimizing ventilation, and with failure to identify secondary etiologies (e.g., pneumothorax), the surgeon should be informed and temporary ventilation of the operative lung resumed. It is crucial to recognize that patient safety should never be jeopardized by allowing surgery to continue with a collapsed lung in the presence of severe, life-threatening hypoxemia. Slow, small intermittent breaths to the collapsed lung or the application of CPAP to the operative lung will almost always improve arterial oxygenation while allowing the operation to proceed. These solutions are impractical during video-assisted thoracoscopic (VATS) procedures, an increasingly popular surgical approach for operations on the thoracic spine.[22,23] The surgical field during a VATS procedure will be obscured by a partially expanded lung. For the experienced thoracic anesthesiologist, selective lobar CPAP or high-frequency jet ventilation may be employed, but these maneuvers are not widely recommended.

Lung separation for the patient undergoing spine surgery

Airway management in the patient undergoing spine surgery may be challenging because of spinal deformity or instability. Postoperatively, airway extubation may have to be delayed owing to airway edema, neuromuscular weakness, or pulmonary restriction. This is highlighted by a case series reporting a 38% re-intubation rate following cervicothoracic procedures.[24] Re-intubation in this setting can be especially challenging, and is associated with an unacceptably high morbidity.[25]

For procedures requiring lung collapse, there is little difference in the operative conditions produced by bronchial blockers and double-lumen tubes. Blockers are more easily placed in the setting of a difficult airway. A single-lumen tracheal tube can be placed by any route (oral, nasal, via a tracheostomy) and then a bronchial blocker can be advanced through it. Intubation with a single-lumen tube in the scenario of a difficult airway will result in less trauma to the glottis. For pediatric patients, airway intubation with a single-lumen tube and then placement of a bronchial blocker remains the only means of safely providing lung collapse. When postoperative ventilation is required for the high-risk patient, use of a single-lumen tube and bronchial blocker can avoid the danger of changing from a double-lumen tube to a single-lumen tracheal tube at the completion of surgery. Considering these points, bronchial blockers are the preferred device for providing lung isolation in spine surgery, particularly procedures on children and in the trauma patient with spinal column injury (Fig. 11.9).

Acute lung injury and respiratory failure may occur in up to 15% of patients following major intrathoracic spine surgery.[26] Following anterior/posterior spine fusions, patients often have evidence of an acute inflammatory pulmonary injury. Several etiologies exist including injury from massive blood and fluid infusions, direct trauma to the lung, systemic inflammatory response, and the embolization of fat and bone-marrow debris. Although medical evidence to guide preventative ventilator measures is sparse, adopting a low-tidal volume, pressure-limited strategy in combination with moderate levels of PEEP during one-lung ventilation seems rational for these patients who are already prone to postoperative lung injury.

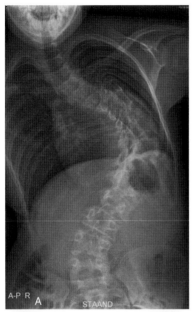

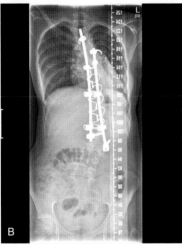

Figure 11.9 (A) The preoperative radiograph of an 11-year-old child with severe spinal deformities is shown. An EZ-Blocker® was placed through an endotracheal tube to collapse her lung allowing a transthoracic spinal correction procedure with instrumentation to be performed. At the completion of the operation, the blocker was removed, the endotracheal tube was kept in place, and the patient was ventilated overnight. (B) This radiograph shows the same patient postoperatively, demonstrating correction of her spinal deformity.

References

1. Brodsky JB. The evolution of thoracic anesthesia. *Thorac Surg Clin* 2005; **15**: 1–10.

2. Lammers CR, Hammer GB, Brodsky JB, Cannon WB. Failure to separate and isolate the lungs with an endotracheal tube positioned in the bronchus. *Anesth Analg* 1997; **85**: 946–7.

3. Conacher ID, Velasquez H, Morrice DJ. Endobronchial tubes – a case for re-evaluation. *Anaesthesia* 2006; **61**: 587–90.

4. Neustein SM. The use of bronchial blockers for providing one-lung ventilation. *J Cardiothorac Vasc Anesth* 2009; **23**: 860–8.

5. Ghosh S, Falter F, Goldsmith K, Arrowsmith JE. The Papworth BiVent tube: a new device for lung isolation. *Anaesthesia* 2008; **63**: 996–1000.

6. Mungroop HE, Wai PT, Morei MN, Loef BG, Epema AH. Lung isolation with a new Y-shaped endobronchial blocking device, the EZ-Blocker. *Br J Anaesth* 2010; **104**: 119–20.

7. Campos JH. Update on tracheobronchial anatomy and flexible fiberoptic bronchoscopy in thoracic anesthesia. *Curr Opin Anaesthesiol* 2009; **22**: 4–10.

8. Campos JH. Which device should be considered the best for lung isolation: double-lumen endotracheal tube versus bronchial blockers. *Curr Opin Anaesthesiol* 2007; **20**: 27–31.

9. Brodsky JB, Macario A, Mark JB. Tracheal diameter predicts double-lumen tube size: a method for selecting left double-lumen tubes. *Anesth Analg* 1996; **82**: 861–4.

10. Brodsky JB, Lemmens HJ. Left double-lumen tubes: clinical experience with 1,170 patients. *J Cardiothorac Vasc Anesth* 2003; **17**: 289–98.

11. Campos JH, Hallam EA, Van Natta T, Kernstine KH. Devices for lung isolation used by anesthesiologists with limited thoracic experience: comparison of double-lumen endotracheal tube, Univent torque control blocker, and Arndt wire-guided endobronchial blocker. *Anesthesiology* 2006; **104**: 261–6.

12. Anantham D, Jagadesan R, Tiew PE. Clinical review: Independent lung ventilation in critical care. *Crit Care* 2005; **9**: 594–600.

13. Brodsky JB. Lung separation and the difficult airway. *Br J Anaesth* 2009; **103**: 166–75.

14. Slinger P. Pro: Low tidal volume is indicated during one-lung ventilation. *Anesth Analg* 2006; **103**: 268–70.

15. Gal TJ. Con: Low tidal volumes are indicated during one-lung ventilation. *Anesth Analg* 2006; **103**: 271–3.

16. Desiderio DP, Birt M, Kolker AC, *et al.* The effects of endo-bronchial cuff inflation on double-lumen endobronchial tube movement after lateral decubitus positioning. *J Cardiothorac Vasc Anesth* 1997; **11**: 595–8.

17. Knoll H, Ziegeler S, Schreiber JU, *et al.* Airway injuries after one-lung ventilation: a comparison between double-lumen tube and endobronchial blocker: a randomized, prospective, controlled trial. *Anesthesiology* 2006; **105**: 471–7.

18. Zhong T, Wang W, Chen J, Ran L, Story DA. Sore throat or hoarse voice with bronchial blockers or

double-lumen tubes for lung isolation: a randomised, prospective trial. *Anaesth Intensive Care* 2009; **37**: 441–6.

19. Fitzmaurice BG, Brodsky JB. Airway rupture from double-lumen tubes. *J Cardiothorac Vasc Anesth* 1999; **13**: 322–9.

20. Karzai W, Schwarzkopf K. Hypoxemia during one-lung ventilation: prediction, prevention and treatment. *Anesthesiology* 2009; **110**(6): 1402–11.

21. Roush TF, Crawford AH, Berlin RE, Wolf RK. Tension pneumothorax as a complication of video-assisted thorascopic surgery for anterior correction of idiopathic scoliosis in an adolescent female. *Spine* 2001; **26**: 448–50.

22. Krasna MJ, Jiao X, Eslami A, Rutter CM, Levine AM. Thoracoscopic approach for spine deformities. *J Am Coll Surg* 2003; **197**: 777–9.

23. Al-Sayyad MJ, Crawford AH, Wolf RK. Early experiences with video-assisted thoracoscopic surgery: our first 70 cases. *Spine* 2004; **29**: 1945–51.

24. Hart RA, Tatsumi RL, Hiratzka JR, JU Yoo. Perioperative complications of combined anterior and posterior cervical decompression and fusion crossing the cervico-thoracic junction. *Spine* 2008; **33**: 2887–91.

25. Kwon B, Yoo JU, Furey CG, Rowbottom J, Emery SE. Risk factors for delayed extubation after single-stage, multi-level anterior cervical decompression and posterior fusion. *J Spinal Disord Tech* 2006; **19**: 389–93.

26. Urban MK, Jules-Elysee KM, Beckman JB, *et al.* Pulmonary injury in patients undergoing complex spine surgery. *Spine J* 2005; **5**: 269–76.

Chapter

12

Anesthesia for lumbar spine surgery

Mariel R. Manlapaz, Ajit A. Krishnaney, and Zeyd Ebrahim

Key points

- Indications for surgery in the lumbar spine are quite varied covering degenerative, traumatic, neoplastic, vascular, infectious, congenital, and idiopathic pathologies.
- Among several techniques used in spine surgery, the use of aminocaproic acid and tranexamic acid has been shown to be effective in decreasing blood loss and transfusion requirements.
- Multimodality neuromonitoring techniques are used in lumbar surgery for complex instrumentation cases and resection of intradural tumors, requiring limitations in anesthetic choices for improved data acquisition.
- An anesthesiologist must be versatile in dealing with lumbar spine surgeries as they vary in complexity and urgency, involvement of intraoperative neuromonitoring, susceptibility to hemodynamic instability, and multiple intraoperative and postoperative catastrophic complications.

Surgical indications

The indications for surgery on the lumbar spine are varied. In general they include degenerative, neoplastic, infectious, traumatic, vascular, and congenital/idiopathic conditions. Indications for surgical intervention in these cases include pain reduction, decompression of neurological structures (e.g., spinal cord, cauda equina, and nerve roots), spinal stabilization, deformity correction, or resection of a pathologic lesion (e.g., tumor, vascular malformation). It is important to note that these indications are not mutually exclusive and that any one patient may have multiple indications for surgery.

Degenerative

Degenerative conditions of the lumbar spine are generally present in the 6th and 7th decade of life. Most present with a combination of lower back pain, radiculopathy, and claudication symptoms. Back pain may be the result of facet arthropathy, degenerative disc disease, or degenerative instability (spondylolisthesis). In the absence of overt instability, surgery is reserved as a last resort for the treatment of low back pain.[1]

Neurogenic claudication is characterized by activity-related lower extremity pain or weakness. It is associated with narrowing of the central canal due to disc bulges, buckling of the ligamentum flavum, and/or facet arthropathy and hypertrophy. Symptoms are usually progressive, developing over months to years. Although physical therapy and pain management interventions have been shown to be helpful in treating the symptoms of lumbar stenosis, the "gold standard" for therapy is surgical decompression of the affected neural elements. Decompression with the addition of fusion may be considered in cases of segmental instability or deformity.[2,3]

Lumbar radiculopathy is characterized by pain, weakness, and/or sensory disturbance in a dermatomal distribution. Most commonly this presents as pain in the buttock or lower extremity. Degenerative causes of radiculopathy include disc herniation, lumbar lateral recess stenosis or foraminal stenosis from spondylolisthesis. Surgical intervention for radiculopathy is reserved for patients who have failed "conservative therapy" including physical therapy, analgesics, anti-inflammatory agents, or epidural steroid injections. The goal of surgical intervention is decompression of the affected nerve root(s). Common operations for the treatment of radiculopathy include hemilaminectomy, laminectomy, and microdiscectomy. Fusion may be considered if there is any evidence of segmental instability.[4,5]

Anesthesia for Spine Surgery, ed. Ehab Farag. Published by Cambridge University Press. © Cambridge University Press 2012.

Tumors

Spinal neoplasms can be divided into primary neoplasms of the spine and spinal cord and secondary neoplasms.[6] The indications for surgery vary based upon the tumor type and location.

Common metastatic lesions include those arising from lung, breast, prostate, and renal cancers. Surgery for metastatic disease of the spine is directed at preserving neurologic function or for palliation of pain. In cases of soft tissue compressing the spinal cord or nerve roots, decompression via laminectomy and tumor debulking may be sufficient. However, in cases where the integrity of the spinal column is compromised, stabilization with instrumentation and/or ventral reconstruction may be required.[7]

When palliation of pain is the goal of surgery other less invasive options may exist. These include vertebral augmentation, percutaneous instrumentation, or placement of an intrathecal pain pump.

Primary tumors of the spine include tumors of the vertebral body and tumors of the neural elements. Neural origin tumors may be extradural, intradural extramedullary, intradural intramedullary, or intra- and extradural tumors. The indications for surgical intervention include obtaining pathologic tissue for diagnosis, decompression of the neural elements, and in some cases cure. These tumors are accessed via a laminectomy approach. Intraoperative neurologic monitoring may be indicated during tumor resection. In cases where the facet joint is compromised, instrumented fusion may be indicated.

For primary bony tumors of the spine, indications for surgical intervention include diagnosis, decompression of neural elements, spinal stabilization, and in some cases cure. In cases where the tumor is confined to the osseous elements, cure of even malignant lesions may be possible. In these cases en bloc vertebrectomy or spondylectomy may be indicated. These approaches generally require staged operations incorporating both ventral and dorsal approaches for resection of the vertebral body and spinal reconstruction.[8]

Trauma

Traumatic injuries to the lumbar spine may result in fractures, dislocations, or soft tissue disruption/dislocation. Surgical intervention is typically reserved for injuries that are considered unstable, injuries that result in significant spinal deformity, or injuries that result in neurologic compression. Surgical intervention, therefore, may consist of decompression via laminectomy, discectomy or corpectomy to decompress the neural elements, and/or instrumented fusion to restore stability to the spine. Stabilization may be performed via a dorsal, ventral, or combined approach based on the degree of instability and the need for dorsal or ventral decompression.

Deformity correction

Spinal deformities may be congenital or acquired. Acquired deformities may be traumatic, degenerative or iatrogenic in origin. Indications for surgery include compression of neurologic structures, resulting in either myelopathy or radiculopathy, progressive deformity in the case of scoliosis, back pain, and cosmesis.

Surgical intervention for deformity is directed at restoring normal sagittal and coronal balance of the spinal axis via reduction of the abnormal curvature of the spine. This correction may be accomplished via a number of techniques all of which require multilevel segmental instrumentation and fusion of the spinal column to maintain the new alignment. In the case of rigid deformities, anterior releases (e.g., discectomies or osteotomies) may be needed to adequately correct the deformity.

Preoperative management

The complexity of lumbar spine surgeries ranges from simple single-level microdiscectomy to multilevel deformity correction. The acuity can also vary from chronic back pain to acute cauda equina syndrome. Thus, preoperative optimization for a lumbar spine surgery depends on the complexity and urgency of the surgery. Standardization of care for high-risk patients in spine surgery is presently being piloted to improve outcomes. Northwestern University has a multidisciplinary protocol to provide comprehensive care in the pre-, peri-, and postoperative periods for patients undergoing high-risk spine procedures. Patients are placed in this protocol if the surgeon anticipates >6 hours of surgery time, plans >6 levels of surgery, or plans a staged procedure. The presence of high-risk medical conditions including coronary artery disease, congestive heart failure, cirrhosis, dementia, emphysema, renal insufficiency, cerebrovascular disease, pulmonary hypertension, or age >80 years also places patients in this protocol.[9] A dedicated multidisciplinary team comprised of an internist, surgeon, anesthesiologist, neuromonitoring technologist, and intensivist follow a set of protocols throughout the pre-, intra-, and postoperative care of these high-risk spine surgery patients. The overall objective of the study is to determine whether protocol-based care in spine surgery leads to reduced complications and better outcomes.

Several studies report favorable outcomes in patients with comorbidities and age >70 years undergoing spine decompression surgery.[10–12] In one study the ASA physical classification system was reported to be a poor predictor of postoperative complications in this population.[12] With an expanding elderly population, lumbar decompression surgery for spinal stenosis in the elderly can be expected to increase.

Intraoperative management

Regional anesthesia

Regional anesthesia has been shown to be a safe and effective alternative to general anesthesia for lumbar spine surgery of short duration. Such procedures include discectomies, laminectomies, and foraminotomies. There is evidence to suggest that single-level or two-level laminectomy/discectomy under spinal anesthesia is associated with less blood loss, less nausea and vomiting, and improved postoperative pain scores.[13] Regional anesthesia allows for an awake patient who can help gauge a comfortable position, one that would prevent nerve pressure and injury. In prolonged cases or less than adequate spinal anesthesia, anesthesia could be augmented with an intrathecal injection by the surgeon.

There are several considerations that must be taken into account with regional anesthesia. Exacerbation of preexisting neurologic disease has been estimated to occur in 0.5% to 0.8% of patients after spinal anesthesia.[14] In patients with severe spinal stenosis not undergoing lumbar surgery, spinal anesthesia has been associated with an increased risk of new neurologic deficit.[15] Furthermore, spinal anesthesia could be variable and may miss coverage for skin incision and muscle/bone dissection. Sedation must be carefully titrated not only for airway protection but also for surgical field optimization. Deep breathing associated with deep sedation could pose a significant disturbance to the surgeon especially during microdissection. Finally, prone position for a long duration is a challenge to the many patients. Short-duration lumbar surgeries lasting 2 hours or less and patients in the kneeling position are optimal candidates for spinal anesthesia.

Positioning

The goal of positioning in major spine surgery is to avoid abdominal compression for surgical field optimization. When abdominal compression occurs, the inferior vena cava (IVC) is somewhat obstructed, impeding the epidural veins from draining well. When these thin-walled veins become engorged, poor surgical exposure and increased blood loss are common consequences. Many authors have hypothesized oxygenation improvement in the prone position due to an increase in functional residual capacity and improved ventilation/perfusion matching.[16,17] However, with abdominal compression, abdominal contents push against the diaphragm, decreasing respiratory compliance. Very high airway pressures may be required to ensure adequate oxygenation and ventilation.

Several prone positioning systems are used in major spine surgery. These include the Siemens positioning system, the Andrews frame, the Wilson frame, the Jackson spine table, and the longitudinal bolster. These systems differ in their abdominal compression, chest, and pelvis support, and leveling of lower extremities compared with the heart. The Jackson spine table (Fig. 12.1) and longitudinal bolsters have been shown to best preserve cardiac function.[18] In these systems, the abdomen hangs free and the lower extremities are at the level of the heart, allowing blood from the IVC and femoral veins to stay in the circulating volume and maintain preload to the heart. The Andrews frame and Jackson table also allow the abdomen to hang free, optimizing respiratory function in the prone position.[18]

In addition to the prone position, other positions seen in lumbar spine surgery include supine, lateral, and kneeling positions. The lateral position (Fig. 12.2) is used to access the ventral lumbar spine from the thoracolumbar junction to L4. Direct ventral access to these levels is often challenging due to the intra-abdominal viscera and vasculature. This position does not allow for a wide view of the intervertebral discs and may make it more difficult to control bleeding. Moreover, the great vessels and segmental vessels are in close proximity to the spine and need to be mobilized, which may lead to increased risk of bleeding. The supine position may be used to access the spine via either a retroperitoneal or transperitoneal approach from L4 to the sacrum. The limits of exposure via this approach are defined by the bifurcation of the great vessels rostrally and the angle of the pelvis caudally. As with the lateral position, mobilization of the iliac vessels

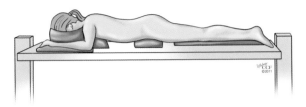

Figure 12.1 Jackson table.

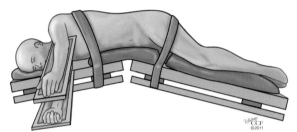

Figure 12.2 Lateral position.

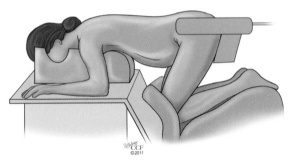

Figure 12.3 Kneeling position.

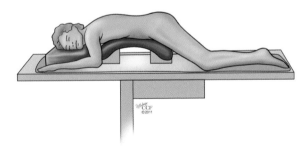

Figure 12.4 Wilson frame.

is required, increasing the risk of bleeding. Retraction of the iliac veins is often necessary for exposure, which could increase the risk of postoperative venous thrombosis and/or thromboembolism. The kneeling position (Fig. 12.3) is a prone position variant often used when fusion is not required. This position has the advantage of opening the interlaminar space and enlarging the spinal canal by placing the lumbar spine in flexion,

thereby making decompression easier. In this position the abdomen hangs freely, thereby minimizing intra-abdominal pressure. A significant portion of the patient's weight rests on the knees in the kneeling position; hence it is generally avoided in patients with significant knee or hip pathology. The Wilson frame (Fig 12.4) may be used in such instances. This frame may be attached to a Jackson table or standard electric operating table. It allows for flexion of the lumbar spine; however, the abdomen does not hang freely in this position.

Anesthetic choices

Hemodynamic management

Controlled hypotension, which was once in vogue in spine surgery, is thought to directly reduce bleeding from injured arterioles and arteries. Blood pressure reduction by venous dilatation also decreases venous pressure and bleeding from bony sinuses. A number of prospective clinical trials have shown a decrease in blood loss and need for transfusion with controlled hypotension.[19–21]. More recent studies, on the other hand, report that controlled hypotension does not consistently result in blood loss and blood transfusion reduction.[22] Due to the risk of end organ hypoperfusion secondary to perfusion pressure dependency, risks versus benefits of controlled hypotension should be carefully weighed in patients susceptible to ischemic complications. These are patients with hypertension, diabetes, coronary artery disease, carotid stenosis, cerebral ischemia, or chronic renal failure. Although the pathology in ischemic optic neuropathy is still poorly understood, it should be remembered that the posterior part of the optic nerve and the anterior part in some individuals are not capable of autoregulation and are dependent on systemic perfusion for adequate flow.[23] In the American Society of Anesthesiology Postoperative Visual Loss (POVL) Registry, among the 23 cases of patients with POVL, controlled hypotension was used in 42% of the cases.[24]

In patients who are believed to be at high risk for neurologic injury such as patients presenting for intradural tumor resection, anesthetic management may include induced hypertension to improve spinal cord perfusion especially during dissection near the cord.

Evoked potentials

The use of intraoperative neuromonitoring (IOM) has become more popular to help avoid neurologic complications and improve outcomes. Common high-risk spine surgeries that employ IOM include but are not limited to congenital kyphosis or scoliosis, large or rigid spine curves, intradural spine tumors, and complex instrumentation cases. Currently, approaches for neuromonitoring include the wake-up test, somatosensory evoked potentials (SSEPs), transcranial motor-evoked potentials (tcMEPs), spontaneous electromyography (sEMG), and triggered electromyography (tEMG).[25]

The wake-up test provides a gross assessment of the components of the motor system. When properly administered this test is estimated to have a 100% accuracy in detecting gross motor changes.[26] To facilitate the wake-up test, anesthetic agents chosen are easily titratable with short duration or reliable reversibility. Although a valuable intraoperative test, the wake-up test has disadvantages that include potential awareness and discomfort, dislodgement of the endotracheal tube and intravenous access, risk of embolism on deep inspiration, self-induced contamination, and lack of nerve root injury information.[18] The wake-up test also provides a one-time measure rather than continuous measure of function. According to Malhotra and Shaffrey, with repetition of the test, the risks multiply but interperformance reliability decreases.[25] The wake-up test is generally used now as a supplement to other intraoperative neuromonitoring techniques.

SSEP is a continuous monitor that can help assess the integrity of the focal posterior column and/or the global condition of the spinal cord. In scoliosis repair, it is considered an indicated monitoring technique by the Scoliosis Research Society to reduce risk of neurologic injury.[27] Motor tract injury, however, can easily occur without changes in SSEPs. When analyzing changes in SSEPs, a decrease in amplitude of 50% or greater and/or an increase in latency of 10% from baseline are considered significant signs of neurologic injury.[28] All volatile anesthetics and nitrous oxide cause a dose-dependent decrease in amplitude and increase in latency of SSEP while opioids cause minimal changes. Therefore, anesthesia with low-dose inhalational agents in combination with opioid infusions or complete total intravenous anesthesia (TIVA) is beneficial in providing a good environment for SSEP monitoring. The use of muscle relaxants also reduces movement artifact and may improve waveform analysis. Physiologic parameters that can alter SSEP signals include hypothermia, hypocapnia, hypoxia, hypotension, and anemia.[28]

tcMEPs monitor the anterior pathways of the spinal cord. Stimulation is at the motor cortex of the brain or the spinal cord. The signal is obtained either from the spinal cord (D wave) or from the end muscle (CMAP).[25] Volatile anesthetics, because of their inhibitory effect on neurotransmission, have a much more significant effect on tcMEPs (more synapses) than SSEPs. Thus, there has been a shift toward use of TIVA to improve MEP data acquisition.[29] In contrast to D waves, muscle relaxants are avoided in CMAP because neuromuscular blockade will ablate the signals. In a study of patients undergoing scoliosis surgery, Schwartz *et al.* report that a 65% decrease in MEP amplitude always predicted postoperative motor deficit, while SSEP monitoring was only sensitive 43% of the time.[30] SSEP warning signals also lagged behind MEP signals by 5 minutes.[25]

Spontaneous EMG is used for selective nerve root monitoring in the setting of segmental spinal instrumentation, while triggered EMG is employed to assess cortical bone perforation during placement of pedicle screws.[25] For optimal analysis, muscle relaxants are avoided for either technique.

There is not a single intraoperative monitor that can detect the onset of deficit for both sensory and motor pathways.[26] With multimodality intraoperative monitoring methods, however, there has not been a reported case of false-negative monitoring.[31]

Blood loss and transfusion in spine surgery

Blood loss and transfusion are commonly encountered in multilevel spine surgery. Without using preventive measures to decrease hemorrhage, the rate of transfusion in adult spine surgery ranges from 50% to 81%.[32] The incidence of allogenic red blood cell (RBC) transfusion and coagulation factors transfusion have been reported as 36.1% and 13.9% respectively, rates that are similar to other surgical procedures considered high risk for blood transfusion.[33] Nuttall *et al.* report that the predictors for increased allogenic RBC transfusion include low preoperative hemoglobin, history of pulmonary disease, surgery for tumors, increased number of levels fused, less availability of autologous RBC, and nonuse of the Jackson table.[33] Serious consideration must be given to allogenic transfusion because of the persistent possibility of transfusion reactions, costs involved, and shortage of blood products. In cardiac surgery, transfusion of packed red blood cells (pRBCs) has been associated with an increase in hospital morbidity and mortality and reduction in survival beyond postoperative recovery phase.[34–36]

Several techniques are currently in use to reduce blood loss and transfusion requirements for spine surgeries. These include preoperative autologous blood donation, acute normovolemic hemodilution, perioperative antifibrinolytic agents, cell salvage, and recombinant factor VIIa (FVIIa).

In preoperative autologous donation, blood is obtained from the patient 3–5 weeks before surgery. Relative contraindications include severe aortic stenosis, coronary artery disease, anemia, and body weight less than 50 kg (110 lbs).[37] Benefits of pre-donated autologous blood include decreasing the risks associated with allogenic blood transfusion. There are reports that indicate 50% reduction of such risks after spinal surgery.[33,38,39] A study by Cha et al., however, shows a 37% rate of allogenic blood transfusion in addition to autologous blood transfusions in patients undergoing posterior lumbar fusions.[39] Several studies have also pointed out the wasting of pre-donated autologous blood. Bess and Lenke report that at least one unit is wasted in up to 50% of patients undergoing scoliosis correction.[40]

When acute normovolemic hemodilution is utilized, the patient's blood is withdrawn early in the operative period and immediately replaced by crystalloid or colloid to maintain blood volume. As a result, the blood lost early during surgery will have a lower hematocrit. Autologous blood can then be returned to the patient when transfusion becomes necessary.

Antifibrinolytic agents are also used to decrease blood loss in spine surgery. As a class, these drugs inhibit fibrin and fibrinogen degradation. In five randomized controlled trials the antifibrinolytic agents, aprotinin, tranexamic acid, and aminocaproic acid, have been shown to reduce blood loss and the need for transfusion in adult spine surgery.[22] Because aprotinin is associated with long-term mortality and renal dysfunction, Elgafy et al. did not recommend the use of this drug in spine surgery. The lysine analogs, tranexamic acid and aminocaproic acid, based on their available efficacy and safety to date, are recommended for use to reduce major hemorrhage in adult spine surgery.[22]

Intraoperative cell salvage is a popular technology currently employed in spine surgeries to reduce allogenic blood transfusion. In this system, blood is collected from the surgical field, anticoagulated, filtered, and stored in a reservoir. Stored blood is then separated into RBCs and plasma components using a centrifuge.

RBCs are washed with a crystalloid solution and reinfused into the patient.[41] The average recovery rate of RBCs with cell salvage in spine surgery has been estimated to be 38%.[42] This is lower than the rates reported in cardiovascular surgery. Possible causes include smaller suction tips that lead to lysis during collection, contamination with bone and fat, and liberal use of sponges. Potential complications associated with cell salvage include paradoxical increase in blood loss, electrolyte abnormalities, metabolic acidosis, and hematuria.[41,43] After the analysis of the three available retrospective cohort studies evaluating the efficacy of cell salvage in preventing blood loss and transfusion, Elgafy et al. concluded that cell salvage to date has low evidence for effectiveness in preventing significant hemorrhage.[22] In terms of cost analysis, cell salvage is at $512 per patient, pre-donation is at $270 per individual, and allogenic blood replacement is at $250 per unit transfused.[42]

The use of factor VIIa in spine surgery has also been investigated. In one randomized controlled trial, factor VIIa was given to patients undergoing multilevel spinal fusion when estimated blood loss was at 10% of blood volume.[44] In this series, factor VIIa was shown to be effective in decreasing blood loss and transfusion. However, in the same study, there was one thromboembolic stroke and one death in the group that received factor VIIa and none in the control group. Thus, Elgafy et al. concluded that there is still insufficient evidence for the effective and safe use of factor VIIa in spine surgery patients.[22]

Other techniques that have been used to reduce blood loss and transfusion in spine surgery include the administration of erythropoietin-alpha, application of induced hypotension, and use of the Jackson table. The latter two have been discussed previously. The preoperative administration of erythropoietin-alpha can increase the number of autologous units that could be collected. When used alone, erythropoietin-alpha is effective in patients undergoing procedures with lower intraoperative blood loss.[45] For patients undergoing spine procedures with considerable blood loss, it does not reduce transfusion requirements.[46]

Postoperative pain management

Postoperative epidural analgesia is an alternative to intravenous patient-controlled analgesia (PCA) in patients undergoing complex lumbar spine surgeries. The epidural catheter is placed under direct vision by the surgeon before wound closure, provided no dural tears occurred during surgery. For posterior spinal correction, the catheter can be inserted directly through the ligamentum flavum by the surgeon. For anterior spinal surgery, the epidural catheter can be inserted percutaneously or under direct vision and tunneled to the skin. There are studies that show comparable analgesia provided by intravenous PCA for patients following spine surgery. Furthermore, different reports indicate some advantages of epidural analgesia including absence of opioid-induced side effects, earlier return of bowel function, and low complication rates.[47-50] Concerns related to epidural analgesia in spine patients include the possibility of superficial skin infection, epidural abscess and epidural hematoma, dural puncture, and intrathecal catheter placement. In addition epidural infusions may make the neurologic assessment of patients after spinal surgery difficult.[51,52]

Other effective techniques for pain control after spine surgery include local anesthetic wound infiltration, wound catheters with infiltration of local anesthetic, and preoperative and postoperative oral controlled-release narcotics.[53-55]

Complications in lumbar spine surgery

Perioperative neuropathy

The etiology of perioperative peripheral nerve injury is believed to be complex and multifactorial. Preexisting patient conditions, positioning, and surgical conditions are associated with such injuries.[56] Pathologic mechanisms for perioperative neuropathy include stretch, compression, ischemia, and metabolic/environmental abnormalities. In the most recent American Society of Anesthesiologists (ASA) closed claims analysis, nerve injuries comprised about 15% of the claims.[57] Except for cardiac surgery, no clear association is established between surgical services and perioperative neuropathy. In a large retrospective study, Welch *et al.* report an association of perioperative peripheral nerve injury and general surgery, orthopedic surgery, and neurosurgery.[58] These investigators hypothesize the frequent use of the prone position in orthopedic and neurosurgery to be a causative factor.[58]

A characteristic of lumbar spine surgery is the surgical need to operate with the patient in prone, supine, or lateral position. In 2000, the ASA Task Force on Prevention of Perioperative Peripheral Neuropathies released a practice advisory on positioning. As one of the recommendations, the patient's ability to tolerate the anticipated operative position must be ascertained before induction of anesthesia. To avoid brachial plexus injury in any surgical position, arm abduction must be limited to 90°. All vulnerable pressure points should be padded.

Postoperative vision loss

Postoperative vision loss is a rare but devastating complication of spine surgery with an estimated incidence of 0–0.1% of cases.[59-61] It can be secondary to central retinal artery occlusion, cortical blindness, or ischemic optic neuropathy (IOP).

Central retinal artery occlusion is the second most common cause of POVL. It is usually the result of an embolic event or external compression of the ocular globe.[23] Symptoms are unilateral and are often noted within 24 hours of surgery.[62] Funduscopic results comprise retinal pallor combined with cherry red spot at the macula.[63] Cortical blindness is also a result of an embolic event in the visual areas of the occipital lobe and more commonly associated with cardiac surgery.[23]

Ischemic optic neuropathy is the most common cause of POVL after lumbar spine surgery.[23] In two recent analyses, the incidence of ION was estimated to be 0.13% overall and 0.36% for spine surgery, and 0.0235% and 0.0309% respectively.[64,65] The two forms of ION include anterior ischemic optic neuropathy (AION) and posterior ischemic optic neuropathy (PION), the latter being the most common cause of POVL in spine surgery. In AION, the anterior portion of the optic nerve is involved. Visual loss can be delayed up to more than a week after surgery. On symptom onset, funduscopic examination shows optic disc edema and hemorrhages. In PION, the infraorbital portion of the optic nerve is involved. Visual loss is reported upon awakening within 24 hours. At the onset of symptoms, the optic disc is usually normal by examination.[66]

Possible factors for ION in spine surgery include patient factors (age >55 years, male, low cup-disc ratio, abnormal autoregulation of optic nerve circulation, anatomic variants in optic nerve blood supply, systemic vascular risk factors, hypercoagulability), prone positioning, length of surgery (>6 h), blood loss, anemia, arterial hypotension, hemodilution, use of vasopressors, and increased intraocular or intraorbital venous pressure.[66] Such risk factors remain speculative, however.

Because the pathophysiology of ION in spine surgery remains unclear, undisputed preventive strategies have yet to be developed. The American Society of Anesthesiologist Task Force on Perioperative Blindness published a practice advisory regarding anesthetic and surgical care of patients undergoing spine surgery. There are a few general recommendation often made.[67] Eye compression should be avoided either with the use of a headrest with a cutout portion for the eyes or with a Mayfield holder. The head is maintained at neutral position relative to the back and at a higher level than the heart if possible. The blood pressure is maintained within the patient's normal limits. Use of vasopressors should be limited. Although anemia is considered one possible risk factor for ION, according to the ASA Task Force, there is no transfusion threshold recommended that eliminates risk of ION. Because substantial use of crystalloids can further increase periorbital edema, combined use of colloids and crystalloids for intravascular volume repletion is recommended. A practice advisory published by ASA Task Force also includes consideration of staged spine procedures for high-risk patients.

There is still inadequate evidence for treatment of ION. Common treatment options include increasing blood pressure and hematocrit, using mannitol and intravenous steroids, and elevating the head to decrease venous congestion.[23]

Vascular injuries

Vascular injury is uncommon but not a rare complication of several lumbar spine surgeries. Anterior lumbar interbody fusion (ALIF), lumbar disc arthroplasty, lumbar discectomy, and posterior lumbar spine surgery have all been associated with vascular injury. During such surgeries, significant vascular disruption is manifested by major vessel laceration, DVT formation, and later complications including pseudoaneurysm and AVF formation. In ALIF procedures, venous laceration is the most common type of vascular injury, with the left common iliac vein being most commonly affected. The injury is associated with retraction of the great vessels. Because the abdominal aorta and iliac artery are more elastic and movable than veins, they are less likely to be injured during dissection, mobilization, and retraction.[68] In lumbar disc arthroplasty, the surgical approach to the lumbosacral disc space is similar and thus, the same vascular injury is likely.[69] During lumbar discectomy, the cause of vascular injury is often a deep bite with the rongeur beyond the anterior spinal ligament.[70, 71] Because the aortic bifurcation and IVC confluence are separated from the 4–5 disc space only by the

anterior spinal ligament, these major vessels become susceptible to injury during discectomy. In posterior interbody fusion of the lumbar spine, vascular injury may occur during lumbar discectomy and placement of interbody graft.[68]

In many cases, significant vascular injuries are recognized during surgery when massive blood loss and hemodynamic instability are noted. During such events, mortality rates have been reported to range between 15% and 65%.[72] Hypotension and dropping hematocrit postoperatively also require exploration. Blood leakage from injured vessels will have the tendency to accumulate in the retroperitoneal space or into an artery in case of an arteriovenous fistula (AVF),[73] two possible paths of least resistance. AVF can be formed immediately when laceration involves both artery and vein. Because no blood leaves the vascular compartment, AVF may remain unrecognized for a long time.[74] Chronic fistula can present as high-output cardiac failure and/or lower leg edema.[70] If acute bleeding is observed in the surgical field, temporizing measures include local compression, aortic clamping, or endovascular placement of an occlusion balloon while the arterial injuries are repaired. For permanent vascular repair, techniques that have been used include direct suturing, endovascular stent graft, aortic reconstruction, and IVC ligation.[72]

Embolism

Three forms of embolism have been reported in spine surgery: air embolism, cement embolism, and thromboembolism.

Venous air embolism (VAE) is a rare complication of multilevel spine surgery.[75] It has a reported incidence of 1–2% in prone lumbar or thoracic procedures.[76] Air entry is through intraosseous vessels or open epidural veins when intravascular pressure is low. There is a higher chance of air entry with low central venous pressure, hypotension, extensive blood loss, increased tidal volume, and kyphosis.[77] VAE can present in different degrees of cardiovascular compromise. With a large VAE, right ventricular (RV) outlet tract obstruction occurs, impeding RV outflow and subsequent left ventricular outflow and thereby leading to cardiovascular collapse. Immediate treatment recommendations include 100% oxygen, patient in Trendelenburg position, flooding of the operative site with saline, inotropic and pressure support, aspiration of air from a multi-orifice central line, and advanced cardiovascular life support (ACLS) as needed.

Most reports of cement leaks and cement embolization involve vertebroplasty and kyphoplasty. The cement used in these procedures, polymethylmethacrylate (PMMA), is applied before complete polymerization. With vertebroplasty, stability is restored through a percutaneous bone cement injection via high-pressure filling. In kyphoplasty low-pressure filling is achieved by first producing a void with a balloon and then creating an internal cast. A fundamental difference between the two is that in vertebroplasty filling is done until the cement leaks, making the volume and pattern unpredictable. For kyphoplasty, filling is done until the cavity is full, making the volume and pattern more predictable. In a study by Choe et al., cement pulmonary embolism was seen in 4.6% of a pool of 65 patients who had percutaneous vertebroplasty or kyphoplasty.[78] Causes of cement embolism include insufficient polymerization of PMMA at the time of injection, poor needle position with respect to the basivertebral vein, or overfilling of the vertebral body. This then allows migration of the embolus into the IVC and the venous system.

Multiple reports have been published on deep venous thrombosis (DVT) and pulmonary embolism (PE) following spine surgery. The latest systematic review by Glotzbecker et al. indicates that the rate of DVT and PE are 2.2% and 0.3%, respectively.[79] Although much rarer, there has been a reported case of massive thromboembolism during an elective thoracolumbar spine surgery for idiopathic scoliosis.[80] Because of the low risk of DVT associated with spine surgery, compression stockings with pneumatic sequential compression devices starting in surgery have been recommended. Furthermore, there is insufficient evidence for chemical anticoagulants or prophylactic filters for patients undergoing elective spine surgery.[79]

Patients undergoing lumbar spine surgery are diverse in their spine pathologies, surgical treatment, and perioperative risks. For optimal management, an anesthesiologist must be versatile in the variations involved, including the levels of complexity and urgency, involvement of intraoperative neuromonitoring, susceptibility to hemodynamic instability, and multiple intraoperative and postoperative catastrophic complications.

References

1. Ruetten S, Komp M, Merk H, Godolias G. Surgical treatment for lumbar lateral recess stenosis with the full-endoscopic interlaminar approach versus conventional microsurgical technique: a prospective randomized controlled study. *J Neurosurg Spine* 2009; **10**: 476–85.

2. Caputy AJ, Luessenhop AJ. Long term evaluation of decompressive surgery for degenerative lumbar stenosis, review. *J Neurosurg* 1992; **77**: 669–76.

3. Herkowitz HN. Degenerative lumbar spondylolisthesis with spinal stenosis. *J Bone Joint Surg* 1991; **73A**: 802–8.

4. Jacobs WC, van Tulder M, Arts M, et al. Surgery versus conservative management of sciatica due to a lumbar herniated disc: a systematic review. *Eur Spine J* 2011 Apr; **20**(4): 513–22.

5. Osterman H, Seitsalo S, Karppinen J. Effectiveness of microdiscectomy for lumbar disc herniation: a randomized controlled trial with 2 years follow-up. *Spine* 2006; **31**: 2409–14.

6. Boriani S, Weinstein JN. Oncologic classification of vertebral neoplasms In: Dickman CA, Fehlings MG, Gokasalan ZL, eds. *Spinal Cord and Spinal Column Tumors: Principles ad Practice.* New York: Thieme Medical Publishers; 2006: 24–40.

7. Boriani S, Weinstein JN, Biagini R. Primary bone tumors of the spine. Terminology and surgical staging. *Spine* 1997; **22**: 1036–44.

8. Gallia GL, Sciubba DM, Bydon A, et al. Total L-5 spondylectomy and reconstruction of the lumbosacral junction. *J Neurosurg Spine* 2007; **7**: 103–11.

9. Halpin RJ, Sugrue PA, Gould RW, et al. Standardizing care for high-risk patients in spine surgery. *Spine* 2010; **35**(25): 2232–8.

10. Sanderson PL, Wood PL. Surgery for lumbar spinal stenosis in old people. *J Bone Joint Surg* 1993; **75**: 393–7.

11. Silvers HR, Lewis PJ, Asch HL. Decompressive lumbar laminectomy for spinal stenosis. *J Neurosurg* 1993; **78**: 695–701.

12. Ragab AA, Fye MA, Bohlman HH. Surgery of lumbar spine for spinal stenosis in 118 patients 70 years of age or older. *Spine* 2003; **28**(4): 348–53.

13. Jellish WS, Thalju Z, Stevenson K, Shea J. A prospective randomized study comparing short and intermediate term perioperative outcome variables after spinal or general anesthesia for lumbar disc and laminectomy surgery. *Anesth Analg* 2004; **98**: 1184–6.

14. Vandam, LD, Dripps, RD. Exacerbation of pre-existing neurologic disease after spinal anesthesia. *N Engl J Med* 1956; **255**: 843–9.

15. Yuen EC, Layzar RB, Weitz SR, Olney RK. Neurologic complications of lumbar epidural anesthesia and analgesia. *Neurology* 1995; **45**: 1795–1801.

16. Douglas WW, Rehder K, Beyman F, et al. Improved oxygenation in patients with acute respiratory failure: the prone position. *Annu Rev Respir Dis* **1151**: 559–66.

17. Rehder K, Knapp TS, Sessler AD. Regional intrapulmonary gas distribution in awake and anesthetized paralyzed prone man. *J Appl Physics* 1978; **45**: 528–35.

18. Langen KE, Jellish WS, Ghanayem AJ. Anesthetic considerations in spine surgery. *Contemp Spine Surg* 2006; **7**: 1–8.

19. Malcolm-Smith NA, McMaster MJ. The use of induced hypotension to control bleeding during posterior fusion for scoliosis. *J Bone Joint Surg Br* 1983; **65**: 255–8.

20. Khambatta HJ, Stone JG, Matteo RS, *et al.* Hypotensive anesthesia for spinal fusion with sodium nitroprusside. *Spine* 1978; **3**: 171–4.

21. Mandel RJ, Brown MD, McCollough NC, *et al.* Hypotensive anesthesia and autotransfusion in spinal surgery. *Clin Orthop Relat Res* 1981; **154**: 27–33.

22. Elgafy H, Bransford RJ, McGuire RA, *et al.* Blood loss in major spine surgery. *Spine* 2010; **35** Suppl: S47–56.

23. Goepfert CE, Ifune C, Tempelhoff R. Ischemic optic neuropathy: are we any further? *Curr Opin Anesthesiol* 2010; **23**: 582–7.

24. Lee, LA. Postoperative visual loss data gathered and analyzed. *ASA Newsletter* 2000; **64**(9): 25–7.

25. Malhotra NR, Shaffrey CI. Intraoperative electrophysiological monitoring in spine surgery. *Spine* 2010; **35**(25); 2167–79.

26. Owen JH. The application of intraoperative monitoring during surgery for spinal deformity. *Spine* 1999; **24**: 2649–62.

27. Nuwer MR, Dawson EG, Carlson EG, *et al.* Somatosensory evoked potential signal spinal cord monitoring reduces neurologic deficits after scoliosis surgery: Results of a large multicenter survey. *Electroencephalogr Clin Neurophysiol* 1995; **96**: 6–11.

28. Banoub M, Tetzlaff JE, Schubert A. Pharmacologic and physiologic influences affecting sensory evoked potentials. *Anesthesiology* 2003; **99**: 716–37.

29. Sloan TB, Heyer EJ. Anesthesia for intraoperative neurophysiologic monitoring of the spinal cord. *J Clin Neurophysiol* 2002; **19**: 430–43.

30. Schwartz DM, Aerbach JD, Dormans JP, *et al.* Neurophysiological detection of impending spinal cord injury during scoliosis surgery. *J Bone Join Surg Am* 2007; **89**: 2440–9.

31. Delitis V, Sala F. Intraoperative neurophysiologic monitoring of the spinal cord during spinal cord and spine surgery: a review focus on the corticospinal tracts. *Clin Neurophysiol* 2008; **119**: 248–64.

32. Elgafy H, Bransford RJ, McGuire RA, Dettori JR, Fischer D. Blood loss in major spine surgery. *Spine* 2010; **35**(95): S47–56.

33. Nuttall GA, Horlocker TT, Santrach PJ, *et al.* Predictors of blood transfusions in spinal instrumentation and fusion surgery. *Spine* 2000; **25**(5); 596–601.

34. Engoren M, Habib R, Zacharias A, *et al.* Effect of blood transfusion on long-term survival after cardiac operation. *Ann Thorac Surg* 2002; **74**: 1180–6.

35. Michalopoulos A, Tzelepis G, Dafni U, Geroulanos S. Determinants of hospital mortality after coronary artery bypass grafting. *Chest* 1999; **115**: 1598–603.

36. Leal-Noval S, Rincon-Ferrari M, Garcia-Curiel A, *et al.* Transfusion of blood components and postoperative infection in patients undergoing cardiac surgery. *Chest* 2001; **119**: 1461–8.

37. Langen KE, Jellish WS, Ghanayem AJ. Anesthetic considerations in spine surgery. *Contemp Spine Surg* 2006; **7**: 1–8.

38. Murray D, Forbes R, Titone MB, *et al.* Transfusion management in pediatric and adolescent scoliosis surgery: efficacy of autologous blood. *Spine* 1997; **22**: 2735–40.

39. Cha CW, Debbie C, Muzzonigro T, *et al.* Allogenic transfusion requirements after autologous donations in posterior lumbar surgeries. *Spine* 2002; **27**: 99–104.

40. Bess RS, Lenke LG. Blood loss minimization and blood salvage techniques for complex spine surgery. *Neurosurg Clin N Am* 2006; **17**: 227–34.

41. Halpern NA, Alicea M, Seabrook B, *et al.* Cell saver autologous transfusion: metabolic consequences of washing blood with normal saline. *J Trauma* 1996; **41**: 407–15.

42. Reitman CA, Watters WC, Sassand WR. The cell saver in adult lumbar fusion surgery. *Spine* 2004; **9**(14): 1580–4.

43. Keverline JP, Sanders JO. Hematuria associated with low volume cell saver in pediatric orthopedics. *J Pediatr Orthop* 1998; **18**: 594–7.

44. Sachs B, Delacy D, Green J, *et al.* Recombinant activated factor VII in spinal surgery. A multicenter, randomized, double-blind, placebo controlled, dose escalation trial. *Spine* 2007; **32**: 2285–93.

45. Shapiro GS, Boachie-Adjei O, Dhawlikar SH. The use of Epoetin alfa in complex spine surgery. *Spine* 2002; **27**: 2067–71.

46. Vitlae MG, Privitera DM, Matsumoto H, *et al.* Efficacy of preoperative erythropoietin administration in pediatric neuromuscular scoliosis. *Spine* 2007; **32**: 2662–7.

47. Cassedy JF Jr, Lederhaas G, Cancel DD, Cummings RJ, Loveless EA. A randomised comparison of the effects of continuous thoracic epidural analgesia and intravenous patient-controlled analgesia after posterior spinal

fusion in adolescents. *Reg Anesth Pain Med* 2000; **25**: 246–53.

48. Shaw BA, Watson TC, Merzel DI, Gerardi JA, Birek A. The safety of continuous epidural infusion for postoperative analgesia in pediatric spine surgery. *J Pediatr Orthop* 1996; **16**: 374–7.

49. Kanamori M, Ohmori K, Yasuda T, *et al.* Postoperative enteroparesis by patient-controlled analgesia combined with continuous epidural block for patients after posterior lumbar surgery. *J Spinal Disord* 2000; **13**: 242–6.

50. Van Boerum DH, Smith JT, Curtin MJ. A comparison of the effects of patient-controlled analgesia with intravenous opioids versus epidural analgesia on recovery after surgery for idiopathic scoliosis. *Spine* 2000; **25**: 2355–7.

51. Raw DA, Beattie JK, Hunter JM. Anaesthesia for spinal surgery in adults. *Br J Anaesth* 2003; **91**: 886–904.

52. Wang LP, Hauerberg J, Schmidt JF. Incidence of spinal epidural abscess after epidural analgesia. *Anaesthesiology* 1999; **91**: 1928–36.

53. Bianconi M, Ferraro L, Ricci R, Zanoli G, *et al.* The pharmacokinetics and efficacy of ropivacaine continuous wound instillation after spine fusion surgery. *Anesth Analg* 2004; **98**(1): 166–72.

54. Blumenthal S, Min K, Marquardt M. Postoperative intravenous morphine consumption, pain scores, and side effects with perioperative oral controlled-release oxycodone after lumbar discectomy. *Anesth Analg* 2007; **105**: 233–7.

55. Ersayli DT, Gurbert A, Uckunkaya N, *et al.* Effects of perioperatively administered bupivacaine and bupivacaine-methylprednisolone on pain after lumbar discectomy. *Spine* 2006; **31**: 2221–6.

56. Dylewsky W, McAlpine FS. Peripheral nervous system. In: Martin JT, Warner MA, eds. *Positioning in Anesthesia and Surgery*, 3d ed. Philadelphia: WB Saunders; 1997: 299–318.

57. Cheney FW, Domino KB, Caplan RA, Posner KL. Nerve injury associated with anesthesia: a closed claims analysis. *Anesthesiology* 1999; **90**: 1062–9.

58. Welch MB, Brummett CM, Welch TD, *et al.* Perioperative peripheral nerve injuries: a retrospective study of 380,680 cases during a 10-year period at a single institution. *Anesthesiology* 2009; **111**: 490–7.

59. Stevens WR, Glazer PA, Kelley SD, Lietman TM, Bradford DS. Ophthalmic complications after spine surgery. *Spine* 1997; **22**: 1319–24.

60. Myers MA, Hamilton Sr, Bogosian AJ, Smith CH, Wagner TA. Visual loss as a complication of spine surgery. A review of 47 cases. *Spine* 1997; **22**: 1329.

61. Cheng MA, Todorov A, Tempelhoff R, *et al.* The effect of prone positioning on intraocular pressure in anesthetized patients. *Anesthesiology* 2001; **95**: 1351–5.

62. Roth S. Postoperative blindness. In: Miller RD, ed. *Anesthesia*, 6th ed. New York: Elsevier; 2005: 2991–3021.

63. Myers MA, Hamilton SR, Bogosian AJ, *et al. Spine (Phila Pa 1976)* 1997 Jun 15; **22**(12): 1325–9.

64. Holy SE, Tsai JH, McAllister RK, *et al.* Perioperative ischemic optic neuropathy: a case control analysis of 126,666 surgical procedures at a single institution. *Anesthesiology* 2009; **110**: 246–253.

65. Shen Y, Drum M, Roth SY. The prevalence of perioperative visual loss in the United States: a 10 year study from 1996 to 2005 of spinal, orthopedic, cardiac, and general surgery. *Anesth Analg* 2009; **109**: 1534–45.

66. Tempelhoff R, Warner DS, RothS, Young WL. *ASA Refresher Courses in Anesthesiology* 2007; **35**(1): 195–207.

67. American Society of Anesthesiologists Task Force on Perioperative Blindness: Practice advisory for perioperative visual loss associated with spine surgery. *Anesthesiology* 2006; **104**: 1319–28.

68. Inamasu J and Guiot BH. Vascular injury and complication in neurosurgical spine surgery. *Acta Neurochir* (2006) **148**: 375–87.

69. Zigler JE. Lumbar spine arthroplasty using ProDisc II. *Spine J* **4**(6 Suppl): 260S–7S.

70. Papadoulas S, Konstantinou D, Kourea HP, *et al.* Vascular injury complicating lumbar disc surgery. A systematic review. *Eur J Vasc Endovasc Surg.* 2002; **24**: 189–95.

71. Faciszewski T, Winter RB, Lonstein JE, Denis F, Johnson L. The surgical and medical perioperative complications of anterior spinal fusion surgery in the thoracic and lumbar spine in adults. A review of 1223 procedures. *Spine* 1995; **20**: 1592–9.

72. Kopp R, Beisse R, Weidenhagen R, *et al.* Strategies for prevention and operative treatment of aortic lesions related to spinal interventions. *Spine* 2007; **32**: 753–60.

73. Ewah B, Calder I. Intraoperative death during lumbar discectomy. *Br J Anaesth* 1991; **66**: 721–3.

74. Freischlag AJ, Sise M, Quinones-Baldrich JW, *et al.* Vascular complications associated with orthopedic procedures. *Surg Gynecol Obs* 1989; **169**: 147–52.

75. Wills J, Schwend R, Paterson A, Albin M. Intraoperative visible bubbling of air may be the first sign of venous air embolism during posterior surgery for scoliosis. *Spine* 2005; **30**(20): E629–35.

76. Black S. Anesthesia for spine surgery. *ASA Refresher Course in Anesthesiology* 2009; **37**(1): 13–23.

77. McCarthy RE, Lonstein JE, Mertz JD, *et al.* Air embolism in spinal surgery. *J Spinal Disord* 1990; **3**: 1–5.

78. Choe DH, Marom EM, Ahrar K, *et al.* Pulmonary embolism of polymethyl methacrylate during percutaneous vertebroplasty and kyphoplasty. *AJR. Am J Roentgenol* 2004; **183**(4): 1097–102.

79. Glotzbecker MP, Bono CM, Wood KB, Harris MB. Thromboembolic disease in spinal surgery. A systematic review. *Spine* 2009; **34**(3): 291–303.

80. Maurtua M. Zhang W. Deogaonkar A. Farag E. Ebrahim Z. Massive pulmonary thromboembolism during spine surgery. *J Clin Anesth* 2005; **17**(3): 213–7.

Chapter

13

Anesthetic management of spinal cord trauma

Brian P. Lemkuil and Piyush M. Patel

Key points

- Functional neurologic deficits associated with acute spinal cord injury are the results of the primary mechanical injury and the secondary processes initiated by the primary injury. The anesthetic goals specific to acute spinal cord injury include prevention of further mechanical injury with an unstable spine and limitation of secondary neurologic injury through optimum medical management.

- Although hemodynamic targets are poorly defined, hypotension should be avoided and mean arterial pressure (MAP) should be maintained at or above 85 mmHg for the first 5–7 days following spinal cord injury.

- Awake fiberoptic intubation (AFI) minimizes cervical movement and allows neurologic assessment and awake positioning before induction of anesthesia. AFI should be considered in cooperative patients with known cervical spine instability at risk for neurologic deterioration, particularly in the presence of ongoing cord compression. In emergent situations, direct laryngoscopic endotracheal intubation with manual in-line stabilization is an appropriate route for securing the airway.

- No anesthetic has been shown to be superior to another or result in neuroprotection in the setting of acute spinal cord injury. The choice of anesthetic may be dictated more by concurrent neurophysiologic monitoring than consideration of the potential neuroprotective effects of anesthetics. Pharmacologic agents have not been shown to have neuroprotective efficacy. In terms of limiting further injury, emphasis should be placed on the maintenance of physiologic homeostasis:

avoidance of hypoxemia, anemia, extreme blood glucose fluctuation, hyperthermia, and hypotension.

- Pulmonary complications are the primary cause of morbidity and mortality following spinal cord injury. The degree of respiratory impairment and risk of pulmonary complications depends on both the level of injury and the resulting severity of muscle weakness. Therefore, pulmonary morbidity is generally greater with higher segmental spinal cord injury.

- Clinical investigations aimed at neuroprotective strategies have failed to demonstrate clinical significance in primary outcome measures. Methylprednisolone, the best known and most extensively investigated neuroprotective therapy, is currently considered a therapeutic option with data supporting a greater likelihood of complications than clinical benefit.

Introduction

Traumatic spinal cord injury (SCI) devastates thousands of otherwise healthy individuals each year, resulting in various degrees of functional impairment (motor, autonomic, bowel/bladder). It imposes an enormous economic and emotional burden on patients and on society at large. Although only minimal advances have been made in neuroprotection and neuroregenerative therapies, more SCI patients are surviving, living longer, and reporting a good quality of life than in previous decades.[1] Improvements in prehospital care, radiologic evaluation, intensive care management, early fracture-dislocation reduction, and early surgical intervention may be partially responsible for these advances. Therefore, it is important for anesthesiologists involved in the acute care of these patients to understand their role in limiting the

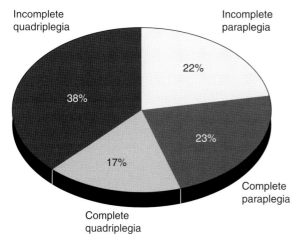

Incomplete quadriplegia

Incomplete paraplegia

38%

22%

23%

17%

Complete quadriplegia

Complete paraplegia

Figure 13.1 Neurologic category distribution at time of hospital discharge following acute spinal cord injury. At time of hospital discharge nearly 55% of spinal cord injury patients are categorized with injury involving the cervical region (complete and incomplete quadriplegia). Since 2005, the most frequent neurologic category at time of hospital discharge has been incomplete quadriplegia.

extent of neurologic injury, while facilitating early surgical intervention.

Epidemiology

Approximately 12 000 Americans with various degrees of functional impairment are discharged from hospitals each year (Fig. 13.1). Since 2005, the average age at time of SCI has increased to 40.2 years and continues to disproportionately affect white males. The most common causes include motor vehicle accidents (41.3%), falls (27.3%), violence (15%), and sports (7.9%). The economic cost associated with SCI approximates $9 billion annually and represents a lifetime cost per individual ranging from $700 000 to over $3 000 000 depending on the degree of functional impairment and age at time of injury.[2]

Anatomy and physiology

Traumatic injuries to the spine predictably occur in regions of high flexibility that are closely approximated with areas of greater stability. The stability afforded the thoracic spine by the rib cage and intercostal muscles creates susceptibility both above and below this region at the cervical–thoracic and thoracic–lumbar junctions. Approximately 55% of all SCI occurs in the cervical spine (Fig. 13.1), the region associated with the greatest functional impairment.

The cervical spine may be classified into upper cervical and subaxial segments. The upper cervical spine

consists of two anatomically unique vertebrae, the atlas and the axis, without an intervening disc, that are stabilized by extrinsic membranes as well as intrinsic spinal ligaments (Fig. 13.2A). The unique bony anatomy and complex ligamentous stabilization in this region allows weight transfer between the head and trunk while simultaneously facilitating neck mobility and protecting both the spinal cord and vertebral arteries. The occipitoatlantal junction is primarily designed for flexion-extension (25°) with minimal lateral bending or rotation, whereas the unique atlas–axis junction allows up to 40° of rotation and an additional 20° of flexion-extension.[3] Ligamentous constraint to subluxation and dislocation of the occipitoatlantal junction is largely provided by the paired alar ligaments and the superior continuation of the posterior longitudinal ligament, the tectorial membrane. Ligamentous constraint at the atlantoaxial junction is provided primarily by the transverse ligament, which is largely responsible for limiting posterior translation of the odontoid process (dens) within the spinal canal at C1 (Fig. 13.2B). Secondary support is provided by the paired alar ligaments. Survival after acute traumatic ligamentous disruption in the upper cervical spine is characteristically poor, although reports of survival are readily available.

Much has been written about radiologic evaluation of upper cervical injuries including various measurements indicative of instability (atlanto-dens interval, posterior atlanto-dens interval, Powers ratio, etc.) that may occur without bony involvement.[4] As a result of the unique anatomy in the upper cervical spine, a large spectrum of bony and ligamentous injuries with various degrees of instability may occur. A detailed review of injury descriptions and classifications is beyond the scope of this chapter.

The subaxial cervical spine is composed of five vertebrae (C3–C7) of relatively consistent anatomic structure stabilized by a discoligamentous complex (DLC): the intervertebral disc and extrinsic spinal ligaments, including facet joints with their capsular ligaments. Two-thirds of all cervical spine fractures occur in the subaxial spine, most frequently involving C6 and C7.

The remaining 45% of spine fractures are found within the thoracic and lumbar spine. Like the subaxial cervical spine, stability is provided by the DLC, including well-developed articulating facet joints. Unstable thoracolumbar injuries are almost always associated with a vertebral fracture.[5]

The spinal cord itself emerges from the foramen magnum at the base of the skull and terminates near the

A

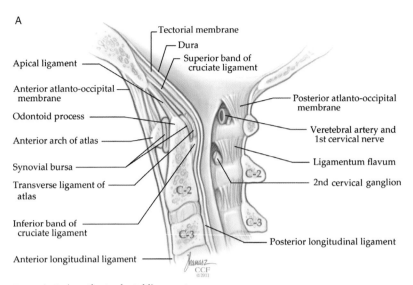

Tectorial membrane

Dura

Superior band of cruciate ligament

Apical ligament

Anterior atlanto-occipital membrane

Odontoid process

Anterior arch of atlas

Synovial bursa

Transverse ligament of atlas

Inferior band of cruciate ligament

Anterior longitudinal ligament

Posterior atlanto-occipital membrane

Veretebral artery and 1st cervical nerve

Ligamentum flavum

C-2

2nd cervical ganglion

C-2

C-3

C-3

Posterior longitudinal ligament

B

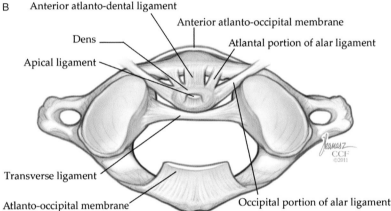

Anterior atlanto-dental ligament

Dens

Apical ligament

Anterior atlanto-occipital membrane

Atlantal portion of alar ligament

Transverse ligament

Atlanto-occipital membrane

Occipital portion of alar ligament

Figure 13.2 (A) Upper cervical spine anatomy. Note the unique anatomic structure of the upper cervical vertebrae. Stability is provided by a combination of membranes as well as intrinsic and extrinsic spinal ligaments. (B) Ligamentous support at the atlantoaxial junction. The transverse ligament is the primary constraint to posterior subluxation of the odontoid process within the spinal canal of C1. Secondary support is provided by the paired alar ligaments.

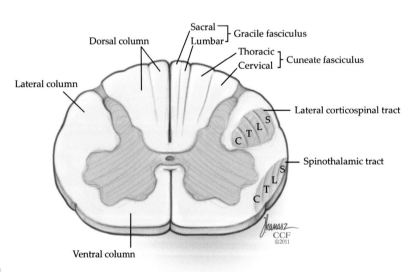

Dorsal column

Lateral column

Sacral
Lumbar — Gracile fasciculus

Thoracic
Cervical — Cuneate fasciculus

Lateral corticospinal tract

S
L
T
C

Spinothalamic tract

S
L
T
C

Ventral column

Figure 13.3 Cross-section of the spinal cord. Note the characteristic inner gray matter surrounded by the myelinated white matter. Dorsal column, lateral corticospinal tract and spinothalamic tract are the three white matter tracts readily evaluated by neurologic examination. Motor testing reflects the integrity of the descending posterolateral corticospinal tracts. Pain and temperature sensation reflects the integrity of the ascending anterolateral spinothalamic tracts. Vibration and proprioceptive sensation is transmitted to the brain by way of the dorsal columns. The somatotopic organization of the lateral corticospinal tract is demonstrated by the labels C, T, L, and S corresponding to cervical, thoracic, lumbar, and sacral motor neurons.

L1–L2 junction in adults. A cross-section of the cord reveals the characteristic inner H-shaped gray matter surrounded by ascending and descending white matter tracts (Fig. 13.3). Of the many white matter tracts, only three are readily evaluated by neurologic examination: (1) the posterolateral corticospinal tracts responsible for motor function; (2) the anterolateral spinothalamic tracts responsible for pain, temperature, and pressure; and (3) the posterior columns responsible for fine touch, vibration, and proprioception.

Perfusion to the spinal cord occurs via one anterior and two posterior spinal arteries with segmental augmentation by radicular arteries that enter the spinal canal along the nerve roots through the neural foramina. Radicular artery compromise, particularly in the watershed regions of the middle and lower thoracic spine, may contribute to secondary ischemic injury.

Spinal cord blood flow is regulated in a fashion similar to cerebral blood flow. Blood flow to the spinal cord is heterogeneous, with a similar 5:1 gray matter–white matter flow ratio. Normal blood flow is approximately 50 ml/100 g/min. Spinal cord blood flow is autoregulated in the range of mean arterial pressure (MAP) of 60–150 mmHg (Fig. 13.4). Mean blood flow is altered by neuronal electrical activity, vasoactive drugs including anesthetics, P_aCO_2, P_aO_2, and temperature.[6] As in the cerebrum, microcirculatory dysfunction and loss of autoregulatory capacity occur following traumatic injury, which predisposes the spinal cord to secondary ischemic injury.

Radiologic evaluation

The incidence of cervical spine injury (CSI) in blunt trauma victims is estimated at 1–3% but may increase to nearly 10% in patients with a Glasgow Coma Score <8.[7] Radiologic evaluation is intended to identify patients with spinal instability; a missed or delayed diagnosis is associated with up to 10 times the rate of secondary neurologic injury.[8] Despite the potentially devastating complications of a missed diagnosis, withholding radiologic evaluation is considered safe when the criteria found in Table 13.1 are met.[9]

The initial radiologic evaluation of the cervical spine in at-risk patients typically consists of three radiographs (cervical series: cross table, AP, open mouth). Under ideal conditions in which the entire cervical spine is adequately visualized, including the body of T1, sensitivity of detection of fractures approaches 90% when the radiographs are read by an expert radiologist.[10]

Table 13.1 Criteria for withholding radiologic evaluation following blunt trauma

1. No midline cervical tenderness
2. No focal neurologic deficit
3. Normal alertness
4. No intoxication
5. No painful distracting injury

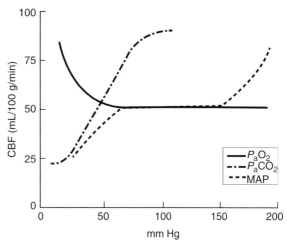

Figure 13.4 The approximate independent effects of P_aCO_2, P_aO_2, and mean arterial pressure (MAP) on spinal cord blood flow (CBF).

Inadequate visualization, radiologic abnormality, or a high clinical suspicion despite adequate films necessitates directed computed tomography (CT) imaging of the region in question. Plain radiographs and CT are complementary modalities with a combined negative predictive value that exceeds 99%.[11] If a physical examination is unattainable or unreliable, a complete cervical spine CT should be considered as an adjunct to the cervical series. Likewise, a high-resolution CT scan of the entire cervical spine with reconstruction is indicated following detection of any upper cervical spine injury because of the high incidence (80%) of concomitant cervical injury.[12]

Routine use of MRI is discouraged in the initial evaluation because of the high false-positive rate for ligamentous injury and decreased sensitivity for bony injuries compared with CT.[13] MRI is well suited for characterizing acute cord injury and should be considered in the presence of a neurologic deficit.

The thoracolumbar spine is far easier to visualize with plain films compared with the cervical spine; thus AP and lateral radiographs are usually sufficient for initial evaluation. However, inadequately visualized segments, plain film abnormalities, or a high clinical suspicion warrant further evaluation with CT imaging.

Biomechanics of spinal injury

The mechanism of spinal injury is often inferred, accurately or not, from the radiologic injury morphology (Fig. 13.5). In reality, multiple mechanisms, or combinations thereof, are likely responsible for any given morphology.

Axial compression injuries

Compressive forces with a neutral spine position may result in a simple axial compression fracture with loss of vertebral body height. More worrisome are burst fractures, involving compressive fracture to the posterior cortical boundary of the vertebral body, often involving retropulsion of bone or disc material into the spinal canal. Simple compression fractures are typically considered stable fractures and are often treated conservatively, whereas burst fractures are considered unstable. Early surgical decompression may be performed for ongoing cord compression and neurologic deterioration.

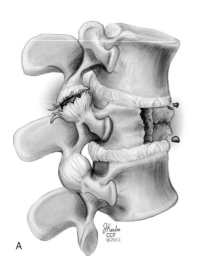

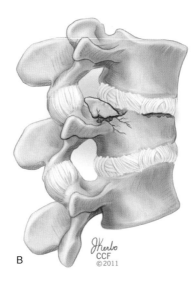

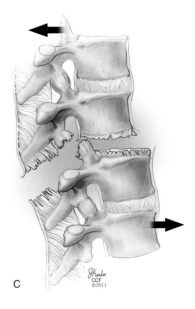

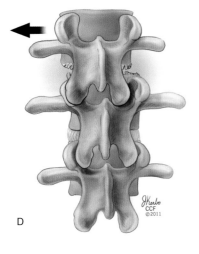

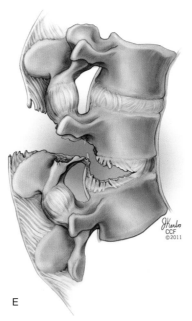

Figure 13.5 Basic morphologic categories of spinal injury. (A) Compression fracture of the vertebral body. (B) Burst fracture of the vertebral body. Note the involvement of the posterior cortical margin with retropulsion of bony material into the spinal canal. (C) Translation injury. Translation, horizontal movement of one vertebra on another, with disruption of various portions of the discoligamentous complex. (D) Rotational injury with malalignment of spinous processes. (E) Distraction injury resulting in abnormal separation of bony elements of adjacent vertebrae.

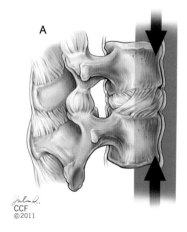

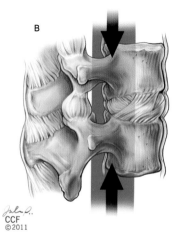

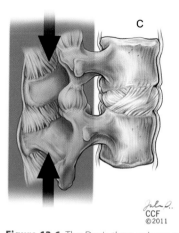

Figure 13.6 The Denis three-column spine classification model. (A) Anterior column: the anterior two-thirds of the vertebral body and annulus including the anterior spinal ligament. (B) Middle column: the posterior one-third of the vertebral body and annulus along with the posterior longitudinal ligament. (C) Posterior column: all elements posterior to the posterior longitudinal ligament.

Flexion injuries

Flexion injuries are thought to result in compression of the anterior column (Fig. 13.6) with or without posterior column distraction (abnormal bony element separation of adjacent vertebrae). Although isolated compression fractures are typically stable, concomitant disruption of the posterior ligamentous complex (ligaments posterior to the posterior longitudinal ligament) may cause instability. Instability may also arise from the acute-flexion or "teardrop" fracture-dislocation in which compression of the vertebral body results in a small anteriorly displaced fragment (teardrop) with posterior displacement of the larger segment into the spinal canal (Fig. 13.7).

Hyperextension injuries

Hyperextension injuries result in compression of the posterior column with possible distraction of the anterior column. When combined with compressive forces, there is a high incidence of cord compression injury from disruption of the lateral masses, pedicles, and lamina.

Rotational injuries

Rotational forces are often combined with flexion or extension, resulting in facet subluxation, dislocation, or fracture-dislocation. Anatomically, the spine is configured to resist significant rotation, thus altered alignment of either spinous processes or pedicles suggests considerable anatomic destruction and instability.

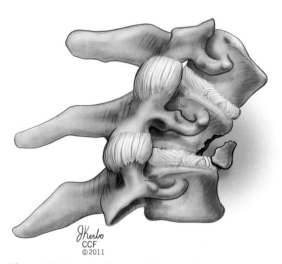

Figure 13.7 Teardrop fracture-dislocation also known as acute-flexion injury. Compression of the anterior vertebral body results in anterior displacement of a bony fragment that may resemble a drop of water with displacement of the posterior-inferior segment into the spinal canal.

Translation (shear) injuries

Translation, horizontal movement of one vertebra on another, denotes significant ligamentous disruption and instability. Neurologic injury may result from cord compression or shear injury from repeated segmental translation with "to and fro" motion.

Distraction injuries

Pure distraction injuries (increased distance between bony elements of adjacent vertebrae) are rare and are often combined with other forces resulting in profound ligament disruption and instability.

Determining spinal stability

Since Bohler first proposed his injury classification in 1929, a number of attempts have been made to define and predict spinal instability with various classifications systems. These classifications have included anatomic- and morphologic-based systems, two- and three-column-based models, mechanistic models, and points-based systems. Unfortunately, even the most popular systems have been shown to have insufficient validity and reproducibility and are unable to direct clinical decision-making or predict outcomes.

> Spinal instability has been defined as
>
> a loss in the ability of the spine under physiologic loads to maintain relationships between vertebrae in such a way that there is neither damage nor subsequent irritation to the spinal cord or nerve roots. In addition there is no development of incapacitating deformity or pain due to structural changes.[14]

This definition is comprehensive but lacks the precision required for making important clinical decisions.

More recently, the Spine Trauma Study Group has developed two comprehensive points-based spinal injury classification systems (Subaxial Cervical Injury Classification and Thoracolumbar Injury Classification and Severity Score) to identify patients with spinal instability who may benefit from acute surgical stabilization to prevent early neurologic deterioration. The panel unanimously agreed upon and numerically graded three injury characteristics (morphology; posterior ligamentous complex or discoligamentous complex integrity; neurologic status) considered to be most important in determining injury severity, mechanical instability, and neurologic risk (Table 13.2). The numerical score of each of the three injury characteristics is summed to produce an injury severity score. A score ≥5 suggests significant instability such that surgical treatment should be considered, whereas a score ≤3 suggests limited instability that may be treated conservatively. Early data demonstrate excellent reliability and validity, but long-term prospective studies will be needed to validate the grading methodology and assess reliability for predicting outcomes.[15] It should be emphasized that no injury classification system will be completely reliable in determining mechanical instability and neurologic risk; however, these more recent classification systems may assist anesthesiologists and surgeons in their assessment of structural injury and potential neurologic risk in the clinical management of the patient.

Neurologic assessment and classification

A thorough neurologic assessment and accurate documentation of baseline neurologic function is important in the management of SCI patients. The American Spinal Injury Association (ASIA) dermatome chart standardizes and facilitates accurate neurologic examination and documentation (Fig. 13.8). The examination evaluates and scores 10 key muscle groups and 28 dermatomes for both light touch and pinprick. It also ensures accurate assessment and documentation of sacral function critical for determining the completeness of spinal injury. Incomplete spinal injury is defined at minimum by preservation of distal sacral nerve root function (S4-S5 motor and/or sensation) and carries a more favorable prognosis with a greater likelihood of functional recovery.

Injury severity is most commonly communicated using the ASIA impairment scale. This scale, formerly the Frankel scale, combines deficit severity with completeness of injury to stratify injury into five classes that correlate with outcome (Table 13.3). Incomplete injuries may fall into one of the clinically defined incomplete spinal cord injury syndromes (Table 13.4).

Pathophysiology of injury

Functional neurologic deficits related to acute SCI represent the collective effects of primary and secondary injury processes. Anesthetic goals specific for management of acute spine injury patients include prevention of further mechanical injury to the cord as well as limiting deterioration related to secondary injury processes.

Table 13.2 Spinal injury classification systems
a: Subaxial cervical injury classification and severity scale (SLIC)

Injury characteristic	Points
Morphology	
Compression	1
Burst	2
Distraction (facet perch, hyperextension)	3
Rotation/translation (facet dislocation, teardrop)	4
Discoligamentous complex	
Intact	0
Indeterminate	1
Disrupted (wide anterior disc space, facet perch, dislocation)	2
Neurologic status	
Intact	0
Root injury	1
Complete cord injury	2
Incomplete cord injury	3
Ongoing cord compression	+1

Reproduced with permission from *Spine* 2010;35: S228–34.

b: Thoracolumbar injury classification and severity score (TLICS)

Injury characteristic	Points
Morphology	
Compression	1
Burst	2
Translation/rotation	3
Distraction	4
Posterior ligamentous complex	
Intact	0
Indeterminate	1
Disrupted (wide anterior disc space, facet perch, dislocation)	2
Neurologic status	
Intact	0
Nerve root injury	2
Spinal cord/conus medullaris complete	2
Incomplete	3
Cauda equina	3

Reproduced with permission from *J Neurosurg Spine* 2009;10:201–6.

Table 13.3 American Spinal Injury Association (ASIA) Impairment Scale

ASIA grade	Injury type	Definition of injury type
A	Complete	No motor or sensory function preserved in sacral segments S4–S5.
B	Incomplete	Sensation is preserved without motor function below the neurologic level and includes S4–S5.
C	Incomplete	Motor function is preserved below the neurologic level. More than half of the key muscles below the neurologic level cannot overcome gravity (motor grade <3/5).
D	Incomplete	Motor function is preserved below the neurologic level. At least half of the key muscle groups have full range of motion against gravity (motor grade 3/5 or greater).
E	Normal	Motor and sensation are normal.

Table 13.4 Incomplete spinal cord injury syndromes

Central cord syndrome	The most common incomplete spinal cord injury syndrome, typically due to hyperextension injury.
	Motor deficit is disproportionately greater in distal upper extremities with variable degrees of sensory impairment below the level of injury. Usually associated with significant bladder function involvement.
Anterior cord syndrome	Due to anterior spinal artery or anterior cord compression. Results in impaired pain and temperature sensation with preservation of proprioception. Motor impairment may be variable.
Brown–Séquard syndrome	Spinal cord hemisection resulting in ipsilateral loss of motor and proprioception with contralateral loss of pain and temperature sensation. Usually due to penetrating trauma.
Posterior cord syndrome	Incomplete injury with loss of fine touch, vibration, and proprioception but preservation of motor function.

Primary injury

Primary injury is the initial and immediate damage imparted to axons and cell bodies by way of energy transfer to the spinal cord through various biomechanical mechanisms. The presence of neurologic injury itself attests to the severity of structural damage to the spinal column and indicates a potential risk for further mechanical injury.

Secondary injury

Secondary injury is defined as neurologic deterioration (dysfunction and cell death) that occurs subsequent

Patient Name

Examiner Name

Date/Time of Exam

INTERNATIONAL STANDARDS FOR NEUROLOGICAL CLASSIFICATION OF SPINAL CORD INJURY

AMERICAN SPINAL INJURY ASSOCIATION

ISCoS

MOTOR
KEY MUSCLES
(scoring on reverse side)

R   L

C5   Elbow flexors
C6   Wrist extensors
C7   Elbow extensors
C8   Finger flexors (distal phalanx of middle finger)
T1   Finger abductors (little finger)

UPPER LIMB TOTAL
[ ] + [ ] = [ ]
(MAXIMUM) (25) (25) (50)

Comments:

L2   Hip flexors
L3   Knee extensors
L4   Ankle dorsiflexors
L5   Long toe extensors
S1   Ankle plantar flexors

(VAC) Voluntary anal contraction (Yes/No)

LOWER LIMB TOTAL
[ ] + [ ] = [ ]
(MAXIMUM) (25) (25) (50)

SENSORY
KEY SENSORY POINTS

0 = absent
1 = impired
2 = normal
NT = not testable

Palm
Dorsum
• Key Sensory Points

C2, C3, C4, C5, C6, C7, C8, T1, T2, T3, T4, T5, T6, T7, T8, T9, T10, T11, T12, L1, L2, L3, L4, L5, S1, S2, S3

S4-5

(DAP) Deep anal pressure (yes/No)

PIN PRICK SCORE   (max: 112)
LIGHT TOUCH SCORE (max: 112)

LIGHT TOUCH   PIN PRICK
R   L   R   L

C2
C3
C4
C5
C6
C7
C8
T1
T2
T3
T4
T5
T6
T7
T8
T9
T10
T11
T12
L1
L2
L3
L4
L5
S1
S2
S3
S4-S5

TOTALS { (56) (56) (56) (56)
(Maximum) (56) (56) (56) (56)

NEUROLOGICAL LEVEL
The most caudal segment with normal function

        R   L
SENSORY [ ] [ ]
MOTOR   [ ] [ ]

SINGLE NEUROLOGICAL LEVEL
[ ]

COMPLETE OR INCOMPLETE?
Incomplete = Any sensory or motor function in S4-S5

ASIA IMPAIRMENT SCALE (AIS)
[ ]

(In complete injuries only)
ZONE OF PARTIAL PRESERVATION
Most caudal level with any innervation

                R   L
SENSORY [ ] [ ]
MOTOR   [ ] [ ]

Rev 04/11

This form may be copied freely but should not be altered without permission from the American Spinal Injury Association.

Muscle Function Grading

0 = total paralysis

1 = palpable or visible contraction

2 = active movement, full range of motion (ROM) with gravity eliminated

3 = active movement, full ROM against gravity

4 = active movement, full ROM against gravity and moderate resistance in a muscle specific position.

5 = (normal) active movement, full ROM against gravity and full resistance in a muscle specific position expected from an otherwise unimpaired peson.

5* = (normal) active movement, full ROM against gravity and sufficient resistance to be considered normal if identified inhibiting factors (i.e. pain, disuse) were not present.

NT = not testable (i.e. due to immobilization, severe pain such that the patient cannot be graded, amputation of limb, or contracture of >50% of the range of motion).

ASIA Impairment (AIS) Scale

☐ **A = Complete.** No sensory or motor function is preserved in the sacral segments S4-S5.

☐ **B = Sensory Incomplete.** Sensory but not motor function is preserved below the neurological level and includes the sacral segments S4-S5 (light touch, pin prick at S4-S5: or deep anal pressure (DAP)), AND no motor function is preserved more than three levels below the motor level on either side of the body.

☐ **C = Motor Incomplete.** Motor function is preserved below the neurological level**, and more than half of key muscle functions below the single neurological level of injury (NLI) have a muscle grade less than 3 (Grades 0-2).

☐ **D = Motor Incomplete.** Motor function is preserved below the neurological level**, and at least half (half or more) of key muscle functions below the NLI have a muscle grade ≥ 3.

☐ **E = Normal.** If sensation and motor function as tested with the ISNCSCI are graded as normal in all segments, and the patient had prior deficits, then the AIS grade is E. Someone without an initial SCI does not receive an AIS grade.

**For an individual to receive a grade of C or D, i.e. motor incomplete status, they must have either (1) voluntary anal sphincter contraction or (2) sacral sensory sparing with sparing of motor function more than three levels below the motor level for that side of the body. The Standards at this time allows even non-key muscle function more than 3 levels below the motor level to be used in determining motor incomplete status (AIS B versus C).

NOTE: When assessing the extent of motor sparing below the level for distinguishing between AIS B and C, the **motor level** on each side is used; whereas to differentiate between AIS C and D (based on proportion of key muscle functions with strength grade 3 or greater) the **single neurological level** is used.

Steps in Classification

The following order is recommended in determining the classification of individuals with SCI.

1. Determine sensory levels for right and left sides.

2. Determine motor levels for right and left sides.
   Note: in regions where there is no myotome to test, the motor level is presumed to be the same as the sensory level, if testable motor function above that level is also normal.

3. Determine the single neurological level.
   This is the lowest segment where motor and sensory function is normal on both sides, and is the most cephalad of the sensory and motor levels determined in steps 1 and 2.

4. Determine whether the injury is Complete or Incomplete.
   (i.e. absence or presence of sacral sparing)
   If voluntary anal contraction = No AND all S4-5 sensory scores = 0 AND deep anal pressure = No, then injury is COMPLETE. Otherwise, injury is incomplete.

5. Determine ASIA Impairment Scale (AIS) Grade:

   Is injury Complete? If **YES**, AIS=A and can record ZPP (lowest dermatome or myotome on each side with some preservation)

   NO

   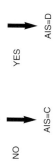

   Is injury motor Incomplete? If **NO**, AIS=B
   (Yes=voluntary anal contraction OR motor function more than three levels below the motor level on a given side, if the patient has sensory incomplete classification)

   YES

   Are at least half of the key muscles below the single neurological level graded 3 or better?

   NO → AIS=C   YES → AIS=D

   If sensation and motor function is normal in all segments, AIS=E
   Note: AIS E is used in follow-up testing when an individual with a documented SCI has recovered normal function. If at initial testing no deficits are found, the individual is neurologically intact; the ASIA Impairment Scale does not apply.

Figure 13.8 American Spinal Injury Association (ASIA): International standards for neurologic classification of spinal cord injury, revised 2011. This dermatome chart outlines and standardizes the comprehensive neurologic evaluation of spinal cord injury patients. Motor function is evaluated by scoring 5 key muscle groups in the upper extremities and 5 key muscle groups in the lower extremities on a scale of 1 to 5. Sensation to both light touch and pinprick is evaluated in 28 dermatomes (C2–S4–5) with a scale of 0 to 2. Used with permission.

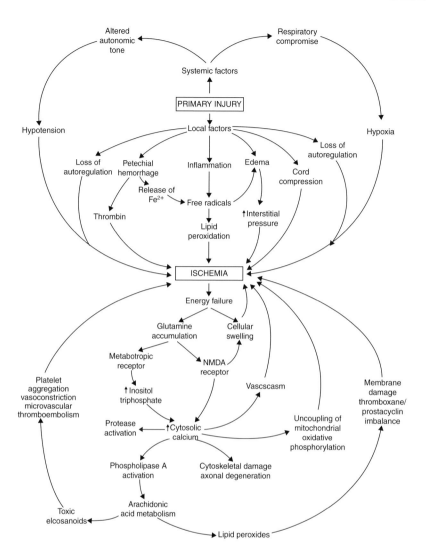

Figure 13.9 Schematic representation of key processes involved in secondary neurologic injury. Note the significant role of ischemia as emphasized in this figure. From Amar AP, Levy ML, Pathogenesis and pharmacological strategies for mitigating secondary damage in acute spinal cord injury. *Neurosurgery* 1999;44:1027–39. Reproduced with permission.

to the initial injury by means other than mechanical energy transfer. Complex biochemical cascades responsible for secondary neurologic injury are triggered within minutes of the primary insult and evolve over many months. Although still poorly understood and characterized, key processes contributing to secondary injury include the inflammatory cascade, immune system, free radical production resulting in lipid peroxidation and impaired ionic homeostasis, neurotransmitter-induced neurotoxicity, and microcirculatory dysfunction (Fig. 13.9). Many of these cascades converge and ultimately contribute to tissue ischemia and further neuronal injury. These processes are often dominant early in the postinjury period, with peak activity during the first few days. Modulation of these biochemical cascades in the early postinjury

stage as a means of providing neuroprotection has been extensively investigated with disappointing clinical results.

Tissue ischemia may act as a trigger for some of the secondary injury processes and as a final common pathway of others. In light of this, an emphasis should be placed on the role of ischemia in secondary neurologic injury and directing clinical focus toward interventions that minimize tissue ischemias.

Anesthetic management of acute spinal cord injury

Anesthetic management of acute SCI patients requires integrating knowledge of anatomy, pathophysiology, pharmacology, radiology, and electrophysiology, as

Table 13.5 Systemic effects of spinal cord injury

System	Physiologic effects
Cardiovascular	Neurogenic shock Autonomic dysreflexia
Respiratory	Ventilatory failure Pneumonia Atalectasis Mucous plugging bronchoconstriction
Hemostasis	Deep venous thrombosis Pulmonary embolus
Gastrointestinal	Gastric atony/distension Stress ulcer Ileus
Urinary	Urinary retention Urinary tract infections
Skin	Decubitus ulcers
Psychiatric	Depression Anxiety Suicide

well as knowledge of the medical-surgical treatments and their associated risks. The anesthetic goals specific to acute SCI include preventing further mechanical injury secondary to spinal instability as well as limiting secondary neurologic injury through optimal medical management.

Preoperative evaluation

A thorough anesthetic preoperative evaluation with focus on associated injuries, airway examination, cardiopulmonary status including assessment of intravascular volume, and radiologic studies and neurologic examination should be conducted. The radiologic evaluation should be assessed specifically for the morphology of injury (Fig. 13.5), the integrity of stabilizing ligaments, segmental level of injury, and presence of ongoing cord compression. The initial or most recent neurologic evaluation should also be carefully reviewed and repeated to the extent that clinically significant neurologic deterioration may be detected and documented, while gaining an appreciation for the completeness of injury. Together, the radiologic and neurologic evaluation will help predict mechanical instability and risk of further neurologic injury, as well as help anticipate systemic sequelae (Table 13.5) of spinal cord injury.

As with any complex case, communication is critically important. Preoperative discussion should specifically address the surgical plan including patient positioning, perceived spinal stability, utility of neurophysiologic monitoring, postoperative management, and any procedure-specific concerns. Following a thorough preoperative evaluation and discussion with the surgical team, an anesthetic plan will be tailored to the clinical scenario. The anesthetic plan must account for a number of factors including: risk of airway complications; risk of neurologic injury during airway management and positioning; the need for intraoperative neurophysiologic monitoring; the likelihood of trauma-related hemorrhage or neurogenic shock requiring hemodynamic support and invasive monitoring; desire for postoperative neurologic examination; and necessity of postoperative ventilatory assistance.

Spine immobilization

Spine immobilization should be initiated outside the hospital in at-risk patients and continued by all medical providers until a proper physical and/or radiologic evaluation has ruled out unstable spinal injury. Spine immobilization is best achieved by the sandbag–tape–backboard technique in conjunction with a hard cervical collar. Together, these maneuvers have been shown to limit cervical motion to approximately 5% of baseline.[16] Hard collars alone are insufficient to prevent cervical spine movement but may serve as a visual reminder of potential spinal injury.[17] During airway management, hard cervical collars have been shown to reduce inter-incisor distance by greater than 10 mm.[18] Therefore, replacement of the anterior cervical collar with manual in-line immobilization (MILI) is recommended for direct laryngoscopy.

Manual in-line immobilization: The goal of MILI is to keep the head and neck in a neutral position without applying traction by using forces equal and opposite to those exerted by direct laryngoscopy. MILI is typically applied by an assistant at the head of the bed who grasps the mastoid processes with the fingertips while cradling the occiput between their palms (Fig. 13.10). MILI appears to reduce overall spinal movement during laryngoscopy but may only be minimally effective at stabilizing the site of injury.[19] That said, direct laryngoscopy with MILI has an excellent clinical safety record worldwide since routine use began in the 1990s.[20] Compared with other immobilization methods, MILI has the least detrimental effect on glottic visualization, although laryngoscopic grade will be increased by 1 in 35% of patients and by 2 grades in 10% of patients.[21]

Airway maneuvers and spinal movement: The effect of basic and advanced airway maneuvers on the

239

Airway management

When it comes to known or suspected acute spinal injury and airway management, there are no established practice guidelines with which to guide clinical care. In fact, there is very little evidence for an association between airway management and neurologic deterioration. Therefore, it is impossible to demonstrate superiority of one technique over another. The anesthesiologist must consider the sum of the case-specific clinical factors as well as their experience/skill with various techniques in making clinical decisions.

Urgent intubation: Immediate airway management may be necessary for a variety of reasons including acute head injury, intoxication, cardiopulmonary insufficiency, or airway compromise. These patients are often immobilized or are uncooperative. Securing the airway may well take precedence over radiologic evaluation. In addition to having unknown spine status and incomplete airway examinationss, they likely have "full stomachs" and may have trauma-related injuries resulting in increased intracranial pressure or hemodynamic instability. In this setting, rapidly securing the airway with direct laryngoscopy using MILI and cricoid pressure may provide the greatest benefit with the least clinical risk. During direct laryngoscopy, only the minimum force required for adequate visualization and successful intubation should be applied with the laryngoscope. After ensuring proper endotracheal tube placement and ventilation, the anterior cervical collar should be replaced unless specifically contraindicated, and attention should then be focused on maintaining adequate tissue perfusion pressure.

Regardless of the airway management technique utilized, the following goals should be sought: (1) prevent hypoxia and hypercarbia; (2) minimize potential neurologic injury by limiting spine movement; (3) secure the airway expediently and in such a way as to reduce the risk of aspiration and pulmonary complication; and (4) prevent hypotension.

Controlled intubation: Alternate methods of airway management may offer certain advantages and should be considered in cooperative patients with known cervical spine instability, with or without neurologic injury, particularly in the presence of ongoing cord compression. Awake fiberoptic intubation (AFOI) has the least effect on spinal movement (compared with other methods of endotracheal intubation) and allows for neurologic assessment and awake positioning prior

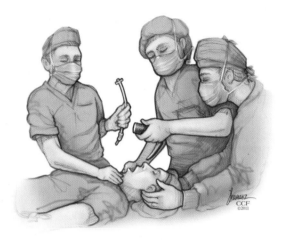

Figure 13.10 Urgent intubation of an acute trauma patient with incomplete spine evaluation. One assistant maintains manual in-line immobilization (MILI) of the spine. Note that the anterior portion of the cervical collar has been removed to "optimize" laryngoscopic grade while the posterior portion remains in place to minimize atlantoaxial extension. A second assistant applies cricoid pressure.

cervical spine has been studied in numerous human cadaver models with a variety of surgically induced unstable cervical injuries. The cumulative results of these studies indicate that basic maneuvers such as chin lift, jaw thrust, oral airway placement, and mask ventilation result in cervical movement that is equal to or greater than movement associated with direct laryngoscopy with MILI.[19] In total, human cadaver studies suggest that cervical spine movements associated with basic and advanced airway maneuvers are small and consistently within the physiologic range. The question remaining is whether physiologic movement is appropriate in the setting of acute spinal cord compression and/or injury and how these movements relate to further neurologic deterioration.

Alternate methods of airway management in cases of difficult direct laryngoscopy have also been evaluated in cadaver models. Video laryngoscopes (e.g., Glidescope) appear to reduce spinal movement in segments C2–C5 but not at the craniocervical junction.[22] Use of a laryngeal mask airway as a conduit for endotracheal intubation results in posterior displacement at C2–C5 during insertion as well as substantial pressure on upper cervical vertebrae while in situ.[23,24] Spinal movements created by these devices again are small and within the normal physiologic range. However, the significance of these movements and their effect on neurologic outcome are unknown.

to induction of anesthesia. Although a neurologic outcome benefit of this technique has not been demonstrated, even small physiologic movements of the spine associated with direct laryngoscopy may place the cord at risk if normal anatomic relationships have been disrupted. In patients considered to be at high risk for neurologic deterioration during airway management or surgical positioning, our practice is to limit spine movement as much as possible by performing AFOI. The patient is then positioned awake (if indicated) followed by a brief neurologic examination prior to induction of anesthesia. Despite these measures, unwanted spine movement may still occur during application of topical anesthesia of the airway or intubation (if topical anesthesia is insufficient).

Surgical positioning

Surgical positioning in the setting of acute spinal cord injury is critical, especially if injury has reduced the cross-sectional area of the spinal canal. Subtle flexion or extension may be sufficient to change the spinal canal–cord relationship, resulting in cord compression or stretching, and thus further attenuate spinal cord perfusion and increase neurologic injury.

The *Poisson effect* describes a phenomenon whereby the spinal canal cross-sectional area is reduced as the canal is axially lengthened. Therefore, spine flexion over the vertebral body should lengthen the canal and reduce the cross-sectional area, whereas extension should axially shorten the canal and increase the area. However, results by Ching *et al.*, in a study conducted to assess the impact of positioning on canal area in a cervical spine burst fracture model, ran counter to those predicted by the *Poisson effect*. Spine extension increased canal occlusion to degrees associated with nerve injury while flexion did not.[25] Similarly, Blease Graham *et al.* demonstrated that neck extension associated with prone positioning results in more severe cervical stenosis.[26] These findings are explained by encroachment into the spinal canal by buckling of the ligamentum flavum. These data suggest that hyperextension of the cervical spine should at least be done with caution in the clinical setting of reduced canal cross-sectional area.

Hyperflexion of the neck also carries certain risks. Unfortunately, the anesthesiologist's goals for patient positioning may at times be at odds with those of the surgeon. Hyperflexion of the spine may be required for surgical exposure of the upper cervical vertebrae. However, flexion of the cervical spine may stretch the cervical cord, particularly in the setting of ongoing cord compression, and thus contribute to ischemic injury. Also, aggressive cervical flexion may result in restricted venous drainage of the head and face, and possibly result in macroglossia or contribute to intracranial hypertension. To help guard against spinal cord ischemia or restricted venous drainage, a minimum of two finger-breadths should comfortably fit between the anterior mandible and the sternal notch. Hyperflexion may also result in increased peak airway pressures related to kinking of the endotracheal tube in the posterior pharynx or from endobronchial intubation resulting from tube advancement that occurs with neck flexion.

Electrophysiologic monitoring

Surgical management itself may cause neurologic compromise by decreasing tissue perfusion during instrumentation via distraction or direct compression. Electrophysiologic monitoring of somatosensory evoked potentials (SSEPs) and motor evoked potentials (MEPs) may help detect reversible neurologic dysfunction due to either surgical interventions or positioning. SSEPs monitor the ascending sensory tracts in the posterior columns with 92% sensitivity for new-onset cord dysfunction.[27] MEPs monitor the anterior cord by way of the anterolateral and posterolateral corticospinal tracts. Although quite sensitive for detecting acute cord dysfunction, physiologic variables that interfere with monitoring, such as anesthetics, hypothermia, hypotension, and anemia, may result in a high false-positive rate.[28] The anesthesiologist must be aware of these confounding variables and work closely with the neurophysiologist to minimize their impact.

Hemodynamic management

As previously mentioned, ischemia is a key component of the secondary injury cascade because of microcirculatory dysfunction and loss of autoregulatory capacity following acute SCI. Although there is a lack of strong scientific data to support its practice, maintenance of MAP with maintenance of intravascular volume and judicious use of vasopressors may be of benefit. A prospective clinical case series involving 77 acute spine injury patients who were treated with aggressive fluid and pharmacologic therapy to maintain MAP greater than 85 mmHg for the first 7 days following injury, reported improved neurologic outcomes

241

at 1 year compared with historical controls.[29,30] The target MAP was arbitrarily set at 85 mmHg and was achieved using a combination of invasive monitoring (Swan–Ganz catheter, arterial line), fluid resuscitation, and vasopressor support (dopamine/norepinephrine). Although precise therapeutic targets remain ill defined, it is reasonable to avoid hypotension (SBP <90 mmHg) and target MAPs of 85 mmHg during the first week following injury. Further systematic evaluation is needed to validate and better define these targets.

Avoidance of hypotension in the setting of acute SCI may be difficult because of pathophysiology associated with SCI or coexisting trauma-related injuries. Neurogenic shock is a diagnosis of exclusion in the setting of acute traumatic injury and it should be considered when other correctible causes of hypotension have been treated.

Neurogenic shock: Neurogenic shock is caused by interruption of sympathetic output from the spinal cord and unopposed parasympathetic activity. The severity and duration of neurogenic shock is related to the level and completeness of SCI. Neurogenic shock secondary to cord injuries at the midthoracic level (T6) or below results from loss of sympathetic tone to arterioles and veins, affecting both systemic vascular resistance and preload, respectively, in the lower extremities. With higher cord injuries, vascular effects are compounded by loss of sympathetic output to the heart (T1–T5), resulting in bradycardia and decreased contractility, and by loss of sympathetic tone in the splanchnic vasculature. The latter results in an increase in vascular capacitance in the splanchnic circulation, thereby reducing venous return and cardiac preload. First-line therapy includes invasive blood pressure monitoring and volume resuscitation with crystalloids, colloids, and blood products as needed to restore preload and oxygen-carrying capacity. Additional invasive monitors such as CVP, Swan–Ganz catheter, or transesophageal echocardiography (TEE) should be considered based on injury location, severity of hypotension, and clinical response to initial fluid resuscitation. If target MAPs are not quickly achieved, pharmacologic therapy should be initiated without further delay. For lesions below T6, a peripheral vasoconstrictor with pure alpha agonist activity such as phenylephrine may be appropriate. However, lesions above T6 may warrant use of pharmacologic therapy with both beta and alpha agonist activity such as dopamine or norepinephrine.[31]

Table 13.6 Muscles of respiration

Respiratory phase	Muscle	Spinal level of innervation
Inspiration	Sternocleidomastoid/trapezius	XI, C1, C2
	Diaphragm	C3–C5
	Scalenes	C4–C8
	Parasternal intercostal	T1–T7
	Lateral external intercostals	T1–T12
Expiration	Pectoralis major	C5–C7
	Lateral internal intercostals	T1–T12
	Rectus abdominis	T7–L1
	External/internal obliques	T7–L1
	Transversus abdominis	T7–L1

Anesthetic choice

No anesthetic has been shown to be superior to another or to result in neuroprotection in the setting of acute SCI. It is far more important to prevent hypoxemia, anemia, extreme blood glucose fluctuation, hyperthermia, or hypotension than to administer any specific anesthetic agent. The choice of anesthetic may be dictated more by concurrent neurophysiologic monitoring than anything else.

Muscle relaxation: By 24 hours after a denervation injury, proliferation of extrajunctional acetylcholine receptors may occur at the neuromuscular junction, thus increasing the risk of a hyperkalemic response to succinylcholine.

Ventilation

Respiratory mechanics: The respiratory cycle typically involves an active inspiratory phase followed by a passive expiratory phase. Muscles involved in inspiration include the diaphragm, parasternal intercostals, and lateral external intercostals. The scalenes, sternocleidomastoid, and trapezius may also be recruited as accessory muscles of inspiration. Although mostly passive, the lateral internal intercostals (T1–T12), pectoralis major, and abdominal musculature (T7–L1) are required to various degrees for reserve expiration, cough, and clearance of secretions.

The degree of respiratory impairment and risk of pulmonary complication depends on both the level of injury and the resulting severity of muscle weakness (Table 13.6). Therefore, pulmonary morbidity is generally greater with higher segmental spinal cord injury as well with injuries that that are more complete. Spinal cord injury above C5 will likely compromise diaphragm function and may require early intubation. However, spinal cord injury involving the lower cervical or upper thoracic region may also significantly compromise respiratory mechanics, without directly effecting diaphragm function. Flaccid paralysis of intercostal muscles may decrease forced vital capacity and maximal inspiratory force by 70%, while paralysis of the abdominal muscles will prevent forced exhalation and the ability to clear secretions.[32] The clinical result is a pattern of rapid, shallow breathing that is quite inefficient and promotes atelectasis, mucus retention, and pulmonary infections, and culminates in significant morbidity and mortality.

Secondary injury cascades initiated by the primary mechanical insult may not result in maximal clinical deficits for a number of days. Progressive respiratory muscle weakness reflecting evolving secondary neurologic injury may continue during the first week. Repeated evaluation of respiratory function may be required during the early post-injury period. Patients should be assessed carefully for signs of respiratory fatigue such as increasing respiratory rate and rising P_aCO_2. Declining serial bedside measurements of vital capacity approaching 1 liter are also indicative of significant pulmonary deterioration and need of mechanical ventilatory assistance.

Extubation: Pulmonary complications are the number one cause of morbidity and mortality in SCI patients. The decision to extubate or not at the end of surgery is based on both the preoperative clinical condition and factors related to the surgical procedure/intraoperative course.

Preoperative respiratory mechanics, ability to clear secretions, time from injury, along with the level and completeness of injury, may collectively help determine the appropriateness of postoperative extubation.

Intraoperative factors that may affect postoperative airway management decisions include the operative procedure performed, duration, and patient position. Further considerations include the volume of fluid resuscitation required during the procedure, hemodynamic stability, concomitant injuries, and deterioration of neurophysiologic signals. Specific concerns related to procedures performed in the prone position include development of facial edema, which may include swelling of the lingual and periglottic areas

sufficient to compromise airway patency. Procedural concerns related to anterior cervical spine surgery include injury to nerves responsible for airway protection (recurrent laryngeal/hypoglossal) and tissue manipulation-induced edema of perilaryngeal structures.

Neuroprotection and repair

Methods of limiting secondary injury following an acute neurologic insult have been extensively investigated with a number of the most promising preclinical therapies brought to clinical trial over the last 20 years. The largest multicenter prospective randomized controlled trials have investigated the neuroprotective effects of methylprednisolone (MP), ganglioside GM1 (Sygen), thyrotropin-releasing hormone, gacyclidine (GK-11), naloxone, and nimodipine. Unfortunately, none of these therapies convincingly demonstrated clinical efficacy in primary clinical outcome measures.

Methylprednisolone: Perhaps the most widely known therapy investigated for neuroprotection to date has been the corticosteroid MP. Neuroprotective effects attributed to corticosteroids are thought to include antioxidant properties, enhancement of spinal cord blood flow, reduced cellular calcium influx, reduced posttraumatic axonal dieback, and attenuated lipid peroxidation.[33] Encouraging preclinical results with MP led to three landmark clinical trials (NASCIS I, II, III) that have undergone intense scientific scrutiny and have been the subject of contentious debate. Primary outcomes were negative in all three trials with a significant increase in (NASCIS I) and trending towards (NASCIS II, III) higher complication rates in MP-treated patients. Post hoc analysis revealed the possibility of a small neurologic benefit of questionable clinical significance (no difference in Functional Independence Measure) in a small subset of patients. However. concerns over incomplete reporting of data (only one side of the body and exclusion of muscle groups), inappropriate statistical methodology, and arbitrary subgroup analysis have brought into question the clinical relevance. Because at the present time the evidence for therapy-induced complications is stronger than any clinical benefit, both the American Association of Neurologic Surgeons and the Congress of Neurologic Surgeons consider it a treatment option "that should be undertaken only with the knowledge that the evidence suggesting harmful side effects

243

is more consistent than any suggestion of clinical benefit."[34]

Future/ongoing clinical trials

More promising pharmacologic and nonpharmacologic therapies have been brought to clinical trial in recent years with results forthcoming. Promising pharmacologic neuroprotective therapies currently under investigation include minocycline, a synthetic tetracycline with microglial inhibitory properties as well as antiapoptotic effects, and riluzole, a benzothiazole anticonvulsant with inhibitory effects on both voltage-gated sodium channels and presynaptic glutamate release. Other pharmacologic strategies currently under clinical investigation aim to encourage CNS axonal regeneration through targeting of myelin-associated inhibitors of axon regeneration or downstream signaling of this inhibition (ATI-355 and Cethrin).

Nonpharmacologic therapies under current clinically investigation in human trials include cerebrospinal fluid (CSF) drainage and systemic hypothermia. In the setting of thoracic aortic aneurysm surgery, evidence suggests that CSF drainage may improve spinal cord perfusion and attenuate neurologic ischemic injury.[35] Investigators at the University of British Columbia have initiated a study investigating the safety and feasibility of CSF drainage after acute SCI via lumbar intrathecal catheters. At present, the efficacy of these interventions cannot be considered to be proven.

Although it is not a novel neuroprotective strategy, renewed interest in hypothermia has emerged with improvements in intravascular heat exchange catheters. Early clinical trials investigated cold irrigant-induced local hypothermia on exposed spinal cord segments with inconsistent results. Enthusiasm has re-emerged following encouraging preclinical data from a variety of animal models demonstrating the efficacy of systemic hypothermia. In a recently published study by Levi et al., the feasibility and safety of maintaining tightly regulated systemic hypothermia was demonstrated with the use of an FDA-approved heat exchange catheter.[36] Compared with age- and injury-matched controls, induction of moderate hypothermia resulted in a comparable incidence of potential complications. At present time, there is insufficient evidence to make any recommendations regarding hypothermia as a neuroprotective therapy and further investigation will be needed to establish both the efficacy and safety.

Cell transplantation therapies

Another frontier for improving neurologic function following SCI involves cell transplantation. Cell transplantation therapies aim to introduce specific cell types into the injured spinal cord by various mechanisms during the postinjury phase to improve functional recovery. Some investigators are attempting to create the regeneration potential seen in the peripheral nervous system (PNS) through transplantation of autologous macrophages into the injured spinal cord. The macrophages seen in in abundance the PNS are thought to promote regeneration by rapid clearance of myelin debris and secretion of nerve growth factor.[37] Other investigators are attempting to transplant cells that integrate into existing neuronal networks (stem cells) or enhance recovery of dysfunctional axons through re-myelination (Schwann cells, olfactory ensheathing cells). Although these therapies have shown potential in multiple experimental models, progress has been slow with only modest improvements in functional recovery.

References

1. Fisher CG, Noonan VK, Dvorak MF. Changing face of spine trauma care in North America. *Spine* 2006; **31**(11 Suppl): S2–8; discussion S36.

2. National Spinal Cord Injury Statistical Center: Spinal Cord Injury Facts and Figures at a Glance [database on the Internet] February 2010. Available from: https://www.nscisc.uab.edu (accessed November 2010).

3. Jackson RS, Banit DM, Rhyne AL, 3rd, Darden BV, 2nd. Upper cervical spine injuries. *J Am Acad Orthop Surg.* 2002; **10**(4): 271–80.

4. Bono CM, Vaccaro AR, Fehlings M, *et al.* Measurement techniques for upper cervical spine injuries: consensus statement of the Spine Trauma Study Group. *Spine* 2007; **32**(5): 593–600.

5. Morris CG, McCoy E. Clearing the cervical spine in unconscious polytrauma victims, balancing risks and effective screening. *Anaesthesia* 2004; **59**(5): 464–82.

6. Hickey R, Albin MS, Bunegin L, Gelineau J. Autoregulation of spinal cord blood flow: is the cord a microcosm of the brain? *Stroke* 1986; **17**(6): 1183–9.

7. Demetriades D, Charalambides K, Chahwan S, *et al.* Nonskeletal cervical spine injuries: epidemiology and diagnostic pitfalls. *J Trauma.* 2000; **48**(4): 724–7.

8. Reid DC, Henderson R, Saboe L, Miller JD. Etiology and clinical course of missed spine fractures. *J Trauma* 1987; **27**(9): 980–6.

9. Hoffman JR, Mower WR, Wolfson AB, Todd KH, Zucker MI. Validity of a set of clinical criteria to rule out injury to the cervical spine in patients with blunt trauma. National Emergency X-Radiography Utilization Study Group. *N Engl J Med* 2000; **343**(2): 94–9.

10. Mower WR, Hoffman JR, Pollack CV, Jr., *et al*. Use of plain radiography to screen for cervical spine injuries. *Ann Emerg Med* 2001; **38**(1): 1–7.

11. Schenarts PJ, Diaz J, Kaiser C, Carrillo Y, Eddy V, Morris JA, Jr. Prospective comparison of admission computed tomographic scan and plain films of the upper cervical spine in trauma patients with altered mental status. *J Trauma*. 2001 Oct; **51**(4): 663–8; discussion 668–9.

12. O'Dowd JK. Basic principles of management for cervical spine trauma. *Eur Spine J;* **19** Suppl 1: S18–22.

13. Klein GR, Vaccaro AR, Albert TJ, *et al*. Efficacy of magnetic resonance imaging in the evaluation of posterior cervical spine fractures. *Spine* 1999; **24**(8): 771–4.

14. White III AA, ed. *Clinical Biomechanics of the Spine.* Philadelphia: JB Lippincott; 1978.

15. Whang PG, Vaccaro AR, Poelstra KA, *et al*. The influence of fracture mechanism and morphology on the reliability and validity of two novel thoracolumbar injury classification systems. *Spine* 2007; **32**(7): 791–5.

16. Podolsky S, Baraff LJ, Simon RR, *et al*. Efficacy of cervical spine immobilization methods. *J Trauma* 1983; **23**(6): 461–5.

17. Majernick TG, Bieniek R, Houston JB, Hughes HG. Cervical spine movement during orotracheal intubation. *Ann Emerg Med* 1986; **15**(4): 417–20.

18. Goutcher CM, Lochhead V. Reduction in mouth opening with semi-rigid cervical collars. *Br J Anaesth* 2005; **95**(3): 344–8.

19. Crosby ET. Airway management in adults after cervical spine trauma. *Anesthesiology* 2006; **104**(6): 1293–318.

20. Manoach S, Paladino L. Manual in-line stabilization for acute airway management of suspected cervical spine injury: historical review and current questions. *Ann Emerg Med* 2007; **50**(3): 236–45.

21. Nolan JP, Wilson ME. Orotracheal intubation in patients with potential cervical spine injuries. An indication for the gum elastic bougie. *Anaesthesia* 1993; **48**(7): 630–3.

22. Turkstra TP, Craen RA, Pelz DM, Gelb AW. Cervical spine motion: a fluoroscopic comparison during intubation with lighted stylet, GlideScope, and Macintosh laryngoscope. *Anesth Analg* 2005; **101**(3): 910–15, table of contents.

23. Kihara S, Watanabe S, Brimacombe J, *et al*. Segmental cervical spine movement with the intubating laryngeal mask during manual in-line stabilization in patients with cervical pathology undergoing cervical spine surgery. *Anesth Analg* 2000; **91**(1): 195–200.

24. Keller C, Brimacombe J, Keller K. Pressures exerted against the cervical vertebrae by the standard and intubating laryngeal mask airways: a randomized, controlled, cross-over study in fresh cadavers. *Anesth Analg* 1999; **89**(5): 1296–300.

25. Ching RP, Watson NA, Carter JW, Tencer AF. The effect of post-injury spinal position on canal occlusion in a cervical spine burst fracture model. *Spine* 1997; **22**(15): 1710–15.

26. Blease Graham C, 3rd, Wippold FJ, 2nd, Bae KT, *et al*. Comparison of CT myelography performed in the prone and supine positions in the detection of cervical spinal stenosis. *Clin Radiol* 2001; **56**(1): 35–9.

27. Nuwer MR, Dawson EG, Carlson LG, Kanim LE, Sherman JE. Somatosensory evoked potential spinal cord monitoring reduces neurologic deficits after scoliosis surgery: results of a large multicenter survey. *Electroencephalogr Clin Neurophysiol* 1995; **96**(1): 6–11.

28. Noonan KJ, Walker T, Feinberg JR, *et al*. Factors related to false- versus true-positive neuromonitoring changes in adolescent idiopathic scoliosis surgery. *Spine* 2002; **27**(8): 825–30.

29. Levi L, Wolf A, Belzberg H. Hemodynamic parameters in patients with acute cervical cord trauma: description, intervention, and prediction of outcome. *Neurosurgery* 1993; **33**(6): 1007–16; discussion 1016–7.

30. Vale FL, Burns J, Jackson AB, Hadley MN. Combined medical and surgical treatment after acute spinal cord injury: results of a prospective pilot study to assess the merits of aggressive medical resuscitation and blood pressure management. *J Neurosurg* 1997; **87**(2): 239–46.

31. Early acute management in adults with spinal cord injury: a clinical practice guideline for health-care professionals. *J Spinal Cord Med* 2008; **31**(4): 403–79.

32. Ball PA. Critical care of spinal cord injury. *Spine* 2001; **26**(24 Suppl): S27–30.

33. Hawryluk GW, Rowland J, Kwon BK, Fehlings MG. Protection and repair of the injured spinal cord: a review of completed, ongoing, and planned clinical trials for acute spinal cord injury. *Neurosurg Focus* 2008; **25**(5): E14.

34. Pharmacological therapy after acute cervical spinal cord injury. *Neurosurgery* 2002; **50**(3 Suppl): S63–72.

35. Coselli JS, Lemaire SA, Koksoy C, Schmittling ZC, Curling PE. Cerebrospinal fluid drainage reduces paraplegia after thoracoabdominal aortic aneurysm

repair: results of a randomized clinical trial. *J Vasc Surg* 2002; **35**(4): 631–9.

36. Levi AD, Green BA, Wang MY, *et al.* Clinical application of modest hypothermia after spinal cord injury. *J Neurotrauma* 2009; **26**(3): 407–15.

37. Perry VH, Brown MC, Gordon S. The macrophage response to central and peripheral nerve injury. A possible role for macrophages in regeneration. *J Exp Med* 1987; **165**(4): 1218–23.

Chapter

14

Anesthesia for patients with spinal cord tumors

Stacie Deiner and Jeffrey Silverstein

Key points

- Spinal cord tumors are an uncommon cause of back pain.
- Spinal cord tumors may be primary tumors of the spinal cord or secondary to metastases.
- It is critical that the anesthesiologist communicates with the surgical team to understand the type of tumor and planned procedure in order to choose appropriate venous access and invasive monitoring.
- Information gathered from intraoperative neuromonitoring is often an important part of the surgical procedure and the anesthesiologist needs to create a conducive anesthetic plan.
- Many patients with spinal cord tumors have postoperative pain and therefore intra- and postoperative pain management may be complicated.

Introduction

The majority of spinal surgery is precipitated by a painful condition or neurologic deficit. Although spinal cord tumors are an unlikely cause of back pain, anesthesia for patients with a spinal cord tumor for surgical resection has specific considerations. Both primary and metastatic tumors of the spine can require surgical resection. The etiology and location of the tumor defines its treatment and prognosis. Anesthetic considerations are based primarily on the nature of the spinal involvement, (e.g., breast cancer with metastases to the spine), the impact of comorbid disease on the anesthetic plan, intraoperative neuromonitoring of the spinal cord, the need for a smooth and rapid emergence to facilitate neurologic examination, and the management of acute or chronic pain.

In this chapter we will begin with a description the different types of spinal cord tumors and their treatment and prognosis. We will discuss in depth the preoperative evaluation and intraoperative and postoperative management of the patient presenting with a spinal cord tumor for surgical resection.

Etiology of spinal tumors

Spinal cord tumors are classified according to their location: intramedullary, intradural-extramedullary, and extradural. Extradural tumors are the most frequent type of spinal cord tumors, the most common of which are secondary metastatic lesions arising from the vertebral bodies. In contrast, primary extradural tumors are less common; an example is a chordoma.

The majority of intramedullary tumors are subtypes of gliomas (referring to their histologic resemblance to normal glial cells). These include ependymomas, astrocytomas, and oligodendrogliomas. Intradural-extramedullary refers to tumors within the dura but outside of the spinal cord. Examples of these are meningiomas and nerve sheath tumors. Meningiomas arise from arachnoid cells and are sometimes found in association with neurofibromas.

Presentation

Spinal cord tumors cause symptomatology consistent with disruption of neural pathways through extrinsic or intrinsic compression of normal neural tissue. Symptoms may be localized to the site of the tumor or have distant effects. In the case of benign tumors, patients may have localized pain for months or years prior to diagnosis. Classically the pain is described as gnawing and unremitting and may result in nocturnal awakening.[1] Distal effects include dysfunction due to interruption of the spinal cord pathways and may be either sensory or motor. Often the symptoms are unilateral and then may progress to bilateral disease. In severe cases, cauda equina syndrome may occur.

Treatment options for spinal cord tumors

The treatment for almost every spinal cord tumor involves surgical resection; the type of tumor determines whether adjunctive therapy with chemotherapeutic agents or radiation is indicated.

In all cases, complete resection is rarely a guarantee of cure, and although in many of the primary tumours 5-years survival is >70%, recurrence is likely.

Treatment options for spinal cord tumors resulting from metastases

Several cancers are likely to result in metastases to the spine; 90% of patients dying of prostate cancer and 75% of those dying of breast cancer have metastases to the spine. Metastatic cancer of the spine may require surgical treatment when it results in a pathologic fracture causing pain and instability or epidural spinal cord compression (ESCC) resulting in a neurologic deficit or cauda equina syndrome. Vertebral metastases are significantly more common than ESCC. The three most common tumors are prostate, breast cancer, and lung cancer. Use of radiation or chemotherapy is dependent on the type of tumor. Because of their potential for invasion of local tissues and generous blood supply, the resection of metastatic lesions of the spine can have significant potential for intraoperative blood loss.

Treatment options for primary tumors of the spinal cord

Chordomas are rare tumors that are locally invasive and frequently recur. Wide local excision is attempted, although complete resection is often not possible.[2] Postoperative radiation therapy is frequently employed.[3] Chemotherapeutic agents with activity include imatinib plus or minus cisplatin, sirolimus, sunitinib, and erlotinib.[4] If the patient has received any chemotherapeutic agent the anesthesiologist should familiarize themselves with the side effects so that they may investigate whether these have occurred and will impact the anesthetic. For example, cisplatin is associated with nephrotoxicity and electrolyte disturbance, and sirolimus is associated with thrombocytopenia. Sarcomas and lymphomas (which may be primary or secondary in the spine) are generally treated with a multimodal approach, which includes surgical resection, radiation, and chemotherapy. Finally, there are

several benign primary bone lesions that may occur in the spine and are treated with resection alone. These include osteoid osteomas, osteoblastomas, osteochondromas, chondroblastomas, giant cell tumors, vertebral hemangiomas, and aneurysmal bone cysts.

Intramedullary tumors

Intramedullary gliomas are preferentially treated surgically.[5] The initial step is attempt at curative resection. There have been no randomized trials of radiation therapy. The role of radiotherapy and chemotherapy has been as adjuvants to surgery in the case of noncurative resections or recurrence. The most recent guidelines suggest that patients who have had curative resections should not receive radiation.

Intradural-extramedullary tumors

These tumors include meningiomas, schwannomas, and ependymomas and are preferably treated with surgery. Radiation may be used for recurrence that is not amenable to resection; chemotherapy is not indicated.[6,7]

Preoperative care

All of the standard issues associated with preparation of any patient for anesthesia apply to patients with spinal tumors, including an underlying understanding of their physical status, their medication regimens, any potential allergies, and their surgical history. In addition, preparation for anesthetic care of patients with spinal tumors starts with an understanding of the chief complaint that brought the patient to surgery. Pain is the most common complaint but this is frequently associated with varying levels of neurologic deficit. These two primary areas should be explored and understood by the anesthesia team. The pain associated with spinal cord tumors may be acute, chronic, or acute-on-chronic. When eliciting a history of pain symptomatology, the anesthesiologist should ask about duration, location, and quality. Use of pain medications should be noted, including current medications and medications used previously. The schedule of medications is relevant as well. This history will help the anesthesia team instruct the patient how to manage their medication regimen prior to surgery, will influence the intraoperative approach, particularly for narcotic usage, and will assist in managing acute postoperative pain.

The patient should be instructed to take all of their pain medications on their usual schedule. Use of transdermal systems, e.g., fentanyl patches should also be continued, although not necessarily initiated.

Continuation of adjunctive medications like gabapentin is recommended; however, use of nonsteroidal anti-inflammatory agents (NSAIDS) should be discussed with the surgeon because of the potential for postoperative bleeding. Beginning gabapentin immediately prior to surgery is controversial. While gabapentin has been shown to decrease postoperative morphine requirements, effective dosages can be associated with significant side effects, most notably dizziness.[8] If a narcotic-tolerant patient is unable or does not take their pain medication on the morning of surgery, then the patient's daily narcotic consumption should be calculated and converted into the equivalent intravenous morphine dosage. This calculation will provide the anesthesiologist with an approximate idea of the patient's daily narcotic intake, some of which will have to be given intravenously during the surgery. The details of converting the patient's oral narcotics to an intravenous dose are somewhat controversial, but the underlying principle is correct – namely that surgical patients who are narcotic tolerant will require narcotic dosing based on their previous consumption.[9] A recent study found that beginning a preoperative multimodal regimen of medications, including gabapentin, acetaminophen, and an oral narcotic, continued into the perioperative period was associated with better pain control and fewer side effects than intravenous morphine PCA.[10]

Some patients with spinal cord tumors will have been taking extremely high doses of opioid medication for an extended period of time. The perioperative period is not a good time to attempt to wean a patient from such medication. For patients with drug-seeking behavior, it is ill-advised to attempt to minimize analgesic consumption in the perioperative period. Changing or altering addictive behaviors should be delayed until after the immediate postoperative period.

Neurologic deficits and their province are important for the anesthesia team. The presence of muscle weakness or loss should be explored and documented in the preoperative record. The neurologic history will direct aspects of the patient's management, including how the patient is manipulated and positioned as well as the expectations of the monitoring team. The anesthesiologist can usually depend on the neurologic examination performed and documented by either a neurologist or a neurosurgeon. Patients may be worried about their functional status following surgery. To the extent possible, the anesthesia team should have an understanding of the surgeon's expectations for the patient's postoperative outcome.

Location and etiology of the tumor is important as well, since some types of tumors may be located at the skull base or cervical cord and be associated with a syrinx. In these cases, particular attention should be paid to the stability of the cervical spine and any concerns related to manipulating the cervical spine during endotracheal intubation. The anesthesia team should be aware of the primary cancer when metastatic disease is suspected, including an appreciation of the therapies that have been received to date, including surgery, chemotherapy, and/or radiation. The presence of metastatic disease in other areas of the body may raise important considerations. Breast and lung cancer may also have concomitant metastases to the brain, potentially resulting in space-occupying lesions. Patients with prior breast cancer who have had surgery may have limitations of the use of the ipsilateral arm for either intravenous access and infusion or noninvasive blood pressure monitoring.

Finally, the ideal preoperative preparation would optimize patient outcomes with a multidisciplinary approach. Although the relevance to patients with spinal tumors will vary depending upon the urgency of the surgery, in more elective cases there has been some success reported with active efforts of prehabilitation. One such regimen included an intensive exercise and nutrition program, and optimization of the analgesic treatment. In addition, protein drinks were given the day before surgery. The early postoperative rehabilitation included balanced pain therapy with self-administered epidural analgesia, doubled intensified mobilization, and protein supplements.[11] In this small study, patients in the intervention group reached the recovery milestones faster than the control group (1–6 days versus 3–13), and left hospital earlier (5 (3–9) versus 7 (5–15) days).

Intraoperative management

Induction and maintenance

The plan for induction and maintenance of anesthesia should be established with respect to the patient's medical comorbidities and in concert with the neuromonitoring plan. While standard of care for neuromonitoring during spinal cord tumor surgery has not been established, multimodality monitoring with MEPs, SSEPs, and EMG is common. The use of intraoperative somatosensory evoked potentials (SSEPs), motor evoked potentials (MEPs), and electromyography (EMG) allows for continual intraoperative assessment of the dorsal columns, anterior spinal cord, and nerve roots, respectively. In both deformity surgery and tumor surgery, several studies have demonstrated that no single modality monitors the entire spinal cord.[12,13] When used in combination with SSEPs, MEPs are associated with a higher sensitivity and specificity of motor tract injury than single-modality monitoring.[14] Utility of monitoring for spinal tumor surgery specifically includes dorsal column mapping during intramedullary surgery and evaluation of temporary clipping of spinal nerve roots in thoracic tumor resection.[15,16]

An anesthetic technique compatible with consistent intraoperative monitoring (IOM) needs to be established well in advance to obtain monitoring signals. This is important because the transition from the relatively rapid dissipation of inhalational agents to the relatively slower onset of steady-state blood levels of drug infusion may take significantly longer than several minutes when not temporally associated with an induction dose. The anesthesiologist should select a combination of agents with a favorable effect profile and start maintenance infusion around the time of induction. Examples include the addition of ketamine to a propofol infusion and the use of dexmedetomidine to decrease propofol and opioid requirements. If it is necessary to use inhalational agents (e.g., propofol shortage, patient history of adverse reaction, expense of total intravenous anesthesia [TIVA]), then there must be clear communication with the monitoring team. A single gas, either a halogenated agent or nitrous oxide, should be used. In any case, whichever technique used during the acquisition of baseline signals must be continued throughout the case to avoid loss of signals at the critical portions of the procedure.

Management of TIVA during spine surgery and neuromonitoring for the patient with a spinal cord tumor has several goals, which may be challenging to achieve simultaneously. Often the patient needs to be immobile without the use of paralytic medication, have steady-state anesthesia compatible with neuromonitoring, and maintain adequate blood pressure to avoid blindness, loss of neuromonitoring signals, and perfusion pressure to the vital organs. In addition, rapid awakening after surgery is desirable to facilitate a neurologic examination. The anesthesiologist should be well aware of the context-sensitive half-time of the agents they are using, and whether their patient has any renal or hepatic insufficiency, which may further complicate the recovery from intravenous anesthetic infusions.

Often MEP and SSEP signal baselines will be established immediately after induction and intubation of the trachea therefore it is important for the anesthesiologist to understand the neuromonitoring plan and be prepared to immediately create a conducive anesthetic. The anesthesiologist should be aware of the relative contraindications for evoked potential monitoring, which include implanted pacemaker, functioning implanted defibrillator, implanted metal in the cranial vault (aneurysm clips, etc.), epilepsy, increased intracranial pressure, and convexity defects of the skull. The manufacturer of commonly used neuromonitoring equipment (Digitimer Ltd., Welwyn, Herts, UK) currently advises against motor evoked potentials with convexity skull fracture or craniotomy because of the possibility of high local current density, which could cause injury to the brain tissue.[17] However, these are all relative contraindications, and the risk of the surgical procedure must be weighed against the risk of arrhythmia, seizure, or thermal injury. For example, in a high surgical risk patient with an implanted defibrillator, the antitachyarrhythmia function can be disabled and the case may proceed with MEP monitoring.

The anesthesiologist must be aware of which monitoring modalities will be utilized during the surgery, since each has anesthetic implications. SSEPs and MEPs are sensitive to all anesthetic agents (inhalational >> intravenous), while MEPs and EMGs are sensitive to paralytic drugs. Although initial studies suggested that <0.5 MAC (minimum alveolar concentration) of inhalational agent still allows for adequate monitoring of signals, a recent study suggests that this may not be the case for older patients with diabetes and/or hypertension.[18]

Optimization of the acquisition of evoked potentials is derived from the basic understanding that all anesthetics affect conduction along neural pathways, as demonstrated by their effects on EEG. The magnitude of the effect increases with the number of synapses in the pathway. Anesthetics may affect the evoked responses by either direct inhibition of synaptic pathways or indirectly by changing the balance of inhibitory and excitatory influences.

Most anesthetics depress evoked response amplitude and increase latency. Inhalational agents accomplish this by altering specific receptors or through nonspecific effects on cell membranes that alter the conformation structure of the receptor or ion channel. The effect of halogenated agents on SSEP signals

Table 14.1 Effects of anesthesia on evoked potentials
http://www.elsevier.com/wps/find/supportfaq.cws_home/permissionusematerial

Drug	SSEPs		BAEPs		VEPs		Transcranial MEPs	
	LAT	AMP	LAT	AMP	LAT	AMP	LAT	AMP
Isoflurane	Yes	Yes	No	No	Yes	Yes	Yes	Yes
Enflurane	Yes	Yes	No	No	Yes	Yes	Yes	Yes
Halothane	Yes	Yes	No	No	Yes	Yes	Yes	Yes
Nitrous oxide	Yes	Yes	No	No	Yes	Yes	Yes	Yes
Barbiturates	Yes	Yes	No	No	Yes	Yes	Yes	Yes
Etomidate	No	No	No	No	Yes	Yes	No	No
Propofol	Yes	Yes	No	No	Yes	Yes	Yes	Yes
Droperidol	No	No	No	No	–	–	Yes	Yes
Diazepam	Yes	Yes	No	No	Yes	Yes	Yes	Yes
Midazolam	Yes	Yes	No	No	Yes	Yes	Yes	Yes
Ketamine	No	No	No	No	Yes	Yes	No	No
Opiates	No	No	No	No	No	No	No	No
Dexmedetomidine	No	No	No	No	No	ND	ND	No

From: *Miller's Anesthesia*, 7th ed. Table 46–3. Churchill Livingstone/Elsevier.

directly correlates with potency: isoflurane > enflurane > halothane. Studies suggest that sevoflurane and desflurane are similar to isoflurane.[19] Nitrous oxide reduces SSEP cortical amplitude and increases latency alone or with halogenated inhalational agents or opioid agents. The greatest effect is seen in the waveforms recorded over the cortex, and less in the Erb's point and cervical waveforms. When compared with equipotent halogenated anesthetic concentrations, nitrous oxide produces more profound changes in cortical SSEPs.[19]

The effect of intravenous agents on evoked potentials is related to their affinity for neurotransmitter receptors (e.g., GABA, NMDA, glutamate, etc.). The effect varies with the specific receptor and pathways affected. Propofol, benzodiazepines, and barbiturates cause significant depression of the amplitude waveforms. Benzodiazepines and barbiturate infusions are out of favor as maintenance anesthetics for spine surgery for various reasons including their extremely long context-sensitive half life, potential for hyperalgesia (barbiturates), and prolonged depression after a bolus induction dose. While induction bolus doses of propofol cause depression of SSEPs, its context-sensitive half-time is significantly more favorable, and therefore its titratability makes it an important component of a maintenance anesthetic during monitored spine surgery, especially in combination with other favorable drugs.

Opioids affect SSEP signals less than inhalational agents, making them an important component of evoked potential monitoring. Bolus doses of opioids can be associated with mild depression of amplitude and an increase of latency in responses recorded from the cortex. Infusion doses are generally conducive to monitoring, and many neuroanesthesiologists have taken advantage of extremely short-acting narcotics such as remifentanil to supplement intravenous maintenance anesthetic. Some intravenous anesthetics which do not depress SSEP waveform amplitude include etomidate and ketamine. These drugs increase signal amplitude, potentially by attenuating inhibition.[19] In addition to its beneficial effects on neuromonitoring signals, ketamine is powerfully analgesic and may be especially helpful in opioid-tolerant patients.[20] Recent studies have examined the effect of dexmedetomidine on the acquisition of neuromonitoring signals. Several studies have found that the use of dexmedetomidine is compatible with acquisition of SSEPs.[21] The effect of inhalational and intravenous agents on SSEP monitoring, with suggested dosage range is summarized in Table 14.1.

Neuromuscular blocking agents have their affect at the neuromuscular junction and therefore do not negatively affect the acquisition of SSEP signals. If anything, this class of drugs improves the acquisition of SSEP signals by decreasing movement artifact. However, if EMG or MEP signals are planned, then neuromuscular blockade should be avoided, or at least attempted with caution and the use of a twitch monitor with an accelerometer.

Maintenance of intraoperative blood pressure

The ventral portion of the spinal cord is particularly vulnerable to injury because of its relatively tenuous blood supply; a single anterior spinal artery supplies 75% of the entire cord which includes the motor tracts. Therefore, the anterior portion of the cord is more susceptible to hypoperfusion injury due to anemia, hypotension, or blood vessel compression. Motor evoked potentials monitor the anterior spinal cord directly and can be exquisitely sensitive to changes in blood pressure, especially in susceptible patients – i.e., those with myelopathy or certain medical comorbidities such as diabetes or hypertension.[18] Anesthesiologists should strive to maintain normotension throughout the surgery, and if the motor evoked signals decline the patient's blood pressure should be additionally augmented to ensure adequate blood flow to areas of the cord that have been chronically compressed.

Access

Prior to the surgical procedure, a discussion regarding the surgical plan and tumor type will give the anesthesiologist an understanding of the need for large bore venous access and invasive monitoring. Patients with metastatic disease may have indwelling venous access for administration of chemotherapy. In general this access can be used for administration of drugs provided there is venous return, the appropriate volume is aspirated if the access has been flushed with heparin, and that the external access will not cause soft tissue injury if the patient is prone. Of note, these lines are rarely adequate for volume resuscitation, which if anticipated requires placement of a large-bore peripheral cannula or central access. Discussion of the surgical plan also allows appropriate ordering of blood and blood products. Resection of primary tumors of the spinal cord (intramedullary tumors and extradural-intramedullary tumors) rarely involves large-volume blood loss.

Choice of opioids

Appropriate management of chronic pain during spinal cord tumor surgery involves "big picture" planning for postoperative pain control. As mentioned above, continuation of the patient's chronic medications,

preoperative administration of oral adjunctive medication, and calculation of daily opioid requirements helps assist in finding the appropriate dosage.

Short-acting narcotics like remifentanil should be used with care in this population, especially if they have not taken their daily opioids. While still controversial, the use of high-dose remifentanil has been associated with the development of acute tolerance, higher morphine requirements in the recovery room, and hyperalgesia.[22,23] One study suggested that use of a propofol infusion for maintenance as opposed to sevoflurane prevents the development of hyperalgesia.[24] Another suggested that ketamine infusion may be effective in preventing remifentanil-induced hyperalgesia.[25] With these studies in mind, the use of remifentanil for spine surgery should be carefully considered especially in patients who are tolerant to narcotics prior to surgery. These patients should receive an anesthetic that includes sufficient longer-acting narcotics to avoid withdrawal and facilitate pain control. Administration of 0.2 mg/kg of methadone given as an intravenous bolus at the beginning of complex spine surgery is associated with lower opioid requirements and lower VAS scores, without additional side effects.[26]

In chronic pain patients, the intraoperative use of ketamine (0.5 mg/kg as a loading dose, and then an infusion of 10 µg/kg/min) has been associated with lower 48-hour postoperative morphine requirements; it also facilitates signal acquisition, and was not associated with an increase in side effects.[20]

Emergence

If the patient is to awaken in a timely fashion at the end of the procedure, it is extremely important that the anesthesiologist is aware of the context-sensitive half life of the drugs they are using to maintain amnesia. Context-sensitive half life is the time for the plasma concentration to decrease by 50% from an infusion that maintains a constant concentration; context refers to the duration of the infusion. Time to 50% decrease in plasma concentration was chosen because a 50% reduction in drug concentration appears to be necessary for recovery after the administration of most intravenous hypnotics (Fig. 14.1). During a long spine surgery this knowledge must be used to aggressively taper the intravenous anesthetic at the appropriate time, often more than 40 minutes prior to surgical finish. Fortunately, often during closure of the incision, the neuromonitoring team will stop monitoring and inhalational gas can be added if necessary.

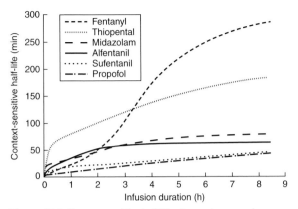

Figure 14.1 Context-sensitive half-life of several commonly used anesthetic agents. Reproduced with permission from: Hughes MA, Glass PSA, Jacobs JR, Context-sensitive half-time in multicompartment pharmacokinetic models for intravenous anesthetic drugs. *Anesthesiology* 1992;76:334–41.

Processed EEG monitoring may be somewhat helpful in determining when infusions can be tapered, although it is not an index of immobility. Studies have shown that sevoflurane and propofol affect movement to noxious stimuli differently. At an equivalent depression of BIS, sevoflurane suppresses the blink reflex more than propofol, indicating different pharmacodynamic properties of these anesthetics at brainstem level.[27] The differential level of immobility at similar levels of hypnosis makes titration of TIVA during spine surgery, without use of paralytic drugs, somewhat complex.

Care should be taken to avoid prolonged coughing and bucking on the endotracheal tube since this will stress the dural repair. Strategies to manage this include allowing the patient to return to spontaneous ventilation prior to emergence, titration of intravenous narcotics at the end of the procedure, and use of drugs like dexmedetomidine during emergence which may blunt the discomfort associated with intubation.

Postoperative management

Comprehensive postoperative care

Because the invasiveness of spinal cord tumor surgery varies so widely, it is impossible to say that a single strategy is appropriate for all patients. While there is no literature regarding the specific postoperative care of spinal cord tumor patients, it is intuitive that healthy patients having smaller surgeries can be treated like simple laminectomy patients, and that patients having larger surgeries may be more akin to complicated deformity surgery. More research is needed regarding the identification and optimization of postoperative care of the complex spine patient.

A recent study was published which elaborated one institution's experience in risk-stratifying spine patients and implementing protocolized interdisciplinary care for those patients who were deemed high risk. The program began with an identification of individuals prior to surgery with the following characteristics: more than 6 h of surgical time, more than 6 levels of surgery, plans for a staged procedure, and/or presence of high-risk medical conditions, e.g., coronary artery disease, congestive heart failure, cirrhosis, dementia, emphysema, renal insufficiency, cerebrovascular disease, pulmonary hypertension, or age greater than 80 years. This program included a preoperative multidisciplinary conference where surgeons, anesthesiologists, and critical care personnel discuss fluid management, transfusion parameters, pain control, and optimization of comorbid medical conditions.[28] The group also emphasized standardized communication for signout to the intensive care unit and use of a mechanical ventilation weaning protocol. Unfortunately, outcomes from this care plan have not yet been published.

Analgesia

There is scant literature devoted primarily to postoperative analgesia of the patient with spinal cord tumors, so the anesthesiologist can best adopt approaches used for other spinal cord procedures.[29] One approach is to use multiple analgesics from several different pharmacologic classes (e.g., opioid, GABA, NMDA receptors). Whether or not scoliosis patients are an appropriate comparison group for spinal cord tumor surgery depends on the invasiveness of the surgery. Surgery for a primary tumor of the spine might involve a laminectomy of just a few levels, whereas a metastatic tumor could involve many levels and involve comorbid surgery like en bloc resection of the chest wall and extensive instrumentation.

Postoperative analgesia for patients following spinal tumor surgery will be variably challenging depending on whether the patient had chronic pain prior to surgery and/or is narcotic tolerant. Patients who have received significant pain medications prior to surgery are likely to have even higher analgesic needs in the immediate postoperative period.

An interesting but under-studied area is the use of epidural or subarachnoid analgesia for patients following spinal surgery for tumor. Surgeons may express some concern about the implications of an epidural catheter, which can be left in place at the end of surgery,

253

or a subarachnoid injection in the sense that there may be a spread of tumor or add a risk factor for infection, or dural leak in the case of an injection. There is no literature to confirm or deny this suspicion. For non-tumor surgery, a meta-analysis of studies comparing epidural anesthesia for adolescent scoliosis surgery with morphine PCA found that average pain scores, scaled from 0–100, were lower in the epidural group, ranging from on average 15 points less on POD1 and about 10 points less on POD2, 3. Patient satisfaction scores, rated 1–10 were on average 1 point less in the epidural group. However, it is unclear whether these differences were clinically relevant. None of the studies examined in the meta-analysis were adequately designed to show whether patients who received epidural anesthesia experienced better outcomes (e.g., less respiratory depression, shorter length of ICU stay, or mortality). Studies showed mixed results regarding whether there was a difference between PCA and epidural infusion in terms of nausea, return of bowel function, pruritis, or use of rescue analgesics. The studies did not find that hypotension was associated with the need to terminate epidural anesthesia, although hypotension was not a specific end point. All of the studies suffered from some obvious flaws: lack of blinding of the groups due to the dubious ethics of placing a sham epidural catheter, and inconsistency between outcome variables between studies (total morphine dosage, formally tracking epidural complications such as hypotension and paresthesias). The authors concluded that while there is sufficient evidence to suggest the use of epidural catheters in clinical practice, better quality studies are needed to be able to track outcomes for each modality.[30]

Conclusion

Providing anesthesia for the patient undergoing resection of a spinal tumor requires an understanding of the tumor type and location. The anesthesiologist needs to discuss the planned procedure with the surgeon, including the need for intraoperative monitoring. Because many patients with spinal cord tumors have chronic pain back pain related to their tumor, it is also important to understand the patient's pain history. This information will guide the preoperative evaluation, choice of intraoperative technique, need for venous access and invasive monitoring, and challenges for postoperative management. While outcomes studies for specific perioperative management of spinal cord tumor patients are lacking, it is likely that high-risk patients will benefit from multidisciplinary comprehensive care.

References

1. Welch WC, Jacobs GB. Surgery for metastatic spinal disease. *J Neurooncol* 1995; **23**: 163–70.

2. Stacchiotti S, Casali PG, Lo Vullo S, *et al.* Chordoma of the mobile spine and sacrum: a retrospective analysis of a series of patients surgically treated at two referral centers. *Ann Surg Oncol* 2010; **17**: 211–19.

3. Park L, Delaney TF, Liebsch NJ, *et al.* Sacral chordomas: Impact of high-dose proton/photon-beam radiation therapy combined with or without surgery for primary versus recurrent tumor. *Int J Radiat Oncol Biol Phys* 2006; **65**: 1514–21.

4. Stacchiotti S, Marrari A, Tamborini E, *et al.* Response to imatinib plus sirolimus in advanced chordoma. *Ann Oncol* 2009; **20**: 1886–94.

5. Abdel-Wahab M, Etuk B, Palermo J, *et al.* Spinal cord gliomas: a multi-institutional retrospective analysis. *Int J Radiat Oncol Biol Phys* 2006; **64**: 1060–71.

6. Pica A, Miller R, Villa S, *et al.* The results of surgery, with or without radiotherapy, for primary spinal myxopapillary ependymoma: a retrospective study from the rare cancer network. *Int J Radiat Oncol Biol Phys* 2009; **74**: 1114–20.

7. Bagley CA, Wilson S, Kothbauer KF, Bookland MJ, Epstein F, Jallo GI. Long term outcomes following surgical resection of myxopapillary ependymomas. *Neurosurg Rev* 2009; **32**: 321–34; discussion 334.

8. Van Elstraete AC, Tirault M, Lebrun T, *et al.* The median effective dose of preemptive gabapentin on postoperative morphine consumption after posterior lumbar spinal fusion. *Anesth Analg* 2008; **106**: 305–8, table of contents.

9. Anderson R, Saiers JH, Abram S, Schlicht C. Accuracy in equianalgesic dosing. conversion dilemmas. *J Pain Symptom Manage* 2001; **21**: 397–406.

10. Rajpal S, Gordon DB, Pellino TA, *et al.* Comparison of perioperative oral multimodal analgesia versus IV PCA for spine surgery. *J Spinal Disord Tech* 2010; **23**: 139–45.

11. Nielsen PR, Jorgensen LD, Dahl B, Pedersen T, Tonnesen H. Prehabilitation and early rehabilitation after spinal surgery: randomized clinical trial. *Clin Rehabil* 2010; **24**: 137–48.

12. Tsirikos AI, Howitt SP, McMaster MJ. Segmental vessel ligation in patients undergoing surgery for anterior spinal deformity. *J Bone Joint Surg Br* 2008; **90**: 474–9.

13. Sala F, Bricolo A, Faccioli F, Lanteri P, Gerosa M. Surgery for intramedullary spinal cord tumors: the role of intraoperative (neurophysiological) monitoring. *Eur Spine J* 2007; **16** Suppl 2: S130–9.

14. Hyun SJ, Rhim SC, Kang JK, Hong SH, Park BR. Combined motor- and somatosensory-evoked potential monitoring for spine and spinal cord surgery: correlation of clinical and neurophysiological data in 85 consecutive procedures. *Spinal Cord* 2009; **47**: 616–22.

15. Eleraky MA, Setzer M, Papanastassiou ID, *et al.* Role of motor-evoked potential monitoring in conjunction with temporary clipping of spinal nerve roots in posterior thoracic spine tumor surgery. *Spine J* 2010; **10**: 396–403.

16. Yanni DS, Ulkatan S, Deletis V, Barrenechea IJ, Sen C, Perin NI. Utility of neurophysiological monitoring using dorsal column mapping in intramedullary spinal cord surgery. *J Neurosurg* Spine 2010; **12**: 623–8.

17. MacDonald DB. Safety of intraoperative transcranial electrical stimulation motor evoked potential monitoring. *J Clin Neurophysiol* 2002; **19**: 416–29.

18. Deiner SG, Kwatra SG, Lin HM, Weisz DJ. Patient characteristics and anesthetic technique are additive but not synergistic predictors of successful motor evoked potential monitoring. *Anesth Analg* 2010; **111**: 421–5.

19. Sloan TB, Heyer EJ. Anesthesia for intraoperative neurophysiologic monitoring of the spinal cord. *J Clin Neurophysiol* 2002; **19**: 430–43.

20. Loftus RW, Yeager MP, Clark JA, *et al.* Intraoperative ketamine reduces perioperative opiate consumption in opiate-dependent patients with chronic back pain undergoing back surgery. *Anesthesiology* 2010; **113**: 639–46.

21. Anschel DJ, Aherne A, Soto RG, *et al.* Successful intraoperative spinal cord monitoring during scoliosis surgery using a total intravenous anesthetic regimen including dexmedetomidine. *J Clin Neurophysiol* 2008; **25**: 56–61.

22. Guignard B, Bossard AE, Coste C, *et al.* Acute opioid tolerance: intraoperative remifentanil increases postoperative pain and morphine requirement. *Anesthesiology* 2000; **93**: 409–17.

23. Schmidt S, Bethge C, Forster MH, Schafer M. Enhanced postoperative sensitivity to painful pressure stimulation after intraoperative high dose remifentanil in patients without significant surgical site pain. *Clin J Pain* 2007; **23**: 605–11.

24. Shin SW, Cho AR, Lee HJ, *et al.* Maintenance anaesthetics during remifentanil-based anaesthesia might affect postoperative pain control after breast cancer surgery. *Br J Anaesth* 2010; **105**: 661–7.

25. Joly V, Richebe P, Guignard B, *et al.* Remifentanil-induced postoperative hyperalgesia and its prevention with small-dose ketamine. *Anesthesiology* 2005; **103**: 147–55.

26. Gottschalk A, Durieux ME, Nemergut EC. Intraoperative methadone improves postoperative pain control in patients undergoing complex spine surgery. *Anesth Analg* 2011 Jan; **112**(1): 218–23.

27. Sadean MR, Glass PS. Pharmacokinetic-pharmacodynamic modeling in anesthesia, intensive care and pain medicine. *Curr Opin Anaesthesiol* 2009; **22**: 463–8.

28. Halpin RJ, Sugrue PA, Gould RW, *et al.* Standardizing care for high-risk patients in spine surgery: the Northwestern high-risk spine protocol. *Spine (Phila Pa 1976)* 2010; **35**: 2232–8.

29. Borgeat A, Blumenthal S. Postoperative pain management following scoliosis surgery. *Curr Opin Anaesthesiol* 2008; **21**: 313–6.

30. Taenzer AH, Clark C. Efficacy of postoperative epidural analgesia in adolescent scoliosis surgery: a meta-analysis. *Paediatr Anaesth* 2010; **20**: 135–43.

Chapter

15

Complications

15.1 Postoperative visual loss

Lorri A. Lee and Raghu Mudumbai

Key points

- Major spine surgery in the prone position is associated with an increased risk of postoperative visual loss (POVL), and clinicians should consider informing patients of this risk preoperatively.

- Patients who are suspected of having POVL should have a full ophthalmologic examination as soon as possible, preferably by a neuro-ophthalmologist, to rule out rare treatable causes of POVL. No effective treatments for the most common causes of POVL have been identified.

- POVL caused by globe compression can be prevented by careful and frequent checking to ensure that the eyes are free of pressure in the prone position.

- Ischemic optic neuropathy (ION) after major spine surgery is associated with the prone position, male sex, use of the Wilson surgical spine frame, prolonged duration in the prone position, large blood loss, and use of a decreased percentage of colloid in the nonblood volume administration.

- Avoiding or minimizing identified risk factors for ION may decrease the occurrence of this complication. The ASA Practice Advisory for perioperative visual loss associated with spine surgery provides some guidance on these issues, though definitive controlled studies are lacking.

Introduction

Blindness or debilitating loss of vision is one of the most devastating complications that can occur in patients undergoing major spine surgery. Vision impairment coupled with preexisting mobility impairment from spinal disease can have a profound impact on productivity and the quality of life. The incidence of POVL after spine surgery varies among institutions and ranges from 0.03% to 0.2% using national databases and multicenter studies.[1-3] It is unclear whether this variation is caused by differences in patient characteristics, perioperative management, or the types of spine operations performed at various centers. Recent studies from national databases have suggested that the prevalence of all types of POVL may be decreasing.[1]

POVL is most common after cardiac bypass, prone spine, and head and neck procedures.[1,4] It is also increased relative to abdominal procedures in other major orthopedic procedures such as hip and knee replacements.[1] For reasons that are unclear, children appear to have an increased prevalence of POVL associated with spine surgery, primarily from cortical blindness.[1] The suggested causes of POVL are numerous and include globe compression, emboli, anemia, hypotension, prolonged venous congestion/prone position, volume or type of fluid administration, and patients' preexisting disease or aberrant physiology and anatomy.[4] Despite this long list of potential etiologies, only globe compression has been shown to reproducibly cause central retinal artery occlusion (CRAO) in a primate model.[5] The paucity of evidence-based medicine on this topic is primarily due to the low incidence of this complication; the multiple different types of POVL; the multiple different perioperative physiologic derangements that occur in different procedures; the inability to perform randomized controlled trials given the severity of the outcome; and the technical difficulties involved in measuring optic nerve blood flow or optic nerve function under anesthesia in humans or in experimental animal models.

Evaluation and differential diagnosis for POVL after major spine surgery

The vast majority of POVL cases associated with major spine surgery are caused by CRAO, anterior and posterior ischemic optic neuropathy (AION, PION), and cortical blindness. Other extremely rare diagnoses that are possible in this setting include central retinal vein occlusion, acute angle closure glaucoma, posterior reversible encephalopathy syndrome (PRES), retinal detachment, direct globe injury, and intracranial hemorrhage.[4] Evaluation for POVL should be done as soon as possible after the initial complaint with a full ophthalmologic work-up with dilated funduscopic examination. Although the most common causes of POVL after major spine surgery have no known beneficial treatment, a complete ophthalmologic examination, which may include dilated funduscopic examination, should eliminate very rare but potentially treatable conditions from the differential diagnosis such as acute angle closure glaucoma, direct globe injury, and retinal detachment.[4,7] Significant delay in the dilated funduscopic examination may also preclude the ability to distinguish AION from PION, as these two injuries have a similar appearance many weeks to months after the injury.[4,7] Specific funduscopic findings can diagnose CRAO related to emboli or globe compression. Computed tomography or magnetic resonance imaging of the head are frequently performed to rule out acute intracranial processes such as cortical emboli, occipital infarction, or intracranial hemorrhage, including previously unsuspected pituitary apoplexy leading to a compressive optic neuropathy.[4,6] The technology in these neuroimaging examinations is currently unable to reliably detect optic nerve infarction. Electroretinograms to assess retinal function, fluorescein angiograms to assess filling of the retinal vasculature, and visual evoked potentials to assess optic nerve function may be useful for further confirmation of specific diagnoses or when patient cooperation is suboptimal. Transcranial Doppler and carotid duplex

Doppler may be useful for detecting embolic phenomena and assessing the extent of any carotid disease.[4,7]

Central retinal artery occlusion (CRAO)

CRAO after spine surgery was originally described in 1954 by Hollenhorst, an ophthalmologist, in association with eight cases of unilateral visual loss in the prone position on the horseshoe headrest.[5] He then replicated this injury in primates by compression of the globe. Consequently, it has also been referred to as the "Hollenhorst" or "headrest" syndrome. The mechanism in this setting is increased intraocular pressure causing occlusion of the inner retinal blood supply (Fig. 15.1). Experimental studies in monkeys have demonstrated that irreversible damage can occur within approximately 105 minutes.[6] CRAO can also be caused by emboli or hypercoagulable states, particularly in the nonoperative setting.[4,7] CRAO is typically unilateral with severe or total loss of vision (Table 15.1). Because the visual loss is severe, patients usually complain of it as soon as they are lucid after awakening from anesthesia. Patients frequently have associated ipsilateral periorbital trauma such as bruising, ophthalmoplegia, proptosis, erythema, or abrasions when caused by globe compression.[4,7,8] The pupillary light reflex will be absent or sluggish, with a relative afferent pupillary defect if unilateral. A classic cherry-red spot at the fovea with a whitened ischemic retina is found on funduscopic examination (Fig 15.2A). The fovea is the thinnest part of the retina. The cherry-red spot is "created" by a separate blood supply under the fovea, the choriocapillaris, which continues to perfuse this area after the central retinal artery has become occluded.[4,7] Electroretinograms will be abnormal with a depressed "b" wave.[4] Fluorescein angiograms will show a marked delay in filling of the central retinal artery, and slowed filling of the venous circulation as a result. Visual recovery is poor and there is no known beneficial treatment to date. Within 1–2 months, a pale optic disc can be found on funduscopic examination as a result of antegrade degeneration of the optic nerve subsequent to death of the inner retinal layers.[4,7] Arterial collaterals may develop and the white retina and cherry-red spot will disappear.

Anterior ischemic optic neuropathy (AION)

AION is divided into arteritic and nonarteritic forms. Arteritic AION secondary to temporal arteritis is extremely rare perioperatively, and will not be discussed further in this chapter. Nonarteritic AION is a form of POVL that occurs in the community more commonly

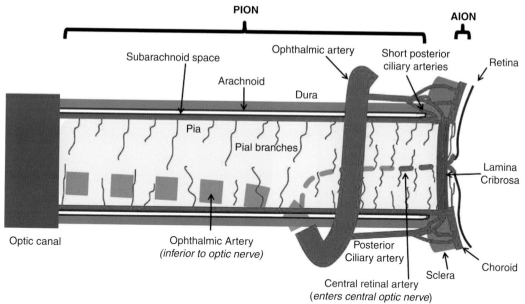

Figure 15.1 Schematic drawing of the optic nerve and blood supply. Central retinal artery occlusion (CRAO) from globe compression occurs through elevated intraocular pressure compressing the inner retinal blood supply anteriorly. It can also be caused by embolic occlusion of the central retinal artery posterior to the globe. Brackets denote areas of the optic nerve affected by anterior ischemic optic neuropathy (AION) and posterior ischemic optic neuropathy (PION).

than the other causes of POVL, and is the most common cause of sudden loss of vision in patients older than 50 years. In the community-acquired form, advanced age, chronic obstructive pulmonary disease, nocturnal hypotension, hypercoagulable disease, diabetes, cerebrovascular and cardiac atherosclerotic disease, and hypertension are associated with its occurrence, although the exact etiology is unknown.[9,10] Patients also typically exhibit a small cup:disc ratio (optic disc measurements from funduscopic examination), which increases their vulnerability to the vasculopathic risk factors.[10] Less commonly, it can occur in healthy individuals. Perioperative AION is more frequent after cardiac bypass procedures than after major spine surgery, and has also been reported after major vascular procedures, abdominal compartment syndrome, liposuction, prostatectomies, and other miscellaneous procedures. Suggested predisposing factors for this perioperative injury from case reports and case series include hypotension, anemia, large fluid shifts with a high volume resuscitation, high crystalloid volume resuscitation, coexisting vascular disease, and a small cup:disc ratio.[4,7] Because of confounding factors with patient populations, perioperative characteristics, and specific procedures, actual risk factors cannot be determined from case reports and case series where denominator data of unaffected patients is not provided. AION affects

the optic nerve head anterior to the lamina cribrosa, a sievelike piece of connective tissue through which the optic nerve and central retinal vessels pass on their way to the globe. Some experts have conjectured that this injury is caused by swelling at the optic nerve head that constricts the blood supply of the optic nerve at the semirigid lamina cribrosa (Fig 15.1).[4,7]

Onset of visual loss can occur immediately on awakening up to several days postoperatively (Table 15.1). Patients may have seemingly normal vision for a few days, and then have sudden onset of visual loss that progresses over a few days. Altitudinal field cuts, central scotoma, or complete loss of vision can occur either unilaterally or bilaterally. Light reflexes are diminished to absent in affected eyes. If the disease is unilateral, there may be a relative afferent pupillary defect.[4,7] An edematous optic disc with blurring of the disc margin is present on funduscopic examination. Splinter or peripapillary flame-shaped hemorrhages may be present in the periphery (Fig. 15.2B). These features of optic disc edema and peripheral hemorrhages distinguish AION from PION, as the latter displays a normal optic disc in the early postoperative period. Visual evoked potentials will be abnormal with significant visual loss. Both the swelling of the optic disc and the hemorrhages subside over several weeks to months, and the optic disc becomes pale. Attenuated arterioles may be

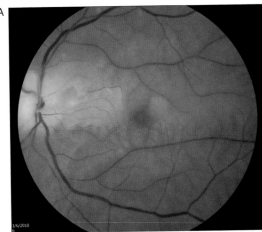

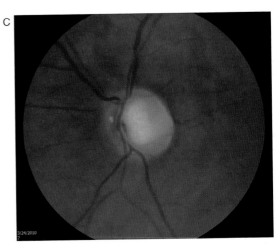

Figures 15.2A–D. Funduscopic photographs of central retinal artery occlusion (CRAO), and anterior and posterior ischemic optic neuropathy (AION, PION) at various stages. (Photographs courtesy of Raghu Mudumbai, M.D., University of Washington, Seattle, WA, USA)

Figure 15.2A Resolving CRAO. Note the prominent central cherry-red spot resulting from the unaffected vascular blush of the choriocapillaris circulation at the fovea, the thinnest area of the retina. Reperfused retina can be seen along with whitened ischemic retina.

Figure 15.2C Resolving AION. Note the optic nerve pallor with attenuation of retinal arterioles. Both AION and PION demonstrate a normal retina with optic nerve pallor several months after the injury.

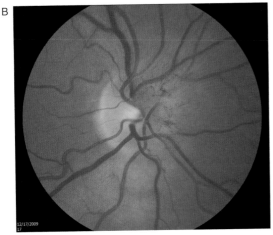

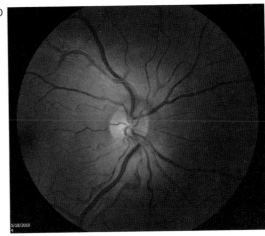

Figure 15.2D Normal fundus and early fundoscopic appearance of PION

Figure 15.2B Acute AION. Blurring of the optic disc margin is from edema. Peripheral hemorrhage is noted superiorly and to the right of the disc.

present. At this point, AION and PION appear identical on examination, with optic disc pallor (Fig 15.2C). No treatment has currently been proven beneficial for this injury. Recovery of vision is typically poor.[4,7]

Posterior ischemic optic neuropathy (PION)

PION is rarer in the community than AION and is typically associated perioperatively with procedures that increase the venous pressure in the head such as prone spine surgery, bilateral head and neck surgery, cardiac operations, and operations performed in steep Trendelenburg position such as the newer robotic-assisted laparoscopic prostatectomies.[4,7,11,12] PION occurs posterior to the lamina cribrosa where the blood supply to the optic nerve has poor collateral supply and is supplied by tiny threadlike pial vessels. It can occur anywhere in the intraorbital component of the optic nerve (Fig. 15.1).[4,7] Suggested predisposing factors for PION from case reports and case series include operations or positions with prolonged duration of elevated venous pressure of the head, hypotension, anemia, large fluid shifts with high volume resuscitation, high crystalloid volume resuscitation,

Table 15.1 Most common causes of postoperative visual loss after major spine surgery

	CRAO	AION	PION	Cortical blindness
Associated procedures	Prone spine surgery; head and neck surgery	Cardiac bypass; prone spine surgery; miscellaneous cases such as prostatectomy, major vascular cases, liposuction, abdominal compartment syndrome	Prone spine surgery, head and neck surgery, cardiac bypass procedures	Cardiac bypass, major orthopedic surgery, events with profound and prolonged hypotension
Postoperative symptom onset[a]	Immediate	Can be immediate, but frequently after first postoperative day	Mostly immediate	Immediate
No. of affected eyes	Unilateral	Slightly more bilateral	Mostly bilateral	Bilateral visual field deficits
Visual field	Usually severe to complete loss of vision	Altitudinal field cuts; central scotoma; or complete loss of vision	Altitudinal field cuts; central scotoma; or complete loss of vision	Homonymous hemianopsia to complete bilateral loss of vision
Pupillary light reflex	Very sluggish to absent; RAPD if unilateral	Sluggish to absent; RAPD if unilateral	Sluggish to absent; RAPD if unilateral	Normal. Never associated with a RAPD
Early funduscopic examination	Cherry-red spot; ischemic whitened retina	Edematous optic disc with blurred disc margin; splinter or peripapillary flame-shaped hemorrhages	Normal	Normal
Late funduscopic examination	If recanalized, then see retinal arterial narrowing; optic nerve pallor; possible neovascularization of iris or disc (rare)	Optic disc pallor; normal retina with attenuated arterioles. (Hemorrhage and edema subsides)	Optic disc pallor; normal retina with attenuated arterioles	Normal
Recovery	Poor	Poor	Poor	Fair depending on cause
Proven treatment	None	None	None	None
Suggested predisposing factors[b]	Globe compression; emboli, hypotension	Coexisting vascular disease; small cup:disc ratio; hypotension; anemia; large volume resuscitation; large crystalloid volume resuscitation	Elevated venous pressure of the head; hypotension; anemia; large volume resuscitation; large crystalloid volume resuscitation; coexisting vascular disease; male sex	Emboli; severe hypotension; anemia
Risk factors identified from experimental animal models or large case control studies for spine surgery	Globe compression[5]	Male sex; obesity; use of Wilson frame; greater blood loss; longer duration; lower percent of colloid in the nonblood fluid administration[22]		

CRAO, central retinal artery occlusion; AION, anterior ischemic optic neuropathy; PION, posterior ischemic optic neuropathy; RAPD, relative afferent pupillary defect.
[a] When the patient is lucid and able to communicate.
[b] Suggested predisposing factors not proven except for globe compression for CRAO.

and coexisting vascular disease.[4,7] The exact mechanism of this injury is unknown, but the leading theory is that the elevated venous pressures, inflammation, and large volume administration result in severe interstitial fluid accumulation and edema. This edema causes a compartment syndrome of the optic nerve, compromising both inflow and outflow of the blood supply and resulting in critical reductions in perfusion pressure and oxygen delivery. Ischemia and eventual infarction of the optic nerve result.[4,7,8]

Onset of visual loss from PION is immediate on awakening from anesthesia, but complaints may be delayed because of postoperative mechanical ventilation with sedation, delirium, or occasionally, patients' mistaken belief that they are experiencing a "normal" temporary side effect of anesthesia (Table 15.1).

PION symptoms do not usually worsen after the initial complaint.[13] The lack of progression of disease may be caused by two factors. First, the severity of PION after major spine surgery is typically quite severe, so there may be less remaining vision to lose.[13] Second, the prone position and venous congestion appear to be precipitators of PION. Completion of surgery and returning the patient to the supine position may immediately remove or lessen this physiologic stress. Patients with complete or near-complete visual loss from any cause may experience flashes of light or other visual disturbances or hallucinations for many weeks to months. Bilateral PION after major spine surgery is more common than unilateral involvement.[13] Similarly to AION, visual field deficits may manifest as altitudinal field cuts, central scotoma, or complete loss of vision. Pupillary responses are sluggish to absent. A relative afferent pupillary defect may be present with unilateral involvement. As noted above, PION has a normal funduscopic examination early (Fig. 15.2D), but many weeks to months later, optic disc pallor develops and attenuated arterioles may be present (Fig. 15.3C). Visual evoked potentials will be abnormal with significant visual loss. No known beneficial treatment has been demonstrated for PION, and visual recovery is poor.[4,7]

The distinction between AION and PION can be difficult to make on funduscopic examination because the subtleties of optic disc swelling can be challenging to identify for all but the most experienced neuro-ophthalmologists. It is particularly difficult when examinations are not performed close to the time of injury. Moreover, Sadda and colleagues documented one patient who developed perioperative PION in one eye and AION in the other eye.[13] However, when the perioperative characteristics and the coexisting diseases of patients are very similar or nearly identical, the distinction between perioperative AION and PION may be less relevant when trying to ascertain etiology.[7]

Cortical blindness

Cortical blindness is associated with events or procedures in which there are large showers of pulmonary emboli, such as cardiac bypass and major orthopedic surgery, or with profound hypotension where watershed infarctions may occur.[4,7] Either etiology is possible during major spine surgery, though this injury is much less common after major spine surgery than are AION, PION, or CRAO. One transesophageal echo study has shown that many emboli are released during major spine surgery, especially during pedicle screw insertion.[14] The presence of a right-to-left shunt such as a patent foramen ovale would allow passage of these emboli to the arterial circulation. Some clinicians have advocated preoperative closure of known patent foramen ovale prior to major spine surgery, but the risk:benefit ratio of this practice has not been studied with adequately powered trials. Visual loss from cortical blindness is usually noted on awakening from anesthesia or when the patient is first lucid (Table 15.1). Visual field defects range from a homonymous hemianopsia with unilateral lesions to complete blindness with bilateral lesion that may spare small islands of central fixation. Pupillary light reflexes and funduscopic examination are normal. Computed tomography or magnetic resonance imaging will demonstrate occipital infarction(s) from emboli, or parieto-occipital watershed infarctions when profound hypotension is the presumed etiology. Recovery from cortical blindness is better than from CRAO, AION, or PION.[4]

The ASA POVL Registry

The ASA POVL Registry was created in 1999 in response to a perceived increase in the number of cases of POVL, particularly after spine surgery.[3,8] At this time, there was little knowledge in the fields of surgery and anesthesiology about the multiple different types of POVL, the differences in the light reflexes and funduscopic examination for these diagnoses, the importance of timing of the examination, and the multiple different possible causes of the different POVL diagnoses. As with many rare diseases, it was primarily the specialists in the field, neuro-ophthalmologists, who began to educate anesthesiologists and surgeons regarding these differences. In fact, it appeared that the most frequent cause of POVL after major spine surgery in adults was ION. Though AION was known to occur in the community, most of the cases were diagnosed with PION. This finding indicated there was something unique about spine surgery in the prone position that was precipitating this acute injury.

The ASA POVL Registry began accepting voluntary submissions of POVL cases occurring within 2 weeks after nonocular surgery in 1999. Although the voluntary nature of the registry introduced the possibility of bias in submission, this complication was relatively uncommon, and would require an extremely large number of centers to produce a meaningful number of cases with a prospective study. A detailed data collection form was created to collect all variables considered potentially relevant to the etiology of the injury. With surgeons, anesthesiologists, and neuro-ophthalmologists working together, the ASA POVL Registry was able to collect 93 cases of POVL occurring after major spine surgery and to provide a perioperative profile of the types of POVL diagnoses encountered and their perioperative characteristics.[8]

Of the 93 cases reported in 2006 by the ASA POVL Registry, 83 cases were diagnosed with ION (19 AION, 56 PION, 8 unspecified ION), and 10 cases with CRAO. A subset analysis of the AION and PION cases did not reveal any significant differences in the perioperative profile with respect to coexisting conditions, hemodynamics, fluid or transfusion management, type of procedure, number of eyes affected, or severity of disease. Because of this homogeneity of groups in collected data, AION and PION groups were combined for this analysis.[8]

Perioperative profile comparison of CRAO and ION patients

When the perioperative characteristics of the 10 CRAO cases were compared with the 83 ION cases, several distinct differences emerged. CRAO cases had a significantly shorter operative time (mean 6.5 ± 2.2 hours for CRAO compared with 9.8 ± 3.1 hours for ION); decreased estimated blood loss (EBL) (median 0.75 liters with a range of 0.5–1.8 liters for CRAO compared with 2.0 liters with a range of 0.1–25 liters for ION); decreased crystalloid administration (mean 4.6 ± 1.7 liters for CRAO compared with 9.7 ± 4.7 liters for ION); no bilateral disease (0 for CRAO compared with 66% for ION); decreased use of Mayfield pins (0 for CRAO compared with 19% for ION); and an increased presence of ipsilateral periorbital trauma (70% for CRAO compared with 1% for ION).[8] These differing patterns between groups are consistent with globe compression causing CRAO, where the injury takes less time to develop and blood loss and volume administration may be less relevant. The associated ipsilateral periorbital trauma and unilateral disease are also consistent with an external mechanical compressive etiology. The high proportion of bilateral disease in the ION group, the large fluid shifts, and the occurrence of ION with patients' heads being in Mayfield pins is consistent with a systemic physiologic etiology.

Coexisting conditions of ION patients

The relatively rare occurrence of this complication with similar procedures and anesthetic management

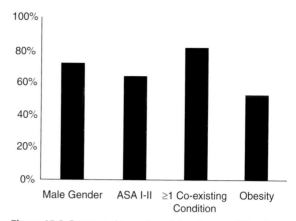

Figure 15.3 Demographics and coexisting diseases of 83 patients with ischemic optic neuropathy associated with major spine surgery. From the American Society of Anesthesiologists POVL Registry.[8]

in the same institutions or across institutions implies intrinsic predisposing factors for ION. Demographic characteristics revealed a higher proportion of men (72%) with ION in the ASA POVL Registry than in the National Inpatient Sample (NIS) data for spinal fusion operations for corresponding years where there was a relatively equal proportion between the sexes.[1,8] The predilection for this injury in men is reminiscent of perioperative ulnar nerve injuries, which had a similar preponderance (70%).[15] Some experimental evidence suggests that animal estrogens may have a protective effect on mitochondrial dysfunction in a specific optic neuropathy disease with a higher male prevalence.[16] Mean age of the ASA POVL Registry patients was 50 ± 14 years with a range of 16–73 years. Though 82% of the 83 ION cases had at least one coexisting vascular condition, 64% of this group were ASA I–II (Fig. 15.3).[8] Unlike community-acquired AION and PION cases, these patients appeared to be somewhat healthier.[13] Approximately half of the ION cases were associated with obesity (53%).

Predetermined procedural factors of ION patients

Surgical procedures were noted to have 89% instrumented operations with just over one-third (39%) as revision cases. More than one level was fused in 77% of cases (11% one level; 12% an unknown number of levels).[8] Only 4 of the 83 ION cases (5%) had the operation confined to the cervical location, whereas 69% were in the lumbar or lumbosacral region. The most common type of surgical frame utilized for ION cases was the Wilson frame (30%), where the head is typically in a

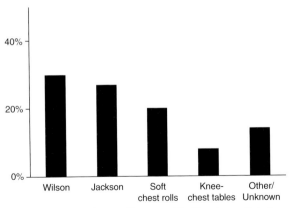

Figure 15.4 Type of surgical frame used for 83 patients with ischemic optic neuropathy associated with major spine surgery. From the American Society of Anesthesiologists POVL Registry.[8]

dependent position relative to the heart (Fig. 15.4). This frame combined with the prone position may greatly elevate the venous pressure in the head. The Jackson frame (27%) and soft chest rolls (20%) were the next most common frames associated with ION cases. Ten of the 83 ION cases (12%) were performed with an anterior–posterior approach, 2 cases were anterior only, and 71 cases (86%) were performed with the posterior approach only. The type of headrest most commonly used was a soft foam cushion (57%) followed by Mayfield pins (19%), where the head is suspended in air with the face free of pressure, and donut or gel pads (8%).[8] This finding provided irrefutable evidence that ION occurs in the absence of pressure on the globe, and that the etiology of this injury most likely arises systemically, not by direct external forces.

Intraoperative procedural factors of ION patients

The mean anesthetic time was 9.8 ± 3.1 hours with a mean prone duration of 7.7 ± 3.1 hours. Only 6% of cases involved less than 6 hours anesthetic time.[8] This finding is consistent with the theory that this injury is precipitated by elevated venous pressures in the head resulting in a compartment syndrome with a critical reduction in perfusion pressure to the optic nerve. Ischemic injuries caused by a compartment syndrome require a considerably longer time to develop than acute reductions in arterial inflow. Median estimated blood loss (EBL) was 2.0 liters with a range of 0.1–25 liters. Only 18% of cases had an EBL < 1.0 liter. Given this large EBL, anemia was common and the mean nadir hematocrit (Hct) was 26 ± 5%, yet 17% of cases never had a Hct below 30%.[8]

Fluid management of ION patients

Fluid replacement varied, with 30% of cases using colloid (albumin or hydroxyethyl starch). Crystalloid replacement was 9.7 ± 4.7 liters. Cell saver (54%) and packed red blood cells (57%) were used in approximately half of the ION cases.[8] Despite seemingly adequate volume replacement, urine output was < 0.5 ml/kg/h in almost one-quarter of cases. Creatinine increased postoperatively in 6 cases and rhabdomyolysis occurred in 3 cases.

Management of volume resuscitation is frequently criticized in ION cases without regard for the EBL or degree of hypotension. Failure to infuse volume with ongoing large blood loss will result in cardiovascular collapse. Further, the physiology of the prone position with increased intra-abdominal and intrathoracic pressure in that position results in decreased venous return and decreased cardiac output. Large volume shifts will increase the degree of inflammation, capillary leak, and edema formation, particularly when performed with elevated venous pressures in the prone position. Some anesthesiologists advocate the use of colloid and limiting the amount of crystalloid in an attempt to minimize the interstitial tissue edema, but controlled studies have not been performed in this setting. Recent evidence indicates that certain types of colloid such as hydroxyethyl starch, gelatin, and dextran are harmful in critically ill patients in a dose-related manner.[17] Albumin has also been shown to increase mortality in traumatically brain-injured patients.[18] and many studies have demonstrated the hazards of blood transfusion in ICU patients. However, none of these fluids – crystalloids, colloids, or blood – has been studied in randomized controlled trials for major spine surgery. The clinical scenario of acute major blood loss over a finite period is very different from the critically ill patient in the ICU. Further research on the optimal fluid and transfusion management strategy for these patients is needed.

Blood pressure management of ION patients

Significant variation existed for blood pressure values measured as absolute values or as percent below a patient's baseline values for a minimum of 15 consecutive or nonconsecutive minutes. Extremes existed on both the high and low ends, with 13% of ION cases having their lowest systolic blood pressures greater than 100 mmHg, while 20% of cases had their lowest systolic blood pressure at 80 mmHg or lower. The remainder of patients had their lowest blood pressure between 81 and 100 mmHg (unknown 4%).[8] Deliberate hypotension was utilized in one-quarter of cases, but this value was not strictly defined in the study.

What is clear from these data is that ION can develop in the absence of significant hypotension. Deliberate hypotension has been utilized in spine surgery for many decades with the goal of reducing blood loss and transfusion. Despite this long history of using deliberate hypotension, uniform agreement on its precise definition is lacking. Some clinicians define it as 20–30 mmHg below baseline awake systolic blood pressures, some describe it as 30–40% below baseline awake values, while others use an absolute number varying anywhere from a mean arterial blood pressure of 50–70 mmHg.[19–21] Several studies have demonstrated reduced blood loss and transfusion with the use of deliberate hypotension, but the benefit in reduced operating time is equivocal.[19–21] One of the few randomized controlled trials found that 5 of 24 patients had somatosensory evoked potential monitoring changes that prompted reversal of hypotension.[20] The majority of the prospective studies on deliberate hypotension in spine surgery had very small numbers of patients (< 25 per group) and were not powered to detect low-incidence complications such as ION or spinal cord damage. Further, many of these studies were performed more than 25 years ago and the duration of operations was approximately 3–4 hours.[21] Thus, the risk:benefit ratio of this technique for major spine surgery with prolonged duration remains undetermined.

Ophthalmologic findings of ION patients

The median time from the end of surgery to reporting of symptoms was 15 hours, excluding one patient with prolonged mechanical ventilation. Two-thirds of ION patients (66%) had both eyes affected, and 57% of patients had complete blindness in the affected eye(s). Some recovery of vision occurred in 42% of patients, although the extent of recovery was often minimal.[8] No patients returned to baseline vision. Treatment varied and included hyperbaric oxygen, mannitol, vasopressors to increase perfusion pressure, transfusion to increase the hematocrit to 30% or greater, and steroids.[8] No discernible pattern of improvement based on treatment was detectable in this study. The bilateral involvement of this injury in two-thirds of patients implicates a systemic etiology. The severity of injury on presentation frequently precluded measurable progression of disease and was a poor prognostic indicator of recovery for an ischemic injury.

The ASA POVL Registry case–control study

Using cases from the ASA POVL Registry, the largest case–control study to date of ION associated with major spine surgery was performed with controls undergoing similar spine operations who did not develop ION from 17 academic centers in North America.[22] This study was unique in that it had the largest number of ION cases from the same type of procedure and it used detailed perioperative data from hospital records, thus allowing control of potential confounding factors. Each case was matched to four controls from a total database of controls of 43 410 who underwent spinal fusion surgery. Cases and controls were matched for year of surgery to avoid effects of changes in practice over time. Inclusion criteria were age >18 years; spinal fusion operation between 1991 and 2006 as the first or only spine operation on the index admission; surgical site including the thoracic, lumbar, or sacral region; surgery in the prone position for at least a portion of the procedure; and anesthetic duration of 4 or more hours. Exclusion criteria were incomplete medical records, history of perioperative cardiopulmonary resuscitation or stroke, or multiple staged procedures preceding ION on the index admission. Controls were also excluded for any POVL. A total of 80 ION cases were matched to 315 controls.

Using stepwise multivariate logistic regression, independent risk factors for ION associated with spinal fusion surgery were male sex, obesity, use of the Wilson surgical spine frame, increasing anesthetic duration, increasing blood loss, and use of a decreased percentage of colloid in the nonblood volume administration (Table 15.2).[22] Although significant in the univariate analysis ($p < 0.05$), blood pressure less than 40% below baseline for a minimum of 30 minutes, and lowest hematocrit were not independent risk factors in the multivariate logistic regression. This finding indicates that hypotension and anemia were correlated with other risk factors with a stronger effect such as blood loss, duration, or fluid administration. This analysis with detailed perioperative information emphasizes the limitations of national databases that utilize billing records to ascertain perioperative factors contributing to a physiologic complication.

Other outcome studies

Ho and coworkers performed a literature search in 2005 of all cases of ION after spine surgery and found

Table 15.2 Risk factors associated with ischemic optic neuropathy after spinal fusion surgery: multivariate regression model[22]

Variable	Odds ratio (OR)	95% Confidence interval	p value
Male sex	2.53	1.35–4.91	0.005
Obesity	2.83	1.52–5.39	0.001
Wilson frame use	4.30	2.13–8.75	<0.001
Estimated blood loss (liters), OR per liter	1.34	1.13–1.61	0.001
Anesthetic duration (hours), OR per hour	1.39	1.22–1.58	<0.001
Colloid as % of nonblood replacement, OR per 5%	0.67	0.52–0.82	<0.001

Risk factors associated with ischemic optic neuropathy (ION) after spinal fusion surgery identified from a case-control study utilizing 80 ION cases from the American Society of Anesthesiologists POVL Registry and matched by year to 315 control patients who underwent similar spinal fusion procedures without visual loss.[22]

22 cases (5 AION and 17 PION).[23] Their analysis was similar to the ASA POVL Registry in that the cases were associated with prolonged duration (mean operative time 450 minutes) and large blood loss (1.7 liters for AION and 5 liters for PION). The lowest mean Hct was 27%, and the lowest mean arterial blood pressure was 64 mmHg. Resuscitation volumes were large because of large EBL, with mean crystalloid/colloid volumes of 6.6/0.8 liters for AION and 8.0/2.2 liters for PION.[23] Although the type of colloid is not specified, these results demonstrate that large amounts of colloid will not prevent the occurrence of ION. This finding by itself may indicate that the composition of the fluid may be less important than the total volume shift, the duration in the prone position, and other factors that may promote swelling in the head.

Myers and colleagues published the first case–control study of POVL after spine surgery in 1997 by gathering cases of POVL with medical records from the Scoliosis Research Society.[24] The perioperative characteristics of a group of 28 patients who developed POVL after major spine surgery in the prone position were compared with a matched group of 28 patients who were of similar age and underwent similar spine procedures but did not develop POVL. The authors found that the lowest hematocrit and lowest systolic blood pressure did not differ between groups. However, the POVL group had a significantly longer operative time (430 minutes for the POVL group compared with 250 minutes for the control group, $p < 0.05$) and larger EBL (3600 ml for the POVL group compared with 880 ml for the control group).[24] This study was performed before there was good dissemination of knowledge regarding the multiple different POVL diagnoses and their different etiologies. Consequently, all POVL diagnoses were combined in the POVL group, thereby preventing correlation with specific POVL diagnoses. Further,

the durations of the lowest blood pressures were not specified. Despite these limitations, the results from this study are very consistent with the findings from the POVL Registry, where the affected ION cases also had very long procedures with large EBL.

Holy and coworkers published a more recent case–control study from a single institution.[25] They identified 17 patients who developed ION from multiple different procedures from a database of 126 666 surgical procedures. ION patients were each matched with two control patients who had similar procedures but did have POVL. Further, the researchers were able to obtain ophthalmologic examinations on 20 of the 34 control patients. The authors found no significant difference in any of the variables examined between groups including coexisting conditions, body mass index, cup:disc ratio, operative duration, EBL, lowest mean arterial blood pressure, lowest hematocrit, transfusion amount, and use of vasopressors.[25] Subgroup analysis of AION, PION, and CABG groups also revealed no differences between POVL and control groups. The authors did note that they had an exceptionally high preponderance of men affected by ION in their study (94%), consistent with findings from the ASA POVL Registry[8] and Shen's study using National Inpatient Sample (NIS) data.[1] However, the combination of different procedures with strikingly different physiologic perturbations, and the low number of patients in each subgroup, may have prevented the detection of significant differences between ION patients and controls.

Two studies using NIS data are notable for their different findings. Patil's study examining POVL after spine surgery from 1993 to 2002 revealed an overall POVL incidence of 0.094%, with the highest incidence in posterior lumbar fusion (0.28%) and scoliosis reconstruction (0.14%).[2] They found that both extremes of age, <18 years and >84 years, had heightened risks for developing non-ION, non-CRAO POVL. Coexisting conditions such as hypertension and peripheral vascular disease also increased the odds of developing non-ION, non-CRAO POVL, as did blood transfusion. For ION, they identified hypotension, peripheral vascular disease, and anemia as risk factors with high odds ratios favoring its occurrence. [2] However, the accuracy of the NIS database is unverifiable, and although routine demographic variables and some procedural factors are recorded consistently for each patient, many variables such as coexisting diseases and perioperative events such as anemia and hypotension may not be identified or may be entered inconsistently. Moreover, complications may engender a more rigorous search for specific conditions. For example, a patient who develops POVL may have his or her anesthetic record examined thoroughly for signs of hypotension, whereas a patient who does not develop POVL or other complications will be unlikely to have his or her intraoperative blood pressure examined. Although the two anesthetics may have had similar blood pressures that fell below an arbitrary definition of hypotension, only the patient with POVL would have this listed as a diagnosis for entry into the NIS database. Therefore, the findings of hypotension, anemia, and peripheral vascular disease as risk factors for developing POVL may be a result of inconsistent and biased data reporting. Additionally, other important variables for ION were not available from the NIS data, such as surgical frame type, operative time, EBL, and type of fluid administration. The findings of anemia and hypotension may be a confounding factor that serves as a surrogate marker for some of these other variables, as noted in the ASA POVL Registry case–control study.[22]

Shen and coworkers avoided analysis of variables such as hypotension that were unlikely to be examined thoroughly for all cases.[1] Their analysis confirmed an increased risk of POVL for cardiac, spinal fusion, and orthopedic surgery compared with abdominal surgery. Using demographic data for spinal fusion surgery, they found that patients <18 years old had an OR of 18.3 of developing POVL ($p < 0.0001$), primarily caused by cortical blindness. Male sex conferred an OR of 1.65 ($p = 0.002$) of developing POVL, and prone position an OR of 4.16 ($p = 0.0001$) for POVL occurrence.[1] Anemia had an OR of 1.65 ($p = 0.03$) for POVL complications, but as noted above, this may reflect the tendency of these cases to be of long duration and involve large blood loss.

Intraoperative monitoring for optic nerve injury

Many observational studies have been performed using intraocular pressure (IOP) as a surrogate marker of vascular congestion in the head during major spine surgery. These studies have consistently demonstrated a significant increase in IOP immediately on turning prone, and then a gradual increase with time in that position. These results are consistent with Goldman's equation, whereby IOP = rate of aqueous humor formation divided by the outflow of aqueous humor + episcleral venous pressure, and the fact that central venous pressure increases in the prone position. The observation that IOPs continue to increase over time in the prone position while central venous pressure is relatively stable after turning indicates that other localized effects influence the IOP. Most studies have reported $\geq 100\%$ increase in IOP from baseline after 3 or more hours with fairly symmetric values between eyes.[26] On the patient turning supine, IOP values decrease sharply again, but not to baseline values. Despite studies demonstrating mean IOPs as high as 40 mmHg by the end of surgery,[26] no ION injuries were reported in any of these studies. It is unclear how IOP correlates with the venous or interstitial pressure of the posterior optic nerve where most of the ION injuries occur. Given the shape, most dependent position, and vasculature of the globe, it is very possible that the engorgement and back pressure are much greater in the anterior compartment than farther posteriorly. Although unlikely to offer a useful monitor for detection of optic nerve injury in individual patients, these studies do provide useful information regarding the ocular physiological changes during prone spine surgery. Similar IOP findings have been demonstrated in robotically assisted laparoscopic prostatectomies in which the patient is positioned in a steep head-down position.[27] Interestingly, these patients also appear to be at risk of developing ION as three cases of PION have already been reported to the ASA POVL Registry from this relatively new procedure.[28]

Visual evoked potentials (VEPs) have been utilized with limited success in neurosurgical procedures involving the optic nerve, though the use of total intravenous anesthesia has improved their reliability somewhat. One study using VEPs during noncranial procedures under anesthesia with total intravenous anesthesia reported that only 4 of 30 patients had stable intraoperative VEP recordings, and that 14 of 30 patients had fewer than half of their recordings with identifiable waveforms.[29] Further research on this monitoring modality is needed before it can be recommended for routine clinical practice. Other groups are currently attempting to use pupillometry to measure changes in the pupillary light reflex as a means of detecting optic nerve dysfunction under anesthesia. However, the standard use of moderate- to high-dose opioids that alter pupillary size during major spine surgery may inhibit its usefulness.

The major difficulty with developing a new intraoperative monitor to detect optic nerve dysfunction is that the sensitivity will need to be tested in procedures where there is a higher incidence of optic nerve injury, such as intracranial tumors or aneurysms that affect the optic nerves and cortical pathways. The highest reported incidence of ION after spine surgery is 1:1000, which makes prospective studies difficult and expensive to perform. This same dilemma is true for interventional or treatment studies of ION after major spine surgery.

The ASA Practice Advisory for perioperative visual loss associated with spine surgery

In 2006, the ASA Task Force on Perioperative Blindness examined the issue of POVL associated with major spine surgery and published a practice advisory, which was recently updated.[30] The recommendations were put forth as an advisory instead of more formal guidelines because of the significant lack of controlled trials on this topic. Case reports, large case series such as the ASA POVL Registry data, one case control study, expert opinion from neuro-ophthalmologists, neuroanesthesiologists, and spine surgeons, open forum commentary, and consensus surveys from relevant professional societies were utilized to develop this advisory. The original advisory was supported or endorsed by the North American Neuro-ophthalmological Society (NANOS) and the North American Spine Society (NASS). For major spine surgery of prolonged duration and/or with substantial blood loss, the advisory addressed the following issues:

1. Patients undergoing procedures in the prone position either for prolonged duration or with substantial blood loss, or both, are at increased risk for developing POVL.
2. Consider informing patients who are considered high risk that there is a small unpredictable risk of POVL.
3. Continually monitor blood pressure.
4. Position patients so that their head is in a neutral position, and level with or higher than the heart to minimize venous congestion of the head.
5. Colloids should be used along with crystalloids for patients who have substantial blood loss.
6. Consider staging procedures in high risk patients.

The Task Force neither endorsed nor could find evidence that the use of deliberate hypotension was associated with POVL. Similarly, no evidence could be found suggesting a transfusion threshold that would eliminate the risk of POVL.[30]

Summary

Major spine surgery in the prone position carries an increased risk for POVL. Children undergoing major spine surgery have a greatly elevated risk of developing POVL, primarily from cortical blindness, for unidentified reasons. Clinicians should consider informing patients at high risk that there is a small but unpredictable risk of POVL associated with their procedure. Patients who are suspected of having POVL should be examined as soon as possible to rule out rare treatable causes of POVL, preferably by a neuro-ophthalmologist. Careful and frequent checking of the eyes during major spine surgery in the prone position can eliminate cases of CRAO caused by globe compression.

ION after major spine surgery appears to be a systemic insult to the optic nerve associated with the prone position, male sex, obesity, use of the Wilson surgical spine frame, prolonged duration in the prone position, large blood loss, and use of a decreased percentage of colloid in the nonblood volume administration. The leading theory regarding ION associated with major spine surgery in the prone position maintains that it is caused by prolonged venous congestion of the head, leading to interstitial edema formation and decreased perfusion of the optic nerve The exact mechanism of how these changes cause irreversible damage to the optic nerve is undetermined. Preventive strategies for ION after major spine surgery should include avoiding or minimizing modifiable risk factors when possible. The ASA practice advisory for perioperative visual loss associated with spine surgery provides some guidance on these issues, though definitive controlled studies are lacking.

References

1. Shen Y, Drum M, Roth S. The prevalence of perioperative visual loss in the United States: A 10-year study from 1996 to 2005 of spinal, orthopedic, cardiac, and general surgery. *Anesth Analg* 2010; **109**: 1534–45.

2. Patil CG, Lad EM, Shivanand PL, *et al.* Visual loss after spine surgery. A population-based study. *Spine* 2008; **33**: 1491–6.

3. Stevens WR, Glazer PA, Kelley SD, *et al.* Ophthalmic complications after spinal surgery. *Spine* 1997; **22**: 1319–24.

4. Roth S. Postoperative blindness. In: Miller RD, ed. *Miller's Anesthesia.* 6th ed. New York: Elsevier; 2005: 2991–3020.

5. Hollenhorst RW, Svien JH, Benoit CF: Unilateral blindness occurring during anesthesia for neurosurgical operations. *AMA Arch Ophthalmol* 1954; **52**: 819–80.

6. Hayreh SS, Weingeist TA. Experimental occlusion of the central retinal artery of the retina. IV: Retinal tolerance time to acute ischaemia. *Br J Ophthalmol* 1980; **64**: 818–25.

7. Lee LA, Newman NJ, Wagner TA, *et al.* Postoperative ischemic optic neuropathy. *Spine* 2010; **35**: S105–16.

8. Lee LA, Roth S, Posner KL, *et al.* The American Society of Anesthesiologists Postoperative Visual Loss Registry: analysis of 93 spine surgery cases with postoperative visual loss. *Anesthesiology* 2006; **105**: 652–9.

9. Hayreh S, Joos K, Podhajsky P, *et al.* Systemic diseases associated with nonarteritic anterior ischemic optic neuropathy. *Am J Ophthalmol* 1994; **118**: 76–80.

10. Buono LM, Foroozan R, Sergott RC, *et al.* Nonarteritic anterior ischemic optic neuropathy. *Curr Opin Ophthalmol* 2002; **13**: 357–61.

11. Pazos GA, Leonard DW, Blice J, *et al.* Blindness after bilateral neck dissection: case report and review. *Am J Otolaryngol* 1999; **20**: 340–5.

12. Weber ED, Colyer MH, Lesser RL, *et al.* Posterior ischemic optic neuropathy after minimally invasive prostatectomy. *J Neuroophthalmol* 2007; **27**: 285–7.

13. Sadda SR, Nee M, Miller NR, *et al.* Clinical spectrum of posterior ischemic optic neuropathy. *Am J Ophthalmol* 2001; **132**: 743–50.

14. Takahashi S, Kitagawa H, Ishii T. Intraoperative pulmonary embolism during spinal instrumentation surgery. A prospective study using transoesophageal echocardiography. *J Bone Joint Surg Br* 2003; **85**: 90–4.

15. Warner MA, Warner ME, Martin JT. Ulnar neuropathy. Incidence, outcome, and risk factors in sedated or anesthetized patients. *Anesthesiology* 1994; **81**: 1332–40.

16. Giordano C, Montopoli M, Perli E, *et al.* Oestrogens ameliorate mitochondrial dysfunction in Leber's hereditary optic neuropathy. *Brain* 2011; **134**: 220–34.

17. Hartog CS, Bauer M, Reinhart K. Review article: the efficacy and safety of colloid resuscitation in the critically ill. *Anesth Analg* 2011; **112**; 156–64.

18. SAFE Study Investigators; Australian and New Zealand Intensive Care Society Clinical Trials Group; Australian Red Cross Blood Service; George Institute for International Health, *et al.* Saline or albumin for fluid resuscitation in patients with traumatic brain injury. *N Engl J Med* 2007; **357**: 874–84.

19. Mandel RJ, Brown MD, McCollough NC 3rd, *et al.* Hypotensive anesthesia and autotransfusion in spinal surgery. *Clin Orthop Relat Res* 1981; **154**: 27–33.

20. Grundy BL, Nash CL Jr, Brown RH. Deliberate hypotension for spinal fusion: prospective randomized study with evoked potential monitoring. *Can Anaesth Soc J* 1982; **29**: 452–62.

21. Malcolm-Smith NA, McMaster MJ. The use of induced hypotension to control bleeding during posterior fusion for scoliosis. *J Bone Joint Surg Br* 1983; **65**: 255–8.

22. The Postoperative Visual Loss Study Group. Risk factors associated with ischemic optic neuropathy after spinal fusion surgery. *Anesthesiology* 2012; **116**: 15–24.

23. Ho VT, Newman NJ, Song S, *et al.* Ischemic optic neuropathy following spine surgery. *J Neurosurg Anesthesiol* 2005; **17**: 38–44.

24. Myers MA, Hamilton SR, Bogosian AJ, *et al.* Visual loss as a complication of spine surgery. A review of 37 cases. *Spine* 1997; **22**: 1325–9.

25. Holy SE, Tsai JH, McAllister RK, *et al.* Perioperative ischemic optic neuropathy: a case control analysis of 126,666 surgical procedures at a single institution. *Anesthesiology* 2009; **110**: 246–53.

26. Cheng MA, Todorov A, Tempelhoff R, *et al.* The effect of prone positioning on intraocular pressure in anesthetized patients. *Anesthesiology* 2001; **95**: 1351–5.

27. Awad H, Santilli S, Ohr M, *et al.* The effects of steep Trendelenburg positioning on intraocular pressure during robotic radical prostatectomy. *Anesth Analg* 2009; **109**: 473–8.

28. Lee LA, Posner KL, Bruchas R, *et al.* Visual loss after prostatectomy. *Proceedings of the 2010 Annual Meeting of the American Society of Anesthesiologists*: A1132, 2010.

29. Wiedemayer H, Fauser B, Sandalcioglu IE, *et al.* Observations on intraoperative monitoring of visual pathways using steady-state visual evoked potentials. *Eur J Anaesthesiol* 2004; **21**: 429–33.

30. Apfelbaum JL, Roth S, Connis RT, *et al.* Practice advisory for perioperative visual loss associated with spine surgery. An updated report by the American Society of Anesthesiologists task force on perioperative visual loss. *Anesthesiology* 2012; **116**: 274–85.

15.2   Other Complications

Lorri A. Lee and Karen B. Domino

Key points

- Cardiopulmonary or stroke complications associated with spine surgery increase with increasing number of levels fused, increasing age, increasing comorbidities, prior hospitalization, and prior spine surgery.
- Hypovolemia with inadequate fluid resuscitation and coagulopathy are frequent complications associated with major spine surgery. Careful assessment of blood loss, volume status, and coagulation parameters is essential for good outcomes.
- Embolic complications from air, bone marrow, fat, or cement during instrumented spine surgery are common, and occasionally result in severe cardiovascular collapse.
- Positioning injuries associated with spine surgery are more common in the prone than in the supine position and preventative measures should be employed. Pressure sores, brachial plexopathy, and other peripheral nerve injuries are more common than rhabdomyolysis, globe compression, ischemic optic neuropathy, cerebral vascular occlusion, macroglossia, and cardiovascular compromise from right ventricular compression associated with pectus excavatum.
- Postoperative pancreatitis associated with pediatric scoliosis operations has been reported in 30% of patients with cerebral palsy. Superior mesenteric artery syndrome and celiac trunk occlusion are much rarer complications after pediatric scoliosis operations and can result in intra-abdominal catastrophes.
- Spine surgery has a greater proportion of medical malpractice claims against anesthesiologists for eye damage and nerve injury than other types of surgical procedures. Air embolism, inadequate fluid therapy, and positioning injuries are more common in spine surgery claims. These events emphasize the importance of adequate fluid resuscitation, careful positioning, and timely treatment of adverse intraoperative events in the prevention of adverse outcomes after spine surgery.

Introduction

This chapter will review general (e.g., mortality, cardiopulmonary) complications and some rare specific complications associated with spine surgery (e.g., air and particulate embolism, complications of excessive blood loss and inadequate fluid resuscitation, peripheral nerve injuries, rhabdomyolysis, and pancreatitis and superior mesenteric artery syndrome [Table 15.3]), as well as briefly mentioning medicolegal sequelae. Postoperative visual loss, discussed in detail in Chapter 17, is another rare complication. Spinal cord injury and airway complications associated with cervical spine procedures are addressed in other chapters.

Life-threatening complications of spine surgery

Complications following spine surgery are dependent upon patient age, comorbidities, as well as complexity of the spine surgery. In a randomized study of surgical treatment compared with nonsurgical treatment for lumbar disc herniation, Weinstein et al.[1] found no perioperative deaths and the absence of postoperative complications in 95% of patients. Superficial wound complications occurred in 4%. Similarly, the risk of perioperative complications was extremely low in a randomized study of surgical versus nonoperative treatment for lumbar spinal stenosis.[2]

However, the surgical trend for increasing complexity of surgery with spinal fusion is associated with increasing morbidity and mortality after surgery for lumbar spinal stenosis.[3] Life-threatening cardiopulmonary complications occurred in 2.3% of Medicare beneficiaries after simple decompression, whereas 5.6% of patients having complex spine fusions had life-threatening complications (Table 15.4).[3] Cardiopulmonary complications or stroke increased with advanced age, increased comorbidity, previous hospitalization, previous spine surgery, and number of disc levels fused

Table 15.3 Specific complications of spine surgery

- Air and particulate embolism
- Excessive blood loss and inadequate fluid resuscitation
- Peripheral nerve injuries
- Rhabdomyolysis
- Pancreatitis/superior mesenteric artery syndrome
- Postoperative visual loss

(Table 15.4). Thirty-day mortality ranged from 0.3% to 1.4%, with higher mortality for 3 or more levels fused, the presence of multiple comorbidities, and age >80 years (Table 15.4). Wound complications were also increased by complex fusion and previous spine surgery. After adjustment for age, comorbidity, previous spine surgery, the likelihood of in-hospital cardiopulmonary or stroke complications after complex fusion almost tripled compared with decompression alone (odds ratio [OR] =2.98 (95% confidence interval [CI] = 2.51–3.54).[3] Mortality within 30 days after complex fusion was also increased to a similar degree (OR = 2.56; 95% CI = 1.61–4.09).[3] Simple fusion also had elevated risk compared with decompression alone. These data emphasize that complex spinal fusion is associated with significant cardiopulmonary morbidity and mortality in the elderly population. Incidence data are lacking concerning adverse outcomes from specific complications described subsequently in this chapter.

Embolic complications associated with spine surgery

Emboli during spine surgery can be composed of air, fat, bone marrow, or cement. They typically arise from instrumentation, insertion of cement, and entrainment of air at the operative site, and less commonly from intravenous lines. Takahashi and colleagues reported an 80% incidence of moderate- to severe-grade emboli in 40 instrumented spine operations documented by transesophageal echocardiography.[4] Insertion of pedicle screws generated the largest numbers of emboli, while the surgical approach, laminectomy, and discectomy were associated with few emboli. They found no emboli in 20 noninstrumented spine operations.[4] Despite these alarming numbers, no patients in this study developed any significant changes in blood pressure, heart rate, electrocardiography, end-tidal carbon dioxide, or oxygen saturation; nor did they develop any clinical sequelae postoperatively. Consistent with this study, Rodriquez and coworkers found that 92%

(n = 13) of pediatric scoliosis surgery patients had high-intensity transient signals (HITS) by transcranial Doppler in the middle cerebral arteries suggestive of brain microembolization, and 2 of the 11 patients with right-to-left atrial shunts had very high numbers of HITS.[5] No patients had any new neurologic deficits after surgery. The pulmonary vasculature appears to be able to tolerate large loads of microemboli for most patients, as intramedullary nailing of femoral shaft fractures has similar effects and outcomes with respect to pulmonary emboli.[6]

However, fatal pulmonary emboli from air, fat, and bone marrow have been reported many times, and vertebroplasty has an especially high rate of embolization of both fat/bone marrow and cement.[7-12] Although kyphoplasties can also be associated with cement and fat/bone marrow embolization, the incidence appears to be less than for vertebroplasties. This difference in rate of embolization is most likely related with a rate of the 4–10% rate of cement leakage for kyphoplasty compared with a rate of up to 20–70% for vertebroplasty.[13] Cement leakage is associated with the viscosity of the cement at the time of injection and the amount of pressurization of the injectate.

Prevention of these potentially fatal emboli is primarily in the hands of the surgeon when placing pedicle screws and injecting cement. Venous air emboli could potentially be reduced by ensuring that patients are euvolemic throughout the procedures so that venous pressures will not favor entrainment of air at the surgical site. However, entrainment of air may also occur during placement of pedicle screws and cement. Clear communication with the surgeon and attention to the operative field will alert the anesthesiologist when portions of the procedure at high risk for embolization take place. As all pulmonary emboli cause varying degrees of pulmonary hypertension, use of inotropic and right ventricular afterload-reducing drugs may be useful if significant hemodynamic compromise ensues after a suspected pulmonary embolus.

Excessive blood loss and inadequate fluid resuscitation

Hypovolemia with inadequate fluid resuscitation is a common complication of spine surgery. The prone position reduces venous return and cardiac output. Blood loss can be difficult to quantify due to pooling on drapes. Massive blood loss may occur during complex spine fusions. Coagulopathy can develop, further exacerbating blood loss. Untreated hypovolemia

Table 15.4 Major medical complications, wound complications, and mortality following surgery for lumbar spinal stenosis (patients 66 years or older, 2007)

		No. (%) of patients		
	No. of patients	Cardiopulmonary complications or stroke	Wound complication	30-day mortality
Overall	32 152	984 (3.1)	398 (1.2)	128 (0.4)
Age (years)				
66–70	8 554	215 (2.5)[a]	98 (1.1)	27 (0.3)[a]
71–74	7 383	208 (2.8)	87 (1.2)	22 (0.3)
75–79	8 667	286 (3.3)	120 (1.4)	32 (0.4)
≥80	7 548	275 (3.6)	93 (1.2)	47 (0.6)
Sex				
Women	17 243	512 (3.0)	219 (1.3)	56 (0.3)[a]
Men	14 909	472 (3.2)	179 (1.2)	72 (0.5)
Race/ethnicity				
White	30 182	913 (3.0)[a]	374 (1.2)	116 (0.4)[a]
Nonwhite	1970	71 (3.6)	24 (1.2)	12 (0.6)
Quantitative comorbidity score				
0	16 631	412 (2.5)[a]	199 (1.2)[a]	43 (0.3)[a]
1	9 731	304 (3.1)	111 (1.1)	36 (0.4)
2	3 432	138 (4.0)	45 (1.3)	23 (0.7)
≥3	2 358	125 (5.3)	43 (1.8)	26 (1.1)
Chronic pulmonary disease				
Yes	5 525	272 (4.9)[a]	77 (1.4)	35 (0.6)[a]
No	26 627	712 (2.7)	321 (1.2)	93 (0.3)
Previous spine surgery				
Yes	2 196	87 (4.0)[a]	101 (4.6)[a]	[b]
No	29 956	897 (3.0)	297 (1.0)	121 (0.4)
Nonlumbar hospitalizations in previous year				
0	24 597	700 (2.8)[a]	288 (1.2)[a]	82 (0.3)[b]
1	4 836	164 (3.4)	63 (1.3)	19 (0.4)
2	1 689	68 (4.0)	22 (1.3)	13 (0.8)
≥3	1 030	52 (5.0)	25 (2.4)	14 (1.4)
Type of surgical procedure				
Decompression	21 474	458 (2.1)[a]	196 (0.9)[a]	72 (0.3)[a]
Simple fusion	6 082	285 (4.7)	100 (1.6)	28 (0.5)
Complex fusion	4 596	241 (5.2)	102 (2.2)	28 (0.6)
No. of disc levels fused				
None or unknown	21 960	508 (2.3)[a]	216 (1.0)[a]	77 (0.4)[a]
1–2	8 386	356 (4.2)	133 (1.6)	31 (0.4)
≥3	1 806	120 (6.6)	49 (2.7)	20 (1.1)

[a] Differences among subgroups significant, $p < 0.05$.
[b] Suppressed for cell count of 10 or less.

predisposes to cardiovascular and renal complications. Transfusion reactions, such as TRALI (transfusion-related acute lung injury), can develop. The detection and management of hypovolemia and blood loss during spine surgery are discussed in detail in chapters on fluid resuscitation (Chapter 9), hemodynamic monitoring (Chapter 8), and blood conservation strategies (Chapter 11).

Risk factors for intraoperative cardiac arrest in the prone position are hypovolemia, poor positioning with occluded venous return, air embolism, wound irrigation with hydrogen peroxide, and major spine surgery in the high-risk cardiac patient.[14] Cardiopulmonary resuscitation (CPR) is most effectively accomplished in the supine position due to the improvement in venous return. However, turning a patient may not be immediately feasible in some cases, such as with protruding metal instrumentation and ongoing blood loss. While preparing to turn the patient, resuscitation, including fluid administration and correction of hypovolemia, may need to be started in the prone position. Successful cardiopulmonary resuscitation has been described in the prone position.[14–16] Cardiac compression from the back is performed either as a one-handed procedure centrally over the vertebra or as a two-handed procedure over both sides of the chest, lateral to the spine. Counter-pressure on the sternum has also been described. Reverse CPR (back-pressure with sternal counter-pressure) generated higher systolic and mean arterial blood pressures during cardiac arrest than standard CPR.[17] The rigid thoracic costovertebral joints allow more forceful compression than the sterno-costo-chondral junctions, thus generating higher pressures in intrathoracic veins and arteries and compressed ventricles, improving forward flow.[17] However, prone CPR should be considered as only temporizing while the patient is prepared to be turned supine.

Injuries associated with positioning

Positioning injuries during spine surgery are relatively frequent and range from minor skin pressure sores in the prone position to brachial plexus and ocular injuries. Injuries result from compression or stretching of nerves, blood vessels, skin, muscles, or other organs during surgery. The severity of injury will be related to the force applied to the stretch or compression, the duration of insult, the degree of interruption of blood supply to the injured tissue, and any preexisting pathology of the injured tissue. The incidence of positioning injuries varies depending on the specific type of injury, the definition of the injury and the method used to detect it, and institution/provider-specific differences in positioning devices and methods.

Brachial plexus injuries

Brachial plexopathy is one of the most dreaded peripheral nerve injuries associated with spine surgery because of its potential to affect quality of life. These injuries can be severely debilitating, with motor dysfunction and/or chronic neuropathic pain. The long, relatively superficial course of the brachial plexus makes it vulnerable to injury, particularly with extremes of positioning.[4] Brachial plexus injuries are thought to occur primarily in three locations: between the anterior and middle scalene muscles in the interscalene space; between the clavicle and first rib in the costoclavicular space; or by stretching of the plexus across the coracoid process and glenohumeral joint in the rectopectoralis minor space.[18,19] Overstretching or compression of the nerves may cause ischemia of the intraneural capillaries and/or direct damage to the axons and myelin.[18,20]

Reports of brachial plexopathy after prone positioning with the arms in the semi-divers (Superman) position are thought to be related to shoulder abduction of more than 90° causing compression of the nerves and subclavian vessels in the costoclavicular space and/or by stretching of the plexus across the coracoid process and glenohumeral joint.[18,20] Additional stretching of the plexus can be caused by turning the head to one side[18,20] as done by some practitioners for positioning of the head in a gel or foam donut in the prone position. The weight of the body on the shoulder area contributes additional force to these compression and stretch injuries. Brachial plexus injuries associated with anterior cervical discectomy and fusion procedures are typically caused by excessive traction on the brachial plexus with taping of the shoulders to provide better exposure for surgery and radiographic imaging.[21]

Little information exists on the incidence of clinical brachial plexus injuries after spine surgery, but numerous studies have documented the prevalence of patients with significant decrements in upper extremity somatosensory evoked potential (SSEP) amplitudes with resolution after positioning changes.[21–26] SSEPs typically have low sensitivity (52%) and high specificity (100%) for detecting new neurologic deficits during spine surgery.[22] Because of their highly specific nature, SSEP amplitude changes below a predetermined percent of the baseline value are thought to reflect evolving upper extremity nerve injuries. The threshold for

273

Table 15.5 Detection of impending upper extremity nerve injuries from positioning by SSEP monitoring during spine surgery

	Schwartz et al., 2000	Labrom et al., 2005	Kamel et al., 2006	Chung et al., 2009
N	500	434	1109	232
SSEP amplitude reduction criterion	≥30%	≥30% (or ≥10% increased latency)	≥ 50%	≥50% (or ≥10% increased latency)
Percentage patients with significant SSEP amplitude reduction (total)	15/500 (3.6%)	27/434 (6.2%) All prone	68/1 109(6.8%) overall; 2/110 (1.8%) supine-arms tucked; 1/31 (3.2%) supine-arms out; 27/359 (7.55) lateral decubitus; 36/514 (7.0%) prone Superman; 2/95 (2.1%) prone-arms tucked	10/232 (4.3%)
Percentage patients in prone position – arm position unspecified		272/434 (62.3%) posterior; 128/434 (29.5%) lat decub→posterior		
Percentage patients in prone position – arms Superman	500/500 (100%)	Unknown	514/1109 (46.3%)	232/232 (100%)
Percentage patients in prone position – arms tucked		Unknown	95/1109 (8.6%)	
Percentage patients in lateral decubitus position	NA	34/434 (7.8%) lat decub only; 128/434 (29.5%) lat decub→posterior	359/1109(32.4%)	
Percentage patients in supine position – arm position unspecified	NA	NA		
Percentage patients in supine position with tucked arms	NA	NA	110/1109 (9.9%)	
Percentage patients in supine position with arms out	NA	NA	31/1109(2.8%)	
Percentage patients with return of SSEP amplitude after repositioning	15/15 (100%)	25/27 (92.6%)	68/68 (100%, by definition)	10/10 (100%)
% pts w/SSEP changes intraoperatively with new neurologic deficit on awakening	0	1/27 (3.7%)	0	0

alerting the anesthesiologist and surgeons for SSEP changes varied in four studies with a total of 2164 patients from ≥30% to ≥50% reduction from baseline SSEP amplitude (Table 15.5).[23–26] Out of 120 patients with significant SSEP decrements from baseline from these four studies, repositioning of the arms restored the SSEP amplitudes to acceptable levels in all but 2 patients. One of these patients had a brachial plexus palsy after awakening, and the other had no injury.[17]

Kamel et al. demonstrated that significant SSEP decrements from baseline (≥50%) in the median and/or ulnar nerves during spine surgery were more common in the lateral decubitus position (7.5%) and prone position with arms in the Superman position (7.0%) compared with the supine position with arms either tucked or out (1.8–3.2%, p <0.001, Table 15.5).[25] In contrast, the study by Labrom and colleagues in scoliosis surgery did not detect any significant SSEP decrements from baseline (≥30%) in the ulnar nerve in the lateral decubitus position, but did find that 6.2% of patients with prone positioning had significant changes.[24]

Kamel's study of over 1000 patients found that the lowest incidence of impending nerve injury of the upper extremities in the prone position, as detected by

SSEP amplitude reduction, was with the arms tucked (2.1%).[25] However, surgeons frequently need the arms placed cephalad for better access to the spine and for better intraoperative fluoroscopy imaging. Availability of the arms for additional vascular access or trouble-shooting existing vascular catheters is an added benefit of having the arms placed in the semi-divers position. Many experts recommend positioning the shoulders at no more than 90° of abduction with the arms supinated (palms down) when the semi-divers or Superman position is utilized in the prone position.[18,20,25] However, there is considerable disagreement among anesthesiologists and consultants as to the exact degree of allowable abduction in the prone position, as demonstrated by the surveys performed for the most recent American Society of Anesthesiologists (ASA) update for prevention of perioperative peripheral neuropathies.[27] Some modifications of position may be required for patients with limited shoulder rotation or elbow extension. The head should be positioned neutrally to avoid any additional stretch on the brachial plexus. Careful attention should be paid to adequate padding of bony prominences and for protection from the firm edges of surgical spine frames.

Meralgia paresthetica (lateral femoral cutaneous nerve injury)

Meralagia paresthetica refers to injuries to the lateral femoral cutaneous nerve that arises from the lumbar plexus at the L2–3 nerve roots and courses downward in the pelvis along the lateral border of the psoas muscle. It runs through a tunnel formed by the lateral inguinal ligament and the anterior superior iliac spine to innervate the anterolateral thigh. This nerve injury is thought to be related to either iliac crest bone harvesting or prone positioning with compression of the nerve anteriorly. Three separate studies in a total of 467 patients undergoing spine surgery identified 94 patients with meralgia paresthetica with symptoms of numbness, pain, or other paresthesia with an incidence of 12–24%.[28–30] Risk factors included prolonged operative time >3.5 hours and degenerative spinal disease with likely preexisting nerve injury, but there was disagreement as to whether lean body mass or obesity was a risk factor. Other possible risk factors cited were hypotension and blood loss. Recovery was complete in the majority of patients (≥91%) within 2 to 6 months without specific treatment. These injuries are typically self-limiting. Preventative measures are aimed at increased padding of the pelvic supports and

modifying the surgical approach for iliac crest bone graft harvesting.

Other rare injuries associated with prone spine surgery and positioning

There are many other rare injuries associated with spine surgery in the prone position reported only as case reports. Brainstem, cerebellar, and cerebral infarcts have been reported after prone spine surgery from occlusion or stretching of the vertebral and carotid vessels when the head was placed in a nonneutral position.[31–34] Carotid dissection and vertebral artery occlusion were thought to be responsible for infarctions. Elevated venous pressure in the prone position has also been postulated to have been the cause in several reports of spinal cord injury during posterior spine surgery in combination with mild arterial hypotension.[35] These injuries are so rare that risk factors cannot be reliably identified, but suggested contributory factors include low perfusion pressure caused by either deliberate or unintentional hypotension; venous congestion; and kinking, shearing, or direct compression of vessels causing low arterial inflow, low venous outflow, or trauma to the vessel wall, particularly when the head is in a nonneutral position. Theoretically, placing the head in as neutral a position as possible should eliminate vascular injuries caused by kinking, compression, or occlusion of vessels.

Several case reports of macroglossia after posterior fossa surgery or posterior cervical decompression have been reported and are thought to be caused by venous congestion and interstitial edema from the dependent position and turning the head to a nonneutral position.[36–38] Additionally, the tongue may become ischemic when it is allowed to protrude between the teeth, causing additional swelling postoperatively.[39] Placing a soft bite block between the molars should prevent tongue injuries from the teeth.

Near-cardiac collapse in the prone position has been reported twice with right ventricular compression from the sternum confirmed by transesophageal echocardiography in children with pectus excavatum.[40,41] One child had the body supports placed longitudinally with successful completion of surgery, while the other had surgical correction of the pectus excavatum prior to having spine surgery. For patients with pectus excavatum, careful attention should be paid to hemodynamics when positioning patients prone, and a high degree of suspicion should be maintained for mediastinal compression in this scenario.

Ophthalmic injuries associated with spine surgery are discussed in Chapter 17.

Rhabdomyolysis

Rhabdomyolysis has been reported after spine surgery.[42–46] Necrosis of skeletal muscle releases myoglobin and other contents, which can cause myoglobinuria and acute renal failure. Although serum creatine phosphokinase (CPK) is commonly elevated after various spine procedures, elevated CPK values generally reflect the degree of surgical invasiveness.[42,47,48] Posterolateral fusion is associated with increased serum CPK levels compared with interlaminar procedures.[49] While direct surgical muscle destruction results in an increase in CPK postoperatively, this elevation does not cause rhabdomyolysis. In contrast, the most common cause of rhabdomyolysis is muscle ischemia caused by muscle compression with resulting ischemia during a prolonged procedure. Obese patients and procedures associated with prolonged operative times are at greatest risk, because of the pressure of the weight on the muscle mass during prolonged immobility.[46] Lagandre et al.[50] showed that surgery duration >4 hours and BMI >40 kg/m² were associated with rhabdomyolysis after bariatric surgery. Minimally invasive lateral spine surgery is associated with rhabdomyolysis due to the prolonged surgical durations.[46]

Clinical signs and symptoms are myoglobinuria and a massive increase in CPK level. Acute renal failure occurs in up to a third of patients and is associated with a mortality of 20–50%.[45] Acute renal failure after myoglobinuria may be prevented by aggressive hydration and possibly alkalinization of the urine. If acute renal failure develops, dialysis may be necessary to prevent acute pulmonary edema and hyperkalemic cardiac arrest. Generally, CPKs in acute renal failure are in the range of >15 000–30 000 U/L.[51] Rhabdomyolysis is also associated with disseminated intravascular coagulation.[52]

Postoperative pancreatitis and superior mesenteric artery syndrome

Both postoperative pancreatitis and superior mesenteric artery (SMA) syndrome are complications associated with surgery for correction of scoliosis, and are more common in the pediatric population than in adults. The incidence of postoperative pancreatitis after spinal fusion in adolescents and young adults varies from 9% to 14%, but has been reported as high as 30.1% in patients with cerebral palsy.[53–55] Pancreatitis has been documented after isolated anterior, isolated posterior, and combined anterior–posterior fusions without a clear association for surgical approach. Laplaza and colleagues identified 7 of 80 (9%) adolescent patients with postoperative pancreatitis after surgical scoliosis correction during a 3-year period.[53] Significant differences between the 7 pancreatitis patients and the other 73 patients included older age, increased height, and lower body BMI.[53] They had an average of 2 days' increase in hospital days. A smaller series of patients described by Leichtner and coworkers had 6 of 44 patients (14%) with elevated lipase and amylase levels postoperatively after scoliosis surgery in patients aged 3.7–35.7 years, but only 4 had signs or symptoms consistent with acute pancreatitis.[54] They identified higher intraoperative blood loss as the only risk factor associated with this complication.[54]

The retrospective cohort study by Borkhuu et al. identified 109 of 355 patients with postoperative pancreatitis after surgical correction of scoliosis over a 12-year period ending in 2006.[55] These patients were aged 5.6–21.0 years with neuromuscular scoliosis from cerebral palsy. They based the definition of pancreatitis on a serum amylase or lipase level >3 times normal, pancreatic ultrasonography findings consistent with pancreatitis, and clinical findings consistent with pancreatitis. The multivariable model identified gastroesophageal reflux disease with feeding difficulties (adjusted RR 1.52, 95% CI, 1.01–2.29) and reactive airway disease (adjusted RR 1.49, 95% CI, 1.10–2.04) as risk factors for pancreatitis.[55] Preoperative Cobb angle, age, and intraoperative blood loss did not differ significantly between groups. Their patients with pancreatitis stayed an average of 7.5 days longer than the patients who did not develop pancreatitis.[55] Despite these studies, the etiology of postoperative pancreatitis remains elusive and suggested risk factors include end organ hypoperfusion, medications, infections, pancreatic duct abnormalities, hypercalcemia, hyperlipidemia, intraoperative positioning, degree of correction of Cobb angle, and increased intraoperative blood loss with complement activation.[53–55]

Interestingly, another complication related to surgical pediatric scoliosis correction, and perhaps related to postoperative pancreatitis, is SMA syndrome. It has also been documented after body casting for correction of scoliosis. SMA syndrome is caused by extrinsic compression of the third portion of the duodenum between the aorta and SMA. The SMA originates from the aorta

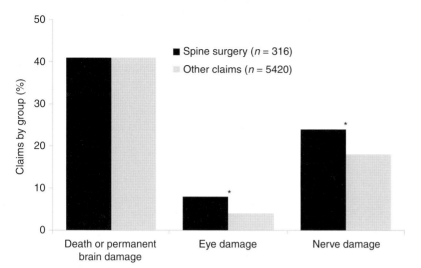

Figure 15.5 Complications associated with spine surgery claims compared with other surgical claims. Claims for craniotomy excluded. Based upon findings reported in Lee LA, *et al.* (Anesthesiology 2003; 99:A362, with permission of Wolters Kluwer/Lippincott.
*p <0.05 spine vs. other surgical claims.

at a 45–60° angle in normal patients. The third portion of the duodenum is suspended between the aorta and SMA by the ligament of Treitz, and any traction on these ligaments or vessels may cause obstruction of the duodenum. The highest reported incidence of SMA syndrome after spinal deformity correction was 4.8% by Braun and colleagues.[56] They identified 17 out of 364 patients over a 5-year period who developed SMA syndrome after surgical correction for scoliosis. Risk factors for postoperative SMA syndrome identified after multivariate regression included a staged procedure (OR 31.0), a Lenke lumbar modifier of B or C instead of A (a classification system from A to C with increasing misalignment of the lumbar spine from the central sacral vertebral line) (OR 9.06), lower BMI (OR 7.75), and thoracic stiffness (OR 6.67).[56] A smaller series of 5 SMA syndrome cases identified over a 4-year period found that a BMI <18 was the most significant risk factor for SMA syndrome.[57]

It has been hypothesized that lumbar hyperextension or hyperlordosis can increase traction on the mesentery and aorta and SMA vessels and cause obstruction of the duodenum.[58] The SMA and celiac trunk supply both the duodenum and the head of the pancreas. It is unclear whether postoperative pancreatitis and SMA syndrome are related complications after pediatric scoliosis surgery. Similarly, celiac trunk stenosis or occlusion with hepatic ischemia, perforated gallbladder, splenic infarction, and/or gastric perforation has been reported after surgical correction of spinal deformities.[59–61] Emergent laparotomy with release of the arcuate ligament restored blood flow in one patient

with full recovery.[59] The other two cases required extensive abdominal surgery, with good recovery in one patient.[60,61] Special attention should be paid to pediatric scoliosis patients in the postoperative period who have abdominal pain, ileus, and feeding difficulties.

Medicolegal concerns

Malpractice claims are useful for the study of rare, severe adverse outcomes after anesthesia and surgery.[62,63] Injuries and their causes in spine surgery claims were compared with those in other surgical claims using the American Society of Anesthesiologists Closed Claims database.[64] The Closed Claims database is a structured evaluation of adverse anesthetic outcomes, excluding dental damage, from the closed claims files of 35 US professional liability insurance companies. The data collection process has been previously described in detail.[62,63]

Death or permanent brain damage occurred in 41% of both spine and other surgical claims (Fig. 15.5).[64] The high proportion of these severe injuries reflects the fact that malpractice claims are biased toward severe, permanent injuries. Eye damage occurred more often in spine surgery (Fig. 15.5), due to the increased risk of ischemic optic neuropathy and central retinal artery occlusion in prone spine procedures. In addition, nerve damage was also increased in spine claims (Fig. 15.5), because of the increased risk of brachial plexopathy and spinal cord injuries. The specific causes of injury (i.e., damaging events) were different in spine surgery compared with other claims (Table 15.6). Air embolism, inadequate fluid therapy, and positioning injuries were

Table 15.6 Specific damaging event in spine surgery claims compared with other surgical claims (claims for craniotomy excluded)

	Spine claims (n = 316 %)	Other claims (n = 5420 %)
Positioning	29 (9)*	66 (1)*
Surgical event	22 (7)	232 (4)
Inadequate fluid therapy	16 (5)*	72 (1)*
Air embolism	11 (3)*	13 (0)*

*p <0.05 spine vs other claims.
Based upon findings reported in Lee LA, et al., Anesthesiology 2003; 9:A362, with permission of Wolters Kluwer/Lippincott.

more common in spine claims (Table 15.6). Surgical events accounted for 7% of spine claims. The median payment in spine claims was higher ($167 000) than in other claims ($100 000).

The Closed Claims data highlight the importance of perioperative nerve injury and visual loss, and the influence of positioning, air embolism, and inadequate fluid therapy in rare adverse outcomes associated with spine surgery. Higher payments were made to plaintiffs, reflecting the high severity of injury. Although the Closed Claims database does not contain incidence data due to the lack of denominators of the total number of procedures performed, the data are consistent with the common perception of increased liability in spine procedures.

References

1. Weinstein JN, Tosteson TD, Lurie JD, et al. Surgical vs. nonoperative treatment for lumbar disk herniation: the Spine Patient Outcomes Research Trial (SPORT): a randomized trial. JAMA 2006; 296(20): 2441–50.

2. Weinstein JN, Tosteson TD, Lurie JD, et al. Surgical versus nonoperative treatment for lumbar spinal stenosis four-year results of the Spine Patient Outcomes Research Trial. Spine 2010; 35(14): 1329–38.

3. Deyo RA, Mirza SK, Martin BI, Kreuter W, Goodman DC, Jarvik JG. Trends, major medical complications, and charges associated with surgery for lumbar spinal stenosis in older adults. JAMA 2010; 303(13): 1259–65.

4. Takahashi S, Kitagawa H, Ishii T. Intraoperative pulmonary embolism during spinal instrumentation surgery. A prospective study using transoesophageal echocardiography. J Bone Joint Surg Br 2003; 85: 90–4.

5. Rodriquez RA, Letts M, Jarvis J, et al. Cerebral microembolization during pediatric scoliosis surgery:

a transcranial Doppler study. J Pediatr Orthop 2001; 21: 532–6.

6. Coles RE, Clements FM, Lardenoye JW, et al. Transesophageal echocardiography in quantification of emboli during femoral nailing: reamed versus unreamed techniques. J South Orthop Assoc 2000; 9: 98–104.

7. McCarthy RE, Lonstein JE, Mertz JD, et al. Air embolism in spinal surgery. J Spinal Disord 1990; 3: 1–5.

8. Sutherland RW, Winter RJ. Two cases of fatal air embolism in children undergoing scoliosis surgery. Acta Anaesthesiol Scand 1997; 41: 1073–6.

9. Wills J, Schwend RM, Paterson A, et al. Intraoperative visible bubbling of air may be the first sign of venous air embolism during posterior surgery for scoliosis. Spine 2005; 30: E629–35.

10. Syed MI, Jan S, Patel NA, et al. Fatal fat embolism after vertebroplasty: identification of the high-risk patient. Am J Neuroradiol 2006; 27: 343–5.

11. Monticelli F, Meyer JH, Tutsch-Bauer E. Fatal pulmonary cement embolism following percutaneous vertebroplasty (PVP). Forensic Sci Int 2005; 149: 35–8.

12. Yoo KY, Jeong SW, Yoon W, et al. Acute respiratory distress syndrome associated with pulmonary cement embolism following percutaneous vertebroplasty with polymethylmethacrylate. Spine 2004; 29: E294–7.

13. Bula P, Lein T, Strassberger C, et al. Ballon kyphoplasty in the treatment of osteoporotic vertebral fractures: indications–treatment strategy – complications. Z Orthop Unfall 2010; 148: 646–56.

14. Brown J, Rogers J, Soar J. Cardiac arrest during surgery and ventilation in the prone position: a case report and systematic review. Resuscitation 2001; 50(2): 233–8.

15. Tobias JD, Mencio GA, Atwood R, Gurwitz GS. Intraoperative cardiopulmonary resuscitation in the prone position. J Pediatr Surg. 1994; 29(12): 1537–8.

16. Dooney N. Prone CPR for transient asystole during lumbosacral spinal surgery. Anaesth Intensive Care 2010; 38(1): 212–13.

17. Mazer SP, Weisfeldt M, Bai D, et al. Reverse CPR: a pilot study of CPR in the prone position. Resuscitation 2003; 57(3): 279–85.

18. Uribe JS, Kolla J, Omar H, et al. Brachial plexus injury following spinal surgery. J Neurosurg Spine 2010; 13: 552–8.

19. Linda DD, Harish S, Stewart BG, et al. Multimodality imaging of peripheral neuropathies of the upper limb and brachial plexus. Radiographics 2010; 30: 1373–400.

20. Winfree CJ, Kline DG. Intraoperative positioning nerve injuries. Surg Neurol 2005; 63: 5–18.

21. Schwartz DM, Sestokas AK, Hilibrand AS, et al. Neurophysiological identification of position-induced

neurologic injury during anterior cervical spine surgery. *J Clin Monit Comput* 2006; **20**: 437–44.

22. Kelleher MO, Tan G, Sarjeant R, *et al.* Predictive value of intraoperative neurophysiological monitoring during cervical spine surgery: a prospective analysis of 1055 consecutive patients. *J Neurosurg Spine* 2008; **8**: 215–21.

23. Schwartz DM, Drummond DS, Hahn M, *et al.* Prevention of positional brachial plexopathy during surgical correction of scoliosis. *J Spinal Disord* 2000; **13**: 178–82.

24. Labrom RD, Hoskins M, Reilly CW, *et al.* Clinical usefulness of somatosensory evoked potentials for detection of brachial plexopathy secondary to malpositioning in scoliosis surgery. *Spine* 2005; **30**: 2089–93.

25. Kamel IR, Drum ET, Koch SA, *et al.* The use of somatosensory evoked potentials to determine the relationship between patient positioning and impending upper extremity nerve injury during spine surgery: a retrospective analysis. *Anesth Analg* 2006; **102**: 1538–42.

26. Chung I, Glow JA, Dimopoulos V, *et al.* Upper-limb somatosensory evoked potential monitoring in lumbosacral spine surgery: a prognostic marker for position-related ulnar nerve injury. *Spine J* 2009; **9**: 287–95.

27. Practice advisory for the prevention of perioperative peripheral neuropathies: an updated report by the American Society of Anesthesiologists Task Force on prevention of perioperative peripheral neuropathies. *Anesthesiology* 2011; **114**: 741–54.

28. Mirovsky Y, Neuwirth M. Injuries to the lateral femoral cutaneous nerve during spine surgery. *Spine* 2000; **25**: 1266–9.

29. Gupta A, Muzumdar D, Ramani PS. Meralgia paraesthetica following lumbar spine surgery: a study in 110 consecutive surgically treated cases. *Neurol India* 2004; **52**: 64–6.

30. Yang SH, Wu CC, Chen PQ. Postoperative meralgia paresthetica after posterior spine surgery: incidence, risk factors, and clinical outcomes. *Spine* 2005; **30**: E547–50.

31. Langmayr JJ, Ortler M, Obwegeser A, *et al.* Quadriplegia after lumbar disc surgery. A case report. *Spine* 1996; **21**: 1932–5.

32. Tettenborn B, Caplan LR, Sloan MA, *et al.* Postoperative brainstem and cerebellar infarcts. *Neurology* 1993; **43**: 471–7.

33. Wang LC, Liou JT, Liu FC, *et al.* Fatal ischemia stroke in a patient with an asymptomatic carotid artery occlusion after lumbar spine surgery – a case report. *Acta Anaesthesiol Taiwan* 2004; **42**: 179–82.

34. Gould DB, Cunningham K. Internal carotid artery dissection after remote surgery. Iatrogenic complications of anesthesia. *Stroke* 1994; **25**: 1276–8.

35. Edgcombe H, Carter K, Yarrow S. Anaesthesia in the prone position. *Br J Anaesth* 2008; **100**: 165–83.

36. Pivalizza EG, Katz J, Singh S. *et al.* Massive macroglossia after posterior fossa surgery in the prone position. *J Neurosurg Anesthesiol* 1998; **10**: 34–6.

37. Sinha A, Agarwal A, Gaur A, *et al.* Oropharyngeal swelling and macroglossia after cervical spine surgery in the prone position. *J Neurosurg Anesthesiol* 2001; **13**: 237–9.

38. Tsung YC, Wu CT, Hsu CH, *et al.* Macroglossia after posterior fossa surgery in the prone position – a case report. *Acta Anaesthesiol Taiwan* 2006; **44**: 43–6.

39. Drummond JC. Macroglossia, déjà vu. *Anesth Analg* 1999; **89**: 534–5.

40. Alexianu D, Skolnick ET, Pinto AC, *et al.* Severe hypotension in the prone position in a child with neurofibromatosis, scoliosis and pectus excavatum presenting for posterior spinal fusion. *Anesth Analg* 2004; **98**: 334–5.

41. Bafus BT, Chiravuri D, van der Velde ME, *et al.* Severe hypotension associated with the prone position in a child with scoliosis and pectus excavatum undergoing posterior spinal fusion. *J Spinal Disord Tech* 2008; **21**: 451–4.

42. Davidas JL, Roullit S, Dubost J, *et al.* [Creatine phosphokinases and serum and urinary myoglobin following a procedure in prolonged knee-chest position for the treatment of spondylolisthesis]. [Article in French] *Ann Fr Anesth Reanim* 1986; **5**(1): 31–4.

43. Cruette D, Navarre MC, Pinaquy C, Siméon F. [Rhabdomyolysis after prolonged knee-chest position]. [Article in French] *Ann Fr Anesth Reanim* 1986; **5**(1): 67–9.

44. Jourdan C, Convert J, Terrier A, Tixier S, Bouchet C, Montarry M. [A comparative study of CPK during spinal surgery in the knee-chest position. Apropos of 93 patients]. [Article in French] *Cah Anesthesiol* 1992; **40**(2): 87–90.

45. Papadakis M, Sapkas G, Tzoutzopoulos A. A rare case of rhabdomyolysis and acute renal failure following spinal surgery. *J Neurosurg Spine* 2008 Oct; **9**: 387–9.

46. Dakwar E, Rifkin SI, Volcan IJ, Goodrich JA, Uribe JS. Rhabdomyolysis and acute renal failure following minimally invasive spine surgery. *J Neurosurg Spine* 2011; **14**(6): 785–8.

47. Arts MP, Nieborg A, Brand R, Peul WC. Serum creatine phosphokinase as an indicator of muscle injury after various spinal and nonspinal surgical procedures. *J Neurosurg Spine* 2007; **7**(3): 282–6.

48. Kim K, Isu T, Sugawara A, Matsumoto R, Isobe M. Comparison of the effect of 3 different approaches to the lumbar spinal canal on postoperative paraspinal muscle damage. *Surg Neurol* 2008; **69**(2): 109–13; discussion 113.

49. Suwa H, Hanakita J, Ohshita N, *et al.* Postoperative changes in paraspinal muscle thickness after various lumbar back surgery procedures. *Neurol Med Chir (Tokyo)* 2000; **40**(3): 151–4; discussion 154–5.

50. Lagandre S, Arnalsteen L, Vallet B, *et al.* Predictive factors for rhabdomyolysis after bariatric surgery. *Obes Surg* 2006; **16**: 1365–70.

51. Ettinger JE, de Souza CA, Santos-Filho PV, *et al.* Rhabdomyolysis: diagnosis and treatment in bariatric surgery. *Obes Surg* 2007; **17**: 525–32.

52. Malinosky DJ, Slater MS. Mullins RJ. Crush injury and rhabdomyolysis. *Crit Care Clin* 2004; **20**: 171–92.

53. Laplaza FJ, Widmann RF, Fealy S, *et al.* Pancreatitis after surgery in adolescent idiopathic scoliosis: incidence and risk factors. *J Pediatr Orthop* 2002; **22**: 80–3.

54. Leichtner AM, Banta JV, Etienne N, *et al.* Pancreatitis following scoliosis surgery in children and young adults. *J Pediatr Orthop* 1991; **11**: 594–8.

55. Borkhuu B, Nagaraju D, Miller F, *et al.* Prevalence and risk factors in postoperative pancreatitis after spine fusion in patients with cerebral palsy. *J Pediatr Orthop* 2009; **29**: 256–62.

56. Braun SV, Hedden DM, Howard AW. Superior mesenteric artery syndrome following spinal deformity correction. *J Bone Joint Surg Am* 2006; **88**: 2252–7.

57. Smith BG, Hakim-Zargar M, Thomson JD. Low body mass index: a risk factor for superior mesenteric artery syndrome in adolescents undergoing spinal fusion for scoliosis. *J Spinal Disord Tech* 2009; **22**: 144–8.

58. Marecek GS, Barsness KA, Sarwark JF. Relief of superior mesenteric artery syndrome with correction of multiplanar spinal deformity by posterior spinal fusion. *Orthopedics* 2010; **33**: 519.

59. von Glinski KS, Krettek C, Blauth M, *et al.* Hepatic ischemia as a complication after correction of post-traumatic gibbus at the thoracolumbar junction. *Spine* 2000; **25**: 1040–4.

60. Debnath UK, Sharma H, Roberts D, *et al.* Coeliac axis thrombosis after surgical correction of spinal deformity in type VI Ehlers–Danlos syndrome: a case report and review of the literature. *Spine* 2007; **32**: E528–31.

61. Daniels AH, Jurgensmeier D, McKee J, *et al.* Acute celiac artery compression syndrome after surgical correction of Scheuermann kyphosis. *Spine* 2009; **34**: E149–52.

62. Cheney FW. The American Society of Anesthesiologists Closed Claims Project: what have we learned, how has it affected practice, and how will it affect practice in the future? *Anesthesiology* 1999; **91**: 552–6.

63. Metzner J, Posner KL, Lam MS, *et al.* Closed claims' analysis. *Best Pract Res Clin Anaesthesiol* 2011; **25**: 263–76.

64. Lee LA, Posner KL, Cheney FW, *et al.* ASA Closed Claims Project: an analysis of claims associated with neurosurgical anesthesia. *Anesthesiology* 2003; **99**: A362.

Chapter

16

Postoperative care in the PACU

Maged Argalious

Key points

- Even patients considered as having an "easy airway" in the operating room can pose airway challenges in the postanesthesia care unit (PACU). Factors including surgery close to the airway (cervical spine), intraoperative airway instrumentation or manipulation, previous neck dissection or radiation, prolonged surgery in the prone position, large volumes of intraoperative fluids, and residual anesthetic effects contribute to these difficulties.

- Although the presence of an airway exchange catheter (AEC) does not guarantee success at subsequent re-intubation, oxygen insufflation through an AEC can maintain oxygenation until definitive measures are taken to secure the airway (e.g., tracheal intubation, cricothyroidotomy, tracheostomy).

- Despite advances in chronic hypertension management, acute postoperative hypertension (APH) occurs with a reported incidence of 4–35%. APH may lead to serious neurologic (hemorrhagic stroke, cerebra ischemia, encephalopathy), cardiovascular (myocardial ischemia, cardiac arrhythmia, congestive heart failure, pulmonary edema), renal (acute kidney injury), and surgical site complications (bleeding) and requires prompt intervention and management.

- Postoperative patients after spine surgery require frequent assessment for evidence of motor or sensory deficits. New-onset motor deficits related to the surgical site will prompt emergent imaging and/or surgical exploration for evidence of a compressive hematoma. Patients who are kept intubated

after spine surgery typically require reversal of neuromuscular blockade (if nondepolarizing muscle relaxants have been used) to aid in assessment of extremity motor strength (wake-up test) before sedation can be resumed.

- The emphasis in positioning-related injuries should be on their prevention. This starts with identification of any preoperative motor or sensory deficits; careful positioning and documentation of positioning details; frequent rechecking of position to rule out any pressure-prone areas; avoidance of hypotension, hypothermia, and severe anemia; and postoperative neurologic examination and documentation of new sensory and/or motor deficits.

- It is common for symptoms of nerve injury (sensory and/or motor) to start more than 48 hours postoperatively, indicating that the etiology may also be related to events in the postanesthetic period.

Introduction

Safe, outcomes-oriented, patient-focused postoperative care requires a team-based, evidence-driven approach to the management of patients with spine surgery. The focus of this chapter is to identify the most common postoperative challenges facing the perioperative team in the management of those patients and to describe an evidenced-based approach to their prevention and management. This chapter will provide an in-depth coverage of the management of postoperative airway and hemodynamic issues, the prevention and management of position-related injuries after spine surgery, and a description of the commonly used discharge scoring systems and their limitations.

Anesthesia for Spine Surgery, ed. Ehab Farag. Published by Cambridge University Press. © Cambridge University Press 2012.

Table 16.1 Causes of postoperative hypoxemia

Mechanism	Examples	Alveolar–arterial O_2 gradient	Response to 100% O_2
Decreased partial pressure of inspired oxygen	Hypoxic gas mixture; high altitude	Normal	Increased P_aO_2
Hypoventilation	Obesity–hypoventilation syndrome, neuromuscular disorders, sleep apnea	Normal	Increased P_aO_2
Ventilation–perfusion mismatch	COPD, asthma, interstitial lung disease	Increased	Increased P_aO_2
Shunt	Pulmonary edema, ARDS, atelectasis, pneumonia, pneumothorax	Increased	Minimal if any increase in P_aO_2
Diffusion impairment	Pulmonary embolism	Increased	Increased P_aO_2

ARDS = acute respiratory distress syndrome; COPD = chronic obstructive pulmonary disease; P_aO_2 = partial oxygen tension in arterial blood.

Airway management after spine surgery

Airway management is often challenging in the PACU.[1,2] Factors including surgery close to the airway (cervical spine), intraoperative airway instrumentation or manipulation, previous neck dissection or radiation,[3] prolonged surgery in the prone position, large volumes of intraoperative fluids, and residual anesthetic effects contribute to these difficulties.

Even patients considered as having an "easy airway" in the operating room can pose airway challenges in the PACU.

Airway obstruction and hypoxemia

The most common cause of postoperative airway obstruction is pharyngeal obstruction by the tongue. Simple interventions such as rousing the patient with gentle stimulation, jaw thrust, and, if necessary, insertion of a nasal or oral airway may restore airway patency. Persistence of airway obstruction or signs of laryngospasm mandate the application of positive-pressure ventilation with oxygen via a bag and mask. Small doses of succinylcholine (20–40 mg) may also be necessary to relieve laryngospasm.

Promptly restoring airway patency reduces the likelihood of negative-pressure pulmonary edema and, more importantly, prevents oxygen desaturation and hypoxemia.

Oxygen supplementation during patient transfer to the PACU is reasonable for all patients. Hypoxic drive is inhibited by minimal residual concentrations of inhalational anesthetics.

Patients with stridor may require treatment with nebulized racemic epinephrine and may benefit from a helium–oxygen mixture (70% helium, 30% oxygen), which reduces airway resistance and the work of breathing relative to oxygen or air. Quick recognition of problems is necessary because stridor may advance to total airway obstruction.

Persistent hypoxemia after restoration of airway patency requires evaluation of possible etiologies (Table 16.1). In negative-pressure pulmonary edema, inspiratory efforts against an obstructed airway can cause alveolar-capillary membrane injury.

Such a capillary leak may lead to respiratory failure requiring mechanical ventilation with positive end-expiratory pressure. The most common cause of hypoxemia in the PACU is an increase in right to left shunting (most often from atelectasis). Other common etiologies include pulmonary aspiration and pulmonary edema. An unrecognized pneumothorax, perhaps caused by high inflation pressures during attempts to ventilate the patient, may lead to hemodynamic compromise and render resuscitation attempts useless.

Hypoventilation

Postoperative hypoventilation and apnea can be caused by residual neuromuscular blockade (as a result of overdose, inadequate reversal dosing, hypothermia, or metabolic factors [e.g., hypokalemia] that interfere with adequate reversal).[4] Opioid-induced respiratory depression is also a frequent cause of postoperative hypoventilation.

Opioids not only shift the carbon dioxide response curve to the right (i.e., raise the apneic threshold), but can also decrease the slope of the carbon dioxide response curve (i.e., reduce the minute volume response to a high P_aCO_2). Although the slope of the carbon dioxide response curve is unchanged by opioids in fully awake patients, residual anesthetic effects can shift the carbon dioxide response curve. Splinting resulting from incisional pain can also cause postoperative hypoventilation.

Airway management after cervical spine surgery

Patients undergoing surgery for cervical spine disease have a greater incidence of difficult intubation than matched control subjects.[5,6] Airway complications are common after anterior cervical spine surgery and range from acute airway obstruction (1.2%) to chronic vocal cord dysfunction.[7,8]

Risk factors associated with airway obstruction after cervical spine surgery include:[8,9]

- Advanced age
- Obesity (greater than 100 kg)
- Exposure of three or more vertebral bodies or exposure of C2, C3, or C4
- Estimated blood loss greater than 300 ml
- Requirement for four or more red cell units
- Operative time more than 10 hours
- Combined anteroposterior cervical spine surgery
- Severe preoperative neurologic deficits

Airway complications may also occur after cervical spine surgery in the prone position, most commonly due to macroglossia and laryngeal edema. Decreased venous return from the face and upper neck is also a contributing factor.[10] A plan for re-intubation should be in place before any extubation attempts (Tables 16.2 and 16.3). The presence of external stabilization devices complicates airway management. Removal of the anterior part of a cervical collar during re-intubation attempts improves airway visualization but should be accompanied by manual inline stabilization in patients with an unstable cervical spine. Manual inline stabilization reduces cervical spine motion during intubation attempts in patients with an unstable cervical spine.[11]

Komatsu *et al.*[12] reported a reasonable success rate of intubation with the use of an intubating laryngeal mask airway in patients with rigid neck collars. A recent study on postoperative patients after anterior cervical spine surgery showed a reduced incidence of airway complication with routine postoperative fiberoptic evaluation of the airway for evidence of airway edema.[13] Patients' tracheas were only extubated if there was no reactive swelling or pharyngeal edema. Close communication among surgeons, anesthesiologists,

Table 16.2 Steps in extubating patients after complex cervical spine surgery

1. Adherence to evidence-based extubation criteria (Table 16.3)
2. A preformulated plan for re-intubation should extubation fail
3. Established institutional protocols that guide extubation timing after complex spine surgery with close communication of the perioperative team (surgical, anesthesia, respiratory therapist, nursing)
4. Consideration for routine fiberoptic evaluation prior to extubation for evidence of resolution of pharyngeal edema[13]

Table 16.3 Criteria for extubation

Awake, cooperative
Hemodynamic stability on no or minimal pressors
Absence of surgical bleeding or coagulopathy
Temperature $\geq 36°C$
Mechanical criteria:
Tidal volume ≥ 6 ml/kg
Vital capacity ≥ 15 ml/kg
Negative inspiratory force ≥ 30 cmH$_2$O
Rapid shallow breathing index (respiratory rate/tidal volume) <100
Chemical criteria:
pH ≥ 7.25
P_aO_2/F_IO_2 ratio >300
$P_aO_2 \geq 65$ mmHg on $F_IO_2 \geq 0.4$
Minimal PEEP of 5–8 cmH$_2$O
Acceptable P_aCO_2 (≤ 50 mmHg)
Stable metabolic status (serum HCO$_3^-$ ≥ 20 mmHg)

and respiratory therapists helps in reducing emergency airway complications.

Postoperative expanding neck hematoma

In patients recovering from neck surgery who develop respiratory insufficiency, the possibility of an expanding neck hematoma must be considered. In most instances, airway obstruction ensues quickly as a result of encroachment and distortion of airway anatomy. If the neck hematoma is visible but is not causing respiratory distress, apply pressure to the surgical site to avoid further expansion. After notifying the surgeon, awake intubation (possibly fiberoptic guided according to the American Society of Anesthesiologists difficult airway algorithm[5]) may be prudent to stabilize the patient before drainage of the hematoma. In some cases, airway edema persists despite drainage of the hematoma.

Table 16.4 Management of postoperative neck hematoma

1. Apply pressure to bleeding site

2. Notify surgery and anesthesia team (call for help)

3 Tight blood pressure control

Outcome

A. No further hematoma expansion

- Communication with surgical team

- Mark the boundaries of the hematoma for early identification of further expansion

- Close observation and extended (8–12 h) monitoring in a critical care environment

B. Continuous expansion of hematoma with no airway compromise

- Awake (fiberoptic) intubation either in the PACU or after immediate transfer to the operating room after topical anesthesia to the airway followed by general anesthesia for exploration of wound and drainage of neck hematoma

- Assess neurologic status at the end of the case

- Consider maintaining the patient intubated postoperatively until resolution of reactionary airway edema

C. Expansion of neck hematoma with rapidly progressive airway compromise (dyspnea, stridor, airway obstruction)

- Emergent intubation (ASA algorithm)

- Cannot intubate/can ventilate using face mask, oral or nasal airways, laryngeal mask airway: Consider immediate surgical drainage of the neck hematoma followed by further attempts to secure the airway

- Cannot intubate/cannot ventilate: surgical airway (emergent cricothyroidotomy, percutaneous or surgical tracheostomy)

- Evacuation of hematoma and wound exploration

- Neurologic assessment

- Maintain airway secured postoperatively

If emergent intubation attempts are unsuccessful, the decision to proceed with a surgical airway (emergency cricothyroidotomy or tracheostomy) depends on the ability (vs. inability) to ventilate the patient with a face-mask or laryngeal mask airway. If ventilation is unsuccessful or becomes inadequate despite drainage of the neck hematoma, invasive airway access should proceed.[5] Table 16.4 identifies the steps in management of postoperative neck hematoma.

Role of airway exchange catheters after spine surgery

Although the presence of an airway exchange catheter does not guarantee success at subsequent re-intubation, a high success rate has been reported.[14,15] In addition,

oxygen insufflation through an airway exchange catheter (AEC) can maintain oxygenation until definitive measures are taken to secure the airway (e.g., tracheal intubation, cricothyroidotomy, tracheostomy).

Numerous AECs are available, but these devices must be used correctly because airway complications can develop (e.g., perforation of the tracheobronchial tree, failure to pass the endotracheal tube [ETT] over the AEC, barotrauma) when the wrong size, type, or technique is used.[16–22] Suggestions for success include the following:

- AECs with a very small outer diameter should be avoided because they are prone to kinking, making railroading of the new ETT difficult

- Match the marking of the AEC with the centimeter markings on the ETT to avoid excessive advancement of the AEC, which can irritate the carina and cause bronchial trauma and bleeding

- Use an AEC with an inner hollow lumen that allows oxygen insufflation, whether by jet ventilation or a bag valve device. Two Rapi-Fits adaptors (Cook Medical, Bloomington, IN, USA) usually accompany the AEC for this purpose

- If resistance is encountered during the advancement of the ETT over the AEC, oral laryngoscopy (if feasible) can aid tube advancement. Rotation of the ETT in 90° anticlockwise increments also helps to pass the ETT tip past the arytenoids. ETTs with flexible tips (Parker Flex-Tip) serve the same purpose in that the tube tip is prevented from becoming caught against the arytenoids

- Avoid using force in advancing the AEC and the ETT because it may traumatize airway structures[19]

- Applying a silicone-based spray or a lubricant gel on the outside of the AEC can facilitate tube advancement

- The position of the new ETT should be confirmed before the AEC is withdrawn. This can be done by end-tidal capnography through a flexible bronchoscope adapter.[16]

- Longer AECs are available for double-lumen tubes and can be used with the same precautions

Role of the cuff leak test

A cuff leak test can be performed on a spontaneously breathing patient by deflating the ETT cuff, blocking the ETT opening, and listening for a leak around the cuff while the patient inspires. Because this method cannot quantify the volume of a leak, a cuff leak test is more effective in detecting postextubation stridor while a patient is being mechanically ventilated. With the patient on controlled ventilation assist/control mode, an inspiratory tidal volume (VT) and six subsequent expiratory VT values are recorded after oropharyngeal suctioning and ETT cuff deflation. Six cycles are recorded because it was found that the exhaled VT values decreased decrementally during the first few breaths before reaching a plateau. The leak is measured as the difference between the preset inspiratory VT and the average of the three lowest of the subsequent six expiratory VT values.[23] A leak of less than 110 ml is considered a positive result of the cuff leak test and indicates that the patient is at risk for postextubation stridor secondary to laryngeal edema. Cuff leak tests have been criticized because of their poor sensitivity in detecting postextubation stridor and their low positive predictive value.[24–26]

Postoperative hemodynamic management after spine surgery

Acute postoperative hypertension

Despite advances in chronic hypertension management, acute postoperative hypertension (APH) occurs with a reported incidence of 4–35%.[27] APH may lead to serious neurologic (hemorrhagic stroke, cerebral ischemia, encephalopathy), cardiovascular (myocardial ischemia, cardiac arrhythmia, congestive heart failure, pulmonary edema), renal (acute kidney injury, acute tubular necrosis), and surgical site complications (bleeding, failure of vascular anastomosis) and requires prompt intervention and management.[27,28] Although there is no precise quantification of APH in the literature, APH typically refers to stages I (systolic 140–159 mmHg or diastolic 90–99 mmHg) and II (systolic >160 mmHg or diastolic >100 mmHg) hypertension according to the Joint National Committee classification of hypertension.[29] (Table 16.5). APH can also be defined as a 20% or more increase in systolic blood pressure, diastolic blood pressure, or mean arterial pressure above baseline.

The final common pathway leading to hypertension seems to be the activation of the sympathetic nervous system as evidenced by increased plasma catecholamine concentrations in patients with APH. APH is especially undesirable in postoperative patients

Table 16.5 Classification of blood pressure[29]

Normal <120 and <80 mmHg
Prehypertension 120–139 or 80–89 mmHg
Stage 1 hypertension 140–159 or 90–99 mmHg
Stage 2 hypertension >160 or >100 mmHg

after spine surgery since postoperative bleeding into a closed space (spinal cord, epidural space) can have life-threatening consequences (expanding neck hematoma, paraplegia, quadriplegia.).[30,31]

In the nonoperative setting, hypertensive emergency has been differentiated from hypertensive urgency by the presence of end organ damage.[32] In the postoperative setting, both clinical entities require prompt intervention to prevent the occurrence or progression of end organ damage and surgical site complications.

Identifying baseline blood pressure helps define a target blood pressure to avoid the deleterious consequences of overaggressive treatment. Prospective studies showing clinical benefits of aggressive blood pressure control in the postoperative period are lacking.[28] Whether to titrate to a target mean arterial pressure or systolic blood pressure is still controversial. There are, however, recent reports of the deleterious effects of pulse pressure hypertension on postoperative outcomes, supporting a focus on systolic blood pressure.[33]

Autonomic hyperreflexia

Patients with chronic spinal cord lesions above the level of T7 may develop autonomic hyperreflexia in response to surgical stimulation below the site of the lesion. Surgical stimulation results in intense vasoconstriction below the level of the lesion which is unmodulated by the typical inhibitory supraspinal reflexes resulting in severe hypertension and a reflex bradycardia (as well as cutaneous vasodilation above the level of the lesion).

Typically, patients show signs of autonomic hyperreflexia in the operating room with the onset of surgical stimulation, requiring deepening of the level of anesthesia to suppress the afferent pathways. If hypertension persists in the PACU, direct-acting vasodilators (e.g., nicardipine) can be helpful in controlling the hypertension (Table 16.6).

Postoperative hypotension

Postoperative hypotension is defined as a decrease of 20% from baseline preoperative blood pressure, a systolic blood pressure less than 80 mmHg, or a diastolic

Table 16.6 Algorithm for management of acute postoperative hypertension

1. Appropriate outpatient treatment of chronic hypertension before elective surgical procedures (Table 16.5, definition of hypertension)

2. Avoid discontinuation of oral antihypertensive medications on the day of surgery

3. Identify a baseline blood pressure preoperatively that acts as a reference point for postoperative management

4. Exclude factors associated with APH (e.g., pain, anxiety, hypothermia, hypoxemia, hypercapnia, bladder distension, presence of an ETT on emergence from anesthesia, antihypertensive withdrawal, increased intracranial pressure, hypervolemia)

5. Evaluate for APH and initiate therapy with intravenous short-acting antihypertensive agents after excluding other factors that can cause/exacerbate APH (pain, anxiety)

6. Short-acting intravenous agents are preferable for the initial management of APH (glyceryl trinitrate, nitroprusside, nicardipine, fenoldopam, clevidipine) because their effect can be reversed by the discontinuation of therapy. Esmolol may be appropriate for patients who will also benefit from beta-blockade

7. Avoid abrupt reduction of blood pressure (greater than 20%), especially in patients at no immediate risk (hypertensive urgencies)

8. Resume oral antihypertensive therapy as soon as possible postoperatively to reduce the occurrence of rebound hypertension, especially in patients taking centrally acting alpha-2 agonists or beta-blockers. Initiate additional agents as needed.

Table 16.7 Causes of hypotension and shock after spine surgery

Hypovolemia
Inadequate fluid replacement
Hemorrhage
External: e.g., surgical drain or incision site
Internal: e.g., from epidural veins, retroperitoneal vessels, bones
Mechanical (obstructive):
Pneumothorax
Pericardial effusion
Abdominal tamponade
Excessive PEEP
Cardiogenic
Chronic heart failure
Acute pulmonary edema
Acute myocardial infarction
Pulmonary embolism (venous air embolism, fat embolism)
Distributive (vasoplegia)
Neurogenic with spinal cord transection
Anaphylaxis
Septic

blood pressure less than 50 mmHg, whereas shock refers to multisystem organ hypoperfusion and inadequate oxygen delivery to tissues. Assessment of hypotension is commonly approached in terms of evaluation of cardiac rate, rhythm, contractility, and peripheral resistance and adequacy of intravascular volume.[34,35]

Hypotension in the PACU is often a sign of hypovolemia and often responds to intravenous fluid boluses. In patients with persistent hypotension despite a fluid "challenge," additional fluids may precipitate acute pulmonary edema, especially in patients with reduced left ventricular function. Other causes of hypotension and shock after spine surgery are listed in Table 16.7.

Several studies have documented the value of early goal-directed therapy in patients with shock. Rapid diagnosis and intervention improve outcomes.[34–37]

Several simple tools are used in the initial management of shock, including chest radiography, electrocardiography, serum chemistries, and blood gas analysis. Measurement of central venous pressure may be used to classify the mechanisms of shock (a low CVP in hypovolemic, a low normal CVP in distributive, and a high CVP in cardiogenic and mechanical), but multiple studies fail to show a good correlation between the so-called "filling pressures" and clinical reality. In addition, measurement of central venous oxygen saturation from a central vein or mixed venous oxygen saturation from a pulmonary artery catheter may be useful in diagnosing and monitoring the impact of therapeutic interventions in patients with shock.

PACU discharge readiness

Several scoring systems have been developed to aid in assessment of patient discharge readiness from the PACU, including the Aldrete scoring system and its modifications and the Post Anesthetic Discharge Scoring System[38–40] (Table 16.8). These scoring systems can also help in early identification of patients who require higher levels of postoperative care (intensive or intermediate care), thereby facilitating prompt triaging and appropriate disposition of patients to the next level of care. It is important to note that most published scoring systems do not include all parameters required for disposition to the next level of care. For example,

Table 16.8 Modified Aldrete and Post Anesthetic Discharge Scoring System

Respiration	Vital signs
2 = Able to take deep breath and cough	2 = BP + pluse within 20% preoperative baseline
1 = Dyspnea/shallow breathing	1 = BP + pulse within 20–40% preoperative baseline
0 = Apnea	0 = BP + pluse within >40% preoperative baseline
O$_2$ saturation	**Activity**
2 = Maintains S_pO_2 >92% on room air	2 = Steady gait, no dizziness or meets preoperative level
1 = Needs O$_2$ inhalation to maintain O$_2$ saturation >90%	1 = Requires assistance
0 = O$_2$ saturation >90% even with supplemental oxygen	0 = Unable to ambulate
Consciousness	**Nausea and vomiting**
2 = Fully awake	2 = Minimal/treated with PO medication
1 = Arousable on calling	1 = Moderate/treated with parenteral medication
0 = Not responding	0 = Severe/continues despite treatment
Circulation	**Pain**
2 = BP ± 20 mmHg preoperative	Controlled with oral analgesics and acceptable to patient:
1 = BP ± 20–50 mmHg preoperative	2 = Yes
0 = BP ± 50 mmHg preoperative	2 = No
Activity	**Surgical bleeding**
2 = Able to move four extremities voluntarily or on command	2 = Minimal/no dressing changes
1 = Able to move two extremities	1 = Moderate/up to two dressing changes required
0 = Unable to move extremities	0 = Severe/more than three dressing changes required
Score ≥9 for discharges	Score ≥9 for discharges

patients with hyper- or hypoglycemia will typically be managed in the PACU until their blood sugars are in the specified range.

In addition, most current PACU discharge scoring systems do not include core temperature assessments despite the deleterious effects of hypothermia on patient outcomes.[41,42] Most postoperative care units, however, require patient temperature to exceed 36°C before discharge and initiate forced air warming for temperatures below 36°C.

Finally, patient discharge from the PACU is typically held for a period of 20–30 minutes following any intravenous medications to allow monitoring of medication-related complications that could occur during patient transport to the next level of care.

Postoperative patients after spine surgery require frequent assessment for evidence of motor or sensory deficits in the upper and/or lower extremities. New-onset motor deficits will prompt emergent imaging and or surgical exploration for evidence of a compressive hematoma.

Patients that are kept intubated after spine surgery typically require reversal of neuromuscular blockade (if nondepolarizing muscle relaxants have been used)

Table 16.9 Motor assessment of limb movement

5 = Normal range of motion/muscle strength
4 = Normal range of motion – can be overcome with resistance
3 = Normal range of motion/against gravity only
2 = Visible movement but unable to overcome gravity
1 = Visible or palpable muscle contraction
R = Reflex withdrawal
F = Abnormal flexion
E = Abnormal extension
N = No Motor response
U = Unable to assist

to aid in assessment of extremity motor strength (Table 16.9) before sedation can be restarted (wake-up test). This is typically done in the operating room but can also be done on the patient's arrival to the PACU.

Delayed emergence requires a logical sequence to identify the underlying cause. Most commonly, anesthetics are the cause (inhalational anesthetics, intravenous anesthetics, narcotics, benzodiazepines, muscle relaxants). Metabolic causes can be ruled out by

Table 16.10 Guidelines for management of perioperative nerve injuries

1. Identify any preoperative motor or sensory deficits (history and physical examination)

2. Consider awake intubation and awake positioning of patients with severe or unstable injuries with postpositioning neurologic examination prior to induction of anesthesia

3. Careful positioning of patients and documentation of positioning details

4. Frequent rechecking of position to rule out any pressure-prone areas (eyes, ears, face, elbows, breasts, genitalia, sacrum, heels)

5. Avoidance of hypotension, hypothermia, and severe anemia

6. Postoperative neurologic examination and documentation of preexisting and new sensory and/ or motor deficits

7. Any suspected or confirmed newly diagnosed motor neuropathy requires a neurology consultation. Typically, electromyography is done to distinguish between acute and chronic motor deficits and to assess the location of any acute lesion

8. Sensory deficits (tingling, numbness, paresthesias) are typically self limited and patients should be informed that most sensory deficits resolve within a few days. Follow-up neurologic examination will identify persistent sensory neuropathy and warrant neurologic consultation

measuring blood glucose, serum sodium, blood urea nitrogen, creatinine, and hemoglobin concentrations. If an anesthetic cause is ruled out by waiting for predicted termination of anesthetic action, and by pharmacologic reversal of drug effects (naloxone, flumazenil, reversible anticholinesterase inhibitors), neurologic causes should be ruled out (e.g., brain edema, stroke) and may require a CT scan of the brain.

Positioning injuries after spine surgery

While most of the emphasis should be on the prevention of positioning-related injuries, identification and management of those injuries typically occurs in the postoperative period (recovery unit or nursing floor).[43] It is important to note that it is common for symptoms of nerve injury (sensory and/or motor) to start more than 48 hours postoperatively, indicating that the etiology may also be related to events in the postanesthetic period.

Guidelines for management of perioperative nerve injuries are listed in Table 16.10.

Common position-related injuries according to type of position during spine surgery

Supine (dorsal decubitus) position[43]

Pressure alopecia[44]

Pressure alopecia can occur in the occipital area especially in prolonged surgeries in the Trendelenburg position.

The use of padded head supports (foam) and avoidance of hypothermia and hypotension can help reduce the incidence of pressure alopecia. While frequent turning of the patient's head is sometimes advocated, it may not be practical in cervical pine surgery and may cause more harm in patients with cervical radiculopathy.

Ischemic necrosis

Ischemic necrosis can occur as a result of external pressure on weight-bearing bony prominences such as elbows, heels and sacrum. Proper padding and avoidance of hypotension and hypothermia that impair tissue perfusion can reduce those complications

Upper extremity injuries[45]

In the dorsal decubitus position, the arms are either tucked securely along the torso or secured on padded arm boards. Arms should be positioned to decrease external pressure on the postcondylar (ulnar) groove of the humerus. When the arms are tucked at the side, a neutral forearm position is recommended. When arms are abducted on arm boards, the abduction should be less than 90° and either supination or a neutral forearm position is acceptable.

In both arm positions, padding of the arm boards (if arms are abducted) or the arm sleds used to support the arms (if arms are tucked) may decrease the risk of upper extremity neuropathy. In the former position, care should be taken to avoid external pressure on the arm and padding with soft supports (foam or gel) is advocated. In addition, care should be taken to avoid external pressure of the ulnar nerve in the ulnar groove or distal to the medial epicondyle. If invasive arterial monitoring is used, it can serve as a method for verification of perfusion to one upper extremity while the pulse oximeter is applied to the contralateral upper extremity. Loss of waveform should alert the anesthesiologist to the possibility of insufficient perfusion and should trigger a change in position and identification of the cause.

Backache

Loss of lumbar curvature that occurs in the supine position is exacerbated by ligamentous relaxation under anesthesia. Padding placed under the lumbar spine or a pillow placed under the knees can help maintain the lumbar curvature. Care should be taken to avoid hyperlordosis since it may result in ischemia of lumbar spinal nerves.[46]

Lower extremities[45]

Placing the heels on a foam support and ensuring that the feet are not protruding from the operating room table (may require placement of an extension to the operating room table) can reduce positioning injuries. In addition, care should be taken during any adjustment of operating room table height to ensure that the patient's lower extremities are not crushed under the operating room equipment table.

Prone (ventral decubitus) position[47]

Eyes, ears, face, and chin

Eyes, ears, face, and chin should be maintained free of any external pressure. The eyelids should be closed and eye shields should be used to avoid eyelid separation and corneal scratching.

Maintaining a slight amount of head-up tilt reduces the occurrence of dependent periorbital edema. The prevention, risk factors, and management of perioperative vision loss are detailed in Chapter 15.

Excessive flexion of the head can result in pressure of the chin on the chest which may cause pressure-related ischemic injuries. Maintenance of the head in a neutral position and proper placement of chest rolls prevents this complication.

In addition, care is taken to protect against tongue and lip injuries that may occur during MEP monitoring by placement of soft mouth guards (bite blocks).

Neck

Excessive head and neck rotation can stretch nerves, ligaments, and muscles and contribute to postoperative nerve injuries. In addition, it can cause a reduction in jugular venous drainage and an impairment of flow to the carotid and vertebral systems.

Maintaining the head and neck in a sagittal plane can reduce these complications. This can be done either by foam or gel head supports of through the use of skull pin head clamps.

Brachial plexus injuries

If the arms are tucked alongside the torso, maintain the forearms in neutral position.

Avoid turning the face to one side since the roots of the brachial plexus on the contralateral side to the turned face may be stretched.

If the arms are placed on arm boards alongside the head, avoid backward displacement (hyperextension) of the shoulder joints, which can occur if the excessive padding of the arms raises the level of the arms above the level of the trunk and results in stretching of the brachial plexus.

Padding the armboard reduces the pressure on vulnerable peripheral nerves (ulnar nerve before, within, and beyond the carpal tunnel and radial nerve in spiral groove proximal to elbow).

Breast injuries

Direct pressure should be avoided. Proper padding and maintaining the breasts in a medial and cephalad orientation reduces the stretch on breast tissue that can occur alongside the medial aspects of the breast if lateral and caudad displacement occurs

Abdominal compression

Abdominal compression causes cephalad displacement and restriction of the diaphragm, impairing ventilation and resembling a restrictive process. In addition, the increase in intra-abdominal pressure reduces venous return from the pelvis and lower extremities and results in engorgement of the vertebral venous plexus, thereby increasing surgical bleeding and impairing hemostasis. If direct compression of the inferior vena cava occurs by the supporting pads or operating table frame (typically occurs in the morbidly obese population), complete cardiovascular collapse can occur due to total obstruction of inferior venal caval flow, resulting in pulseless electrical activity. This requires early identification, return of the patient to the supine position to restore venous return, and a change in the position of the supporting frames/pads. If this is unsuccessful, a different surgical operating table that allows a freely hanging abdomen or a different surgical approach should be considered. The aforementioned complications can be prevented by careful patient positioning on the operating room table to allow free cephalad diaphragmatic excursion and avoid direct pressure of the supporting pads and frames on the anterior abdominal wall.

References

1. Hines R, Barash PG, Watrous G, O'Connor T. Complications occurring in the postanesthesia care unit: a survey. *Anesth Analg* 1992; **74**: 503–9.

2. Duncan PG, Cohen MM, Tweed WA, *et al.* The Canadian four-centre study of anaesthetic outcomes: III. Are anaesthetic complications predictable in day surgical practice? *Can J Anaesth* 1992; **39**: 440–8.

3. Burkle CM, Walsh MT, Pryor SG, Kasperbauer JL. Severe postextubation laryngeal obstruction: the role of prior neck dissection and radiation. *Anesth Analg* 2006; **102**: 322–5.

4. Murphy GS, Szokol JW, Marymont JH, *et al.* Residual neuromuscular blockade and critical respiratory events in the postanesthesia care unit. *Anesth Analg* 2008; **107**: 130–7.

5. American Society of Anesthesiologists Task Force on Management of the Difficult Airway: Practice guidelines for management of the difficult airway: An updated report by the American Society of Anesthesiologists Task Force on Management of the Difficult Airway. *Anesthesiology* 2003; **98**: 1269–77.

6. Calder I, Calder J, Crockard HA. Difficult direct laryngoscopy in patients with cervical spine disease. *Anaesthesia* 1995; **50**: 756–63.

7. Manninen PH, Jose GB, Lukitto K, Venkatraghavan L, El Beheiry H. Management of the airway in patients undergoing cervical spine surgery. *J Neurosurg Anesthesiol* 2007; **19**: 190–4.

8. Crosby ET. Considerations for airway management for cervical spine surgery in adults. *Anesthesiol Clin* 2007; **25**: 511–33.

9. Epstein NE, Hollingsworth R, Nardi D, Singer J. Can airway complications following multilevel anterior cervical surgery be avoided? *J Neurosurg* 2001; **94**: 185–8.

10. Sinha A, Agarwal A, Gaur A, Pandey CK. Oropharyngeal swelling and macroglossia after cervical spine surgery in the prone position. *J Neurosurg Anesthesiol* 2001; **13**: 237–9.

11. Lennarson PJ, Smith DW, Sawin PD, *et al.* Cervical spinal motion during intubation: Efficacy of stabilization maneuvers in the setting of complete segmental instability. *J Neurosurg* 2001; **94**: 265–70.

12. Komatsu R, Nagata O, Kamata K, *et al.* Intubating laryngeal mask airway allows tracheal intubation when the cervical spine is immobilized by a rigid collar. *Br J Anaesth* 2004; **93**: 655–9.

13. Terao Y, Matsumoto S, Yamashita K, *et al.* Increased incidence of emergency airway management after combined anterior – posterior cervical spine surgery. *J Neurosurg Anesthesiol* 2004; **16**: 282–6.

14. Mort TC. Continuous airway access for the difficult extubation: The efficacy of the airway exchange catheter. *Anesth Analg* 2007; **105**: 1357–62.

15. Loudermilk EP, Hartmannsgruber M, Stoltzfus DP, Langevin PB. A prospective study of the safety of tracheal extubation using a pediatric airway exchange catheter for patients with a known difficult airway. *Chest* 1997; **111**: 1660–5.

16. Takata M, Benumof JL, Ozaki GT. Confirmation of endotracheal intubation over a jet stylet: In vitro studies. *Anesth Analg* 1995; **80**: 800–5.

17. Benumof JL. Airway exchange catheters: Simple concept, potentially great danger. *Anesthesiology* 1999; **91**: 342–4.

18. Cooper RM. The use of an endotracheal ventilation catheter in the management of difficult extubations. *Can J Anaesth* 1996; **43**: 90–3.

19. Benumof JL. Airway exchange catheters for safe extubation: The clinical and scientific details that make the concept work. *Chest* 1997; **111**: 1483–6.

20. Argalious M, Ritchey M, deUngria M, Doyle DJ. An airway exchange catheter contributing to airway obstruction. *Can J Anaesth* 2008; **55**: 128–9.

21. Argalious M, Doyle DJ. Questioning the length of airway exchange catheters. *Anesthesiology* 2007; **106**: 404.

22. Argalious M. Airway challenges in PACU/ICU. *Anesthesiol News* 2005; **31**: 57–61.

23. Miller RL, Cole RP. Association between reduced cuff leak volume and postextubation stridor. *Chest* 1996; **110**: 1035–40.

24. De Bast Y, De Backer D, Moraine JJ, *et al.* The cuff leak test to predict failure of tracheal extubation for laryngeal edema. *Intensive Care Med* 2002; **28**: 1267–72.

25. Engoren M. Evaluation of the cuff-leak test in a cardiac surgery population. *Chest* 1999; **116**: 1029–31.

26. Jaber S, Chanques G, Matecki S, *et al.* Post-extubation stridor in intensive care unit patients. Risk factors evaluation and importance of the cuff-leak test. *Intensive Care Med* 2003; **29**: 69–74.

27. Haas CE, LeBlanc JM. Acute postoperative hypertension: A review of therapeutic options. *Am J Health Syst Pharm* 2004; **61**: 1661–73.

28. Marik PE, Varon J. Hypertensive crises: Challenges and management. *Chest* 2007; **131**: 1949–62.

29. Chobanian AV, Bakris GL, Black HR, *et al.* The seventh report of the Joint National Committee on Prevention, Detection, Evaluation, and Treatment of High Blood Pressure: The JNC 7 report. *JAMA* 2003; **289**: 2560–72.

30. Prys-Roberts C. Anaesthesia and hypertension. *Br J Anaesth* 1984; **56**: 711–24.

31. Halpern NA, Goldberg M, Neely C, *et al.* Postoperative hypertension: A multicenter, prospective, randomized comparison between intravenous nicardipine and sodium nitroprusside. *Crit Care Med* 1992; **20**: 1637–43.

32. Slama M, Modeliar SS. Hypertension in the intensive care unit. *Curr Opin Cardiol* 2006; **21**: 279–87.

33. Aronson S, Fontes ML. Hypertension: A new look at an old problem. *Curr Opin Anaesthesiol* 2006; **19**: 59–64.

34. Pinsky MR. Hemodynamic evaluation and monitoring in the ICU. *Chest* 2007; **132**: 2020–9.

35. Axler O. Evaluation and management of shock. *Semin Respir Crit Care Med* 2006; **27**: 230–40.

36. Subramaniam B, Talmor D. Echocardiography for management of hypotension in the intensive care unit. *Crit Care Med* 2007; **35**: S401–7.

37. Monnet X, Teboul JL. Volume responsiveness. *Curr Opin Crit Care* 2007; **13**: 549–53.

38. Aldrete JA. The post-anesthesia recovery score revisited. *J Clin Anesth* 1995; **7**(1): 89–91.

39. White PF, Song D. New criteria for fast-tracking after outpatient anesthesia: a comparison with the modified Aldrete's scoring system. *Anesth Analg* 1999; **88**: 1069.

40. Standards for Postanesthesia Care (last amended October 27, 2004). Available at www.asahq.org/publicationsAndServices/standards/36.pdf.

41. Kurz A, Sessler DI, Lenhardt R for the Study of Wound Infection and Temperature Group. Perioperative normothermia to reduce the incidence of surgical-wound infection and shorten hospitalization *N Engl J Med* 1996; **334**: 1209–16.

42. Schmied H, Kurz A, Sessler DI, *et al.* Mild intraoperative hypothermia increases blood loss and allogenic transfusion requirements during total hip arthroplasty. *Lancet* 1996; **347**: 289–92.

43. Practice advisory for the prevention of perioperative peripheral neuropathies: a report by the American Society of Anesthesiologists Task Force on Prevention of Perioperative Peripheral Neuropathies. *Anesthesiology* 2000; **92**: 1168–82.

44. Lawson NW, Mills NL, Ochsner JL. Occipital alopecia following cardiopulmonary bypass. *J Thorac Cardiovasc Surg* 1976; **71**: 342.

45. Warner MA, Warner DO, Matsumoto JY, *et al.* Ulnar neuropathy in surgical patients. *Anesthesiology* 1999; **90**: 54.

46. Amoiridis G, Worhrle JC, Langkafel M, *et al.* Spinal cord infarction after surgery in a patient in a hyperlordotic position. *Anesthesiology* 1996; **84**: 228.

47. Edgcombe H, Carter K, Yarrow S. Anesthesia in the prone position. *Br J Anaesth* 2008; **100**: 165.

Chapter

17

Postoperative care in the neuro-intensive care unit

James K. C. Liu, Dani S. Bidros, and Edward M. Manno

Key points

- The postoperative care of the spine surgery patient requires a multidisciplinary approach between the spine surgeon, the intensive care team, as well as an approach surgeon, if one was involved in the procedure.
- A thorough examination of the postoperative spine patient is vital to elucidate any new deficits that have occurred as a result of a surgical complication and to facilitate rapid treatment.
- The level of prophylaxis for deep vein thrombosis should be tailored depending on the procedure being performed and the patient's comorbidities.
- Airway compromise is a potentially lethal complication following cervical spine surgery and should be closely monitored in the postoperative period.
- Anterior thoracic and lumbar spine procedures can be complicated by respiratory or gastrointestinal related symptoms due to the manipulation of the relevant structures during the approach.

Introduction

Postoperative care of the spine surgery patient can be very complex. Often times, these patients require the attention provided in an intensive care setting. In order for members of the intensive care team to adequately care for the patient, it is imperative that the team is equipped with a baseline understanding of different spinal surgical procedures and how each procedure can uniquely affect the patient in the post-operative setting. In this chapter, a brief overview of the pertinent spinal anatomy will be reviewed. This

will be followed by a review of general considerations for all postoperative spine surgery patients. Finally, segments of the spine will be discussed individually, and the complications related to approaches specific to each segment will be reviewed.

Surgical anatomy of the spine

The spinal column consists of 7 cervical, 12 thoracic, 5 lumbar, and 5 sacral vertebrae, and 1 coccyx. The spinal cord extends from the medulla of the brainstem, beginning prior to the foramen magnum, down to the L1 to L2 levels in adults. There are matching ventral and dorsal nerve roots at each spinal level with the exception of the first cervical level which contains only a ventral nerve root. There are also nerve roots at the C8 level, despite an absence of the C8 vertebra.

The main arterial supply of the spinal cord is derived from three longitudinal spinal arteries, one anterior spinal artery, and a pair of posterior spinal arteries. The anterior spinal artery travels in the median sulcus on the ventral aspect of the spinal cord, and extends from the medulla to the conus medullaris. It is formed by a branch from each of the vertebral arteries and supplies the anterior two-thirds of the spinal cord. Infarction of the anterior spinal artery would manifest predominantly as motor deficits and loss of pain and temperature. Two posterior spinal arteries arising from the vertebral arteries supply the posterior aspect of the spinal cord. They traverse the length of the spinal cord to the conus medullaris just medial to the exiting dorsal nerve roots. These arteries provide the primary blood supply to the posterior columns, infarction of which will lead to loss of vibration sense and proprioception. The spinal arteries are largest in the cervical and lumbar regions, matching the ganglionic enlargements in the spinal cord at those levels.

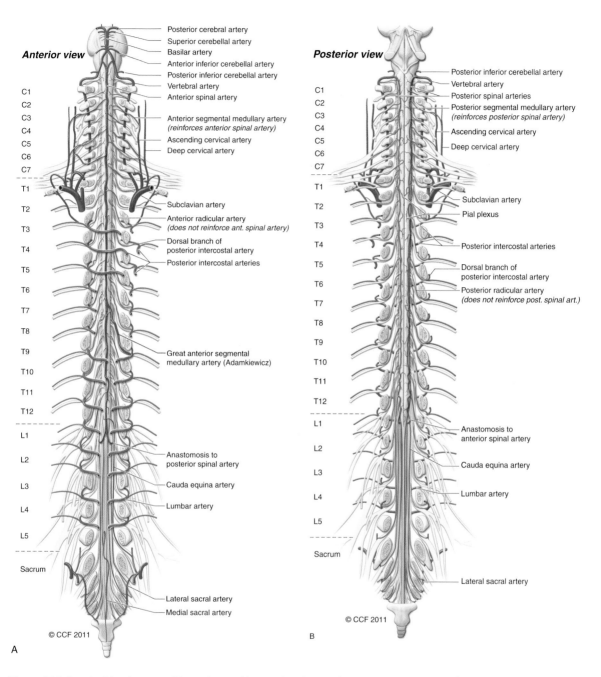

Figure 17.1 Anterior (A) and posterior (B) vasculature of the spinal cord. A singular anterior spinal artery is formed from a branch from each of the vertebral arteries. Segmental arteries from the aorta contribute blood supply to the thoracic and lumbar spinal cord. The artery of Adamkiewicz is a major radicular artery usually feeding from the left side. Two posterior spinal arteries branch from each of the vertebral arteries and travel the distance of the spinal cord just medial to the dorsal nerve roots.

The anterior and posterior spinal arterial supply is supplemented by radicular arteries through the length of the spinal cord. In the cervical region, 80% of the radicular arteries are supplied by the vertebral arteries, whereas in the thoracic and lumbar regions, intercostal arteries that branch off the aorta are the source of the blood supply. The artery of Adamkiewicz, the largest anterior radicular artery, occurs on the left side 80%

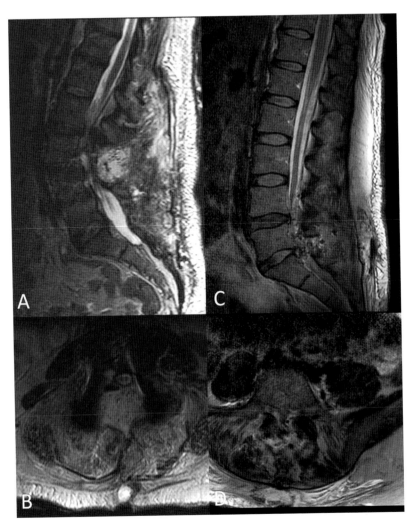

Figure 17.2 Postoperative epidural hematomas. A 62-year-old patient underwent multiple level laminectomy and fusion. The patient presented one week following surgery with back and bilateral lower extremity pain. Sagittal (A) and axial (B) T2W MRI shows an epidural fluid collection with compression on the thecal sac at the level of L3–4, where the previous laminectomy was performed. A 47-year-old patient who underwent a unilateral discectomy returned with recurrent bilateral lower extremity pain. Sagittal (C) and axial (D) T2W MRI shows an epidural collection at the L5–S1 level.

of the time and is commonly seen around the T9 to T11 levels.[1] This artery is believed to contribute greatly to the blood supply to the spinal cord from T8 to the conus. Great care is taken during preoperative planning to avoid ligation of this artery (Fig. 17.1).

Neurologic assessment

Interval neurologic assessments are necessary following spinal surgery in order to detect any deficits that may be present due to a postoperative complication which will require immediate intervention. Although a thorough neurologic assessment should be performed, a basic understanding of the surgical procedure performed will help to focus the examination to elucidate the complications that are more common to that particular type of procedure. Understanding the surgical levels performed and the complications that

can be associated with that particular approach to the spine will allow the physician to be more readily able to detect such complications.

The neurologic assessment of all spine surgery patients should include a detailed upper and lower extremity strength and sensory examination. This should be compared to the patient's preoperative examination to properly assess whether any new deficits have developed since the procedure. In all spine surgery patients, any new and progressive motor or sensory deficits must lead the physician to consider the development of a spinal epidural hematoma (Fig. 17.2). Epidural hematomas are rare but potentially devastating complications following spinal surgery. Reported incidence is approximately 0.2%, with increased risk shown in patients undergoing multilevel procedures or in patients with a preoperative coagulopathy.[2]

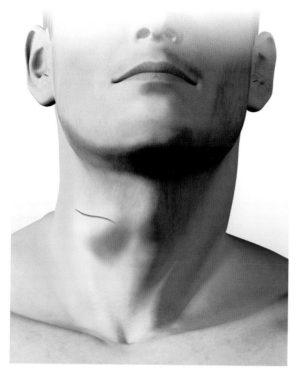

Figure 17.3 Postoperative hematoma following anterior cervical surgery: a patient with neck swelling following anterior cervical discectomy and fusion procedure. Note the right-sided incision with bulging and contralateral tracheal deviation.

Clinical presentations include radicular pain, bladder dysfunction, and motor and sensory deficits. Imaging to confirm diagnosis followed by immediate surgical intervention has been shown to improve neurologic recovery.[3]

For anterior cervical spine surgery, special attention must be given to the neck area to assess for the development of a fluid collection. Assessment of neck size and evaluation for any signs of tracheal deviation should be performed regularly in the postoperative period (Fig. 17.3). Any change in neck size or tracheal deviation may indicate a developing collection of cerebrospinal fluid, CSF or blood. Some surgeons use regular neck circumference measurements to detect for any occult swelling that may result in respiratory compromise.

The presence of postoperative radicular pain or weakness in patients after spinal fusion with instrumentation may indicate nerve root impingement from an errantly placed screw (Figs. 17.4 and 17.5). It may be difficult to delineate postoperative pain and weakness due to transient postoperative inflammation of the nerve root from structural impingement. Radicular pain that matches a dermatomal distribution and is disproportionate to expected postoperative pain suggests a structural etiology. Under these circumstances, one may consider the use of plain radiographs to evaluate any gross abnormalities with the instrumentation. Plain radiographs will only provide an idea of the alignment of the spine and the instrumentation. If suspicion persists, computed tomography (CT) imaging will provide the most accurate depiction of hardware placement in the spine. Magnetic resonance imaging (MRI), which would otherwise be the most effective imaging modality for evaluating neural structures, may be less effective due to artifact from the nearby instrumentation.

The wound should be regularly examined for any evidence of infection, dehiscence, or fluid leakage. Patients who have suffered an incidental dural tear intraoperatively may experience positional headaches that are worse when sitting up or standing and alleviated in the supine position. Compressible distension in the area of the incision implies a fluid collection in the surgical bed.

General considerations

Spinal cord ischemia

Spinal cord ischemia is a relatively rare occurrence that can present either due to a predisposed condition or from a direct iatrogenic injury. An injured spinal cord from chronic spinal canal stenosis, as indicated from signal changes on MRI, can be more susceptible to variations in perfusion. This may result from a decreased ability for autoregulation in the injured spinal cord, making it more susceptible to hypotension during the procedure. An iatrogenic injury to the spinal cord can also disrupt the vascular flow. This may include direct trauma or manipulation of the spinal cord, or from tethering of the cord and/or its vascular supply during deformity correction procedures. Decreased perfusion from a lack of adequate autoregulation can lead to accumulation of intracellular calcium and sodium ions, leading to an excess of glutamate and resulting in the production of free radicals. This can eventually result in edema, inflammation, and – ultimately – cell apoptosis. The thoracic spine is particularly susceptible to such ischemic injury as the T4 through T9 levels are considered a vascular watershed area.[1]

Spinal shock can be a clinical manifestation of severe spinal cord ischemia. Spinal shock is a form of

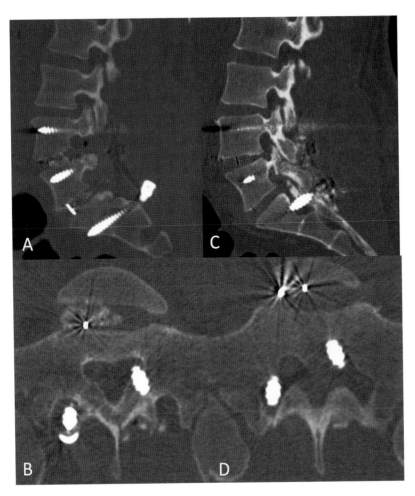

Figure 17.4 Misplaced lumbar pedicle screw. A 39-year-old patient underwent an L4–S1 posterolateral fusion presented with significant right S1 distribution leg pain postoperatively. CT imaging was performed to evaluate the instrumentation which showed both the right (A) and left (C) S1 pedicles screws were placed too inferiorly and traversing the S1 neural foramina. Axial views of the S1 screws (B and D) also show the left screw to be too medial, breaching the lateral border of the spinal canal.

neurogenic shock and consists of the loss of somatic motor, sensory, and sympathetic autonomic function. In the early postinjury period, an upper motor neuron injury manifests itself clinically as a lower motor neuron injury (hyporeflexia). The more severe the cord injury and the higher the level of injury, the greater the severity and duration of spinal shock. Thus, spinal shock is more severe in complete upper cervical cord injuries than in lumbar cord injury. The somatic motor component of spinal shock may consist of paralysis, flaccidity, and areflexia. The sensory component may be completely lost, and the autonomic dysfunction will lead to hypotension, bradycardia, skin hyperemia, and warmth. This phase persists for a variable length of time – usually from several days to several months.

Diagnosis of spinal cord ischemia should come after ruling out other structural causes of neurologic deficit including spinal cord compression from hematoma formation or errant instrumentation. MRI should then be performed in order to detect signal changes indicating ischemic insult. Treatment of cord ischemia includes adequate cord perfusion, generally considered as maintaining a mean arterial pressure of greater than 80 mmHg. Vasopressors should be utilized if necessary, such as dopamine and levophed, avoiding epinephrine as its alpha adrenergic effects can lead to vasoconstriction and possibly decreased spinal cord perfusion.[4] Systemic cooling is another treatment considered in the treatment of postoperative spinal cord ischemia, although the neuroprotective effect of this technique in the spine has not been fully proven.[5] CSF drainage via a postoperatively placed subarachnoid drain is a technique commonly employed following thoracoabdominal aortic aneurysm repair; it can also be utilized for prevention and treatment of spinal cord ischemia. Drainage of CSF is thought to reduce the pressure surrounding the spinal cord, allowing for increased blood flow to the spinal cord.[6]

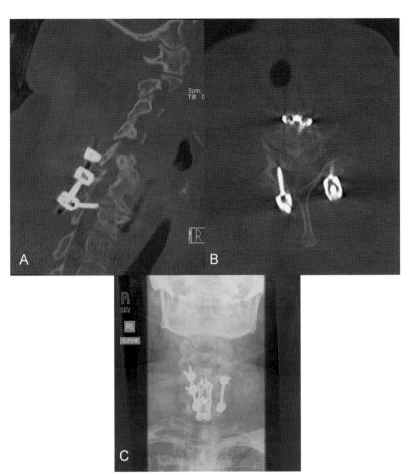

Figure 17.5 Misplaced cervical lateral mass screw. A 51-year-old patient with a previous history of a C5–6 and C6–7 ACDF two years previously presented with neck pain and numbness and tingling in both arms. She underwent a C6 laminectomy with a C5–7 posterior fusion with lateral mass screws in the right C5–7 lateral masses and the left C5 and C7 lateral masses. Postoperatively the patient has right-sided weakness in the upper and lower extremities. Anterior–posterior view radiographs (C) and CT (A and B) scan revealed a medially placed right C7 lateral mass screw extending into the spinal canal. The patient was taken to the operating room for screw repositioning, following which there was improvement in the patient's neurologic examination.

Perioperative blood transfusions

Fluid management in postoperative spine surgery is possibly the most important aspect of the patient's care. Patients undergoing major spine surgery will often experience major blood loss during the procedure and will require blood transfusions intraoperatively, and commonly postoperatively. In a study of 112 patients undergoing posterior lumbar fusions, the authors concluded that predictors for blood transfusions included increased number of levels fused, preoperative anemia, and advanced age.[7] Another retrospective review of 244 patients undergoing spinal fusions with instrumentation also attributed increased transfusions to tumor surgery and in patients with a history of pulmonary disease. Patients with a history of pulmonary disease are likely to require more transfusions to maintain higher hemoglobin concentrations for adequate tissue perfusion. Tumors involving the spinal column are highly vascular and can involve significant blood loss.[8] Management of patients with these risk factors

may include perioperative interventions such as using erythropoietin to elevate preoperative hemoglobin levels.[9]

Venous thromboembolism

The development of deep venous thrombosis (DVT) and pulmonary embolism is a major concern in spine surgery patients. Treatment is controversial. The incidence of DVT and venous thromboembolism (VTE) after elective spinal procedures is low. The risk of VTE increases in patients undergoing prolonged surgical procedures, including circumferential procedures involving combined anterior and posterior approaches, as well as in patients with increased preoperative risks for developing DVT such as hypercoagulable states, malignancy, spinal cord injury, or prolonged immobilization. In 2009, the Antithrombotic Therapies Work Group of the North American Spine Society Evidence-Based Guideline Development Committee published guidelines for the use of antithrombotic therapy

297

following spine surgery. The work group recommended the use of mechanical compression devices in the lower extremities because of their proven effectiveness in decreasing VTE and their low associated complication rates. There is considerable debate considering the use of chemoprophylaxis due to the risk of developing postoperative epidural hematomas. Although the literature supports the use of postoperative low-molecular weight heparin, it was suggested that chemoprophylaxis may not be warranted in commonly performed elective procedures. The use of chemoprophylaxis may be warranted for high-risk patients, and there is literature to support that it is safe to start chemoprophylaxis as early as the day of elective spine surgery. This is merely a consensus provided by the work group and the timing of initiating chemoprophylaxis will vary depending on surgeon preference.[10] In our institution, guidelines for VTE prophylaxis were recently set by stratifying patients into low, intermediate, and high risk. Sequential compression devices are applied to all patients prior to induction of anesthesia until the patient is ambulating independently. For high-risk patients, chemoprophylaxis will be started within 48 hours of the procedure, the exact timing being dependent on surgeon preference and the patient's condition. In our institution, we will consider bi-weekly ultrasound screening only for high-risk patients, primarily in those with a history of malignancy.

Cervical spine surgery

Among the major concerns in the management of patients who have undergone cervical spine surgery is airway compromise, particularly if an anterior approach was taken. Complications that result in airway compromise can be from inadvertent injury to nerve structures or from retraction edema.

One of the most commonly performed procedures is anterior cervical discectomy and fusion (ACDF). This procedure is performed for cervical disc herniations, manifesting as unilateral radicular upper extremity pain. It is performed from a unilateral anterior approach, to access levels between C2 and C7. In addition, the same approach is used for cervical corpectomies, in which an entire vertebral body is removed followed by inserting a graft in its place. In addition to replacement of the intervertebral disc or vertebral body by a graft, a plate is placed anterior to the graft and secured to the adjacent levels with screws in order to help facilitate fusion. Multiple cervical levels can be accessed through a single incision

in this approach, necessitating an increasing amount of retraction.

A rare but potentially lethal complication following anterior cervical surgery is airway obstruction. Airway obstruction typically results from mass effect, such as hematoma formation or CSF collection. Risk of postoperative hematoma formation can be reduced with meticulous intraoperative hemostasis as well as placement of a drain for a short period postoperatively. CSF collections are a result of dural tears, and can be prevented by effective dural closure and possibly the addition of a dural sealant. Another cause of airway obstruction is prevertebral soft tissue swelling. A certain degree of prevertebral soft tissue swelling is unavoidable following anterior cervical procedures. In a study of 87 patients undergoing one- or two-level ACDFs, it was noted that prevertebral soft tissue swelling peaked at the second and third postoperative days.[11] Another study evaluating the same types of procedures noted that the greatest amount of soft tissue swelling occurred in the upper cervical spine, rostral to the C4 level.[12] Respiratory compromise secondary to prevertebral soft tissue swelling is relatively rare but can be difficult to manage due to the insidious nature of the swelling. In a study by Suk et al.,[11] only one patient out of 87 (1.1%) required intubation for respiratory compromise secondary to edema. The risk for respiratory compromise increases with increasing complexity of cases. In a retrospective analysis of 311 anterior cervical procedures, Sagi et al. noted a 6.1% incidence of postoperative airway complications with 1.9% requiring re-intubation. Factors that were associated with increased risk of postoperative airway compromise included exposure of greater than three vertebral bodies, blood loss >300 ml, operative time >5 h, and exposure of C2 through C4 levels.[13] Myelopathy, spinal cord injury, pulmonary pathology, smoking, or anesthetic risk factors were not correlated with postoperative respiratory compromise. Emery et al. evaluated seven patients who underwent multilevel cervical corpectomies and required re-intubation. Four of the seven patients were noted to have severe hypopharyngeal and supraglottic swelling.[14] The authors concluded that the major risk factors for postoperative respiratory distress were multilevel procedures and prolonged operative and retraction times.

These studies indicate that although there is an expected amount of prevertebral soft tissue swelling following anterior cervical procedures, as the complexity of the procedure increases, so does the amount of swelling and likelihood of respiratory compromise. Multilevel discectomies or corpectomies, which require a larger surgical field of view, will likely involve a greater degree of retraction and for longer operative times. Familiarity with the expected course of postoperative prevertebral swelling can assist in the management of these patients. Some surgeons have advocated maintaining intubation of patients undergoing complex procedures and using direct fiberoptic visualization to evaluate for the amount of postoperative tracheal swelling.[15] Delaying extubation can avoid the need for emergent re-intubation, which can put the patient at risk for graft-related complications. Some practitioners use postoperative steroids for reduction of edema, although this practice is unproven. A prospective, randomized, double-blinded study performed by Emery et al. showed that postoperative administration of intravenous steroids following multilevel cervical corpectomies did not have any effect on reducing re-tubation following the procedure.[16]

Thoracic spine surgery

Management of the postoperative thoracic spine surgery patient can be challenging, particularly in patients who undergo anterior approaches. Anterior approaches to the thoracic spine are utilized to obtain access for disc herniations, osteomyelitis, trauma, or spinal deformity. Many spine surgeons prefer to enlist the services of an "approach surgeon," such as a thoracic surgeon, to assist with the approach. Therefore, the postoperative care of the spine patient having undergone an anterior thoracic approach requires a team approach between the intensive care team, thoracic surgeons, and spine surgeons.

The anterior approach to the thoracic spine can pose unique complications due to the manipulation of the respiratory system. Approaches to the thoracic spine can be categorized based on the level of the pathology. The upper thoracic spine, generally T2 or above, is most commonly approached through a straight anterior approach requiring a sternotomy. For pathology involving the mid thoracic spine, a thoracotomy approach is typically utilized. Lesions between T2 and T5 are commonly approached from the right side to avoid the arch of the aorta, while lesions below T5 are approached from the left side to avoid the vena cava (which is more sensitive to manipulation and difficult to repair than the aorta). These categorizations are general guidelines utilized by many surgeons; the exact

approach taken will depend on the type and location of the pathology and the experience of the surgeon.

The transthoracic approach to the mid thoracic spine includes a transpleural dissection. Following a transpleural approach, a chest tube is placed through an incision separate to the primary incision. Management of the chest tube is usually carried out by the team performing the approach. Weaning of the chest tube occurs over the next several days. As expected, pulmonary-related complications predominate in patients following thoracic spine surgery with anterior approaches and should be a concern for these patients. In a study of 117 patients undergoing a thoracotomy for anterior approach to the thoracic spine, 5 suffered postoperative pneumonia and 10 patients required either re-intubation due to hypoxemia, or remained dependent on mechanical ventilation for more than three postoperative days.[17] In another study of 59 patients undergoing anterior thoracic spine surgery, 66% developed pleural effusions, 5% developed atelectasis, and 13% developed evidence of partial or complete lobar collapse.[18]

The postoperative care of a patient having undergone a thoracotomy to approach the anterior thoracic spine should include daily chest radiography to monitor for worsening atelectasis, pleural effusion, or pneumothorax. Chest tube weaning should be based on the results of the daily chest radiography. Adequate pain control is also crucial as there can be significant postoperative pain from a thoractomy approach. Severe chest wall pain may restrict respiratory mechanics and further compound existing atelectasis. Aggressive incentive spirometry in the immediate postoperative period as well as aggressive pain control will help to avoid this complication. Some surgeons advocate the use of intercostal blocks or nonsteroidal anti-inflammatory agents to assist in pain control.[17]

A less commonly encountered but potentially severe complication of anterior thoracic spine surgery is development of a chylothorax due to a thoracic duct injury. This can occur following a right-sided approach to the caudal thoracic spine. Clinical presentation of a chylothorax may vary, depending on when the patient returns to a normal diet, increasing the production of chyle secondary to an increased intake of fatty acids. Dehydration as well as electrolyte abnormalities, particularly hyponatremia, can develop as a result of a chyle leak. Initial treatment of chyle leaks includes pleural drainage as well as reduced oral intake especially of long-chain fatty acids, with intravenous nutritional supplementation. If there is not significant reduction of the loss of chyle with conservative management, surgical ligation of the leak may be necessary.[19]

Lumbar spine surgery

Anterior approaches to the lumbar spine will involve manipulations of organs different from those encountered in the thoracic cavity and therefore pose a slightly different set of postoperative challenges. The thoracolumbar junction and lumbar spine is typically accessed through a left-sided thoracoabdominal approach, consisting of a retroperitoneal approach through a low left-sided thoractomy with division of the diaphragm. The violation of the intrapleural space in this approach dictates the use of a chest tube postoperatively. In Pettiford's study of 91 patients undergoing thoracolumbar approaches, five patients suffered from pneumonia postoperatively. Although there were fewer patients suffering respiratory failure, (8.5% vs. 5.4%) in the thoracolumbar group, postoperative ileus was more prominent in this group.[17] This is likely secondary to manipulation of the bowel through a retroperitoneal approach. The postoperative patient should be kept without oral intake until there is evidence of bowel motility, such as flatus or bowel sounds, at which time the diet can be cautiously advanced.

The lower lumbar spine can be accessed through a retroperitoneal or a transabdominal transperitoneal approach. Because of the proximity to the major vessels in these approaches, many spine surgeons choose to have a vascular surgeon provide the access. Therefore, postoperative care should be coordinated between both the spine and the vascular surgeons. Not unlike the thoracolumbar approach, manipulation of the abdominal contents precludes the patient to postoperative ileus, but fewer pulmonary-related complications are encountered. Bowel rest followed by conservative advancement of diet in the postoperative periods is required. Gastric suctioning is used to prevent overdistension until bowel activity has returned.

Vascular complications are not uncommon following an anterior approach to the lumbar spine given the manipulation of the aorta, vena cava, and iliac arteries and veins encountered during this approach. Iliac artery thrombosis is a complication that may occur in the postoperative period without any obvious injury noted intraoperatively.[20,21] Since this complication is rare, it can be further hidden by the fact that any neurologic deficits noted postoperatively following a spinal procedure would most likely be first attributed to nerve root injury. Therefore, it is important to consider the diagnosis of arterial thrombosis in a patient suffering neurologic deficits following anterior lumbar surgery. Arterial thrombosis typically manifests as limb pain with motor or sensory deficits. Therefore, a careful pulse examination with pulse oximetry of the left lower extremity should be performed, as well as attention to any temperature differences between the two extremities. Arterial thrombosis can be diagnosed with angiography, but if high suspicion of an arterial thrombosis exists, immediate treatment with a thrombectomy or bypass may be warranted to prevent irreversible ischemic injury.

Ureteral injuries can be commonly encountered following anterior lumbar spine approaches, and have been reported from 0.3% to 8%.[22] Ureteral injuries can be occult at the time the procedure, caused by retraction injury during a retroperitoneal approach as the peritoneum is retracted laterally. Clinical signs of a ureteral injury will manifest as flank or abdominal pain. Infection may develop, resulting in fevers or leukocytosis, as well as azotemia or elevated serum creatinine. CT scanning or ultrasound imaging can be utilized for diagnosis of a retroperitoneal collection, but it may be confused with a retroperitoneal hematoma. One study reported performing an ultrasound-guided aspiration of a retroperitoneal fluid collection to diagnose urine, after which the patient was taken for placement of ureteral stents.[23] This strategy can also be utilized to diagnose lymphoceles, which can also develop in the retroperitoneal space.[24]

Conclusion

The intensive care management of the postoperative spine surgery patient can be a very complex undertaking. Advancements in spine surgery have allowed surgeons to exercise more aggressive and radical treatments on a steadily aging patient population. This results in patients undergoing surgical procedures with more numerous comorbidities and a higher risk of complication following the surgical procedure. This has resulted in larger numbers of patients who require intensive medical management following their procedures. An understanding of the anatomy associated with the surgical procedure being performed, as well as the ability to elicit these findings on physical examination, is essential to the early diagnosis and proper treatment of possible complications. A team approach utilizing the experience of the surgical team with the medical care expertise of the intensive care team is vital to successfully treating the complications that may be encountered.

References

1. Dommisse GF. The blood supply of the spinal cord. A critical vascular zone in spinal surgery. *J Bone Joint Surg Br* 1974; **56**: 225–35.

2. Yi S, Yoon DH, Kim KN, *et al.* Postoperative spinal epidural hematoma: risk factor and clinical outcome. *Yonsei Med J* 2006; **47**: 326–32.

3. Lawton MT, Porter RW, Heiserman JE, *et al.* Surgical management of spinal epidural hematoma: relationship between surgical timing and neurological outcome. *J Neurosurg* 1995; **83**: 1–7.

4. H Ahn, Fehlings MG. Prevention, identification, and treatment of perioperative spinal cord injury. *Neurosurg Focus* 2008; **25**: E15.

5. Kwon BK, Mann C, Sohn HM, *et al.* Hypothermia for spinal cord injury. *Spine J* 2008; **8**: 859–74.

6. Coselli JS, Lemaire SA, Koksoy C, *et al.* Cerebrospinal fluid drainage reduces paraplegia after thoracoabdominal aortic aneurysm repair: results of a randomized clinical trial. *J Vasc Surg* 2002; **35**: 631–9.

7. Zheng F, Cammisa FP Jr., Sandhu HS, *et al.* Factors predicting hospital stay, operative time, blood loss, and transfusion in patients undergoing revision posterior lumbar spine decompression, fusion, and segmental instrumentation. *Spine (Phila Pa 1976)* 2002; **27**: 818–24.

8. GA Nuttall, Horlocker TT, Santrach PJ, *et al.* Predictors of blood transfusions in spinal instrumentation and fusion surgery. *Spine (Phila Pa 1976)* 2000; **25**: 596–601.

9. Goodnough LT, Rudnick S, Price TH, *et al.* Increased preoperative collection of autologous blood with recombinant human erythropoietin therapy. *N Engl J Med* 1989; **321**: 1163–8.

10. Bono CM, Watters WC 3rd, Heggeness MH, *et al.* An evidence-based clinical guideline for the use of antithrombotic therapies in spine surgery. *Spine J* 2009; **9**: 1046–51.

11. Suk KS, Kim KT, Lee SH, *et al.* Prevertebral soft tissue swelling after anterior cervical discectomy and fusion with plate fixation. *Int Orthop* 2006; **30**: 290–4.

12. Andrew SA, Sidhu KS. Airway changes after anterior cervical discectomy and fusion. *J Spinal Disord Tech* 2007; **20**: 577–81.

13. Sagi HC, Beutler W, Carroll E, *et al.* Airway complications associated with surgery on the anterior cervical spine. *Spine (Phila Pa 1976)* 2002; **27**: 949–53.

14. Emery SE, Smith MD, Bohlman HH. Upper-airway obstruction after multilevel cervical corpectomy for myelopathy. *J Bone Joint Surg Am* 1991; **73**: 544–51.

15. Epstein NE, Hollingsworth R, Nardi D, *et al.* Can airway complications following multilevel anterior cervical surgery be avoided? *J Neurosurg* 2001; **94**: 185–8.

16. Emery SE, Akhavan S, Miller P, *et al.* Steroids and risk factors for airway compromise in multilevel cervical corpectomy patients: a prospective, randomized, double-blind study. *Spine (Phila Pa 1976)* 2009; **34**: 299–32.

17. Pettiford BL, Shuchert MJ, Jeyabalan G, *et al.* Technical challenges and utility of anterior exposure for thoracic spine pathology. *Ann Thorac Surg* 2008; **86**: 1762–8.

18. Jules-Elysee K, Urban MK, Urquhart BL, *et al.* Pulmonary complications in anterior–posterior thoracic lumbar fusions. *Spine J* 2004; **4**: 312–16.

19. Colletta AJ, Mayer PJ. Chylothorax: an unusual complication of anterior thoracic interbody spinal fusion. *Spine (Phila Pa 1976)* 1982; **7**: 46–9.

20. Kulkarni SS, Lowery GL, Ross RE, *et al.* Arterial complications following anterior lumbar interbody fusion: report of eight cases. *Eur Spine J* 2003; **12**: 48–54.

21. Raskas DS, Delamarter RB. Occlusion of the left iliac artery after retroperitoneal exposure of the spine. *Clin Orthop Relat Res* 1997; **338**: 86–9.

22. Ikard RW. Methods and complications of anterior exposure of the thoracic and lumbar spine. *Arch Surg* 2006; **141**: 1025–34.

23. Isiklar ZU, Lindsey RW, Coburn M. Ureteral injury after anterior lumbar interbody fusion. A case report. *Spine (Phila Pa 1976)* 1995; **21**: 2379–82.

24. Patel AA, Spiker WR, Daubs MD, *et al.* Retroperitoneal lymphocele after anterior spinal surgery. *Spine (Phila Pa 1976)* 2008; **33**: E648–52.

Chapter

18

Postoperative acute pain

Juan P. Cata and Sherif Zaky

Key points

- Multiple factors contribute to poor postoperative pain control, including: inadequate assessment by nursing and physicians and erroneous beliefs that surgical pain is inevitable and acceptable and that it has harmless consequences for the sufferers.
- Postoperative acute pain after spine surgery is usually described as moderate to severe with its maximum within the first 3 days after surgery.
- Postoperative acute pain after spine surgery causes functional interference and is one of the leading causes of readmission after ambulatory spine surgery.
- The importance of achieving successful postoperative acute pain management is due to the fact that postoperative pain is associated with complications such as poor early mobilization, deep venous thrombosis, urinary infection, and delayed return of bowel function.
- Due to the complex physiology behind postoperative acute pain after spine surgery, multimodal analgesia appears to be the most effective approach for pain control.
- Intravenous patient-controlled analgesia (IV PCA) has been shown to be better than "around the clock" administration of analgesic but might not be sufficient for pain control after major spine surgeries.
- Epidural administration of local anesthetics has proven to reduce postoperative acute pain after spine surgery; however, there are still controversies regarding their use because they can potentially mask early symptoms of spinal bleeding.

Introduction

The International Association for Study of Pain defined pain as "an unpleasant sensory and emotional experience associated with actual or potential tissue damage, or described in terms of such damage." Accordingly, the ability to detect pain is essential to avoid further tissue damage. Despite this definition and tremendous efforts from scientific and medical societies, there continue to be barriers to effective postoperative pain management. Poorly controlled postoperative pain is a major impediment to postoperative functional recovery and is a persistent problem in the United States.[1,2] Multiple factors have been identified to contribute to this problem, including its inadequate assessment by nurses and physicians and erroneous beliefs that surgical pain is inevitable and acceptable and that it has harmless consequences for the sufferers.[3]

The absence of reliable physiological indicators of pain, the presence of specific diseases such as diabetes or dementia and/or pharmacological mechanisms, such as beta blockers, and the very subjective nature of it with levels of pain threshold varying from one patient to another and from one type of surgical intervention to another, make the assessment of postoperative surgical pain difficult and most of the time poorly obtained. The tragic consequence of this is that still at the time of this publication there are patients complaining of moderate and severe postoperative pain.

Acute pain physiology

From the peripheral to the central nervous system

Nociceptors are "receptors preferentially sensitive to a noxious stimulus or to a stimulus which would become noxious if prolonged" (International Association for the Study of Pain [IASP] definition) Nociceptors are

Anesthesia for Spine Surgery, ed. Ehab Farag. Published by Cambridge University Press. © Cambridge University Press 2012.

located in sensory afferent neurons responsible for carrying information from the periphery to the spinal cord. Sensory neurons have their cell body in the dorsal root ganglia and send their terminal fibers to different areas of the dorsal horn of the spinal cord. It is important to note that peripheral nociceptive sensory neurons are also responsible for the so-called "axonal reflex" by which neurogenic inflammation takes place and involves the release of peptides in the periphery. The most obvious clinical manifestations of this phenomenon are vasodilation and edema.[4]

Myelinated and unmyelinated sensory fibers

Sensory neurons are classified on the basis of their degree of myelin coverage as unmyelinated (C fibers – small-diameter neurons) or myelinated, and the latter are further subclassified as medium-diameter (Aδ fibers) and large-diameter fibers (Aβ fibers). Aβ fibers have the fastest velocity of conduction of the three types of fiber. They innervate sensory structures such as hair follicles, Merkel cells, and Pacinian corpuscles which do not normally participate in noxious stimuli transmission and project in laminae III, IV, and V of the dorsal horn. Aβ fibers, however, can transmit noxious stimuli in pathologic states such as persistent and chronic pain.[5]

Aδ fibers have a faster velocity of conduction than C fibers but slower than Aβ-fibers; they are responsible for the so-called "well localized fast" pain and bring nociceptive information to laminae I–III of the dorsal horn of the spinal cord. Based on their electrophysiological features Aδ nociceptors can be differentiated into two main classes: type I and type II. Under normal conditions, type I nociceptors respond to both mechanical and chemical stimuli but are relatively insensitive to heat. However, these nociceptors will become responsive to heat stimulus in the presence of tissue injury. Type II nociceptors have lower heat thresholds but are relatively insensitive to mechanical stimulation.[5]

C fibers have the slowest velocity of conduction; they are responsible for the so-called "poorly localized slow" pain and bring nociceptive information to the most superficial laminaa (I and II, also known as substantia gelatinosa) of the dorsal horn of the spinal cord. Traditionally, it has been taught that C-fiber nociceptors respond to heat.[6] Schmidt *et al.* identified a particularly important subtype of C-nociceptors that are responsive to heat but insensitive to mechanical stimulation. However, they are able to evoke stimulation in the presence of tissue injury.[7] Also, a small population of C-nociceptors may even respond to non-noxious stimuli such as a gentle touch on hairy skin.[8]

The dorsal horn

The excitation of primary afferent nociceptors by any strong stimuli will result in the release of glutamate and peptides, including substance P, neurokinin A, and calcitonin gene-related peptide, in the spinal cord dorsal horn, which results in modulation of dorsal horn interneurons.[9–12] The dorsal horn is organized into different laminae, extending from the superficial to the deep dorsal horn. Nociceptive Aδ and C fibers terminate superficially in laminae I–II, whereas Aβ fibers send their terminals into laminae III–VI.[13] Three main types of interneurons can be identified in the dorsal horn of the spinal cord based on their electrophysiological characteristics and pattern of response to different stimuli. The first group of neurons, the so-called nociceptive specific neurons, receive information from C fibers and respond mainly to noxious stimuli. A second group of neurons (low-threshold interneurons) respond to mainly non-noxious information from large myelinated neurons; and the last type of interneurons are called wide dynamic response neurons because they can respond to both nociceptive and innocuous stimulation.[13]

Supraspinal sensory centers

Projection neurons located in the dorsal horn of the spinal cord synapse with primary afferents and interneurons, and transmit nociceptive information through the spinothalamic and spinoreticulothalamic tracts to higher central levels such as the thalamus and brainstem, respectively.[14] From the thalamus the sensory information is sent to the somatosensory cortex, which has discriminative functions. The parabrachial region of the dorsolateral pons plays an important function in the sensory process because it receives information from the spinal cord and sends information to the amygdala, thus participating in the emotional component of pain.[14] Other areas of the brain that are involved in its emotional aspects are the insular cortex and anterior cingulate gyrus.

The TRP receptor family

Under physiological circumstances, not one single substance but an unknown combination of substances (the inflammatory "soup") acts on nociceptors. Thus, peripheral nociceptors are activated by a wide variety of mediators such as heat, cold, glutamate, prostaglandins, cytokines, ATP, chemical irritants, bradykinins, neurokinins, and growth factors.[15–18]

The excitation of many sensory afferent neurons by noxious thermal or chemical stimuli depends on the presence in their surface membranes of transient receptor potential (TRP) receptors.[19] The transduction mechanism involves the opening of nonselective cation channels, allowing the influx of Na^+ and Ca^{2+} ions. Six different TRPV (transient receptor potential vanilloid) receptors are known to respond to various gradations of temperature. The TRPV1, TRPV2, TRPV3, and TRPV4 receptors are excited by temperatures from warming to noxious heating levels; the TRPM8 (transient receptor potential menthol) responds to cooling and menthol and TRPA1 (transient receptor potential acetone) to cold stimulation.[20] TRPV1 receptors produce a sensation of burning pain by causing sensory discharges in cutaneous afferents that can be classified as polymodal C and mechano-heat Aδ-nociceptors.[20] In mice lacking TRPV1 receptors, heat hyperalgesia after plantar incision is significantly lesser than in the wild-type animal. Notably, the thermal heat threshold of mechanically sensitive C fibers was reduced after plantar incision in normal animals compared with TRPV1 knockouts.[21] Moreover, in an incisional pain model resembling postoperative acute pain, the administration of TRPV1 receptor antagonists was effective in treating thermal hyperalgesia.[22]

Cytokines, prostaglandins, and leukotrienes

Cytokines modulate the function of sensory neurons. Tumor necrosis factor (TNF) exerts its actions via its receptors, TNF receptor 1 (TNFR1) and the lower-affinity TNFR2.[23] In physiological conditions, stimulation of TNFR1 but not of TNFR2 induces pain-associated behavior in vivo and ectopic activity in Aβ and Aδ fibers in vitro, and when applied to peripheral nerve fibers it lowers mechanical activation thresholds in C-nociceptors.[24-26] Also, injection of IL-1β induces transient spontaneous discharges in sensory neurons and a brief exposure of the skin to IL-1β facilitates heat-evoked calcitonin gene-related peptide (CGRP) release from peptidergic neurons, which is a direct effect independent of changes in gene expression or receptor upregulation.[24,25,27]

Prostaglandins (PGs) play a significant role in acute pain physiology. PGE_2 is the predominant eicosanoid released after surgical trauma. PGE_2 exerts its actions by acting on a group of G-protein-coupled receptors (GPCRs). There are four GPCRs responding to PGE_2, designated subtypes EP1, EP2, EP3, and EP4, and multiple splicing isoforms of the subtype EP3.[28] TNF, IL-1β, and IL-6 are potent inducers of prostaglandins.[29,30]

C fibers express high levels of G-protein-coupled receptors for prostaglandins and it is through the activation of such receptors that other receptors important in pain transmission, such as the transient receptor potential vanilloid subfamily 1 (TRPV1) receptor and purinergic receptor, are modulated and participate in peripheral sensitization. Central and peripheral release of PGE_2 is diminished by the administration of cyclooxygenase-2 inhibitors.[28,31] This effect has been shown by Stalman et al., who demonstrated that the intra-articular administration of ketorolac decreased the production of PGE_2 in the synovial tissue of patients undergoing knee arthroscopy.[32]

Leukotrienes (LTs) belong to the family of lipid mediators responsible for several effects in inflammatory disorders. The action of LTs is through the activation of four distinct types (BLT1, BLT2, CysLT1, and CysLT2) of G-protein-coupled receptors. Intraplantar injection of leukotriene receptor agonist (LTB4) and 8R-15-diHETE, which are metabolites derived from 5- and 15-lipoxygenase pathways, respectively, evokes a profound hyperalgesic response.[33-35] Inhibition of the lipoxygenase enzyme has been shown to be effective in ameliorating inflammation and pain.[36] More interestingly, the administration of montelukast, an LT receptor antagonist, has shown antinociceptive properties in animal models of pain.[37]

Bradykinins

Bradykinins (BKs) are among the most potent algogenic and inflammatory mediators. Cellular effects of BKs are mediated by specific receptors, B1 and B2.[38] It is believed that the majority of the acute effects of BKs are mediated by B2 receptors, which are G-protein-coupled receptors acting via Gq/11 signaling cascades.[39] A recent study demonstrated that bradykinin receptor activation induces M channel (Kv7 or KCNQ) inhibition and calcium channel activation. Both, in turn, are responsible for neuronal hyperexcitability and nociception.[40] Paradoxically, an animal study did not demonstrate that the administration of B1 and, most importantly, B2 receptor antagonists was effective in ameliorating incisional pain.[41]

Purinergic receptors

Accumulating evidence indicates that nucleotides released from nonexcitable cells as well as neurons are involved in cell-to-cell communication in pain physiology.[42] Tissue pH is decreased by incision and the decrease in tissue pH corresponds to and may contribute to pain.[43] The purinergic receptors P1, P2X, and P2Y are particularly important in acute postoperative pain. P2X receptors belong to a family of ligand-gated ion channels and are cation-selective channels with almost equal permeability to Na^+ and K^+ and significant permeability to Ca^{2+}.[44] P2Y receptors are G-protein-coupled receptors activated by purine or pyrimidine nucleotides or sugar-nucleotides with subtype-dependent heterotrimeric G-proteins.[45] In animal studies during acute inflammation, high concentrations of extracellular ATP (adenosine triphosphate) have been measured at tissue injury sites.[46,47] Furthermore, the ATP released from the damaged peripheral nerve tissue might contribute to initiation of neuronal and glial activation, inducing the synthesis and release of proinflammatory cytokines and nitric oxide (NO).[48–50] In response to peripheral inflammation, mice lacking the ATP-gated P2X4 channel (P2X4R) do not develop pain hypersensitivity and show a complete absence of inflammatory PGE2 in tissue exudates.[51]

Substance P

Substance P (SP) has at least two potential mechanisms in supporting nociception after incision: first, as a neurotransmitter and second as a cytokine and NK (neurokinin) modulator.[52] The release of SP occurs after the activation of peptidergic C-nociceptors.[53] A high proportion of afferent neurons contain SP and the highest concentration of NK1 receptors in the spinal cord is found in the regions concerned with nociceptive processing.[53] The administration of NK-1 and NK-2 antagonists has been shown to prevent central sensitization.[54]

Substabce P also modulates the production of cytokines in skin and skin cells after injury or inflammation.[55] Moreover, the increase in cytokine production triggered by SP and observed during inflammation at the injury site appears to be necessary for adequate wound healing.[56,57] Mice deficient in SP display reduced pain behavior, and NK receptor antagonists have analgesic effects in pain models.[58,59]

Growth factors

Nerve growth factor, brain-derived neurotropic factor (BDNF), neurotropin-3, and neurotropin-4/5 are members of the neurotropin family. Neurotropic growth factor (NGF) is a small protein necessary for the promotion and survival of nociceptors. Intraplantar injection of NGF causes peripheral sensitization and induction of inflammation.[60,61] TNF and IL-1β induce NGF in inflamed tissue.[62] Also, intraplantar injection of SP promotes production of NGF that is blocked by the co-administration of an NK-1 antagonist.[52] Laboratory evidence shows an increase in NGF mRNA and protein levels as soon as 2 hours after skin incision that is maintained for 7 days and coincides with the peak in heat hyperalgesia.[63]

Brain-derived neurotropic factor is a 12.4 kDa basic protein expressed in the small and medium-sized neurons in the dorsal root ganglia (DRG) and transported to the spinal cord where is found in large, dense-cored vesicles in terminals of primary afferent fibers.[64,65] Spinal administration of anti-BDNF antibody has an antiallodynic effect. Moreover, in animal skin incision-induced transient activation of BDNF expression is mainly localized in the nerve terminals and neurons in the lumbar DRG and spinal cord. Remarkably, the exaggerated expression of BDNF was prevented by a sciatic nerve block.[66]

Ion channels

Once nociceptors become active the plasma membrane of sensory neurons depolarizes and the resultant electrical impulse will be transmitted throughout the neuron by the constant activation of sodium channels, which in turn can cause changes in the expression and functional properties of the same and other voltage-gated ion channels.[67,68] Sodium voltage-gated channels are key in the transmission of electrical impulses from the periphery to sensory centers and vice versa. Two main classes of voltage-gated sodium channels are present in sensory neurons: the tetrodotoxin-sensitive and tetrodotoxin-resistant channels. Voltage-gated sodium channels are particularly important for anesthesiologists because they are the sites of action of local anesthetics. Also, antidepressants have demonstrated activity against these channels. Another type of ion channel involved in pain physiology is the voltage-gated calcium channel. Four main subtypes of voltage-gated calcium channels have been described: L, T, N, and P/Q. All calcium channels are composed of α1 pore-forming subunits and the modulatory subunits α2δ, α2β, or α2γ. The α2δ is particularly important because is the site of action of the gabapentinoid class of anticonvulsants such as gabapentin and pregabalin, which are now known to treat acute postoperative pain.[69] Potassium channels are also involved in nociception; they are responsible of maintaining the resting membrane potential in neurons. Thus, inhibition of M currents conducted by Kv7 channels causes neuronal hyperexcitability and pain, whereas Kv7 activation leads to hyperpolarization and analgesia.[70–72]

305

Glutamate

Glutamate is one of main neurotransmitters of nociceptive afferent fibers. The major glutamate receptor subtypes at glutamatergic synapses are currently subdivided into ionotropic glutamate receptors (ion channel-forming) and metabotropic glutamate receptors (G-protein-coupled). The N-methyl-D-aspartate (NMDA) receptor is an ionotropic glutamate receptor that has the form of a channel through which ions can pass (predominantly Ca^{2+}), whereas the α-amino-3-hydroxy-5-methyl-4-isoxazolepropionic acid (AMPA) and kainite receptors are metabotropics. Glutamate-evoked discharges are attenuated by ketamine, a non-competitive NMDA receptor blocker.[73] Both NMDA and AMPA receptors are involved in pain formation and maintenance. Incision of the hindpaw of rats causes an increase in the background activity, mechanosensitivity, and receptive field size of WDR and HT neurons in the dorsal horn. To illustrate the importance of non-NDMA receptors in acute pain, Zahn et al. administered a non-NMDA and a NMDA receptor antagonist in the spinal cord of rodents with incisional pain. Interestingly, only the non-NMDA antagonist inhibited the hyperexcitable features exhibited by dorsal horn neurons.[74] In contrast, Richebe et al. were able to demonstrate that ketamine had antihyperalgesic effects on animals with incisional pain.[75] Clinical data demonstrate that the administration of dextromethorphan (an NMDA antagonist) does ameliorate postoperative pain after cholecystectomy.[76] Also, the epidural co-administration of morphine and ketamine has shown strong analgesic effects compared with placebo.[77] Thus, both studies suggest the participation of NMDA receptors in acute postoperative pain.

Peripheral and central sensitization

The action of the inflammatory soup on peripheral sensory nociceptors causes quantitative and functional changes in sensory neurons, resulting in "peripheral sensitization" (Fig. 18.1). This is usually interpreted as an increased excitability of the neural mechanisms whereby the responses of a given sensory neuron are progressively enhanced following continuous noxious stimulation. Remarkably, the neuron remains in a hyperexcitable state even after the originating stimulus has ceased as may occur in the postoperative period.[78] The tetrodotoxin-resistant sodium channels appear to play a key role in the genesis of peripheral sensitization. Akopian et al. demonstrated that mice carrying a null mutation of tetrodotoxin-resistant Nav1.8 gene revealed a complete absence of responses to a tonic noxious mechanical stimulus and attenuated primary hyperalgesia evoked by intraplantar injection of nerve growth factor.[79] Persistent pain also modifies the expression of voltage-activated calcium channels in sensory neurons. A recent study demonstrated that subcutaneous injection of the irritant complete Freund's adjuvant

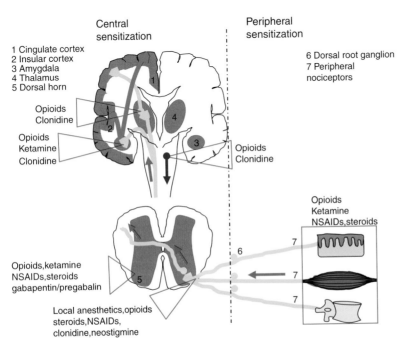

Central sensitization

1 Cingulate cortex
2 Insular cortex
3 Amygdala
4 Thalamus
5 Dorsal horn

Opioids
Clonidine

Opioids
Ketamine
Clonidine

Peripheral sensitization

6 Dorsal root ganglion
7 Peripheral nociceptors

Opioids
Clonidine

Opioids
Ketamine
NSAIDs, steroids

Opioids, ketamine
NSAIDs, steroids
gabapentin/pregabalin

Local anesthetics, opioids
steroids, NSAIDs,
clonidine, neostigmine

Figure 18.1 The physiological changes and pathways involved in postoperative pain. The figure also indicates the potential sites in the peripheral and central nervous system where different analgesics act in order to modulate the generation, transmission, and maintenance (sensitization) of pain. Hence, the figure helps in understanding the role of multimodal analgesia in which analgesics with different mechanisms and site of action can be administered in the perioperative period with the goal of maximizing the decrease in pain intensity by minimizing the side effects of analgesics.

(inflammatory model) in the hindpaw of rats caused an increase in both the α2δ1 and Ca(V)2.2 protein in the dorsal root ganglia.[80] Furthermore, the administration of TROX-1, an inhibitor of the Ca(V)2.2 calcium channel showed analgesic properties in a rodent model of inflammatory pain.[38]

"Central sensitization" results from persistent and augmented afferent sensory nerve firing, which causes the release of mediators such as glutamate, nitric oxide, prostaglandins, and cytokines that modulate the response of a wide dynamic range of neurons located in the dorsal horn, which results in hyperexcitability and wind-up (Fig. 18.1). The latter refers to the frequency-dependent facilitation of the excitability of spinal neurons induced by repetitive electrical stimulation of afferent C fibers.[81] The signal transduction molecules involved in the central sensitization process include several protein kinases, such as Ca^{2+}/calmodulin-dependent protein kinase (CaMKII)[82], protein kinase A (PKA)[83], PKC[84–86], PKG,[83] and PKB/Akt.[87]

Summarizing, features of peripheral and central sensitization include the presence of spontaneous activity (ongoing pain) and of increased responses to noxious stimulation (hyperalgesia) and the acquisition by nociceptor-specific neurons of responses to low-intensity stimulation (allodynia).[88]

Postoperative acute surgical pain after spine surgery

"Postoperative pain is an association of somatic, inflammatory, neuropathic, and – at times – visceral pain."[89] Postoperative acute pain after spine surgery is usually described as moderate to severe with its maximum within the first 3 days after surgery.[90–93] A recent study by Gottschalk et al. reported that the average pain 48 hours after multilevel thoracolumbar spine surgery with instrumentation and fusion was 4.8 out of 10, which was similar to that reported by other studies in patients who underwent cervical spinal fusion, lumbar discectomy, lumbar decompression, or posterior spinal fusion for idiopathic scoliosis.[94–98] It is surprising to observe that these studies involved different surgical techniques (instrumented and noninstrumented) and possibly different degrees of surgical trauma; thus, it is important to obtain pain scores, but what might be more interesting to evaluate is the amount of analgesic consumption or level of activity since patients may adjust the amount of analgesic required or their activity level to a similar "comfort zone" of pain intensity. Also,

striking is the finding by Bianconi et al. who reported mean maximal pain scores at rest, which were 73 (visual analog scale, score 0–100) 4 hours after posterior fusion surgery.[92] Moreover, only half of these patients may report "good" postoperative acute pain control after spine surgery.[99] As an obvious consequence, large amounts of opioids and other analgesics are administered to improve pain control. The importance of understanding postoperative pain control comes from evidence suggesting that higher pain intensity 24 hours after surgery, at rest and with movement, was a predictor of long-term pain.[100]

Remarkably, postoperative acute pain after spine surgery causes functional interference and is one of the leading causes of readmission after ambulatory spine surgery.[101,102] The importance of achieving a successful postoperative acute pain after spine surgery is due to the fact that postoperative pain is associated with complications such as poor early mobilization, deep venous thrombosis, urinary infection, and delayed return of bowel function.[14,91] Kehlet et al. reported that effective treatment of postoperative pain allows for early mobilization.[103,104] Perhaps more important is the fact that the presence of any of these complications can delay leaving hospital and lead to increased economic costs.

Preoperative pain and anxiety have significant implications in the presence and ability of patients to cope with early and persistent postoperative pain. Patients with significant preoperative pain appear to require higher doses of opioids postoperatively.[105] Hickey et al. have shown that patients with poorer outcomes following lumbar discectomy had experienced greater preoperative anxiety.[106] Recently there has been recognition of the interrelationship between acute pain and the effects of psychological and social factors associated with the injury.[107] Severe postoperative pain also exacerbates anxiety and frustration in patients and caregivers, which may further interfere with their participation in postoperative therapy.[108] The Brief Pain Inventory short form (BPI-sf) is a validated, widely used, self-administered questionnaire developed to assess the severity of pain and the impact of pain on daily functions.[109] A recent study demonstrated that even a "small" reduction in postoperative acute pain after spine surgery had a significant impact on BPI-sf scores, highlighting the importance of adequate pain control and its impact on quality of life in the immediate postoperative period.[110] Hence, achieving effective analgesia following spine surgery would result in less anxiety, fewer readmissions after ambulatory surgery, early mobilization of the patient, shorter hospital stay, and potentially lower costs.

Postoperative acute pain after spine surgery is due to the activation of nociceptors located around the surgical wound such as those in the skin, subcutaneous tissue, muscles, blood vessels, ligaments, periosteum, and dura mater. To complicate this matter, there are at least a dozen different surgical techniques that vary according to the location of the surgery (cervical, thoracic, lumbar, or a combination of any of these), the surgical approach (anterior and/or posterior), the number of vertebral segments operated on, the presence or absence of instrumentation, and the degree of surgical invasiveness (minimally invasive procedures or open conventional approach). Even patients undergoing relatively less traumatic surgery such as discectomies complain of poorly controlled postoperative acute pain after spine surgery. This was observed in a recent small randomized-controlled trial by Blumenthal et al., who demonstrated that patients who received intravenous self-controlled analgesia with morphine complained of moderate and severe postoperative acute pain after spine surgery at rest, on coughing, or during motion.[111]

Several pharmacologic and nonpharmacologic modalities targeted to control postoperative have been used in the treatment of postoperative acute pain after spine surgery. Because of the complex physiology behind this type of pain, no single intervention appears to be more effective than others. Hence, this has led several authors to propose the concept of multimodal analgesia (Fig. 18.1).[112,113] The rationale behind this concept is the fact that there is, as previously mentioned, a wide variety of pain nociceptors and intracellular pathways activated at the same time after the initial surgical injury. More important is the concept of using modalities to target peripheral, spinal, and supraspinal pain pathways. For instance, the addition of nonsteroidal anti-inflammatory drugs (NSAIDs) to an opioid-based regimen has been shown to improve postoperative acute pain after spine surgery.[114] Also, the addition of local anesthetics into the epidural space or to nerve roots has been shown to be beneficial in the treatment of postoperative acute pain after spine surgery.[115-117] Multimodal analgesia may also have a positive impact in costs, since a large retrospective study demonstrated that the addition of ketorolac to opioid-based analgesia after spine and orthopedic procedures decreased health care resource utilization and

total per-patient cost of treatment compared with only opioid-based analgesia.[118] Unfortunately, the concept of multimodal analgesia cannot deal with nonmodifiable risk factors such as genetics that affect acute and persistent pain physiology. For instance, humans carrying the haplotype of GCH1 (GTP cyclohydrolase 1) have significantly less risk of developing persistent pain following lumbar discectomy than those not carrying the haplotype.[119]

Opioids

Opioids are among the most common analgesics used in the intra- and postoperative periods. In this section, we will focus on those frequently administered for the treatment of acute surgical pain after spine surgery.

Opioids exert their analgesic action by binding at least four different receptors (mu, kappa, delta, and sigma). Mu receptors are G-protein-coupled proteins widely spread in neurons of the central and peripheral nervous system (Fig. 18.1), and also in other cells such as lymphocytes. Activation of the mu receptors results in decreased levels of cyclic adenosine monophosphate (cAMP), which targets cAMP/kinase, which in turn results in modification of intracellular pathways responsible for short- and long-term action on the exposed cells. Mu receptor agonists cause hyperpolarization of sensory neurons, thus decreasing the release of nociceptive mediators such as glutamate, substance P, and CGRP. Opioids may also exert antagonizing effects on NMDA receptors, activating the descending serotonin and norepinephrine pain pathways from the brainstem that can be involved in descending inhibition and analgesia.[14,120]

Based on their chemical structure, four main groups of opioids (phenanthrenes, benzomorphans, phenylpiperidines, and diphenylheptanes) are part of the daily armamentarium of anesthesiologists and pain physicians. Morphine is a naturally occurring phenanthrene, considered a long-acting narcotic, that has a low lipid solubility compared with synthetic opioids, which confers upon it significantly lesser lung uptake when given intravenously and more rostral spread when given spinally. Morphine is metabolized by the liver into two main metabolites, morphine-3-glucuronide (inactive or antagonistic) and morphine-6-glucoronide (active) which are excreted by the kidney. Thus, precautions should be taken or morphine should be avoided in patients with poor renal function. Morphine is also metabolized into small amounts of codeine and hydromorphone. There are a variety of side effects related to the administration of morphine. Morphine-induced respiratory depression is dose-dependent and is commonly seen in elderly patients, in those with obstructive sleep apnea, and after the co-administration of other depressants of the CNS. Hypotension can be seen after the intravenous administration of morphine and it is due to the release of histamine and the reduction of the sympathetic tone. Other side effects include pruritus, nausea and vomiting, constipation, and urinary retention.[120]

Hydromorphone is a semi-synthetic opioid agonist that also belongs to the phenanthrene family of opioids. It is more lipophilic, has faster onset, and is 7 to 10 times more potent than morphine.[120,121] After intravenous administration the peak effect is 10–20 minutes after injection with a slightly shorter duration of action (2–3 h) than morphine (3–6 h). Hydromorphone is metabolized by the liver into hydromphorne-3-glucoronide (inactive or antagonistic), which is excreted by the kidney; therefore, some authors have suggested that this is the opioid of choice in patients with end-stage renal disease.[122,123]

Fentanyl is a phenylpiperidine synthetic mu-opioid receptor agonist that is significantly more lipid soluble and potent (80 times) than morphine. Its peak effect of action is 3–5 minutes after intravenous administration. The termination of effect is due to redistribution away from the CNS; however, it is important to remember that its high lipophilicity can lead to accumulation after repeated or continuous intravenous administration (mainly in infusions longer than 4 h). Fentanyl is metabolized by the liver into two inactive metabolites: hydroxyfentanyl and norfentanyl.[120,123,124] Importantly, fentanyl appears to be associated with less respiratory depression than morphine (0.67% vs. 2.8%, respectively).[125]

Sufentanil is also a phenylpiperidine synthetic opioid agonist. It is more potent (5–10 times) and lipophilic (partition coefficient of 1770–2842) than fentanyl. It undergoes liver metabolism to N-phenylpropanamide. As with other fentanyl congeners, it appears safe to administer sufentanil in patients with renal failure. Sufentanil might be an interesting alternative to fentanyl or morphine due to the fact that the former does not show a delayed increase in plasma concentration during the elimination phase.[120,123,124] A clinical trial conducted by Ved *et al.* demonstrated that sufentanil caused fewer episodes of hypoxemia than morphine (3.4% vs. 18.9%, respectively) when both were administered as patient-controlled analgesia.[126]

Remifentanil is an ultra-short phenylpiperidine synthetic mu-receptor opioid agonist. It is metabolized by specific esterases, mainly from the muscle.[120] Its role in the management of postoperative acute pain is controversial. Its use in the context of acute pain management has been reported in labor analgesia.[127] A recent concern relates to the development of acute tolerance and/ or hyperalgesia after the use of high doses of remifentanil. In animals, there is a growing bulk of literature suggesting that remifentanil causes dose-dependent hyperalgesia that is speculated to be mediated by several mechanisms such as activation of dorsal horn NMDA systems, inactivation of mu-opioid receptors, spinal dynorphin release, and increased activity of the AMPc pathway.[128–132] Human studies appear to support the laboratory data.[133,134] A recent study in adolescents undergoing spine surgery demonstrated that patients receiving a mean dose of 0.31 µg/kg/min of remifentanil developed acute tolerance and hyperalgesia that was not prevented by the use of ketamine.[133]

Oxycodone is a phenanthrene mu and kappa receptor agonist that is only used for oral administration in the United States, but the intravenous form is available elsewhere. It undergoes liver metabolism into active (oxymorphone, mu agonist) and inactive metabolites that are mainly renally excreted.[120,124,135] It is commonly given when bowel function has returned in the postoperative period, although one clinical study suggests its efficacy when given preoperatively as a single dose of 10 mg PO.[136] The oral dose frequently given is 5–10 mg every 3–4 hours.[120]

Intravenous patient-controlled analgesia (IV PCA) is a commonly used analgesia technique to control postoperative acute pain after spine surgery. It consists of the intravenous administration of analgesics, most commonly opioids, self-controlled by the patient. Morphine, hydromorphone, and fentanyl are the most common opioids used during IV PCA (Table 18.1). This technique has proved to be better than "around the clock" administration of analgesic but may not provide sufficient pain control in the vast majority of patients, mainly to those undergoing complex, extensive spine surgery and those with cognitive problems such as dementia. A potential problem associated with the use of IV PCA is related to the administration of large amounts of opioids. Cata *et al.* showed that the median amount of morphine equivalents administered to patients after complex spine surgery was 35 mg when an IV PCA technique was used as the main analgesia technique.[116] Similarly, Schenk *et al.* reported

Table 18.1 Recommended solutions and schedule of administration of PCA

Route	Solution	Basal rate	Demand bolus	Lock interval
Intravenous	Morphine 2 mg/ml	0–1 mg/h	1–2 mg	10 minutes/6 doses per hour
	Fentanyl 20 µg/ml	0–20 µg/h	20–30 µg	6 minutes/10 doses per hour
	Hydromorphone 0.5 mg/ml	0–0.2 mg/h	0.2–0.5 mg	6 minutes/10 doses per hour
	Sufentanil 2 µg/ml	0–5 µg/h	4–6 µg	6 minutes/10 doses per hour
Epidural	Bupivacaine 0.0625–0.125% +/– fentanyl 1–5 µg/ml	3–7 ml/h	3–5 ml	10–15 minutes/4–6 doses per hour
	Bupivacaine 0.0625–0.125% +/– fentanyl 1–5 µg/ml +/– clonidine 0.4 mg/ml	3–7 ml/h	3–5 ml	10–15 minutes/4–6 doses per hour
	Bupivacaine 0.0625–0.125% +/– sufentanil 2 µg/ml	3–5 ml/h	3–5 ml	10–15 minutes/4–6 doses per hour
	Bupivacaine 0.0625–0.125% +/– hydromorphone 3–10 µg/ml	3–5 ml/h	3–5 ml	10–15 minutes/4–6 doses per hour
	Ropivacaine 0.05–0.2% +/– fentanyl 2–5 µg/ml +/– clonidine 0.4 mg/ml	3–7 ml/h	3–5 ml	10–15 minutes/4–6 doses per hour
	Ropivacaine 0.05–0.2% +/– fentanyl 2–5 µg/ml	3–7 ml/h	3–5 ml	10–15 minutes/4–6 doses per hour
	Ropivacaine 0.05–0.2% +/– sufentanil 2 µg/ml	3–5 ml/h	3–5 ml	10–15 minutes/4–6 doses per hour
	Ropivacaine 0.05–0.2% +/– hydromorphone 3–10 µg/ml	3–5 ml/h	3–5 ml	10–15 minutes/4–6 doses per hour

that patients who underwent major spine surgery had a median amount of morphine consumption of 51 mg and 57 mg in the immediate postoperative period and day 1 after surgery, respectively.[117] A disadvantage of IV PCA is that patients are often exposed to systemic side effects of opioids such as nausea and vomiting (18–31%), sedation (1–8%), pruritus (3–16%), urinary retention (3–16%), and respiratory depression (4–8%).[123] Thus, to avoid the administration of large doses of opioids, several researchers have focused on the role of multimodal analgesia.

Nonsteroidal anti-inflammatory drugs

NSAIDs block the synthesis of prostaglandins by inhibiting cyclooxygenase types 1 and 2. Based on their chemical structure, there are six families of NSAIDs (Table 18.2). Ketorolac belongs to the family of acetic acid derivatives. It is widely used in the perioperative period due to its potency and availability parenterally (15–30 mg IV). Acetaminophen is a *para-aminophenol* derivative that is traditionally administered orally; however, it has recently been approved for intravenous administration in the United States. A preoperative single intravenous dose of 1000 mg of this NSAID has shown to be effective in decreasing

intraoperative opioid requirements and postoperative pain.[137] Postoperative intravenous and oral administration of acetaminophen has been shown to be an effective analgesic.[138,139] For instance, 1000 mg of intravenous acetaminophen reduced opioid consumption and improved pain and sedation scores in patients admitted to the intensive care unit after major surgical procedures.[140] Thus, NSAIDs are an attractive alternative as an adjuvant analgesic for patients undergoing spine surgery.

A retrospective study demonstrated that ketorolac caused a significant improvement in postoperative ambulation and lower postoperative costs in patients after lumbar spine surgery;[141] however, it efficacy is still controversial and depends on factors such as dose and time of administration. Reuben *et al.* demonstrated that 15 mg and 30 mg of intravenous ketorolac were more effective than placebo and 5 mg in patients after spinal fusion.[142] In one study by Mack *et al.* the intraoperative administration of ketorolac was not effective in decreasing postoperative acute pain after spine surgery and opioids, which is in striking contrast to findings reported by Cassinelli *et al.* and Le Roux and Samudrala, who demonstrated that ketorolac not only improved pain control but also reduced the amount

Table 18.2 NSAIDs used for postoperative pain after spine surgery

Name	Class	Dose	Comments	Reference(s)
Acetaminophen	*para*-aminophenol derivative	1000 mg PO/IV preoperatively or postoperatively every 4–6 h. Max. 5 doses	Overdose leads to liver failure	129, 130
Ketorolac	Pyrrolizine carboxylate	15–30 mg IV every 6 h	Potent analgesic Fusion defects Renal impairment	105, 114, 134
Diclofenac sodium	Phenylacetate derivatives	50–75 mg PO/PR preoperatively or postoperatively every 8–12 h	20% incidence of side effects	91
Naproxen	Propionic acid derivative	250–500 mg PO preoperatively or postoperatively every 6–12 h	Delayed onset of effect	135
Rofecoxib	Selective COX-2 inhibitor		No longer commercially available in the USA	137
Parecoxib	Selective COX-2 inhibitor	40 mg IV preoperatively or postoperatively every 12 h	Not approved for use in the USA	99, 136

of morphine equivalents after lumbar decompression surgery.[105,114,143] In Japan, diclofenac sodium, another NSAID, is commonly used as an adjuvant analgesic after spine surgery. Yukawa *et al.* demonstrated that diclofenac sodium provided only a transient favorable effect immediately after surgery.[91] Naproxen has also been shown to decrease opioid consumption after instrumented spinal fusion without evidence of systemic anti-inflammatory effects indicating a site-specific action.[144] Selective cyclooxygenase (COX)-2 inhibitors have also been investigated as adjuvant analgesics in the treatment of postoperative acute pain after spine surgery. Parecoxib was ineffective in providing adequate pain control compared with placebo and performed worse than metamizol after lumbar microdiscectomy.[145] In sharp contrast, another randomized controlled trial demonstrated that rofecoxib did improve pain control and reduced opioid consumption.[146] Also, a clinical study showed that 40 mg of parecoxib improved pain at rest and decreased the total amount of morphine required over 48 hours compared with placebo. Remarkably, the number-needed-to-treat for one patient to have at least 50% pain relief was 3.1 (2.0–4.6).[99]

The discrepancy between studies regarding the effect of different or same class of NSAIDs on postoperative pain control after spine surgery can be explained by the fact that the microsurgical techniques would result in a small degree of tissue trauma compared with more complex surgeries and because once the herniated nucleus pulposus material is surgically removed, mainly with the newer minimally invasive techniques, the major source of pain is expected not

to be present postoperatively. Also, it is important to remark that analgesic potency varies within different NSAIDs, hence caution is recommended when interpreting results from different studies.

Defects in the quality of fusion are common concerns associated with the use of ketorolac and other NSAIDs. In animals, a single dose of ketoprofen did not cause nonunion defects compared with tramadol.[147] A recent meta-analysis and a retrospective study have suggested that high doses of ketorolac in the perioperative period of spine surgery may increase the risk of nonunion after fusion; however, this has been disputed by other studies.[148–152] Lumawig *et al.* demonstrated that diclofenac sodium caused a dose-dependent increase in the incidence of pseudoarthrosis after posterior lumbar interbody fusion (PLIF) and led the authors to recommend that the use of diclofenac sodium be cautious, especially in the immediate postoperative period of PLIF.[153]

Another concern related to the perioperative use of NSAIDs is the risk of intraoperative or postoperative spinal bleeding. A survey among neurosurgeons in Germany demonstrated that over 90% recommended discontinuation of even low doses of aspirin 6.9 days before spinal surgery and 65.5% would use special medical therapy, preferably desmopressin alone or in combination with other blood products or prohemostatic agents, if hemorrhagic complications developed intra- or postoperatively.[154]

Other analgesic adjuvants

Gabapentin, a 3-alkylated analogue of γ-aminobutyric acid, has been shown to play an important role in the prevention of postoperative pain. Gabapentin does not bind to GABA A or GABA B receptor but to the α2-δ subunit of the presynaptic voltage-gated calcium channels responsible for the inhibition of the calcium influx. The bioavailability of gabapentin actually decreases from 60% to 27% with increasing doses due to saturable absorption (900 mg/day versus 4800 mg/day, respectively). In humans, gabapentin is not metabolized and is eliminated unchanged in the urine. Thus, dosage adjustments are needed in patients with renal impairment. Gabapentin-related adverse effects include somnolence, dizziness, asthenia, headache, nausea, ataxia, and weight gain.[155]

Pandey et al. demonstrated that the preoperative administration of gabapentin in patients undergoing single-level lumbar discectomy reduced the consumption of fentanyl by 35% during the postoperative 24 hours.[156] A clinical study from the same group also showed that 600 mg preoperatively was the optimal dose to reduce postoperative pain after lumbar discectomy.[157] Similarly, Turan et al. demonstrated that gabapentin showed short-term efficacy as an adjuvant analgesic in patients undergoing discectomy or spine fusion surgery. Perhaps, more remarkable was that patients randomized to gabapentin complained of less vomiting than those randomized to placebo.[158]

Pregabalin ((S)-(+-3-isobutyl GABA), a structural analog of GABA has a similar mechanism of action to gabapentin but with a better pharmacokinetic profile. Pregabalin has an oral bioavailability of ≥90% and a single oral dose of 300 mg reaches cerebrospinal fluid levels capable of having analgesic effects up to at least 6 hours after surgery.[159] Pregabalin undergoes minimal hepatic metabolism, thus most of the drug is eliminated unchanged through the kidney. Pregabalin is effectively cleared by hemodialysis.[160,161] In nonspine surgery, a single dose of 75 mg of pregabalin has been shown to ameliorate acute pain; however, the administration of 150 mg preoperatively followed by the same dose twice a day was associated with increased sedation.[162,163]

Pregabalin has also shown beneficial effects in patients undergoing spine surgery. In a randomized controlled trial the preoperative administration of 300 mg followed by 150 mg every 12 h during the first 24 h postoperatively improved functional pain outcomes 3 months after surgery compared with placebo.[164] More prospective studies are needed to assess the efficacy of pregabalin in the context of, for instance, complex spine surgery.

Neuraxial analgesic techniques

Neuraxial analgesia has also been used in the management of postoperative acute pain after spine surgery and appears to be superior to intravenous analgesia.[98,116,165,166] Single-dose injections and catheter-based techniques have been described in several studies. A pre-incision single dose of local anesthetics and opioids via caudal epidural injections has been described in patients undergoing lumbar procedures.[98] The placement one or two (cephalad and caudal) epidural catheters has been described and depends on several factors such as provider's preference and extent of the surgical wound. The surgeon commonly places the catheter under direct visualization before wound closure. Usually, thoracolumbar incisions are best managed with two epidural catheters through which solutions of analgesics are administered independently.[93,167–169] Potential problems related to the placement of catheters before wound closure include, first, nonuniform spread of analgesics due to the presence of small clots or hemostatic solutions; second, the presence of draining devices may interfere with the spread of analgesic solutions; and third, failure to provide preemptive analgesia, although this remains controversial. For instance, the preoperative epidural administration of bupivacaine 0.25% plus 1–3 mg of morphine not only reduced the consumption of analgesics intra- and postoperatively but also improved postoperative pain scores, suggesting a potential preemptive analgesic effect.[170]

Epidural solutions consisting of a local anesthetic plus an opioid are routinely used in patient-controlled epidural analgesia and appear to be superior to intravenous patient-controlled analgesia (Table 18.1). Schenk et al. demonstrated that the combination of 0.125% of ropivacaine plus 1 µg/ml of sufentanil provided better pain relief than patient-controlled intravenous analgesia with morphine.[117] Another study that also compared patient-controlled epidural analgesia based on a solution of 0.1% of bupivacaine plus fentanyl 5 µg/ml with fentanyl intravenous patient-controlled analgesia found that the patients randomized to epidural patient-controlled analgesia had significantly lower requirements for opioids but with significantly higher number of side effects and no differences in pain scores. It is important to note that a solution of fentanyl 5 µg/ml is higher than other authors have reported and thus may be responsible for side effects, and more importantly that the study was not of sufficient power to detect a difference in postoperative pain.[171] Yukawa *et al.* also reported that patients randomized to an epidural solution of 0.75% of lidocaine plus morphine had a significantly higher number of side effects and lower postoperative pain scores than those who received diclofenac sodium or subcutaneous lidocaine plus morphine.[91]

The epidural administration of epidural solution based *only* on local anesthetics has been proven to reduce postoperative acute pain and analgesic consumption after spine surgery. Gottschalk *et al.* randomized patients to either an epidural infusion of placebo or 0.1% ropivacaine started at the end of surgery. Those patients treated with ropivacaine 0.1% had significantly lower pain scores and piritramide consumption throughout a period of 72 h. More importantly patients' satisfaction was better in those randomized to the ropivacaine group.[172] There are still controversies regarding this use because they can potentially mask early symptoms of epidural hematoma and make the diagnosis of this neurological complication difficult. Thus, it has been recommended to use a solution with a low concentration of local anesthetics or based on opioids only to avoid marked motor weakness.[172] In adolescents undergoing scoliosis-corrective surgery, the addition of 0.3% of ropivacaine through a double epidural catheter improved postoperative pain, reduced the percentage of patients with nausea and vomiting, pruritus, and accelerated bowel activity compared with placebo.[173] Another potential advantage of using epidural analgesia is an early return of bowel function that has been demonstrated in several clinical studies. There are two possible mechanisms to explain this phenomenon: first, a reduction of opioid consumption and, second, the sympathetic blockade associated with epidural analgesia.

The use of clonidine as an analgesic adjuvant has been shown to reduce the requirements for opioids; however, it may be associated with side effects such as hypotension, sedation, and bradycardia.[174,175] A single dose of clonidine (1.5 µg/kg) followed by an infusion of 25 µg/h in the epidural space just before wound closure reduced the consumption of morphine compared with placebo by 43%.[96] Several authors have recommended the addition of corticosteroids as part of the multimodal approach for pain management during spine surgery. A randomized trial that enrolled patients to placebo or peridural methylprednisolone plus wound infiltration with bupivacaine demonstrated that those who were treated with the corticosteroid had fewer side effects and less pain at rest and postoperative leg pain.[176]

In conclusion, postoperative pain management after spine surgery can be challenging for any anesthesiologist or pain physician because of psychological, physiological, and surgery-related factors. Acute pain after spine surgery is usually moderate to severe and can be associated with distress and care burden. The importance of understanding the complexity of the pain physiology may help anesthesiologists and pain practitioners to develop multimodal analgesic approaches that will not only decrease pain but also improve other outcomes such as ambulation and length of hospital stay.

References

1. Morrison RS, Meier DE, Fischberg D, *et al.* Improving the management of pain in hospitalized adults. *Arch Intern Med* 2006; **166**: 1033–9.

2. Max MB. How to move pain and symptom research from the margin to the mainstream. *J Pain* 2003; **4**: 355–60.

3. Klopfenstein CE, Herrmann FR, Mamie C, Van Gessel E, Forster A. Pain intensity and pain relief after surgery. A comparison between patients' reported assessments and nurses' and physicians' observations. *Acta Anaesthesiol Scand* 2000; **44**: 58–62.

4. Benemei S, Nicoletti P, Capone JG, Geppetti P. CGRP receptors in the control of pain and inflammation. *Curr Opin Pharmacol* 2009; **9**: 9–14.

5. Basbaum AI, Bautista DM, Scherrer G, Julius D. Cellular and molecular mechanisms of pain. *Cell* 2009; **139**: 267–84.

6. Perl ER. Ideas about pain, a historical view. *Nat Rev Neurosci* 2007; **8**: 71–80.

7. Schmidt R, Schmelz M, Forster C, *et al.* Novel classes of responsive and unresponsive C nociceptors in human skin. *J Neurosci* 1995; **15**: 333–41.

8. Olausson H, Cole J, Rylander K, *et al.* Functional role of unmyelinated tactile afferents in human hairy skin: sympathetic response and perceptual localization. *Exp Brain Res* 2008; **184**: 135–40.

9. Sorkin LS, Westlund KN, Sluka KA, Dougherty PM, Willis WD. Neural changes in acute arthritis in monkeys. IV. Time-course of amino acid release into the lumbar dorsal horn. *Brain Res Brain Res Rev* 1992; **17**: 39–50.

10. Dougherty PM, Sluka KA, Sorkin LS, Westlund KN, Willis WD. Neural changes in acute arthritis in monkeys. I. Parallel enhancement of responses of spinothalamic tract neurons to mechanical stimulation and excitatory amino acids. *Brain Res Brain Res Rev* 1992; **17**: 1–13.

11. Sluka KA, Dougherty PM, Sorkin LS, Willis WD, Westlund KN. Neural changes in acute arthritis in monkeys. III. Changes in substance P, calcitonin gene-related peptide and glutamate in the dorsal horn of the spinal cord. *Brain Res Brain Res Rev* 1992; **17**: 29–38.

12. Westlund KN, Sun YC, Sluka KA, *et al.* Neural changes in acute arthritis in monkeys. II. Increased glutamate immunoreactivity in the medial articular nerve. *Brain Res Brain Res Rev* 1992; **17**: 15–27.

13. Todd AJ. Anatomy of primary afferents and projection neurones in the rat spinal dorsal horn with particular emphasis on substance P and the neurokinin 1 receptor. *Exp Physiol* 2002; **87**: 245–9.

14. Wall PD, McMahon SB, Koltzenburg M. Representation pain in the brain. In: McMahon SB, Koltzenburg M, eds. *Wall and Melzack's Textbook of Pain*. 5th ed. Philadelphia, PA: Elsevier; 2006: xviii.

15. Cairns BE, Hu JW, Arendt-Nielsen L, Sessle BJ, Svensson P. Sex-related differences in human pain and rat afferent discharge evoked by injection of glutamate into the masseter muscle. *J Neurophysiol* 2001; **86**: 782–91.

16. Mork H, Ashina M, Bendtsen L, Olesen J, Jensen R. Experimental muscle pain and tenderness following infusion of endogenous substances in humans. *Eur J Pain* 2003; **7**: 145–53.

17. Svensson P, Cairns BE, Wang K, Arendt-Nielsen L. Injection of nerve growth factor into human masseter muscle evokes long-lasting mechanical allodynia and hyperalgesia. *Pain* 2003; **104**: 241–7.

18. Rotto DM, Hill JM, Schultz HD, Kaufman MP. Cyclooxygenase blockade attenuates responses of group IV muscle afferents to static contraction. *Am J Physiol* 1990; **259**: H745–50.

19. Montell C, Jones K, Hafen E, Rubin G. Rescue of the *Drosophila* phototransduction mutation trp by germline transformation. *Science* 1985; **230**: 1040–3.

20. Willis WD Jr. The role of TRPV1 receptors in pain evoked by noxious thermal and chemical stimuli. *Exp Brain Res* 2009; **196**: 5–11.

21. Banik RK, Brennan TJ. Trpv1 mediates spontaneous firing and heat sensitization of cutaneous primary afferents after plantar incision. *Pain* 2009; **141**: 41–51.

22. Tekus V, Bolcskei K, Kis-Varga A, *et al.* Effect of transient receptor potential vanilloid 1 (TRPV1) receptor antagonist compounds SB705498, BCTC and AMG9810 in rat models of thermal hyperalgesia measured with an increasing-temperature water bath. *Eur J Pharmacol*; **641**: 135–41.

23. MacEwan DJ. TNF receptor subtype signalling: differences and cellular consequences. *Cell Signal* 2002; **14**: 477–92.

24. Sorkin LS, Xiao WH, Wagner R, Myers RR. Tumour necrosis factor-alpha induces ectopic activity in nociceptive primary afferent fibres. *Neuroscience* 1997; **81**: 255–62.

25. Fukuoka H, Kawatani M, Hisamitsu T, Takeshige C. Cutaneous hyperalgesia induced by peripheral injection of interleukin-1 beta in the rat. *Brain Res* 1994; **657**: 133–40.

26. Schafers M, Sommer C, Geis C, *et al.* Selective stimulation of either tumor necrosis factor receptor differentially induces pain behavior in vivo and ectopic activity in sensory neurons in vitro. *Neuroscience* 2008; **157**: 414–23.

27. Opree A, Kress M. Involvement of the proinflammatory cytokines tumor necrosis factor-alpha, IL-1 beta, and IL-6 but not IL-8 in the development of heat hyperalgesia: effects on heat-evoked calcitonin gene-related peptide release from rat skin. *J Neurosci* 2000; **20**: 6289–93.

28. Funk CD. Prostaglandins and leukotrienes: advances in eicosanoid biology. *Science* 2001; **294**: 1871–5.

29. Dayer JM, Beutler B, Cerami A. Cachectin/tumor necrosis factor stimulates collagenase and prostaglandin E2 production by human synovial cells and dermal fibroblasts. *J Exp Med* 1985; **162**: 2163–8.

30. Ferreira SH, Lorenzetti BB, Bristow AF, Poole S. Interleukin-1 beta as a potent hyperalgesic agent antagonized by a tripeptide analogue. *Nature* 1988; **334**: 698–700.

31. Buvanendran A, Kroin JS, Berger RA, *et al.* Upregulation of prostaglandin E2 and interleukins in the central nervous system and peripheral tissue during and after surgery in humans. *Anesthesiology* 2006; **104**: 403–10.

32. Stalman A, Tsai JA, Segerdahl M, *et al.* Ketorolac but not morphine exerts inflammatory and metabolic effects in synovial membrane after knee arthroscopy: a double-blind randomized prospective study using the microdialysis technique. *Reg Anesth Pain Med* 2009; **34**: 557–64.

33. Levine JD, Lam D, Taiwo YO, Donatoni P, Goetzl EJ. Hyperalgesic properties of 15-lipoxygenase products of arachidonic acid. *Proc Natl Acad Sci USA* 1986; **83**: 5331–4.

34. Martin HA, Basbaum AI, Kwiat GC, Goetzl EJ, Levine JD. Leukotriene and prostaglandin sensitization of cutaneous high-threshold C- and A-delta mechanonociceptors in the hairy skin of rat hindlimbs. *Neuroscience* 1987; **22**: 651–9.

35. Martin HA, Basbaum AI, Goetzl EJ, Levine JD. Leukotriene B4 decreases the mechanical and thermal thresholds of C-fiber nociceptors in the hairy skin of the rat. *J Neurophysiol* 1988; **60**: 438–45.

36. Masferrer JL, Zweifel BS, Hardy M, *et al*. Pharmacology of PF-4191834, a novel, selective non-redox 5-lipoxygenase inhibitor effective in inflammation and pain. *J Pharmacol Exp Ther* 2010; **334**: 294–301.

37. Singh VP, Patil CS, Kulkarni SK. Differential effect of zileuton, a 5-lipoxygenase inhibitor, against nociceptive paradigms in mice and rats. *Pharmacol Biochem Behav* 2005; **81**: 433–9.

38. Abbadie C, McManus OB, Sun SY, *et al*. Analgesic effects of a substituted N-triazole oxindole (TROX-1), a state-dependent, voltage-gated calcium channel 2 blocker. *J Pharmacol Exp Ther* 2010; **334**: 545–55.

39. Couture R, Harrisson M, Vianna RM, Cloutier F. Kinin receptors in pain and inflammation. *Eur J Pharmacol* 2001; **429**: 161–76.

40. Liu B, Linley JE, Du X, *et al*. The acute nociceptive signals induced by bradykinin in rat sensory neurons are mediated by inhibition of M-type K+ channels and activation of Ca^{2+}-activated Cl- channels. *J Clin Invest* 2010; **120**: 1240–52.

41. Leonard PA, Arunkumar R, Brennan TJ. Bradykinin antagonists have no analgesic effect on incisional pain. *Anesth Analg* 2004; **99**: 1166–72.

42. Burnstock G. Purinergic signalling and disorders of the central nervous system. *Nat Rev Drug Discov* 2008; 7: 575–90.

43. Woo YC, Park SS, Subieta AR, Brennan TJ. Changes in tissue pH and temperature after incision indicate acidosis may contribute to postoperative pain. *Anesthesiology* 2004; **101**: 468–75.

44. Khakh BS, Burnstock G, Kennedy C, *et al*. International union of pharmacology. XXIV. Current status of the nomenclature and properties of P2X receptors and their subunits. *Pharmacol Rev* 2001; **53**: 107–18.

45. Abbracchio MP, Burnstock G, Boeynaems JM, *et al*. International Union of Pharmacology LVIII: update on the P2Y G protein-coupled nucleotide receptors: from molecular mechanisms and pathophysiology to therapy. *Pharmacol Rev* 2006; **58**: 281–341.

46. Gordon JL. Extracellular ATP: effects, sources and fate. *Biochem J* 1986; **233**: 309–19.

47. Verghese MW, Kneisler TB, Boucheron JA. P2U agonists induce chemotaxis and actin polymerization in human neutrophils and differentiated HL60 cells. *J Biol Chem* 1996; **271**: 15597–601.

48. Koizumi S, Fujishita K, Inoue K, Shigemoto-Mogami Y, Tsuda M. Ca^{2+} waves in keratinocytes are transmitted to sensory neurons: the involvement of extracellular ATP and P2Y2 receptor activation. *Biochem J* 2004; **380**: 329–38.

49. Zhao P, Barr TP, Hou Q, *et al*. Voltage-gated sodium channel expression in rat and human epidermal keratinocytes: evidence for a role in pain. *Pain* 2008; **139**: 90–105.

50. Martucci C, Trovato AE, Costa B, *et al*. The purinergic antagonist PPADS reduces pain related behaviours and interleukin-1 beta, interleukin-6, iNOS and nNOS overproduction in central and peripheral nervous system after peripheral neuropathy in mice. *Pain* 2008; **137**: 81–95.

51. Ulmann L, Hirbec H, Rassendren F. P2X4 receptors mediate PGE2 release by tissue-resident macrophages and initiate inflammatory pain. *EMBO* 2010; **J 29**: 2290–300.

52. Sahbaie P, Shi X, Guo TZ, *et al*. Role of substance P signaling in enhanced nociceptive sensitization and local cytokine production after incision. *Pain* 2009; **145**: 341–9.

53. Iversen L. Substance P equals pain substance? *Nature* 1998; **392**: 334–5.

54. Dougherty PM, Palecek J, Paleckova V, Willis WD. Neurokinin 1 and 2 antagonists attenuate the responses and NK1 antagonists prevent the sensitization of primate spinothalamic tract neurons after intradermal capsaicin. *J Neurophysiol* 1994; **72**: 1464–75.

55. Dallos A, Kiss M, Polyanka H, *et al*. Effects of the neuropeptides substance P, calcitonin gene-related peptide, vasoactive intestinal polypeptide and galanin on the production of nerve growth factor and inflammatory cytokines in cultured human keratinocytes. *Neuropeptides* 2006; **40**: 251–63.

56. Delgado AV, McManus AT, Chambers JP. Production of tumor necrosis factor-alpha, interleukin 1-beta, interleukin 2, and interleukin 6 by rat leukocyte subpopulations after exposure to substance P. *Neuropeptides* 2003; **37**: 355–61.

57. Delgado AV, McManus AT, Chambers JP. Exogenous administration of Substance P enhances wound healing in a novel skin-injury model. *Exp Biol Med (Maywood)* 2005; **230**: 271–80.

58. Cao YQ, Mantyh PW, Carlson EJ, *et al*. Primary afferent tachykinins are required to experience moderate to intense pain. *Nature* 1998; **392**: 390–4.

59. Coudore-Civiale MA, Courteix C, Eschalier A, Fialip J. Effect of tachykinin receptor antagonists in experimental neuropathic pain. *Eur J Pharmacol* 1998; **361**: 175–84.

60. Julius D, Basbaum AI. Molecular mechanisms of nociception. *Nature* 2001; **413**: 203–10.

61. Woolf CJ, Safieh-Garabedian B, Ma QP, Crilly P, Winter J. Nerve growth factor contributes to the

generation of inflammatory sensory hypersensitivity. *Neuroscience* 1994; **62**: 327–31.

62. Manni L, Aloe L. Role of IL-1 beta and TNF-alpha in the regulation of NGF in experimentally induced arthritis in mice. *Rheumatol Int* 1998; **18**: 97–102.

63. Wu C, Boustany L, Liang H, Brennan TJ. Nerve growth factor expression after plantar incision in the rat. *Anesthesiology* 2007; **107**: 128–35.

64. Luo XG, Rush RA, Zhou XF. Ultrastructural localization of brain-derived neurotrophic factor in rat primary sensory neurons. *Neurosci Res* 2001; **39**: 377–84.

65. Michael GJ, Averill S, Nitkunan A, *et al.* Nerve growth factor treatment increases brain-derived neurotrophic factor selectively in TrkA-expressing dorsal root ganglion cells and in their central terminations within the spinal cord. *J Neurosci* 1997; **17**: 8476–90.

66. Li CQ, Xu JM, Liu D, Zhang JY, Dai RP. Brain derived neurotrophic factor (BDNF) contributes to the pain hypersensitivity following surgical incision in the rats. *Mol Pain* 2008; **4**: 27.

67. Porreca F, Lai J, Bian D, *et al.* A comparison of the potential role of the tetrodotoxin-insensitive sodium channels, PN3/SNS and NaN/SNS2, in rat models of chronic pain. *Proc Natl Acad Sci USA* 1999; **96**: 7640–4.

68. Roza C, Laird JM, Souslova V, Wood JN, Cervero F. The tetrodotoxin-resistant Na+ channel Nav1.8 is essential for the expression of spontaneous activity in damaged sensory axons of mice. *J Physiol* 2003; **550**: 921–6.

69. Grover VK, Mathew PJ, Yaddanapudi S, Sehgal S. A single dose of preoperative gabapentin for pain reduction and requirement of morphine after total mastectomy and axillary dissection: randomized placebo-controlled double-blind trial. *J Postgrad Med* 2009; **55**: 257–60.

70. Gu N, Vervaeke K, Hu H, Storm JF. Kv7/KCNQ/M and HCN/h, but not KCa2/SK channels, contribute to the somatic medium after-hyperpolarization and excitability control in CA1 hippocampal pyramidal cells. *J Physiol* 2005; **566**: 689–715.

71. Passmore GM, Selyanko AA, Mistry M, *et al.* KCNQ/M currents in sensory neurons: significance for pain therapy. *J Neurosci* 2003; **23**: 7227–36.

72. Blackburn-Munro G, Jensen BS. The anticonvulsant retigabine attenuates nociceptive behaviours in rat models of persistent and neuropathic pain. *Eur J Pharmacol* 2003; **460**: 109–16.

73. Cairns BE, Svensson P, Wang K, *et al.* Activation of peripheral NMDA receptors contributes to human pain and rat afferent discharges evoked by injection of glutamate into the masseter muscle. *J Neurophysiol* 2003; **90**: 2098–105.

74. Zahn PK, Pogatzki-Zahn EM, Brennan TJ. Spinal administration of MK-801 and NBQX demonstrates NMDA-independent dorsal horn sensitization in incisional pain. *Pain* 2005; **114**: 499–510.

75. Richebe P, Rivat C, Laulin JP, Maurette P, Simonnet G. Ketamine improves the management of exaggerated postoperative pain observed in perioperative fentanyl-treated rats. *Anesthesiology* 2005; **102**: 421–8.

76. Yeh CC, Wu CT, Lee MS, *et al.* Analgesic effects of preincisional administration of dextromethorphan and tenoxicam following laparoscopic cholecystectomy. *Acta Anaesthesiol Scand* 2004; **48**: 1049–53.

77. Wu CT, Yeh CC, Yu JC, *et al.* Pre-incisional epidural ketamine, morphine and bupivacaine combined with epidural and general anaesthesia provides preemptive analgesia for upper abdominal surgery. *Acta Anaesthesiol Scand* 2000; **44**: 63–8.

78. Sandkuhler J. Understanding LTP in pain pathways. *Mol Pain* 2007; **3**: 9.

79. Akopian AN, Sivilotti L, Wood JN. A tetrodotoxin-resistant voltage-gated sodium channel expressed by sensory neurons. *Nature* 1996; **379**: 257–62.

80. Lu SG, Zhang XL, Luo ZD, Gold MS. Persistent inflammation alters the density and distribution of voltage-activated calcium channels in subpopulations of rat cutaneous DRG neurons. *Pain* 2010 Dec; **151**(3): 633–43.

81. Herrero JF, Laird JM, Lopez-Garcia JA. Wind-up of spinal cord neurones and pain sensation: much ado about something? *Prog Neurobiol* 2000; **61**: 169–203.

82. Fang L, Wu J, Lin Q, Willis WD. Calcium-calmodulin-dependent protein kinase II contributes to spinal cord central sensitization. *J Neurosci* 2002; **22**: 4196–204.

83. Sluka KA, Willis WD. The effects of G-protein and protein kinase inhibitors on the behavioral responses of rats to intradermal injection of capsaicin. *Pain* 1997; **71**: 165–78.

84. Coderre TJ. Contribution of protein kinase C to central sensitization and persistent pain following tissue injury. *Neurosci Lett* 1992; **140**: 181–4.

85. Palecek J, Paleckova V, Dougherty PM, Willis WD. The effect of phorbol esters on the responses of primate spinothalamic neurons to mechanical and thermal stimuli. *J Neurophysiol* 1994; **71**: 529–37.

86. Sluka KA, Rees H, Chen PS, Tsuruoka M, Willis WD. Capsaicin-induced sensitization of primate spinothalamic tract cells is prevented by a protein kinase C inhibitor. *Brain Res* 1997; **772**: 82–6.

87. Sun RQ, Tu YJ, Yan JY, Willis WD. Activation of protein kinase B/Akt signaling pathway contributes to mechanical hypersensitivity induced by capsaicin. *Pain* 2006; **120**: 86–96.

88. Woolf CJ, Salter MW. Neuronal plasticity: increasing the gain in pain. *Science* 2000; **288**: 1765–9.

89. De Kock M. Expanding our horizons: transition of acute postoperative pain to persistent pain and establishment of chronic postsurgical pain services. *Anesthesiology* 2009; **111**: 461–3.

90. Toroudi HP, Borghei Razavi M, Borghei Razavi H, *et al.* Comparison of the analgesic effect of ibuprofen with mesalamine after discectomy surgery in patients with lumbar disc herniation: a double-blind randomized controlled trial. *Neurol India* 2009; **57**: 305–9.

91. Yukawa Y, Kato F, Ito K, Terashima T, Horie Y. A prospective randomized study of preemptive analgesia for postoperative pain in the patients undergoing posterior lumbar interbody fusion: continuous subcutaneous morphine, continuous epidural morphine, and diclofenac sodium. *Spine* 2005; **30**: 2357–61.

92. Bianconi M, Ferraro L, Ricci R, *et al.* The pharmacokinetics and efficacy of ropivacaine continuous wound instillation after spine fusion surgery. *Anesth Analg* 2004; **98**: 166–72.

93. Cohen BE, Hartman MB, Wade JT, *et al.* Postoperative pain control after lumbar spine fusion. Patient-controlled analgesia versus continuous epidural analgesia. *Spine* 1997; **22**: 1892–6; discussion 1896–7.

94. Gottschalk A, Durieux ME, Nemergut EC. Intraoperative methadone improves postoperative pain control in patients undergoing complex spine surgery. *Anesth Analg* 2011 Jan; **112**(1): 218–23.

95. Elder JB, Hoh DJ, Wang MY. Postoperative continuous paravertebral anesthetic infusion for pain control in lumbar spinal fusion surgery. *Spine* 2008; **33**: 210–18.

96. Farmery AD, Wilson-MacDonald J. The analgesic effect of epidural clonidine after spinal surgery: a randomized placebo-controlled trial. *Anesth Analg* 2009; **108**: 631–4.

97. Poe-Kochert C, Tripi PA, Potzman J, Son-Hing JP, Thompson GH. Continuous intravenous morphine infusion for postoperative analgesia following posterior spinal fusion for idiopathic scoliosis. *Spine* **35**: 754–7.

98. Sekar C, Rajasekaran S, Kannan R, *et al.* Preemptive analgesia for postoperative pain relief in lumbosacral spine surgeries: a randomized controlled trial. *Spine J* 2004; **4**: 261–4.

99. Jirarattanaphochai K, Thienthong S, Sriraj W, *et al.* Effect of parecoxib on postoperative pain after lumbar spine surgery: a bicenter, randomized, double-blinded, placebo-controlled trial. *Spine (Phila Pa 1976)* 2008; **33**: 132–9.

100. Katz J, Jackson M, Kavanagh BP, Sandler AN. Acute pain after thoracic surgery predicts long-term post-thoracotomy pain. *Clin J Pain* 1996; **12**: 50–5.

101. Garringer SM, Sasso RC. Safety of anterior cervical discectomy and fusion performed as outpatient surgery. *J Spinal Disord Tech* 2010 Oct; **23**(7): 439–43.

102. Rajpal S, Gordon DB, Pellino TA, *et al.* Comparison of perioperative oral multimodal analgesia versus IV PCA for spine surgery. *J Spinal Disord Tech* 2010; **23**: 139–45.

103. Kehlet H, Werner M, Perkins F. Balanced analgesia: what is it and what are its advantages in postoperative pain? *Drugs* 1999; **58**: 793–7.

104. Kehlet H. Balanced analgesia: a prerequisite for optimal recovery. *Br J Surg* 1998; **85**: 3–4.

105. Mack PF, Hass D, Lavyne MH, Snow RB, Lien CA. Postoperative narcotic requirement after microscopic lumbar discectomy is not affected by intraoperative ketorolac or bupivacaine. *Spine (Phila Pa 1976)* 2001; **26**: 658–61.

106. Hickey OT, Burke SM, Hafeez P, *et al.* Determinants of outcome for patients undergoing lumbar discectomy: a pilot study. *Eur J Anaesthesiol* 2010; **27**: 696–701.

107. Barratt SM, Smith RC, Kee AJ, Mather LE, Cousins MJ. Multimodal analgesia and intravenous nutrition preserves total body protein following major upper gastrointestinal surgery. *Reg Anesth Pain Med* 2002; **27**: 15–22.

108. Apfelbaum JL, Chen C, Mehta SS, Gan TJ. Postoperative pain experience: results from a national survey suggest postoperative pain continues to be undermanaged. *Anesth Analg* 2003; **97**: 534–40.

109. Mendoza T, Mayne T, Rublee D, Cleeland C. Reliability and validity of a modified Brief Pain Inventory short form in patients with osteoarthritis. *Eur J Pain* 2006; **10**: 353–61.

110. Riest G, Peters J, Weiss M, *et al.* Preventive effects of perioperative parecoxib on post-discectomy pain. *Br J Anaesth* 2008; **100**: 256–62.

111. Blumenthal S, Min K, Marquardt M, Borgeat A. Postoperative intravenous morphine consumption, pain scores, and side effects with perioperative oral controlled-release oxycodone after lumbar discectomy. *Anesth Analg* 2007; **105**: 233–7.

112. Buvanendran A, Kroin JS. Multimodal analgesia for controlling acute postoperative pain. *Curr Opin Anaesthesiol* 2009; **22**: 588–93.

113. White PF. Multimodal analgesia: its role in preventing postoperative pain. *Curr Opin Investig Drugs* 2008; **9**: 76–82.

114. Cassinelli EH, Dean CL, Garcia RM, Furey CG, Bohlman HH. Ketorolac use for postoperative pain

management following lumbar decompression surgery: a prospective, randomized, double-blinded, placebo-controlled trial. *Spine (Phila Pa 1976)* 2008; **33**: 1313–17.

115. Mordeniz C, Torun F, Soran AF, *et al.* The effects of pre-emptive analgesia with bupivacaine on acute post-laminectomy pain. *Arch Orthop Trauma Surg*; **130**: 205–8.

116. Cata JP, Noguera EM, Parke E, *et al.* Patient-controlled epidural analgesia (PCEA) for postoperative pain control after lumbar spine surgery. *J Neurosurg Anesthesiol* 2008; **20**: 256–60.

117. Schenk MR, Putzier M, Kugler B, *et al.* Postoperative analgesia after major spine surgery: patient-controlled epidural analgesia versus patient-controlled intravenous analgesia. *Anesth Analg* 2006; **103**: 1311–17.

118. Gora-Harper ML, Record KE, Darkow T, Tibbs PA. Opioid analgesics versus ketorolac in spine and joint procedures: impact on healthcare resources. *Ann Pharmacother* 2001; **35**: 1320–6.

119. Tegeder I, Costigan M, Griffin RS, *et al.* GTP cyclohydrolase and tetrahydrobiopterin regulate pain sensitivity and persistence. *Nat Med* 2006; **12**: 1269–77.

120. Rosow CD. Pharmacology of opioid analgesics. In: Longnecker DE. ed. *Anesthesiology*. New York: McGraw-Hill; 2008: xxi.

121. Chang AK, Bijur PE, Meyer RH, *et al.* Safety and efficacy of hydromorphone as an analgesic alternative to morphine in acute pain: a randomized clinical trial. *Ann Emerg Med* 2006; **48**: 164–72.

122. Jacobi J, Fraser GL, Coursin DB, *et al.* Clinical practice guidelines for the sustained use of sedatives and analgesics in the critically ill adult. *Crit Care Med* 2002; **30**: 119–41.

123. Palmer PP, Miller RD. Current and developing methods of patient-controlled analgesia. *Anesthesiol Clin* 2010; **28**: 587–99.

124. Longnecker DE. *Anesthesiology*. New York: McGraw-Hill; 2008.

125. Cepeda MS, Alvarez H, Morales O, Carr DB. Addition of ultralow dose naloxone to postoperative morphine PCA: unchanged analgesia and opioid requirement but decreased incidence of opioid side effects. *Pain* 2004; **107**: 41–6.

126. Ved SA, Dubois M, Carron H, Lea D. Sufentanil and alfentanil pattern of consumption during patient-controlled analgesia: a comparison with morphine. *Clin J Pain* 1989; **5** Suppl 1: S63–70.

127. Douma MR, Verwey RA, Kam-Endtz CE, van der Linden PD, Stienstra R. Obstetric analgesia:

a comparison of patient-controlled meperidine, remifentanil, and fentanyl in labour. *Br J Anaesth*; **104**: 209–15.

128. Cabanero D, Campillo A, Celerier E, Romero A, Puig MM. Pronociceptive effects of remifentanil in a mouse model of postsurgical pain: effect of a second surgery. *Anesthesiology* 2009; **111**: 1334–45.

129. Jordan B, Devi LA. Molecular mechanisms of opioid receptor signal transduction. *Br J Anaesth* 1998; **81**: 12–19.

130. Trafton JA, Abbadie C, Marek K, Basbaum AI. Postsynaptic signaling via the [mu]-opioid receptor: responses of dorsal horn neurons to exogenous opioids and noxious stimulation. *J Neurosci* 2000; **20**: 8578–84.

131. Gardell LR, Wang R, Burgess SE, *et al.* Sustained morphine exposure induces a spinal dynorphin-dependent enhancement of excitatory transmitter release from primary afferent fibers. *J Neurosci* 2002; **22**: 6747–55.

132. Borgland SL. Acute opioid receptor desensitization and tolerance: is there a link? *Clin Exp Pharmacol Physiol* 2001; **28**: 147–54.

133. Engelhardt T, Zaarour C, Naser B, *et al.* Intraoperative low-dose ketamine does not prevent a remifentanil-induced increase in morphine requirement after pediatric scoliosis surgery. *Anesth Analg* 2008; **107**: 1170–5.

134. Crawford MW, Hickey C, Zaarour C, Howard A, Naser B. Development of acute opioid tolerance during infusion of remifentanil for pediatric scoliosis surgery. *Anesth Analg* 2006; **102**: 1662–7.

135. Trescot AM, Datta S, Lee M, Hansen H. Opioid pharmacology. *Pain Physician* 2008; **11**: S133–53.

136. Reuben SS, Steinberg RB, Maciolek H, Joshi W. Preoperative administration of controlled-release oxycodone for the management of pain after ambulatory laparoscopic tubal ligation surgery. *J Clin Anesth* 2002; **14**: 223–7.

137. Arici S, Gurbet A, Turker G, Yavascaoglu B, Sahin S. Preemptive analgesic effects of intravenous paracetamol in total abdominal hysterectomy. *Agri* 2009; **21**: 54–61.

138. Macario A, Royal MA. A literature review of randomized clinical trials of intravenous acetaminophen (paracetamol) for acute postoperative pain. *Pain Pract* 2011; **11**(3): 290–6.

139. Toms L, McQuay HJ, Derry S, Moore RA. Single dose oral paracetamol (acetaminophen) for postoperative pain in adults. *Cochrane Database Syst Rev* 2008: CD004602.

140. Memis D, Inal MT, Kavalci G, Sezer A, Sut N. Intravenous paracetamol reduced the use of opioids,

extubation time, and opioid-related adverse effects after major surgery in intensive care unit. *J Crit Care*; **25**: 458–62.

141. Turner DM, Warson JS, Wirt TC, *et al.* The use of ketorolac in lumbar spine surgery: a cost-benefit analysis. *J Spinal Disord* 1995; **8**: 206–12.

142. Reuben SS, Connelly NR, Lurie S, Klatt M, Gibson CS. Dose–response of ketorolac as an adjunct to patient-controlled analgesia morphine in patients after spinal fusion surgery. *Anesth Analg* 1998; **87**: 98–102.

143. Le Roux PD, Samudrala S. Postoperative pain after lumbar disc surgery: a comparison between parenteral ketorolac and narcotics. *Acta Neurochir (Wien)* 1999; **141**: 261–7.

144. Munoz M, Garcia-Vallejo JJ, Sempere JM, *et al.* Acute phase response in patients undergoing lumbar spinal surgery: modulation by perioperative treatment with naproxen and famotidine. *Eur Spine J* 2004; **13**: 367–73.

145. Grundmann U, Wornle C, Biedler A, *et al.* The efficacy of the non-opioid analgesics parecoxib, paracetamol and metamizol for postoperative pain relief after lumbar microdiscectomy. *Anesth Analg* 2006; **103**: 217–22.

146. Bekker A, Cooper PR, Frempong-Boadu A, *et al.* Evaluation of preoperative administration of the cyclooxygenase-2 inhibitor rofecoxib for the treatment of postoperative pain after lumbar disc surgery. *Neurosurgery* 2002; **50**: 1053–7; discussion 1057–8.

147. Urrutia J, Mardones R, Quezada F. The effect of ketoprofen on lumbar spinal fusion healing in a rabbit model. Laboratory investigation. *J Neurosurg Spine* 2007; **7**: 631–6.

148. Li Q, Zhang Z, Cai Z. High-dose ketorolac affects adult spinal fusion: a meta-analysis of the effect of perioperative nonsteroidal anti-inflammatory drugs on spinal fusion. *Spine (Phila Pa 1976)* 2011; **36**(7): E461–8.

149. Pradhan BB, Tatsumi RL, Gallina J, *et al.* Ketorolac and spinal fusion: does the perioperative use of ketorolac really inhibit spinal fusion? *Spine (Phila Pa 1976)* 2008; **33**: 2079–82.

150. Sucato DJ, Lovejoy JF, Agrawal S, *et al.* Postoperative ketorolac does not predispose to pseudoarthrosis following posterior spinal fusion and instrumentation for adolescent idiopathic scoliosis. *Spine (Phila Pa 1976)* 2008; **33**: 1119–24.

151. Glassman SD, Rose SM, Dimar JR, *et al.* The effect of postoperative nonsteroidal anti-inflammatory drug administration on spinal fusion. *Spine (Phila Pa 1976)* 1998; **23**: 834–8.

152. Thaller J, Walker M, Kline AJ, Anderson DG. The effect of nonsteroidal anti-inflammatory agents on

spinal fusion. *Orthopedics* 2005; **28**: 299–303; quiz 304–5.

153. Lumawig JM, Yamazaki A, Watanabe K. Dose-dependent inhibition of diclofenac sodium on posterior lumbar interbody fusion rates. *Spine J* 2009; **9**: 343–9.

154. Korinth MC, Gilsbach JM, Weinzierl MR. Low-dose aspirin before spinal surgery: results of a survey among neurosurgeons in Germany. *Eur Spine J* 2007; **16**: 365–72.

155. Kong VK, Irwin MG. Gabapentin: a multimodal perioperative drug? *Br J Anaesth* 2007; **99**: 775–86.

156. Pandey CK, Sahay S, Gupta D, *et al.* Preemptive gabapentin decreases postoperative pain after lumbar discoidectomy. *Can J Anaesth* 2004; **51**: 986–9.

157. Pandey CK, Navkar DV, Giri PJ, *et al.* Evaluation of the optimal preemptive dose of gabapentin for postoperative pain relief after lumbar diskectomy: a randomized, double-blind, placebo-controlled study. *J Neurosurg Anesthesiol* 2005; **17**: 65–8.

158. Turan A, Karamanlioglu B, Memis D, *et al.* Analgesic effects of gabapentin after spinal surgery. *Anesthesiology* 2004; **100**: 935–8.

159. Buvanendran A, Kroin JS, Kari M, Tuman KJ. Can a single dose of 300 mg of pregabalin reach acute antihyperalgesic levels in the central nervous system? *Reg Anesth Pain Med*; **35**: 535–8.

160. Cada DJ, Levien, T., Baker, D.E.: Pregabalin. *Hospital Pharmacy* 2006; **41**: 157–72.

161. Blommel ML, Blommel AL. Pregabalin: an antiepileptic agent useful for neuropathic pain. *Am J Health Syst Pharm* 2007; **64**: 1475–82.

162. Peng PW, Li C, Farcas E, *et al.* Use of low-dose pregabalin in patients undergoing laparoscopic cholecystectomy. *Br J Anaesth*; **105**: 155–61.

163. Kim SY, Jeong JJ, Chung WY, *et al.* Perioperative administration of pregabalin for pain after robot-assisted endoscopic thyroidectomy: a randomized clinical trial. *Surg Endosc* 2010; **24**: 2776–81.

164. Burke SM, Shorten GD. Perioperative pregabalin improves pain and functional outcomes 3 months after lumbar discectomy. *Anesth Analg*; **110**: 1180–5.

165. Milbrandt TA, Singhal M, Minter C, *et al.* A comparison of three methods of pain control for posterior spinal fusions in adolescent idiopathic scoliosis. *Spine (Phila Pa 1976)* 2009; **34**: 1499–503.

166. Sucato DJ, Duey-Holtz A, Elerson E, Safavi F. Postoperative analgesia following surgical correction for adolescent idiopathic scoliosis: a comparison of continuous epidural analgesia and patient-controlled analgesia. *Spine (Phila Pa 1976)* 2005; **30**: 211–17.

167. Shaw BA, Watson TC, Merzel DI, Gerardi JA, Birek A. The safety of continuous epidural infusion for

319

postoperative analgesia in pediatric spine surgery. *J Pediatr Orthop* 1996; **16**: 374–7.

168. Turner A, Lee J, Mitchell R, Berman J, Edge G, Fennelly M. The efficacy of surgically placed epidural catheters for analgesia after posterior spinal surgery. *Anaesthesia* 2000; **55**: 370–3.

169. Ekatodramis G, Min K, Cathrein P, Borgeat A. Use of a double epidural catheter provides effective postoperative analgesia after spine deformity surgery. *Can J Anaesth* 2002; **49**: 173–7.

170. Yoshimoto H, Nagashima K, Sato S, *et al.* A prospective evaluation of anesthesia for posterior lumbar spine fusion: the effectiveness of preoperative epidural anesthesia with morphine. *Spine (Phila Pa 1976)* 2005; **30**: 863–9.

171. Fisher CG, Belanger L, Gofton EG, *et al.* Prospective randomized clinical trial comparing patient-controlled intravenous analgesia with patient-controlled epidural analgesia after lumbar spinal fusion. *Spine (Phila Pa 1976)* 2003; **28**: 739–43.

172. Gottschalk A, Freitag M, Tank S, *et al.* Quality of postoperative pain using an intraoperatively placed epidural catheter after major lumbar spinal surgery. *Anesthesiology* 2004; **101**: 175–80.

173. Blumenthal S, Min K, Nadig M, Borgeat A. Double epidural catheter with ropivacaine versus intravenous morphine: a comparison for postoperative analgesia after scoliosis correction surgery. *Anesthesiology* 2005; **102**: 175–80.

174. Jellish WS, Abodeely A, Fluder EM, Shea J. The effect of spinal bupivacaine in combination with either epidural clonidine and/or 0.5% bupivacaine administered at the incision site on postoperative outcome in patients undergoing lumbar laminectomy. *Anesth Analg* 2003; **96**: 874–80.

175. Marinangeli F, Ciccozzi A, Donatelli F, *et al.* Clonidine for treatment of postoperative pain: a dose-finding study. *Eur J Pain* 2002; **6**: 35–42.

176. Jirarattanaphochai K, Jung S, Thienthong S, Krisanaprakornkit W, Sumananont C. Peridural methylprednisolone and wound infiltration with bupivacaine for postoperative pain control after posterior lumbar spine surgery: a randomized double-blinded placebo-controlled trial. *Spine (Phila Pa 1976)* 2007; **32**: 609–16; discussion 617.

Chapter

19

Postoperative chronic pain management

Dmitri Souzdalnitski and Jianguo Cheng

Key points

- Inadequate pain control is a common complaint of patients with preexisting chronic pain and may be related to significant adverse outcomes.

- Recent data from structural, functional, and molecular imaging studies support the notion that chronic pain has characteristics of a disease rather than just a constellation of symptoms. It is only possible to differentiate aberrant behavior or drug abuse from pseudo-addiction when the pain is adequately controlled.

- Postoperative management of patients with preexisting chronic pain is extremely challenging mainly because escalation of opioid dose is often required for adequate pain control due to tolerance built up in opioid-dependent patients. It may be required to increase the opioid dose by as much as a factor of 2–4 to control acute surgical pain superimposed on chronic pain.

- Patients who report better effect of one opioid over another should *not* be automatically categorized as "drug seekers." Genetic variations may influence individual responsiveness to pharmacotherapy of acute and chronic pain.

- The increased availability of nonopioid analgesics, adjuncts, peripherally acting opioid receptor antagonists, and regional anesthesia techniques brings up new opportunities for improving the experience of chronic-pain patients after spine surgery.

Introduction

Chronic pain is the leading reason for patients' consent to spine surgery. Not only is the prevalence of chronic pain in the spine surgery patient population high, almost half of these patients are dependent on opioids.[1] One of the major concerns of these patients is whether the pain can be adequately controlled after surgery. These patients are in fact much more prone to exacerbation of their chronic pain condition in the postoperative period.[2] This concern is shared by many surgeons and anesthesiologists. It is often necessary to use large doses of opioids for postoperative pain control due to the high tolerance of these opioid-dependent patients.[3] Consequently, physicians are often faced with increased risks for respiratory depression and other significant side effects of opioids. Postoperative pain control is closely related to clinical outcomes, length of hospital stay, and patient (and family) satisfaction. There is compelling evidence that demonstrates medical, social, and economic benefits of adequate perioperative pain control. Yet there are no existing pain management guidelines regarding the best practice of postoperative control in this patient population.[4] We review in this chapter a variety of techniques and multidisciplinary approaches described in the literature that can be utilized to optimize postoperative pain management in patients with preexisting chronic pain who are undergoing spine surgery. The goal is to help the reader to effectively utilize available pain management options that can provide safe, efficacious, and cost-effective postoperative pain management, better clinical outcomes, and patient satisfaction.

The challenges of postoperative pain management in chronic pain patients

Predictors of postoperative pain in spine surgery

Up to 80% of patients will have acute pain after surgery and moderate to severe pain is experienced in about 30% of patients.[5,6] About 50% of the patients undergoing surgical procedures will develop chronic

Anesthesia for Spine Surgery, ed. Ehab Farag. Published by Cambridge University Press. © Cambridge University Press 2012.

pain, and up to 87% of patients undergoing spine surgery may develop chronic pain.[7] The major predictors of developing chronic postoperative pain are existence of preoperative pain and anxiety, according to a recent meta-analysis of 48 studies that enrolled 23 037 patients.[2] These predictors are commonly present in patients undergoing spine surgery. The patients presenting for spine surgery typically have preoperative pain, accompanied by anxiety and depression, and analgesics intake (41% of them take opioids, 25% take antidepressants, and 9% take anxiolytic mediations regularly).[1] Inadequate pain control is a common complaint in this population of patients and may be related to significant adverse outcomes.

Inadequate control of postoperative pain and related clinical outcomes

Adverse clinical outcomes associated with inadequate pain control include decrease in vital capacity and alveolar ventilation, pneumonia, hypertension, tachycardia, myocardial ischemia and myocardial infarction, poor wound healing, change in mental status, and other physiological and psychological abnormalities. The mechanisms of these complications may include pain-related sympathetic stimulation, hypoventilation, decreased oxygen content in the wound, and a variety of molecular mechanisms associated with peripheral and central sensitization.[5] Inadequate postoperative pain management has been associated with more frequent incidents of chronic postsurgical pain syndrome, which is a significant medical, societal, and economical problem.[6] Adequate postoperative pain control, in contrast, has been associated with early discharges and quicker recovery and rehabilitation after surgery.

Barriers to adequate postoperative chronic pain management

Postoperative chronic pain management can be a difficult task. Opioid tolerance is particularly challenging; it is often complicated by a common belief that a modest increase in preadmission opioid dose should effectively control chronic pain, without the significant opioid dose escalation.[8] The fact is that the majority of hospital patients have inadequate pain relief. Many patients who report severe pain are labeled as "drug-seeking" due to their requests for additional medication. Thus, inadequate training of hospital staff in pain management is one of the barriers that prevents optimal patient care. The fear of prescribing opioid analgesics and related medicolegal consequences often hampers adequate pain control in postsurgical patients,[9] leading to undertreatment of pain and the pseudo-addiction phenomena.[10] It is only possible to differentiate aberrant behavior or drug abuse from pseudo-addiction when the pain is adequately controlled[10] (Table 19.1). This appears to be a challenging task in the perioperative setting and requires close behavioral observations by the medical team. A further barrier to adequate pain control is the potential bias influenced by socio-demographic factors. For example, in some studies the pain was found to be less adequately controlled in certain patient categories such as the pediatric and the elderly populations, African-Americans, young women, and patients with central pain syndromes.[11]

Challenges of postoperative chronic pain management in opioid-tolerant patients

Contrary to common myths, the perioperative management of patients with chronic pain and opioid tolerance often requires escalation of opioid doses by a factor of 2–4, to control acute surgical pain superimposed on chronic pain. While the medical, social, and economic advantages of adequate perioperative pain control have been proven, it is imperative to be aware of immediate and long-term risks associated with opioid dose escalation.[12] Patients on chronic opioid pain therapy have less itching, nausea, and vomiting associated with opioid intake. Opioid-induced respiratory depression may be less severe in patients with chronic pain as suggested by some clinical investigations. However, experts warn that these patients are more prone to respiratory depression than are opioid-naive patients, probably because of the significant opioid dose escalation required for adequate control of their pain.[13] Potential solutions to the problem are opioid rotation, use of adjuvant pain medications, administration of regional anesthesia, and application of a variety of other pain management techniques as discussed later in this chapter. Multimodal strategies in postoperative chronic pain management are often more effective than monotherapy due to the multifactorial nature of chronic pain.

Chronic pain as a disease

Chronic pain has been linked to distinct structural, functional, psychological, and social markers[14] (Fig. 19.1). Certain molecular and genetic aberrations have also been related to chronic pain that possesses characteristics of a chronic disease rather than just a constellation of well-defined structural problems. An injury, acute

Table 19.1 Differentiation of various types of conditions associated with substance use disorder or chronic opioid use

Addiction and pseudo-addiction	"Addiction": a pattern of maladaptive behaviors, including loss control over use, craving and preoccupation with substance use, and continued use despite harm resulting from use (this term is being replaced by the term "substance use disorder with psychological and physical dependence")
	"Pseudo-addiction": addiction-like behavior caused by inadequate pain control
Substance use disorder	"Substance dependence disorder" or/and "substance abuse disorder" with psychological or/and physical dependence
	"Substance-induced" disorders (intoxication, withdrawal, delirium, psychotic disorders, and others)
Dependence	"Psychological dependence": need for a specific psychoactive substance either for its positive effects or to avoid negative psychological or physical effects associated with its withdrawal
	"Physical dependence": a physiologic state of adaptation to a specific psychoactive substance characterized by the emergence of a withdrawal syndrome during abstinence, which may be relieved in total or in part by readministration of the substance
Drugs-seeking behavior	Patient's requests for additional opioids or supply of other psychoactive medications
	"Drug seeking" and other related terms can be only be applied when the patient's pain is adequately controlled as the patient may exhibit an appropriate response to inadequately treated pain
Opioid tolerance and pseudo-opioid tolerance	"Opioid tolerance": habituation or *desensitization* of antinociceptive pathways by opioid medications producing reduction in the analgesic effect of normally efficacious doses of opioids
	"Pseudo-opioid tolerance": patients may exhibit "drug-seeking" behavior despite adequate pain relief in order to prevent reduction in current opioid analgesic dose
Opioid-induced hyperalgesia	"Opioid-induced hyperalgesia": decline in the analgesic effect of normally efficacious doses of opioids, also defined as a state of nociceptive *sensitization* caused by exposure to opioids, a paradoxical response to opioids which decreases the overall pain tolerance, probably resulting from neuroplastic changes in the peripheral and central nervous systems that lead to sensitization of proprioceptive pathways

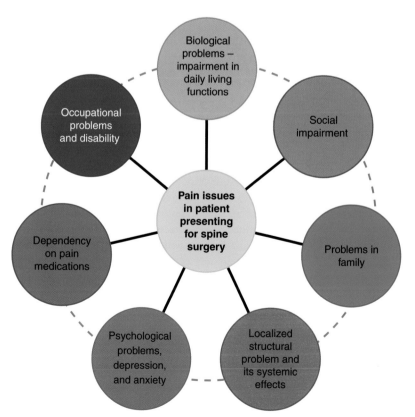

Figure 19.1. Chronic pain in a patient presenting for spine surgery: a complex entity.

inflammation, or neuropathic event typically precedes the development of chronic pain and leads to the release of inflammatory mediators by activated nociceptors or nonneural cells that reside within or infiltrate into the injured area, including mast cells, basophils, platelets, macrophages, neutrophils, endothelial cells, keratinocytes, and fibroblasts. The "inflammatory soup" of signaling molecules includes serotonin, histamine, glutamate, ATP, adenosine, substance P, calcitonin-gene related peptide (CGRP), bradykinin, eicosanoids prostaglandins, thromboxanes, leukotrienes, endocannabinoids, nerve growth factor (NGF), tumor necrosis factor α (TNF-α), interleukin-1β (IL-1β), extracellular proteases, and protons. These factors act directly on the nociceptor by binding to one or more cell surface receptors, including G-protein-coupled receptors (GPCRs), transient receptor potential (TRP) ion channels, acid-sensitive ion channels (ASICs), two-pore potassium channels (K2Ps), and receptor tyrosine kinases (RTKs). For example, nociception may be mediated by activation of B1 and B2 G-protein-coupled receptor complexes by bradykinin. This facilitates Na^+ influx while weakening outward K^+ currents, producing nociceptor excitation. Another mechanism of conversion of noxious stimuli into the generation of action potential is a calcium ion-mediated electrical depolarization. Various types of injuries produce diverse blends of inflammatory milieus, which initiate cascades of different types of neuroplastic changes. For example, 5-hydroxytryptamine (HT) released after thermal injury sensitizes primary afferent neurons and produces mechanical allodynia and thermal hyperalgesia via peripheral 5-HT_{2a} receptors. It produces a state of peripheral sensitization, which serves to protect the body from repeated injury and promote healing. The repeated painful stimulation of peripheral nerve endings propagated to the spinal dorsal horn neurons via Aδ and C-fibers may lead to progressive activation of N-methyl-D-aspartate (NMDA) receptor associated with sustained release of glutamate, substance P, and other molecules in the dorsal horns. The process leads to increased pain from noxious stimuli (hyperalgesia), pain from previously innocuous stimuli (allodynia), or spontaneous pain. The process involves not only the spinal structures but also the brain, collectively termed as "central pain sensitization." Due to these and other incompletely understood mechanisms, irreversible neurochemical and neuropathological changes may occur, leading to a chronic state clinically described as chronic pain disorder. Central pain syndrome may be due to these or other processes that cause direct damage to the spinal cord or brain such as ischemia, spinal cord injury, tumors, trauma, multiple sclerosis, or other conditions.

There are controversies over how different organ systems participate in adapting to a state of chronic pain, including the neurologic, psychiatric, endocrine, immune, cardiovascular, respiratory, metabolic, musculoskeletal, and other pathological changes in patients with chronic pain. However, recent data from structural, functional, and molecular imaging studies support the notion that chronic pain has the characteristics of a disease rather than just a constellation of symptoms. This concept is likely to lead to more widespread acceptance and classification of chronic pain as a disease and promote further research and better understanding of chronic pain, its diagnosis, aberrant pain behavior, and treatments including postoperative chronic pain management.

Effective postoperative chronic pain management begins early

Preoperative period

For optimal perioperative pain management it is imperative to communicate effectively with patients undergoing surgery. The patient history including types of opioids (and any other pain medications), precise dose, previous anesthesia, and presence and type of implanted pain management devices, should be accurately taken. The analgesic plan, which may include regional anesthesia (if applicable) and multimodal pain management techniques, should be discussed with the patient by the surgery and anesthesia/pain management teams. A comprehensive preoperative discussion of postoperative pain control options may be effectively complemented by multimedia information;[15] this information is easily accessible and may help reduce anxiety in patients undergoing surgery, particularly in those with preexisting chronic pain and significant anxiety in the perioperative period. Due to their low pain thresholds and high sensitivity to pain, this group of patients may not be able to tolerate early rehabilitation after the spine surgery without adequate pain control strategies. Thus, a thorough preoperative evaluation and planning of postoperative chronic pain control is required for optimal pain management.[3,12,13] Preemptive analgesia should be considered whenever applicable and all questions should be answered preoperatively (Table 19.2).

Table 19.2 Effective postoperative management of the chronic pain patient begins early

Preoperative period: comprehensive preoperative communication
Identify precise dose, type of opioid (and any other pain management medication), history of substance abuse, quality of previous anesthesia, presence and type of implanted pain management device
Establish a consensus with the surgeon about multimodal postoperative chronic pain management, including regional anesthesia (if applicable)
Details of postoperative chronic pain management and preemptive analgesia (if applicable) should be discussed with patient and all questions should be answered
Complement the preoperative discussion with multimedia information
Preemptive analgesia: the options
Prehabilitation: the augmenting of functional capacity *before* the spine surgery
Premedication: NSAIDs, gabapentin, pregabalin. Some reports: acetaminophen, opioids, ketamine
Preemptive local anesthetic infiltration
Preemptive epidural analgesia
Intraoperative management has impact on postoperative pain in the chronic pain patient
Expect significant pain in the immediate postoperative period with intraoperative use of ultra-short-acting opioids (remifentanil) in opioid-dependent patients
Consider intraoperative propofol infusion (less postoperative pain than with use of sevoflurane), and better patient satisfaction than with inhaled agents (in ambulatory surgery)
Consider intraoperative use of NMDA receptor antagonists (ketamine, methadone, possibly magnesium or nitrous oxide)

Preemptive analgesia and prehabilitation

Preemptive analgesia refers to a pharmacological or regional anesthesia intervention initiated prior to surgical procedure. Additionally, prehabilitation, defined as the augmenting of functional capacity *before* the spine surgery, could be considered as a form of preemptive intervention.[16] The preemptive analgesia is intended to block nociception associated with actual surgical injury. The goals of preemptive intervention are (1) to reduce pain resulting from the activation of inflammatory and nociceptive mechanisms triggered by surgical trauma; (2) to decrease the intensity of pain memory response of the central nervous system; (3) to improve quality of postoperative pain control; and (4) to reduce the risks of development of chronic pain.[17] Although these goals *were* achieved in animal models, meta-analysis of available data has not clearly demonstrated a direct translation of these results into clinical practice. While data on preemptive administration of epidural analgesia, local anesthetic wound infiltration, and NSAIDs are somewhat promising, data on the efficacy of preemptive analgesia with ketamine and opioids appear to be less supportive.[18] There is a growing body of evidence that preemptive analgesia with antiepileptic drugs may be effective in patients undergoing spine surgery. Earlier studies recommended gabapentin at an effective preemptive analgesic dose of 600 mg in spine surgery.[19] A higher median effective gabapentin

dose of 21.7 mg/kg was reported recently.[20] Pregabalin was effective as a preemptive remedy in doses of 300 mg at 90 minutes preoperatively and 150 mg at 12 and 24 hours postoperatively.[21] Local anesthetics,[22] prehabilitation,[16] and transcutaneous neurostimulation[23] have also been reported to be effective as preemptive analgesia tools in spine surgery. Interestingly, cognitive intervention prior to spine surgery failed to improve postoperative pain, or decrease opioid consumption.[24] Although recent publications on preemptive analgesia in spine surgery have not yet been reviewed in the form of meta-analysis or in a systematic manner, some hospitals have adopted preemptive analgesia as a regular component of spine surgery protocols.

General anesthesia and postoperative chronic pain management

Intraoperative anesthetic management is affected by the presence of chronic pain and the consumption of opioids and antidepressants, all of which increase MAC during the surgery. The anesthetic choice may conversely influence *postoperative* pain management. For example, the effects of the ultra-short-acting opioid remifentanil, which is frequently used in spine surgery, wear off very quickly, exposing patients with chronic pain to a sudden drop in opioid concentration and the likelihood of severe pain during emergence from surgery. It has recently been shown that opioid-dependent patients require much higher doses of remifentanil, up to 30 times that of opioid-naive patients, in order to control their pain in outpatient settings.[25] While remifentanil is not associated with the development of opioid-induced hyperalgesia and acute opioid tolerance in opioid-naive patients,[26] it is unclear whether remifentanil increases tolerance and/or opioid-induced hyperalgesia in opioid-dependent patients. Clinical observations suggest that remifentanil may cause acute opioid tolerance in opioid-dependent patients after the surgery, rendering them prone to reduced responsiveness to longer-acting opioids (see Clinical Case Scenario 19.1 at the end of the text).

Some anesthetic agents produce more plausible conditions for postoperative pain management than others. Patients anesthetized with propofol appeared to experience less pain than patients anesthetized with sevoflurane.[27]. Propofol has long been considered as nonanalgesic. However, there is evidence that propofol may modulate pain processing, perception, and central sensitization. It is not certain, though, whether the above finding was attributable to the analgesic properties of propofol or the hyperalgesic effects of sevoflurane. A recent meta-analysis demonstrated that total intravenous anesthesia appeared to produce better patient satisfaction in ambulatory settings when compared with inhalational general anesthesia.[28]. Nitrous oxide, however, was found to be an effective inhibitor of NMDA receptors, even in sub-anesthetic concentrations. As intraoperative administration of a variety of medications with NMDA receptor antagonist properties (ketamine,[29] magnesium,[30] methadone[31]) has been shown to produce postoperative opioid-sparing effect in spine surgery, nitrous oxide may have similar effects.

Regional anesthesia techniques in spine surgery

The benefits of regional anesthesia in postoperative chronic pain management

In addition to the demonstrated opioid-sparing effects and improved pain control, regional anesthesia and analgesia (collectively termed "regional anesthesia" in this chapter) can improve surgical outcomes and reduce morbidity and mortality following major surgeries in high-risk patients. Patients with preexisting chronic pain and multiple comorbidities may particularly benefit from perioperative application of regional anesthesia. For example, those with opioid dependency and a triad of morbid obesity, obstructive sleep apnea, and potentially difficult airway are prone to respiratory compromise in the postoperative setting, especially when opioid escalation is required after surgery. Regional anesthesia, using either spinal or epidural techniques, could be an excellent alternative approach in such cases and should be considered whenever applicable.[32] Although opioid-induced hyperalgesia (OIH) remains controversial in opioid-naive patients, it is well recognized in patients with chronic pain on opioid therapy.[33] Opioid-induced hyperalgesia is defined as a state of abnormal pain sensitization due to repeated administration of opioids. The mechanisms of OIH are an area of an active investigation and may involve reduced expression of opioid receptors in the spinal cord, resulting in a paradoxical response to opioids and sensitization of pro-nociceptive pathways (Table 19.1). In such patients, application of regional anesthesia may help avoid OIH and provide better control of the surgical pain superimposed on top of the chronic pain. In fact, regional anesthesia has been associated with better pain control, opioid-sparing effects, reduced costs, and improved patient satisfaction[32] (Table 19.3).

The risks of regional anesthesia

While there are case reports on regional anesthesia complications, the actual incidence of these complications is not easy to determine. Based on the limited number of cases reported and extensive clinical experiences, the complications appear to be rather rare.[32]

Infection

The incidence of infection associated with spinal anesthesia has been quoted to be as low as 1.1 in 100 000. Infections associated with neuraxial interventions are commonly related to skin and nasal microbial flora, *Staphylococcus aureus*, and *Staphylococcus epidermidis*.[34] Animals that received chronic morphine administration had a significant suppression of angiogenesis and myofibroblast recruitment, a lack of bacterial clearance, and delayed wound healing. Clinically, long-term opioid treatment resulted in a decrease of production of immunoglobulin G. Although patients with preexisting chronic pain may have impaired immune functions, partly because of chronic opioid use, the rate of infections associated with interventional pain management is very low.[35] Neuraxial blocks are considered to be contraindicated in certain categories of patients, such as intravenous drug users, because

Table 19.3 Benefits of regional anesthesia for postoperative management of chronic pain

Benefits	Comments
May provide better pain relief	Patient satisfaction is increased along with fulfillment of professional goals such as: increased satisfaction of anesthesiologists, surgeons, and nurses (increased demand to control pain in patient with preexisting chronic pain)
May promote mobilization and active engagement in physical rehabilitation therapy to improve surgical outcome	Restriction in patient mobility is a known disability factor
Is associated with opioid sparing	Important for patients with chronic pain to prevent the 2- to 4-fold increase in opioid requirements associated with treatment of perioperative pain (potential for compromise of patient safety)
May prevent development of chronic postoperative pain	Patients with preexisting pain and heightened analgesic requirements are among the factors of chronic postsurgical pain development
Prevention of opioid-induced hyperalgesia	May become a significant clinical problem in patients with preexisting chronic pain associated with opioid dose escalation (may not be relevant to opioid-naïve patients)
Decrease stress response in cancer patients	53% of patients with cancer reported preexisting pain. Decreased stress response to surgery has been intensively explored recently as a factor that may potentially prevent dissemination of cancer
Potential for reduced cognitive dysfunction associated with application of regional anesthesia compared with general anesthesia	Important for children and elderly with chronic pain as these patients are more likely to have surgery than individuals without chronic pain
Decrease surgical stress in patients with significant comorbidities (cardiovascular disease, respiratory disease, etc.)	Better acute on chronic pain control may decrease probability of catastrophic cardiovascular events and iatrogenic respiratory depression.
Regional anesthesia and children	Potential benefits in children with preexisting chronic pain are the same as in adults, but are not well described
Regional anesthesia in elderly: improved pain control without opioid-related side effects, hastening of the rehabilitation process (decreased probability of muscle mass loss, venous thromboembolism, and cutaneous pressure ulcers)	Uncontrolled pain may prove detrimental to patients with coronary artery disease, diabetes mellitus, and other comorbidities prevalent in the elderly (67% prevalence of preexisting pain in the elderly). The positive impact of regional anesthesia on morbidity and mortality after hip surgery has been demonstrated
Economic benefits associated with "fast track" surgery: less recovery time, better pain control and opioid sparing	Important for patients with chronic pain as uncontrolled acute pain is a factor of prolonged recovery and overall hospital stay. Avoiding a 2- to 4-fold increase in the opioid dose may prevent the need for telemetry/step down unit admission or other ICU admissions. May decrease the need for hospital admission or re-admission of patients with poorly controlled pain

of a high risk of complications.[36] Prophylactic use of antibiotics may allow application of regional anesthesia in immunocompromised patients with preexisting chronic pain in spine surgery. However, concerns over increased risk of infection with instrumentation among the surgical team often preclude regional anesthesia for preemptive or postoperative pain control. It is therefore good practice to discuss with the surgical team the best approach to postoperative pain management. The observation of strict aseptic precautions is mandatory for regional anesthesia techniques, regardless of whether the procedures are performed before, during, or after the surgery.

Nerve injuries and bleeding

Serious neural injuries are rare in regional anesthesia. Temporary paresthesia after a nerve block may be experienced in 10–15% patients, usually with complete resolution within one year in 99% of the patients.[37] More recent data demonstrate a significantly lower risk, less than 0.5%, of nerve injury with regional anesthesia.[38]

Spinal or epidural hematoma may appear spontaneously or as a result of regional anesthesia intervention. Generally, this complication is linked to anticoagulation treatment. The recently published guidelines are based on case reports, clinical series, pharmacology, hematology, and risk factors for surgical bleeding. They reflect the collective experience of recognized experts in neuraxial anesthesia and anticoagulation. These guidelines emphasize the importance of prevention of spinal hematoma, rapid clinical and imaging diagnosis, and prompt treatment to optimize neurologic outcomes.[39]

Complications associated with medications used in regional anesthesia

Transient neurologic symptoms (TNS) are believed to be one of the most common complications of regional anesthesia, observed in about 3% of patients after spinal anesthesia. This painful condition occurs in the immediate postoperative period in some patients with complaint of pain in the lower extremities after an initial full recovery. This complication is strongly associated with the use of lidocaine, independent of its concentration.[40] While most malpractice claims are associated with temporary injuries after regional anesthesia, the major cause of death/brain damage in these claims is associated with local anesthetic toxicity.[41] Decreased sensitivity, and even insensitivity, to certain local anesthetics is known to exist in some patients with chronic pain;[42] 7.5% of patients were hypoesthetic to mepivacaine, and an additional 3.8% to lidocaine. This phenomenon may be related to changes in sodium channels in the nerve cell membrane. This should be borne in mind when titrating regional anesthesia. Spine surgeons may request the use of a low concentration of local anesthetic in regional anesthesia to reduce the risk of masking important signs of nerve root or spinal cord injury.[43] The advantages and disadvantages of higher doses of opioids in regional anesthesia solution, or their combination with various adjuncts (for example, clonidine), are discussed later in this chapter. Complications have also occurred from accidental *intrathecal* injections of medications prepared for epidural analgesia for spine surgery. This complication is described in association with incidental lumbosacral dural sac widening (typically in children, though sometimes in adults).[44]

Regional anesthesia: intervention failure

Intervention failure of regional anesthesia may have a more profound impact on patients with a chronic pain condition. It is important to differentiate a true technical failure from ones that are "successful" but not perceived in that way by the patient with high pain sensitivity who might be uncomfortable with the regional anesthesia procedure itself. Many of the spine surgery cases may potentially be done under neuraxial anesthesia, including laminectomy for a herniated lumbar disc in levels 1 to 2, discectomy, microdiscectomy, and hemilaminectomy of up to 2 hours' duration. The level of spine surgery under spinal anesthesia should be limited to lower than T10 to minimize cardiac and respiratory effects. Spinal anesthesia may not be successful when used for spinal decompression procedures for spinal stenosis because this condition may not allow for adequate spread of the spinal anesthetic.[45] The advantages of regional anesthesia over general anesthesia are a subject of debate, but patients with preexisting chronic pain frequently have to undergo general anesthesia or require deep sedation, even after a successful neural blockade.[46] Regional anesthesia alone usually creates suboptimal operative conditions due to a higher level of anxiety and fear of worsening pain by the patient. Many anesthesiologists would administer general anesthesia to supplement regional anesthesia in order to decrease opioid requirement that may be associated with life-threatening adverse events.

Regional anesthesia techniques in spine surgery

Spinal anesthesia

Both general anesthesia and neuraxial anesthesia have been shown to be suitable techniques for patients undergoing lower thoracic and lumbar spine surgery. Spinal anesthesia is most frequently used for postoperative pain management. The administration of neuraxial anesthesia in spine surgery differs from a typical general surgical scenario in that it is usually administered by the surgeons, not the anesthesiologists. Opioids are the most commonly administered intrathecal medications in this type of surgery because local anesthetics may mask surgical complications in spine surgery. The advantages of neuraxial anesthesia are related to the fact that intrathecal and epidural doses of opioids are roughly 100 and 10 times more efficacious, respectively, than the same doses administered intravenously.[3] For example, intrathecal morphine (0.2–0.4 mg), administered intraoperatively, is a relatively safe and effective technique for postoperative pain control in spinal surgery that decreases postoperative intravenous opioid consumption.[47]

The doses of neuraxial opioids used for postoperative pain control in patients with chronic pain are 2–3 times higher than in the opioid-naive population. This is because neuraxial opioid analgesia is influenced by the downregulation of spinal opiate receptors, in contrast to local anesthetic blockade. An increased dosage of long-acting opioids for spinal anesthesia may not be safe.[48] The shorter-acting opioid fentanyl (15 μg), administered intrathecally by the surgeon before wound closure in patients undergoing posterior lumbar spine decompression, produced a significant decrease in postoperative pain scores, a significant delay of the first intravenous PCA bolus, and a close to 50% reduction of the total PCA morphine received, compared with the placebo. No patients had respiratory compromise that required treatment.[49] An increased dose of fentanyl may be anticipated in opioid-dependent patients. It is important to note that, even with a successful spinal anesthesia, the baseline opioid requirements should be maintained in opioid-dependent patients. This is because the plasma concentrations and supraspinal receptor binding may decline to a point where acute withdrawal is precipitated unless supplementary opioids are given by other than the spinal route. And, further observations will be needed to verify a safety margin of increase in opioid doses and to establish the optimal combinations of neuraxial and intravenous opioid regimens in postoperative chronic pain management after spine surgery.

The potential role of alpha-adrenergic, GABA, and other spinal receptors has been explored. Neostigmine, a cholinesterase inhibitor, has been investigated for intrathecal use as it potentiates spinal cholinergic receptors that participate in the control of somatic pain. A prospective, double-blind, randomized study found that intrathecal injection of 100 μg of hyperbaric neostigmine effectively reduced pain and postoperative opiate consumption after lumbar disc surgery.[50]

A single preoperative or intraoperative intrathecal injection that will control pain for the first 24 hours after surgery is a standard procedure.[51] Effective postoperative pain control achieved with continuous spinal analgesia, with the use of a 25G spinal catheter after extensive spinal surgery, has been reported. The risks of postdural puncture headaches, infection of the wound and/or meninges, and the optimum drug doses and combinations are yet to be determined.[52] Nonetheless, continuous epidural infusion is a relatively common approach in spine surgery.

Epidural anesthesia and analgesia

Epidural analgesia provided better postoperative pain control, reduced opioid consumption compared with patient-controlled intravenous analgesia, and decreased intravenous use of opioids as rescue analgesia in spine surgery.[53] It offered the longest duration of pain control and allowed for a quicker return to the consumption of solid foods.[51] Pain and nausea scores were significantly lower in the epidural infusion group compared with the group with hypodermic infusion of a local anesthetic. The epidural infusion did not cause any complications.[54]

Spine surgery poses certain limitations on epidural anesthesia; that has to do with the surgical sites being close to the site of epidural anesthesia. The success of epidural infusion depends on the correct placement and maintenance of the catheter in the epidural space. Various techniques, including continuous epidural analgesia through two epidural catheters, were shown to improve the reliability of pain control.[55] When continuous epidural infusion is not applicable, a single-dose epidural administration can be utilized. Epidural injection of levobupivacaine 0.25% (10 ml), 20 minutes before skin closure, led to an opioid-sparing effect of about 1/3 after a two- or three-vertebrae fusion.[56] Higher doses of local anesthetics and opioids may be used in epidural anesthesia solutions for opioid-tolerant patients. However, high doses of local anesthetics may obscure or mimic spine surgery complications and a large opioid dose almost guarantees an increased risk of opioid-associated complications.[57] Other epidural agents have also been explored; a bolus dose of clonidine in a 5 ml solution was administered (via the epidural catheter) just before surgical closure and was repeated in the recovery room. This approach resulted in an almost 50% decrease in morphine consumption, as well as a decrease in nausea, compared with PCA after the spine surgery.[44] The epidural catheter is typically inserted by the surgeon under direct vision before closing the wound. Dural tear is considered a contraindication for epidural analgesia.

Wound and perineural infiltration

Wound infiltration may be used for perioperative pain control in patients with preexisting chronic pain. Perioperative intra- and peri-facet bupivacaine infiltration effectively reduced postoperative IV PCA requirements.[58] Intraoperative bupivacaine infiltration of the nerve roots resulted in delayed requests for postoperative IV analgesia and reduced analgesic consumption, compared with the IV PCA control group.[59] Also, preemptive infiltration with levobupivacaine was superior to at-closure administration in lumbar laminectomy patients.[22] Lidocaine infiltration of the dorsal neural sheath, immediately before retraction of the root, extended the time before analgesia was requested and reduced the total analgesic consumption.[59] Both preemptive wound infiltration with levobupivacaine or bupivacaine alone, or combined with methylprednisolone provided effective pain control with reduced opioid consumption after spine surgery.[60] No complications were associated with the perioperative use of methylprednisolone or the local anesthetic. In contrast, the local administration of morphine 5 mg for analgesia, after autologous anterior or posterior iliac crest bone graft harvesting for spinal fusion, demonstrated no additional benefits.[61]

Perineural and subcutaneous catheters

Perineural catheters may prove to be a good option for patients with preexisting chronic pain. Such a technique appeared to provide effective pain control in the general patient population: compared with IV PCA, continuous infusion of 0.5% bupivacaine via an elastomeric pump into subfascial aspects of the wound resulted in 30–40% lower pain scores and about a 50% decrease in opioid demand within the first 3–4 days after posterior lumbar spine fusion.[62] Also there was a lower incidence of nausea and vomiting, a decreased number of requests for mobility, and increased functional independence. Additional benefits included early ambulation and first bowel movement, reduced IV PCA requirement, and hospital stay shortened by 2 days. No complications were associated with this technique.[63] The use of continuous local anesthetic infusion at the iliac crest site after posterior spinal arthrodesis may help in alleviating graft-related pain, even beyond the perioperative phase.[64]

Surgical techniques as a factor in postoperative chronic pain management

The choice of surgical techniques may affect postoperative chronic pain management. For example, microdiscectomy through a minimally invasive expanding retractor system and operating microscope significantly reduced analgesic requirement and length of stay, with comparable length of surgery, blood loss, complications, and outcome to a traditional open microdiscectomy.[65] Also, postsurgical analgesic consumption was significantly less when a tubular retractor was inserted via a transmuscular approach in open lumbar microdiscectomy, compared with the conventional subperiosteal approach.[66] This is because the conventional approach requires an incision of tendinous insertions of the paraspinal muscles and their retraction from the spinous process. The paravertebral muscles are rich in proprioceptors and are injured by local ischemia when retracted. There is a correlation between the denervation/retraction-ischemia of the muscles and the postoperative pain.[66] Furthermore, one study found that the number of vertebrae involved was associated with the daily IV PCA requirement.[67]

Special surgical techniques can be considered to facilitate postoperative chronic pain management. Epidural application of morphine–vaseline sterile-oil compound at the end of lumbar microdiscectomy proved to be a safe and effective measure to improve postoperative pain control and facilitate the return to normal function.[68] One study demonstrated a significant decrease in postoperative pain after an epidural application of meperidine-impregnated autologous free fat grafts at the end of lumbar disc surgery. These examples demonstrate that the surgeons are an integral part of the pain management team and they can assist with spinal, epidural, perineural, infiltrative, and other pain management techniques. Therefore, effective planning of postsurgical pain management should include the surgical factors whenever possible.

Opioids in postoperative chronic pain management

Clinical estimate of opioid dose

The number of patients with chronic pain treated with opioids has increased dramatically over the last decade, despite feeble evidence of improvement in quality of life or function.[69] Forty-one percent of patients presenting for spine surgery are opioid dependent.[1] Accordingly, the need for complex postoperative opioid management in chronic pain patients in spine surgery is increasing. Anesthesiologists frequently receive requests from spine surgeons for managing opioid-tolerant patients due to lack of responses to conventional pain management in the perioperative period.

Preoperative and intraoperative opioid dose

The morning dose of opioids should be taken on the day of spine surgery. Transdermal fentanyl patch should also be maintained. When patients did *not* take their opioids, they had to be treated with an equivalent loading dose of opioids preoperatively, either by oral medication such as morphine oral elixir (up to 2 h prior to the surgery), or by intravenous opioids during anesthesia induction. The perioperative opioid dose could be estimated by a conversion formula/table[70] (Table 19.4). (The specifics of preoperative opioid management in patients with history of substance abuse, or patients taking opioids in combination with opioid receptor antagonists, will be discussed later in this chapter.) An equivalent intravenous dose of opioid should be given intraoperatively to patients receiving opioid-based IV PCA transferred for surgery from

Table 19.4 Equianalgesic doses, half-life, and dosing intervals of commonly used opioids*

Medication	Equianalgesic dose (mg) (compared with morphine 30 mg PO) IV	Equianalgesic dose (mg) (compared with morphine 10 mg IV) Oral	Half-life (h)	Dosing interval (h) IV	Dosing interval (h) Oral
Morphine	10	30	2–3	1–2	2–4
Morphine CR	10	30	2–3	NA	8–12
Morphine SR	10	30	2–3	NA	24
Oxycodone	NA	20	2–3	NA	3–4
Oxycodone CR	NA	20	2–3	NA	12
Hydromorphone	1.5	7.5	2–3	1–2	2–4
Methadone	varies	varies	12–190	3–4	4–12
Oxymorphone	1	10	2–3	NA	2–4
Oxymorphone ER	NA	10	2–3	NA	12
Fentanyl	0.1 (single dose)	0.6	7–12	1–2	NA
Fentanyl transdermal patch 50 µg/h	30 mg IV morphine	90 mg PO morphine	16–24	NA	48–72 (transdermal)

* Various formulations are not bioequivalent. Conversion factor and potency may change during prolonged use, therefore observe cautions and decrease in the dose suggested on conversion. For example, while 1:100 ratio of morphine to fentanyl applies to an intravenous bolus, intravenous infusion of fentanyl 250 µg/h typically corresponds to 10 mg/h of intravenous morphine infusion. Methadone conversion factors vary even more. For example, while a 1:1 ratio of methadone conversion to morphine can be applied to a single dose or small doses, a 1:10 ratio may be applied for someone taking 1000 mg of morphine a day (= 100 mg of methadone only). The oral to intravenous methadone ratio is thought to be 2:1, but may vary significantly.

an outside hospital or hospice to match their baseline opioid requirement.

The baseline opioid dose should be administered *before* the initiation of either a general or a neuraxial anesthesia, or, though less preferably, during the induction of anesthesia. The opioids may be loaded either during induction, after preoxygenation, or in increments, depending on the length and extent of the operation and anesthesiologist's preferences. It is critical to closely monitor the patient's responses as opioid dose requirements may vary significantly in opioid-dependent patients.[3]

In addition to maintaining a baseline opioid dose throughout the hospitalization for spine surgery, an increased intraoperative requirement of opioids by 30–100% could be anticipated compared with opioid-naive patients, due to a downregulation of opioid receptors in opioid-dependent patients.[3] The dose escalation, however, may be avoided with an intraoperative employment of adjunctive opioid-sparing techniques. Neuraxial anesthesia performed preoperatively and utilized during the surgical procedure, for example, may negate the need for opioid dose escalation.[3,12] Chronic pain patients often experience a severe exacerbation of pain upon transitioning from short-acting intravenous opioids (such as alfentanil and remifentanil) that are commonly used in spine surgery to longer-acting oral opioids. Longer-acting intravenous opioids such as morphine or hydromorphone may be administered prior to emergence from anesthesia to alleviate the acute opioid tolerance and severe pain associated with the intraoperative use of short-acting opioids in the immediate postoperative period. However, this may not completely resolve the problem, even with maintenance of a baseline opioid dose (see Clinical Case Scenario 19.1). Alternatively, sufentanil infusion (0.01–0.1 µg/kg/min) can be administered intraoperatively. One should note that the elimination half-life of sufentanil is 164 minutes in adults.

Postoperative opioid dose

Postoperative use of opioids can be achieved by scheduled IV injection or IV PCA, as a part of the continuum of the perioperative opioid management. Both approaches appeared to be more effective than the "as needed" bolus approach in postoperative pain control in opioid-dependent patients. Early initiation of IV PCA after leaving the operating room lowers the chances of undertreatment. A basal IV PCA opioid infusion, based on the patient's preoperative baseline dose requirement, may be supplemented with or one to two PCA boluses per hour. A higher-than-normal bolus dose is usually required to compensate for opioid tolerance. The total initial IV PCA opioid dose can be up to 200–400% of the baseline dose (conventional conversion tables may be utilized).[12] However, much lower doses could be effectively used with an opioid rotation strategy.

Some prefer not to administer basal infusion via PCA because of safety concerns. This practice, however, often leads to severe postoperative pain when intraoperative anesthesia and analgesia start to wear off. Basal IV PCA infusion has proven to be helpful in improving patient experience postoperatively and should be encouraged. Intravenous PCA settings should be evaluated at least every 4–8 hours, depending on opioids, in the first 24–48 hours after surgery. The ratio of demand to actual delivery of boluses should ideally match. This ratio should not exceed 2 to 1 to avoid undertreatment of postoperative pain. The IV PCA should not be converted to oral opioid analgesia before the acceptable level of postoperative pain control is achieved. The continuing of IV PCA more than 48 hours after the surgery is not advisable, unless the patient cannot take/keep oral medications. PCA should allow titration of oral opioids with small increments until the adequate opioid dose is established. Some experts suggest continuing opioid analgesia, at doses of at least one-half of the preadmission maintenance dose, even in the case of successful continued neuraxial anesthesia.[3,12]

Preoperative opioid challenge and other tests

A variety of nociceptive stimulation methods, including heat injury, pressure algometry, and electrical stimulation, are useful in predicting the intensity of postoperative pain in opioid-naive patients. The predictive value of these tests is much higher than the analysis of demographics and psychological factors.[71] Some of these techniques may predict the probability of developing sustained postsurgical pain.[71] Estimating an effective dose of opioid in the opioid-dependent patient remains a difficult task. Opioid-dependent patients may experience severe postoperative pain and also be at the margin of opioid overdose. A preoperative infusion of fentanyl is found to be a valuable tool for individualizing postoperative chronic pain management; it does so by identifying the safe IV PCA dose while taking into account both effective

postoperative analgesia and the clinical margins of respiratory depression.[70] The test was performed in opioid-dependent patients for an elective multilevel spine fusion. A fentanyl infusion was started at 2 µg/kg/min (based on ideal body weight) and continued until the respiratory rate was <5 breaths/min. This is to define the dose–response relationship for analgesia and respiratory depression. Then pharmacokinetic simulations were used to estimate the dose of fentanyl at the time of respiratory depression and to predict the effective and safe PCA settings. The median arterial pCO_2 level was 41 mmHg (an interquartile range of 39–46 mmHg) in patients who received the postoperative IV PCA in the dose, calculated on the basis of the preoperative test.

Opioid conversion and rotation

It is recommended to continue the same dose of opioids including on the morning of the surgery.[3] However, the conversion and rotation of opioids during the hospitalization for spine surgery is almost inevitable. There are different opinions on the conversion of oral opioids to intravenous and on opioid rotation, and consensus remains to be reached.[72] Differences in the oral to intravenous dose equivalency need to be appreciated, in order to estimate perioperative baseline and supplemental opioid dose requirements. Most intravenous or intramuscular doses of opioids can be adjusted down from oral doses, because parenteral administration bypasses gastrointestinal absorption variables and first-pass hepatic clearance and metabolism. This is particularly the case with intravenous morphine and hydromorphone, which have 3 and 2 times, respectively, greater bioavailability and systemic potency than the equivalent oral doses. One exception is oxycodone and its extended-release preparations that have high oral bioavailability, more than 80% of an intravenous dose; and the baseline oral dose can be approximated by similar doses of intravenous morphine (1.0–1.5 mg oral oxycodone = 1 mg intravenous morphine).[3] Ultimately, variables of individual patients should be taken into consideration when conversion tables are applied. These variables may be pain-related, disease-related, age- and sex-related, and other medical conditions that may alter the metabolism and excretion of drugs.[72,73]

Opioid rotation means a switch from one opioid to another in an effort to improve therapeutic response or reduce side effects.[72] The specific mechanisms by which opioid rotation improves the overall response to therapy are not completely understood but may be related

Table 19.5 Potential problems associated with opioid conversion and opioid rotation

Concerns regarding clinical efficacy and safety of opioid conversion and rotation
Difficulties in prediction of pain responsiveness to postconversion opioid
Errors during conversion and rotation (dose may be miscalculated)
Not enough time provided to assess clinical efficacy before the conversion
Inadequate titration pre- and post-conversion (inadequate pain control versus safety compromise)
Pharmacodynamic and pharmacokinetic issues of conversion and rotation
Conversion of drugs with different half-lives
Safety of the postconversion equianalgesic dose may vary in patients with renal impairment
Certain drugs may impair metabolism of postconversion opioids in the liver
Polypharmacy may affect the new opioid safety after the conversion or rotation
Variable conversion coefficients may affect safety and efficacy of conversion (example: the methadone to morphine conversion may range from 1:1 to 1:10)
Conversion rules for some routes of delivery of opioid delivery systems are not well established (inhalational, intranasal, transbuccal, transdermal, rectal)
Significant difference in potency between different routes of delivery (oral morphine: intrathecal 300:1) may have an impact on patient safety

to incomplete cross-tolerance to different opioid medications that act on different types or subtypes of receptors. Opioid rotation may thus lead to a decrease in tolerance, total dose, and toxicity. For example, in addition to acting on opiate receptors, methadone is also a NMDA receptor antagonist and may be a better choice for opioid-dependent patients. A single bolus of methadone (0.2 mg/kg) before surgical incision was compared with a continuous sufentanil infusion of 0.25 µg/kg/h after a load of 0.75 µg/kg in patients undergoing complex spine surgery. Methadone reduced postoperative opioid requirement and decreased postoperative pain by approximately 50% at 48 hours compared with sufentanil (all patients were on IV PCA after the surgery).[31] While being beneficial, the conversion and rotation of opioids in the perioperative period have notable limitations and may increase the risks of medical errors significantly (Table 19.5). Future research may make opioid rotation safer and more effective in postoperative chronic pain management by revealing the weight of impact of

various factors, such as the genetic and other individual variations, in opioid rotation and conversion.

Genetic variability

Patients who report better effect of one opioid over another ("codeine doesn't work for me") should *not* be automatically categorized as "drug seekers." Genetic variations may influence individual responsiveness to pharmacotherapy of acute and chronic pain. Polymorphisms of the cytochrome P450 enzymes (CYP2D6) are found to influence the metabolism of codeine, tramadol, hydrocodone, and oxycodone. Genomic variants of these genes appeared to be associated with the side effect profiles. Other genes, such as those encoding the configuration of opioid receptors and transporters and other molecules, may become important for postoperative chronic pain management. Although pharmacogenetics, as a diagnostic tool, has the potential to improve patient therapy, well-designed studies are needed to demonstrate superiority to conventional dosing and opioid conversion approaches. This is because genetic factors are only one of many individual variables such as age, comorbidities and organ function, concomitant medications, and patient compliance.[73] Additionally, adequate postoperative chronic back pain management may be associated with inherited pain sensitivity. Recent analysis suggested that pain-relevant genetic markers, such as catechol-*O*-methyltransferase, may provide useful clinical information in terms of predicting the outcome of spine surgery for patients diagnosed with axial chronic back pain.[74] Catechol-*O*-methyltransferase is involved in central pain processing via its direct regulation of dopaminergic pathways. The genetic variation in catechol-O-methyltransferase could have an impact on pain behaviors in patients with chronic pain through the opioidergic compensatory mechanisms.[75] It may potentially also interfere with patients' response to exogenous opioids.

Transdermal and other opioid delivery systems

Opioids can be delivered by different routes and in different forms such as oral, nasal, transmucosal, inhalational, and transdermal delivery (and its variations, including iontophoretic delivery) in various immediate- and extended-release preparations.[3,12] Adverse events associated with the use of the newly developed opioid delivery systems are generally similar to those experienced by patients using traditional opioid analgesia. It is

333

important to note that newly marketed opioids often do not have names that are readily recognizable as opioids, but may represent potent or long-acting preparations that can confer a high degree of opioid tolerance and dependence.[3] Patients should be advised to maintain their preoperative delivery systems of opioid preparations. A transdermal fentanyl patch is not an exception. The date and time of fentanyl patch application should be verified and documented, and the patient should proceed to the operating room *with* the patch. If the fentanyl patch is removed, an intravenous opioid infusion (preferably fentanyl) may be initiated to maintain the baseline plasma opioid concentrations. The opioid dosing in such cases is relatively straightforward; the baseline requirement in patients with a known fentanyl patch dose may be supplied by an equivalent intravenous dose of opioids. A new patch may then be applied intra- or postoperatively. However, it may take 6–12 hours to re-establish the baseline analgesic level.[3,12] The fentanyl infusion may be gradually decreased in rate, and eventually discontinued. If IV PCA is started postoperatively, a basal infusion may not be required if the patient continues to use the same dose of transdermal fentanyl patch postoperatively. Inhalational, intranasal, buccal, or rectal opioid preparations can be used as rescue analgesics for patients whose intravenous access is lost, or when it is difficult to obtain immediately in pediatric, geriatric, agitated, and other patients.

Opioid antagonists with only peripheral action

Opioid analgesics are commonly associated with adverse effects. Constipation and ileus are among the most common and may be devastating in the acute postoperative period. Laxatives or enemas often fail to provide satisfactory relief. The newer opioid antagonists with only peripheral action may help avoid these effects without opposing the opioid analgesic effects. These opioid receptor antagonists function though ether limited systemic bioavailability or a peripherally restricted site of action (they do not the cross blood–brain barrier). Alvimopan, for instance, may shorten the postoperative ileus associated with opioid use. However, its use is recommended for only a short time because patients chronically exposed to opioids may have a significantly increased sensitivity to the blockade of peripheral mu receptors. Alvimopan is therefore contraindicated in patients taking therapeutic doses of opioids for more than 7 days. Methylnaltrexone, another peripherally acting mu-receptor antagonist,

can be effectively used subcutaneously. As the patient resumes oral intake and is getting ready for discharge, a combination of extended-release naloxone with extended-release oxycodone can be used to decrease the degree of opioid-induced motor stasis of the bowels without compromising its analgesic efficacy because there is limited systemic availability of the extended-release naloxone formulation.

Itching is another common side effect of opioids. However, specific control of opioid-induced itching by peripherally acting opioid receptor antagonists is not successful. This is probably because there is a central component in the pathogenesis of opioid-induced pruritus that is not fully understood.

Patient monitoring

Opioid-dependent patients are less susceptible to some side effects of opioids such as itching and nausea. However, respiratory depression and excessive sedation are common. Unusually large doses of opioids in nonmonitored settings are well-known triggers for situations where a rapid response has to be undertaken to save the patient's life. Morbidly obese patients, the elderly, and patients with multiple comorbidities are particularly at high risk. Close monitoring of the patients for complications such as excessive sedation and respiratory depression is mandatory when high doses of opioids are used as the primary form of analgesia for postoperative chronic pain management in opioid-dependent patients. When administering opioids to patients with end-stage organ diseases (of the kidney or liver), depending on the opioid used, monitoring is advisable. Escalating opioid doses in conjunction with increasing doses of sedatives or anxiolytics may also require patient monitoring. Even with careful monitoring, this practice can be associated with serious adverse events. Therefore, opioid-sparing strategies should be routinely employed in postoperative chronic pain management.

Nonopioid medications and supplemental strategies in postoperative chronic pain management

Nonsteroidal anti-inflammatory drugs

Unless contraindicated, patients should continue taking their nonsteroidal anti-inflammatory drugs (NSAIDs) until the surgery (including the morning dose) to reduce

Table 19.6 Adjuncts to opioids in postoperative management of chronic pain patients

Nonsteroidal anti-inflammatory drugs

Advise to continue NSAIDs until the surgery, including the morning dose of the medication, unless contraindicated or opposed by the surgeon

Continue oral or IV NSAIDs (ketorolac) after the surgery unless contraindicated or opposed by the surgeon

NSAIDs can be used along with regional anesthesia

Anti-anxiety medications

Anti-anxiety medications should be continued prior to and after the surgery

When considering clonidine or dexmedetomidine, continue the preadmission dose of benzodiazepines in the postoperative period to avoid withdrawal symptoms

Watch for excessive sedation, potentiated by an escalation in the opioid dose

Antidepressants and antipsychotics

Continue SSRIs, SNRIs, and TCAs in the perioperative period unless contraindicated

Avoid meperidine in combination with SSRIs (paroxetine, fluoxetine, sertraline, citalopram, and others) and MAOI antidepressants (phenelzin, selegiline, tranylcypromine, and others) as these combinations may cause "serotonin syndrome"

Watch for adverse effects of TCAs (sedation, delirium, or other anticholinergic effects, particularly in elderly patients)

Continue antipsychotics, monitor for signs of neuroleptic malignant syndrome in acute postoperative setting (hyperthermia, hypertonicity of skeletal muscles, fluctuating levels of consciousness and autonomic nervous system instability)

Anticonvulsants

Continue anticonvulsants if the patient takes these medications for chronic pain, neuropathy or seizure disorder and if there are no contraindications

Rapid withdrawal from anticonvulsants may trigger seizures, anxiety, and depression

Consider using gabapentin or pregabaline for preemptive analgesia

Other adjuncts to opioids in postoperative chronic pain management

Acetaminophen, PO or IV (now available in the United States)

Alpha-2-receptor agonists, clonidine and dexmedetomidine

NMDA receptor antagonists, ketamine, methadone, and potentially others

Cholinergic receptor agonists, nicotine and neostigmine

Steroids

Early rehabilitation

NSAIDs – nonsteroidal anti-inflammatory drugs; SSRIs – selective serotonin reuptake inhibitors; SNRIs – serotonin/norepinephrine reuptake inhibitors; TCAs – tricyclic antidepressants; MAOIs – monoamine oxidase inhibitors; NMDA – N-methyl-D-aspartate.

inflammatory responses to surgery and to supplement opioid analgesia. It is known that patients are frequently asked to stop NSAIDs prior to spine surgery for fear of blood loss associated with the antiplatelet effects of NSAIDs. However, this fear is not supported by the literature. In fact, there are no identifiable postoperative complications associated with the use of ketorolac in appropriate patient populations. Intravenous ketorolac seems to be a safe and effective analgesic agent following multilevel lumbar decompressive laminectomy.[76] Patients can expect significantly lower opioid requirements and better pain scores throughout the postoperative course.[76] One study demonstrated that parecoxib 40 mg reduced pain by 30% and the total amount of morphine required over 48 hours by 40%

compared with a placebo in lumbar spine surgery. The number needed to treat for at least 50% pain relief was 3.[77] Therefore, it is advised to reinstate the administration of an NSAID maintenance dose as soon as possible if it is not contraindicated by such factors as cardiovascular and kidney diseases. The same applies if neuraxial anesthesia is planned. The recently published guidelines on the application of regional anesthesia techniques confirm the previous statement that NSAIDs can be used along with regional anesthesia in patients who are on antithrombotic therapy[39] (Table 19.6).

Anxiolytic medications

About 1 in 10 patients coming in for spine surgery takes anxiolytic mediations in association with their chronic pain, though these medications are not indicated for pain treatment.[1] Nevertheless, anti-anxiety medications should be continued prior to surgery, as patients with preexisting chronic pain typically exhibit significant anxiety in association with the anticipation of worsening pain in the perioperative period. Additionally, anxiolytic medications are a routine component of various premedication protocols. A recent meta-analysis showed that clonidine is superior to benzodiazepines.[78] Even with alpha-2-agonists, such as clonidine or dexmedetomidine (used for sedation), it is imperative to continue the pre-admission dose of benzodiazepines in the postoperative period to avoid withdrawal symptoms. Patients should be watched for excessive sedation, potentiated by an escalation of opioid dose.

Antidepressants and antipsychotics

One out of 4 patients coming for spine surgery takes antidepressants.[1] Antidepressants are important elements of the multimodal treatment of chronic pain, as chronic pain patients have an increased prevalence of depression compared with the normal population. Selective serotonin reuptake inhibitors (SSRIs), serotonin/norepinephrine reuptake inhibitors (SNRIs), and tricyclic antidepressants (TCAs) are to be continued in the perioperative period. The analgesic potency has been demonstrated for TCAs, duloxetine, milnacipran, and several others that are approved for treatment of chronic neuropathic or myofascial pain. These medications, therefore, may contribute to the overall effects of postoperative chronic pain management. Meperidine should be avoided in combination with SSRIs (paroxetine, fluoxetine, sertraline, citalopram, and others), monoamine oxidase inhibitors (MAOIs), or antidepressant medications (phenelzine, selegiline, tranylcypromine, and others), as these combinations may produce somatic, autonomic, and neuropsychiatric derangements (including hyperreflexia, myoclonus, ataxia, fever, shivering, diaphoresis, diarrhea, anxiety, aviation, confusion, and others, termed "serotonin syndrome").[79] Adverse effects of TCAs are common, and patients on TCAs should be re-evaluated if there is evidence of sedation and delirium, or other anticholinergic effects, particularly in elderly patients. Cardiovascular risks with regular doses of TCAs are extremely low. The TCAs should be continued in the perioperative period with a regular dosage.

It is also recommended that antipsychotics be continued perioperatively.[80] Nonetheless, it has to be kept in mind that fewer than 1% of all patients treated with antipsychotic drugs may develop a neuroleptic malignant syndrome presented as hyperthermia, hypertonicity of skeletal muscles, fluctuating levels of consciousness, and autonomic nervous system instability. Therefore, close monitoring of patients taking antipsychotics in the perioperative period is advisable.

Anticonvulsants

Anticonvulsants are commonly used to treat chronic neuropathic pain. Analgesic, anxiolytic activity, relatively benign side effects, and minimal interactions of gabapentin with other medications made it part of the multimodal perioperative analgesic regimens in some spine surgery protocols.[81] Pregabalin is frequently reported to be a part of the preemptive or postoperative analgesia regimens as well. If the patient takes these medications or any other anticonvulsants for chronic pain or seizure disorder preoperatively and there are no contraindications, they should also be continued. Rapid withdrawal from anticonvulsant drugs may trigger seizures, anxiety, and depression. Patients who started on gabapentin and some other newer anticonvulsants in the perioperative period should be advised about potential side effects, including increased suicidal risks in younger and older patients, patients with mood disorders, and patients with epilepsy or seizures.[82]

Other adjuncts to opioids in postoperative chronic pain management

Acetaminophen

Acetaminophen, the active metabolite of phenacetin, has been used in medicine since 1893. The mechanism of action of this drug remains a subject of debate. It appears to function as a reversible inhibitor of cyclooxygenase (participating in prostaglandin synthesis), and is believed to inhibit synthesis of various chemical mediators in the central neural system that participate in sensitization to pain. Oral acetaminophen is commonly used as an adjunct to opioids in the perioperative period (example: 1 g before and after spine surgery).[42] Intravenous acetaminophen preparations (available in many countries, and now approved by the FDA) combined with opioids showed a higher analgesic effect than opioids acting alone.[83] Patients who received a perioperative multimodal regimen including acetaminophen had significant reduction in opioid consumption, pain scores, nausea, and drowsiness. Patients also experienced less pain interference with walking, coughing, and deep breathing compared with opioid-only IV PCA after spine surgery.[81] This adjunct should be cautiously used in patients with a history of alcohol abuse as these patients have lower threshold for hepatotoxicity or nephrotoxicity secondary to depletion of glutathione associated with the accumulation of metabolites of acetaminophen.

Alpha-2-receptor agonists, clonidine and dexmedetomidine

Clonidine, an alpha-2-adrenoreceptor and imidazoline receptor agonist, can be administered orally, intravenously, or as a transdermal patch (0.1–0.3 mg/day). It can provide effective supplementation in analgesia and sedation if it is used intraoperatively (minimum alveolar anesthetic concentration sparing). Additionally, it is an effective epidural agent in spine surgery. Clonidine at 1.5 μg/kg repeated twice via epidural catheter was found to be effective in opioid sparing. This study was inspired by the desire to avoid masking of important signs of nerve root or spinal cord injury with the application of local anesthetic-based epidural analgesia postoperatively in spine surgery.[42]

There is evidence that a postoperative infusion of dexmedetomidine, another alpha-2 agonist, at 0.4 μg/kg/h for 24 h as an adjunct to morphine-based IV PCA could have a morphine-sparing effect, reducing about 1/3 of the total PCA dose. The increase in morphine use on postoperative day 2 was avoided after dexmedetomidine infusion.[84] While patients receiving alpha-2-agonists have to be watched for the potential side effects (most commonly hypotension), the overall frequency of all perioperative complications is thought to be lower than with opioid-only analgesia.[84]

Ketamine and other NMDA receptor antagonists

The state of hyperalgesia, associated with chronic opioid use and with chronic pain disorder itself, appeared to be a major barrier for adequate postoperative chronic pain management. NMDA receptors have been indicated in the mechanisms of hyperalgesia. Ketamine is a well-known anesthetic drug that is commonly used postoperatively in sub-anesthetic doses. It has been shown to produce an opioid-sparing effect in spine surgery and an antihyperalgesic effect due to its NMDA receptor antagonistic property. A loading dose 1 mg/kg followed by 50–100 μg/kg/h ketamine infusion improved the analgesic effects of opioid-based IV PCA opioids after cervical surgery.[29] Nurses reported that is easier to take care of the opioid-tolerant chronic

pain patient postoperatively if the patient is on a low-dose ketamine infusion.[32]

Ketamine may produce side effects such as changes in mental status and sympathetic stimulation if there is no dedicated intravenous line for the infusion and if a high plasma concentration of the ketamine is produced by the boluses of other perioperative medications pushed through the same IV line.[85] Therefore, when ketamine is used as an adjunct for postoperative pain control, it is recommended to have a dedicated IV line for ketamine to avoid high plasma concentration. Even low-dose ketamine infusion should be used cautiously in patients with advanced cardiovascular conditions.[86] Some of the side effects of ketamine (tachycardia and hypertension) can be utilized intraoperatively to compensate for the intraoperative remifentanil side effects, such as bradycardia and hypotension (300–400 μg/kg/h). The *postoperative* analgesic requirements were also decreased with this regimen.[87] Indeed, intraoperative ketamine reduced perioperative opioid consumption at 24 and 48 hours after the spine surgery in opioid-dependent patients. Intravenous ketamine, 0.5 mg/kg on induction of anesthesia followed by a continuous infusion at 10 μg/kg/min, is usually terminated at wound closure in opioid-dependent chronic back pain patients. Interestingly, the patients who had received ketamine intraoperatively had better chronic back pain control for as long as 6 weeks after the surgery.

Intravenous magnesium and methadone are other drugs known to act as NMDA receptor antagonists and indeed are associated with better perioperative pain control.[30,31] The role in postoperative pain management of nitrous oxide, a commonly used anesthetic gas with recently discovered NMDA antagonistic properties, is to be explored.

Cholinergic receptor agonists, nicotine and neostigmine

There is evidence that cholinergic receptors may be involved in the intrinsic regulation of mediators of pain.[88] Chronic consumption of nicotine, a cholinergic agonist, is associated with a higher prevalence of chronic lower back pain.[89] The nicotine patch should be applied (if not contraindicated) in postoperative chronic pain management to prevent nicotine withdrawal, which may potentially worsen perioperative pain. Nicotine patches were actually found to be an effective adjunct to opioid analgesics in *nonsmokers* in postoperative pain management.[88] The analgesic properties of nicotine were explained by a variety of mechanisms, including central nervous system stimulation and increase of dopamine in the mesolimbic system, activation of alpha-2 adrenergic receptor in a way similar to clonidine, and induction of β-endorphin and enkephalins, which are endogenous analgesic molecules. Morphine and other opioids produce analgesia, in part, by releasing acetylcholine and stimulating acetylcholine receptors. Nicotine stimulates the same receptors.[88] Neostigmine, an acetylcholine esterase inhibitor that prolongs the action of acetylcholine, was found to be an effective adjunct to opioid-based analgesia when 100 µg of neostigmine methylsulfate was administered intrathecally at the end of lumbar disc surgery.[50]

Steroids

The anti-inflammatory properties of corticosteroids, frequently employed in the management of acute and chronic radiculitis, can potentially be employed in postoperative chronic pain management. Steroids or placebos were locally applied to the affected nerve roots in a double-blind study in patients undergoing discectomy, decompression, and/or spinal fusion. Peridural administration of methylprednisolone along with wound infiltration with bupivacaine provided a significant opioid-sparing effect immediately after posterior lumbosacral spine surgery.[60] The study design, however, did not allow verification of the opioid-sparing effects of steroids alone. There are concerns over the potentially increased risks of infections associated with perioperative corticosteroid use, even though no complications were observed in this particular study.

Early rehabilitation

The early postoperative period was suggested to be the best timing of therapeutic intervention targeted at facilitating and reinforcing the acquisition of correct motor patterns in spine surgery.[90] Early postoperative rehabilitation, while having a positive impact on outcomes, may worsen chronic pain and thus decrease patient satisfaction after the spine surgery. Therefore, early rehabilitation should be applied as a part of intensive multimodal postoperative chronic pain management. This approach, employed in patients with degenerative disc disease, demonstrated that patients may reach the recovery twice as fast as with conventional management.[16] The program included prehabilitation, self-administered epidural analgesia, and intensified mobilization and protein supplements. In addition to a shortened hospital stay (from 7 days to 5 days) the early rehabilitation program was associated

with significantly higher patient satisfaction, most likely because their postoperative pain was well controlled during the mobilization exercises.[16] Various other rehabilitation modalities can potentially be applied. An example is postoperative TENS therapy, that may reduce the postoperative demand for analgesics in major spinal surgery. It was found to be a safe and simple way, which is free of systemic side effects, to improve postoperative pain control in patients undergoing spine surgery.[23] Despite reasonable outlook, cognitive intervention (preoperative relaxation) for postoperative pain in patients undergoing lumbar and cervical spine surgery had completely unexpected results: it failed to demonstrate a measurable decrease in pain and narcotic demand postoperatively.[24]

Postoperative chronic pain management in special categories of patients

The elderly and children

As the postoperative chronic pain management in the pediatric population is discussed elsewhere in this book (see Chapter 25), we focus on the elderly here. There are an increasing number of surgical procedures on the elderly, commonly defined as 65 years and older. Surgical treatment of spinal stenosis, severe scoliosis, discs and vertebrae, and other conditions, is performed in order to improve the functional status and the quality of life. There is a high prevalence of chronic pain in the elderly presenting for spine surgery. The pain of these patients also tends to be under-assessed and under-treated. While recognizing that postoperative pain in the elderly has a negative impact on clinical and economic outcomes, aggressive pain control in this patient population is uniquely challenging. A decline in hearing and cognitive function, language barriers, and common myths about "getting addicted" may create significant obstacles in communication with these patients. Furthermore, decreased physiologic reserves increase their risk for perioperative complications, associated with autonomic and immune disregulation secondary to surgical stress and medication management. Polypharmacy is common in the elderly because they commonly have multiple medical conditions; often, this justifies the simultaneous administration of multiple medications. Polypharmacy, however, provokes drug interactions that may have a significant impact on pain management, leading to changes in efficacy, tolerability, and toxicity of analgesics and causing difficulties for both the physicians and the patients. The glomerular filtration rate and the overall kidney function commonly decline with aging, compromising the safety of the elderly taking NSAIDs, opioids, and other pain medications. The elderly have a higher prevalence of cardiovascular, cerebrovascular, respiratory, endocrine, and other diseases that makes them more susceptible to respiratory depression, bradycardia, and hypotension. Constipation, a relatively benign side effect of opioids in healthy adults, may quickly become a life-threatening postoperative situation in the elderly. Additionally, their response to general anesthesia and the drugs used in neuraxial anesthesia can be altered. Postoperative delirium in the elderly is a significant medical condition often associated with a prolonged hospital stay, an increased risk of early and long-term mortality, increased physical dependence, and increased rates of nursing home placement. Careful assessment, however, may reveal a completely different list of causes: it could potentially be the result of a pain medication overdose or due to inadequately treated pain. Thoughtful drug selection, appropriate education of physicians and nurses, effective communication, and family involvement early on may help prevent problems associated with postoperative chronic pain management in the elderly after spine surgery.

History of substance abuse

Managing postoperative chronic pain in patients who have a history of substance abuse is particularly difficult. It is challenging to identify the patients. "Drug user," for example, is a highly sensitive label, with an enormous social stigmatization. This label, if documented in the chart, may place the patient in a position where hospital bills for spine surgery may be turned down by the insurance company, and become the responsibility of the patient. It is not surprising that patients do not want to share this type of information about substance abuse, and so an acceptable degree of confidentiality and privacy should be allowed (Table 19.7). The patient should also be informed that the information regarding substance abuse is important only for clinical safety reasons. One patient, for example, reported that he "did drugs" when he was a kid when substance abuse was suspected. After a discussion on the importance of knowing the details of substance abuse to allow for a better management of postoperative pain, the patient reported that his mother (who lives with this patient)

used "drugs" to treat her headaches, and he tried them too. After repeated questioning about "when was the last time that you treated your pain with "drugs?" the patient replied "last Monday," which was 2 days prior to the evaluation. It is well presented in literature that patients highly addicted to opioids tend to deny it or report lower amounts of drug consumed. Clues to potential substance abuse include general appearance and manners of communication of the patient, relevant notes in the medical records, including history of substance abuse, abnormal laboratory drug screen, repeated early refills, rapid escalation of the opioid dose out of proportion to change in the linical picture, multiple telephone encounters with requests to increase the dose of opioids, prescription problems (lost or stolen medications or prescriptions, etc.), multiple emergency room visits for pain-related issues, and opioid prescription reports demonstrating multiple sourcing. Physical examination findings may demonstrate numerous skin needle marks, skin abscesses, or poor peripheral vein access (because of disseminated superficial vein thrombosis).

Patients who present to the anesthesiologist as "drug seeking," should not automatically be assumed to be "drug abusers." There are multiple and delicate variations in terms used to characterize patients who press unwavering pain medications requests as described earlier. (Table 19.1) The classification of "drug abuser" can only be applied when the patient's pain is adequately controlled, which is a very difficult task. Multimodal approaches may make this task easier. These approaches may be useful, moreover, because drug users commonly present to surgery with multiple comorbidities such as viral or alcohol-related liver disease, HIV, lung disease (as smoking is common in this patient population), encephalopathy, and psychiatric comorbidities. It is of critical importance *not* to attempt detoxification in the perioperative period. The maintenance of the baseline level of opioids is critically important. The intravenous baseline maintenance dose of methadone is typically one-half of the oral methadone dose taken by patients who are participating in outpatient substance-abuse management programs. Participation in these programs, and the methadone dose, should be verified for patient safety reasons. Recovering opioid abusers maintained on buprenorphine may continue on this medication in the IV form for postoperative pain control. If the quality of analgesia provided by buprenorphine is inadequate, supplementation with methadone and morphine can be considered.[3] Of note,

Table 19.7 Postoperative management of pain in patients with history of substance abuse

Identification of patient with history of substance abuse

Discuss privacy, confidentiality, and autonomy

Pay attention to the general appearance and manner of communication

Check for relevant notes in the medical records, including history of abuse, abnormal laboratory drugs screen, repeated early refill, rapid escalation of opioid dose out of proportion to change in clinical picture, multiple telephone encounters with request to increase the dose of opioids, prescription problems (lost or stolen medications or prescriptions, etc.), multiple emergency room visits for pain-related issues

Check, if available, for state or federal opioid prescription reports, demonstrating multiple sourcing

Physical examination data (skin appearing to have numerous needle marks, skin abscesses, poor peripheral vein access because of disseminated superficial vein thrombosis), and others

Repeat laboratory drug screen, pain medications panel

Inform patient that addiction history will not prevent adequate postoperative pain management

Differentiate various types of conditions associated with substance use disorder

"Drug-seeking" patient should not be automatically assumed be "drug user"

Differentiate "addiction" and "pseudo-addiction," "opioid tolerance" and pseudo-opioid tolerance," opioid-induced hyperalgesia," "physical dependence" and "psychological dependence," and other various conditions with substance use disorder

"Drug seeking" and other related terms can be only be applied when the patient's pain is adequately controlled

Maintain baseline opioid dose

Do not attempt detoxification for *any* patient, whether abusing opioids, or taking prescribed opioids

Maintain the baseline level of opioids

Keep in mind that patients may under-report or over-report the opioid doses

Management of patients participating in substance abuse maintenance programs

Verify participation in these programs, and the methadone or buprenorphine doses, for patient safety reasons

The intravenous baseline maintenance dose of methadone is typically one-half the oral methadone dose that is taken by patients who are participating in these programs

Recovering opioid abusers maintained on buprenorphine may continue on this medication in the IV form for postoperative pain control (unless the quality of analgesia provided by buprenorphine is inadequate, supplementation with methadone and morphine may be considered)

Management of patients treated with combined agonist–antagonist agents preoperatively

Combined formulations of opioids and opioid antagonists, including naloxone, should not be used for opioid-dependent patients because postoperative administration may produce withdrawal symptoms

Naltrexone, a long-acting oral opioid antagonist, sometimes used in recovering opioid abusers, should also be discontinued at least 24 h prior to surgery

Use of mixed opioid agonist–antagonist drugs postoperatively

Inform the surgical team that mixed agonist–antagonist opioids should not be used in substance abusers or opioid-dependent patients (such agents as nalbuphine, butorphanol, pentazocine, tramadol, and others)

Consider multimodal regimens but watch for comorbidities

Multimodal approaches may be useful to spare opioids

Consider multiple comorbidities commonly accompanying substance abuse states, including: viral or alcohol-related liver disease, HIV, lung disease (as smoking is common in this patient population), encephalopathy, psychiatric comorbidities, and others

Substances other than opioids

Substances other than opioids may complicate the postoperative chronic pain management

Watch for alcohol abuse and withdrawal

Nicotine patches should invariably be applied to smokers to prevent withdrawal and potentially improve their perception of recovery after surgery

Management of substance use at the time of discharge

Health care providers should address substance abuse issues in a conventional way when the patient is stable and the pain is tolerable

Standard pathways and recovery options should be offered to patients with history of substance abuse, including alcohol and nicotine

Table 19.7 (*cont.*)

Patients suffering from tobacco use disorder should be informed about tight association between chronic nicotine use and chronic back pain

The primary care provider and/or the addiction treatment maintenance program and/or the physician prescribing any opioids and benzodiazepines should be informed about medications given to the patient during hospitalization, because these may show up on routine urine drug screening, and about the doses of these medications to provide effective continuous care

buprenorphine may be the best choice for a hemodialysis patient who needs an opioid, because this medication is not cleared by the hemodialysis, which allows for smooth dose adjustments. However, it may be inappropriately avoided because of stigmata related to its association with substance abuse treatment.

Combined formulations of opioids and opioid antagonists, including naloxone and naltrexone, are gaining popularity in chronic opioid management. However, they should not be used for opioid-dependent patients, because postoperative administration may produce withdrawal symptoms. Naltrexone, a long-acting oral opioid antagonist (sometimes used in recovering opioid abusers), should also be discontinued at least 24 hours prior to surgery.[3]

Mixed agonist/antagonist opioids should not be used either for substance abusers or for opioid-dependent patients. The agents nalbuphine, butorphanol, and pentazocine are commonly used as part of postoperative protocols to decrease the intensity of some side effects of neuraxial opioids such as pruritus and nausea, or just independently. However, these agents can possibly exacerbate pain significantly in patients who receive chronic maintenance opioids, and may even hasten withdrawal. Similar symptoms have been reported in highly dependent patients who were treated with tramadol.[91]

There is a tendency to limit the opioid use or circumvent the use of PCA in substance abusers. These patients should be treated the same way as opioid-dependent patients, and should be provided with adequate opioid coverage in order to overcome opioid tolerance. Avoiding IV PCA for patients with a known history of substance abuse because of the risk of excessive self-administration of opioids is likely unjustified.

Substances other than opioids may complicate postoperative chronic pain management. If a risk of delirium tremens in the 2–4 days after spine surgery is present, some programs would allow the prescription of oral light drinks containing alcohol. Nicotine patches should invariably be applied to smokers to prevent withdrawal, and potentially improve their discomfort perception in the acute postoperative period. None of this information means that health care providers should simply give up and "let the problem be." The substance abuse issues should be addressed in a conventional way when the patient is stable and the pain is tolerable.

Depression and/or anxiety

The presence of depression and/or anxiety has time and again been reported in patients presenting for spine surgery.[1] Spine surgery patients are at a higher risk of suffering from depression and anxiety than the general population. It is known that the rates of depression and anxiety in patients who undergo surgery for a herniated disc are up to 50% before, and rise to 80% after spine surgery. The outcomes of spine surgery, disability, pain experience, behavioral problems, and opioid abuse are critical parameters found to be dependent on the presence of depression and anxiety.[47] While recognizing a link between postoperative chronic pain management and issues related to depression and anxiety, the data on how to manage this association best are still being explored in order to improve postoperative outcomes in patients undergoing spinal surgery. The literature recommends that clinicians be more sensitive to the psychological concerns in patients undergoing spine surgery. Brief psychological screening and, if needed, comprehensive assessment and assistance from mental health professionals should be considered in order to improve the chronic pain patient's experience and that of his/her family during the acute postoperative period.

Implanted pain and spasticity management devices

Spinal cord stimulators, peripheral nerve stimulators, and intrathecal pumps are generally (if they are not explanted before or during spine surgery) maintained in the postoperative period, with parameters kept at a baseline level. It is advised to discontinue/reduce the intrathecal infusion of baclofen during the immediate perioperative period, because the central effects and peripheral skeletal muscle-relaxing effects of this agent may enhance neuromuscular blockade and increase the chance of hypotension and excessive sedation. However,

341

this matter should be managed in consultation with the neurological or other related services to ensure the safety of the patients. Because of the increased number of patients with scoliosis, central or spinal spasticity, and a variety of CNS conditions receiving intrathecal baclofen and requiring spine surgery, anesthesiologists should be aware of baclofen withdrawal symptomatology, particularly where signs and symptoms may be difficult to interpret due to patient population characteristics.[92] Return of baseline level of spasticity and pain associated with spasticity, pruritus, anxiety, and change in mental status may herald the intrathecal baclofen withdrawal syndrome. Hyperthermia, myoclonus, seizures, rhabdomyolysis, disseminated intravascular coagulation, multisystem organ failure, cardiac arrest, or coma have been reported as well. In addition to conventional symptomatic and oral baclofen management, a temporary intrathecal catheter can be placed if needed for prevention of deterioration secondary to intrathecal baclofen withdrawal syndrome.[93]

Chronic pain related to primary localization other than the spine

Special precautions should be taken for patients with a history of complex regional pain syndrome, who present for spine surgery. Patients with this condition may report a worsening of their symptoms after a major stress (a certain attribute of spine surgery). Continuous peripheral nerve block or a tunneled epidural catheter can be used after consultation with the spine surgeon to improve the patient's experience.

Patients with migraines should continue their preventive regimens preoperatively (these are typically anticonvulsants, antidepressants, beta-blockers, magnesium, and other medications). They may experience a worsening of their headaches after being exposed to opioids postoperatively. Multimodal techniques should be adequately utilized in the care of these patients. NSAIDs, triptans, and other headache-abortive medications, may be given postoperatively (if needed, and if not contraindicated).

Summary

Postoperative management of patients with preexisting chronic pain is challenging because opioid dose escalation needed for adequate pain control can compromise patient safety. The increased availability of nonopioid analgesics, adjuncts, and regional techniques brings up new opportunities for improving the experience of chronic pain patients after spine surgery.

These techniques are summarized in Table 19.6. The practical points in the management of opioid-dependent patients and substance abusers are summarized in Tables 19.1, 19.6, and 19.7. These patients, if indicated, should be scheduled for a follow-up visit to the pain management specialists or, even better, to be evaluated in a multidisciplinary chronic pain rehabilitation program, after being discharged from the hospital.

Clinical case scenario 19.1

Preoperative course

A 39-year-old woman with chronic neck pain secondary to C5–C6 spinal stenosis presented for elective anterior cervical discectomy with fusion. Her preadmission medications included venlafaxine, omeprazole, zolpidem, and alprazolam. In addition, she was taking extended-release oxycodone (OxyContin; 10 mg three times a day) and a combination of oxycodone and acetaminophen (Percocet; 5/325 mg three to four times a day) for breakthrough pain.

Intraoperative management

Induction was with propofol (200 mg) and fentanyl (250 μg) following premedication with midazolam (2 mg). Maintenance of anesthesia was provided by infusions of remifentanil (0.1 μg/kg/min) and (propofol 100 μg/kg/min). Long-acting opioids were not used during the procedure. The intraoperative course was uneventful.

Postoperative course

Upon arrival at the postanesthesia care unit the patient complained of intolerable pain in a very disruptive manner. Her extreme discomfort was difficult to control with intravenous administration of hydromorphone (3.6 mg), fentanyl (100 μg), and lorazepam (2 mg). After approximately 45 minutes she noted reduction in pain intensity from 10 to 5 on a ten-point verbal pain scale (VPS). Following this she was attached to an intravenous patient-controlled analgesia (PCA) pump programmed to administer hydromorphone on demand (0.4 mg every 6 min). Following discharge to the surgical care unit, her pain was effectively controlled with the hydromorphone PCA, totaling 4.5 mg overnight.

On rounds the following morning, her VPS was between 3 and 5 on a ten-point scale, equivalent to her preadmission pain scores. She reported satisfaction with the anesthetic and postoperative care that she received. Oral oxycodone and acetaminophen were started, and she was discharged home in the morning of postoperative day 2 with her pain being adequately controlled with her preadmission medications in the same preadmission doses.

Discussion

The magnitude of this patient's immediate discomfort and the amount of opioids required to control her pain suggest that remifentanil may induce significant opioid-induced hyperalgesia (OIH) and acute opioid tolerance (AOT), and probably should not be used in opioid-dependent patients. The pain management physicians and the supporting staff were also affected by this incident as evidenced by the increased time commitment in attempting to manage a screaming patient, and trying to explain to the patient and family why this incident occurred.

A similar case report indicated acute tolerance and OIH after intraoperative remifentanil infusion in a patient treated with fentanyl patch. In the discussion that followed, acute opioid withdrawal was suspected in this patient. As a result, there was a suggestion to use morphine to prevent this. It is not uncommon to use a long-acting opioid along with remifentanil to reduce AOT and OIH effects. However, the available data suggest that concomitant use of morphine does not prevent OIH. Recent psychological studies help to better understand the acute tolerance and OIH with remifentanil in opioid-dependent patients. It was demonstrated that remifentanil can induce acute dysphoria irrespective of its analgesic properties. Initially promising perioperative use of NMDA receptor antagonists, ketamine, tramadol, other opioids, and anti-inflammatory drugs failed to adequately reduce patients' discomfort. In light of these distressing cases we suggest using alternatives to intraoperative remifentanil in opioid-dependent patients.

References

1. Walid MS, Robinson JS 3rd, Robinson ER, *et al.* Comparison of outpatient and inpatient spine surgery patients with regards to obesity, comorbidities and readmission for infection. *J Clin Neurosci* 2010; 17(12): 1497–8.

2. Ip HY, Abrishami A, Peng PW, Wong J, Chung F. Predictors of postoperative pain and analgesic consumption: a qualitative systematic review. *Anesthesiology* 2009; 111(3): 657–77.

3. Mitra S, Sinatra RS. Perioperative management of acute pain in the opioid-dependent patient. *Anesthesiology* 2004; 101(1): 212–27.

4. Practice guidelines for chronic pain management: an updated report by the American Society of Anesthesiologists Task Force on Chronic Pain Management and the American Society of Regional Anesthesia and Pain Medicine. *Anesthesiology* 2010; 112(4): 810–33.

5. Vadivelu N, Mitra S, Narayan D. Recent advances in postoperative pain management. *Yale J Biol Med* 2010; 83(1): 11–25.

6. White PF, Kehlet H. Improving postoperative pain management: what are the unresolved issues? *Anesthesiology* 2010; 112(1): 220–5.

7. Bentsen SB, Rustoen T, Wahl AK, Miaskowski C. The pain experience and future expectations of chronic low back pain patients following spinal fusion. *J Clin Nurs* 2008; 17(7B): 153–9.

8. Alford DP, Compton P, Samet JH. Acute pain management for patients receiving maintenance methadone or buprenorphine therapy. *Ann Intern Med* 2006; 144(2): 127–34.

9. Murnion BP, Gnjidic D, Hilmer SN. Prescription and administration of opioids to hospital in-patients, and barriers to effective use. *Pain Med* 2010; 11(1): 58–66.

10. Bell K, Salmon A. Pain, physical dependence and pseudoaddiction: redefining addiction for 'nice' people? *Int J Drug Policy*. 2009; 20(2): 170–8.

11. Green CR, Hart-Johnson T. The adequacy of chronic pain management prior to presenting at a tertiary care pain center: the role of patient socio-demographic characteristics. *J Pain* 2010; 11(8): 746–54.

12. Kopf A, Banzhaf A, Stein C. Perioperative management of the chronic pain patient. *Best Pract Res Clin Anaesthesiol* 2005; 19(1): 59–76.

13. Carroll IR, Angst MS, Clark JD. Management of perioperative pain in patients chronically consuming opioids. *Reg Anesth Pain Med* 2004; 29(6): 576–91.

14. Tracey I, Bushnell MC. How neuroimaging studies have challenged us to rethink: is chronic pain a disease? *J Pain* 2009; 10(11): 1113–20.

15. Jlala HA, French JL, Foxall GL, Hardman JG, Bedforth NM. Effect of preoperative multimedia information on perioperative anxiety in patients undergoing procedures under regional anaesthesia. *Br J Anaesth* 2010; 104(3): 369–74.

16. Nielsen PR, Jorgensen LD, Dahl B, Pedersen T, Tonnesen H. Prehabilitation and early rehabilitation after spinal surgery: randomized clinical trial. *Clin Rehabil* 2010; 24(2): 137–48.

17. Campiglia L, Consales G, De Gaudio AR. Pre-emptive analgesia for postoperative pain control: a review. *Clin Drug Invest* 2010; 30 Suppl 2: 15–26.

18. Ong CK, Lirk P, Seymour RA, Jenkins BJ. The efficacy of preemptive analgesia for acute postoperative pain

management: a meta-analysis. *Anesth Analg* 2005; **100**(3): 757–73.

19. Pandey CK, Navkar DV, Giri PJ, *et al.* Evaluation of the optimal preemptive dose of gabapentin for postoperative pain relief after lumbar diskectomy: a randomized, double-blind, placebo-controlled study. *J Neurosurg Anesthesiol* 2005; **17**(2): 65–8.

20. Van Elstraete AC, Tirault M, Lebrun T, *et al.* The median effective dose of preemptive gabapentin on postoperative morphine consumption after posterior lumbar spinal fusion. *Anesth Analg* 2008; **106**(1): 305–8.

21. Burke SM, Shorten GD. Perioperative pregabalin improves pain and functional outcomes 3 months after lumbar discectomy. *Anesth Analg* 2010; **110**(4): 1180–5.

22. Gurbet A, Bekar A, Bilgin H, *et al.* Pre-emptive infiltration of levobupivacaine is superior to at-closure administration in lumbar laminectomy patients. *Eur Spine J* 2008; **17**(9): 1237–41.

23. Unterrainer AF, Friedrich C, Krenn MH, *et al.* Postoperative and preincisional electrical nerve stimulation TENS reduce postoperative opioid requirement after major spinal surgery. *J Neurosurg Anesthesiol* 2010; **22**(1): 1–5.

24. Gavin M, Litt M, Khan A, Onyiuke H, Kozol R. A prospective, randomized trial of cognitive intervention for postoperative pain. *Am Surg* 2006; **72**(5): 414–18.

25. Hay JL, White JM, Bochner F, Somogyi AA. Antinociceptive effects of high-dose remifentanil in male methadone-maintained patients. *Eur J Pain* 2008; **12**(7): 926–33.

26. Angst MS, Chu LF, Tingle MS, *et al.* No evidence for the development of acute tolerance to analgesic, respiratory depressant and sedative opioid effects in humans. *Pain* 2009; **142**(1–2): 17–26.

27. Tan T, Bhinder R, Carey M, Briggs L. Day-surgery patients anesthetized with propofol have less postoperative pain than those anesthetized with sevoflurane. *Anesth Analg* 2010; **111**(1): 83–5.

28. Leonova M. Souzdalnitski D. Patient satisfaction is higher with TIVA than with inhalational anesthesia for ambulatory surgery. 2010. http://www.asaabstracts.com (accessed November 30, 2010).

29. Yamauchi M, Asano M, Watanabe M, *et al.* Continuous low-dose ketamine improves the analgesic effects of fentanyl patient-controlled analgesia after cervical spine surgery. *Anesth Analg* 2008; **107**(3): 1041–4.

30. Oguzhan N, Gunday I, Turan A. Effect of magnesium sulfate infusion on sevoflurane consumption, hemodynamics, and perioperative opioid consumption in lumbar disc surgery. *J Opioid Manag* 2008; **4**(2): 105–10.

31. Gottschalk A, Durieux ME, Nemergut EC. Intraoperative methadone improves postoperative pain

32. Souzdalnitski D, Halaszynski TM, Faclier G. Regional anesthesia and co-existing chronic pain. *Curr Opin Anaesthesiol* 2010; **23**(5): 662–70.

33. Bekhit MH. Opioid-induced hyperalgesia and tolerance. *Am J Ther* 2010; **17**(5): 498–510.

34. Pradilla G, Ardila GP, Hsu W, Rigamonti D. Epidural abscesses of the CNS. *Lancet Neurol* 2009; **8**(3): 292–300.

35. Kapoor SG, Huff J, Cohen SP. Systematic review of the incidence of discitis after cervical discography. *Spine J.* 2010; **10**(8): 739–45.

36. Gomar C, Luis M, Nalda MA. Sacro-iliitis in a heroin addict. A contra-indication to spinal anaesthesia. *Anaesthesia* 1984; **39**(2): 167–70.

37. Weeks L, Barry A, Wolff T, Firrell J, Scheker L. Regional anaesthesia and subsequent long-term pain. *J Hand Surg Br* 1994; **19**(3): 342–6.

38. Sorenson EJ. Neurological injuries associated with regional anesthesia. *Reg Anesth Pain Med.* 2008; **33**(5): 442–8.

39. Horlocker TT, Wedel DJ, Rowlingson JC, *et al.* Regional anesthesia in the patient receiving antithrombotic or thrombolytic therapy: American Society of Regional Anesthesia and Pain Medicine Evidence-Based Guidelines (Third Edition). *Reg Anesth Pain Med* 2010; **35**(1): 64–101.

40. Zaric D, Pace NL. Transient neurologic symptoms (TNS) following spinal anaesthesia with lidocaine versus other local anaesthetics. *Cochrane Database Syst Rev* 2009; (2): CD003006.

41. Neal JM, Bernards CM, Butterworth JF 4th, *et al.* ASRA practice advisory on local anesthetic systemic toxicity. *Reg Anesth Pain Med* 2010; **35**(2): 152–61.

42. Trescot AM. Local anesthetic "resistance." *Pain Physician* 2003; **6**(3): 291–3.

43. Farmery AD, Wilson-MacDonald J. The analgesic effect of epidural clonidine after spinal surgery: a randomized placebo-controlled trial. *Anesth Analg* 2009; **108**(2): 631–4.

44. Kanna PR, Sekar C, Shetty AP, Rajasekaran S. Transient paraplegia due to accidental intrathecal bupivacaine infiltration following pre-emptive analgesia in a patient with missed sacral dural ectasia. *Spine (Phila Pa 1976)* 2010; **35**(24): E1444–6.

45. Sadrolsadat SH, Mahdavi AR, Moharari RS, *et al.* A prospective randomized trial comparing the technique of spinal and general anesthesia for lumbar disk surgery: a study of 100 cases. *Surg Neurol* 2009; **71**(1): 60–5.

46. Souza LF, Pereira AC, Lavinas PS. Monetary claims should not influence the practice of anaesthesia. *Acta Anaesthesiol Scand* 2008; **52**(1): 161–71.

344

47. Ziegeler S, Fritsch E, Bauer C, *et al.* Therapeutic effect of intrathecal morphine after posterior lumbar interbody fusion surgery: a prospective, double-blind, randomized study. *Spine (Phila Pa 1976)* 2008; **33**(22): 2379–86.

48. Gehling M, Tryba M. Risks and side-effects of intrathecal morphine combined with spinal anaesthesia: a meta-analysis. *Anaesthesia* 2009; **64**(6): 643–51.

49. Chan JH, Heilpern GN, Packham I, *et al.* A prospective randomized double-blind trial of the use of intrathecal fentanyl in patients undergoing lumbar spinal surgery. *Spine (Phila Pa 1976)* 2006; **31**(22): 2529–33.

50. Khan ZH, Hamidi S, Miri M, Majedi H, Nourijelyani K. Post-operative pain relief following intrathecal injection of acetylcholine esterase inhibitor during lumbar disc surgery: a prospective double blind randomized study. *J Clin Pharm Ther* 2008; **33**(6): 669–75.

51. Milbrandt TA, Singhal M, Minter C, *et al.* A comparison of three methods of pain control for posterior spinal fusions in adolescent idiopathic scoliosis. *Spine (Phila Pa 1976)* 2009; **34**(14): 1499–503.

52. McKenzie A, Sherwood M. Continuous spinal analgesia after extensive lumbar spine surgery. *Anaesth Intensive Care* 2009; **37**(3): 473–6.

53. Cata JP, Noguera EM, Parke E, *et al.* Patient-controlled epidural analgesia (PCEA) for postoperative pain control after lumbar spine surgery. *J Neurosurg Anesthesiol* 2008; **20**(4): 256–60.

54. Ukita M, Sato M, Sato K, *et al.* Clinical utility of epidural anesthesia during and after major spine surgery. *Masui* 2009; **58**(2): 170–3.

55. Blumenthal S, Borgeat A, Nadig M, Min K. Postoperative analgesia after anterior correction of thoracic scoliosis: a prospective randomized study comparing continuous double epidural catheter technique with intravenous morphine. *Spine (Phila Pa 1976)* 2006; **31**(15): 1646–51.

56. Unterrainer AF, Al-Schameri AR, Piotrowski WP, *et al.* Opioid sparing effect of epidural levobupivacaine on postoperative pain treatment in major spinal surgery. *Middle East J Anesthesiol* 2008; **19**(4): 781–8.

57. Meylan N, Elia N, Lysakowski C, Tramer MR. Benefit and risk of intrathecal morphine without local anaesthetic in patients undergoing major surgery: meta-analysis of randomized trials. *Br J Anaesth* 2009; **102**(2): 156–67.

58. Bademci G, Basar H, Sahin S, *et al.* Can facet joint infiltrative analgesia reduce postoperative pain in degenerative lumbar disc surgery? *Neurocirugia (Astur)* 2008; **19**(1): 45–9.

59. Mordeniz C, Torun F, Soran AF, *et al.* The effects of pre-emptive analgesia with bupivacaine on acute post-

60. Jirarattanaphochai K, Jung S, Thienthong S, Krisanaprakornkit W, Sumanonт C. Peridural methylprednisolone and wound infiltration with bupivacaine for postoperative pain control after posterior lumbar spine surgery: a randomized double-blinded placebo-controlled trial. *Spine (Phila Pa 1976)* 2007; **32**(6): 609–16.

61. Wai EK, Sathiaseelan S, O'Neil J, Simchison BL. Local administration of morphine for analgesia after autogenous anterior or posterior iliac crest bone graft harvest for spinal fusion: a prospective, randomized, double-blind, placebo-controlled study. *Anesth Analg* 2010; **110**(3): 928–33.

62. Elder JB, Hoh DJ, Wang MY. Postoperative continuous paravertebral anesthetic infusion for pain control in lumbar spinal fusion surgery. *Spine (Phila Pa 1976)* 2008; **33**(2): 210–18.

63. Elder JB, Hoh DJ, Liu CY, Wang MY. Postoperative continuous paravertebral anesthetic infusion for pain control in posterior cervical spine surgery: a case-control study. *Neurosurgery* 2010; **66**(3 Suppl Operative): 99–106; discussion 106–7.

64. Singh K, Phillips FM, Kuo E, Campbell M. A prospective, randomized, double-blind study of the efficacy of postoperative continuous local anesthetic infusion at the iliac crest bone graft site after posterior spinal arthrodesis: a minimum of 4-year follow-up. *Spine (Phila Pa 1976)* 2007; **32**(25): 2790–6.

65. Harrington JF, French P. Open versus minimally invasive lumbar microdiscectomy: comparison of operative times, length of hospital stay, narcotic use and complications. *Minim Invasive Neurosurg* 2008; **51**(1): 30–5.

66. Brock M, Kunkel P, Papavero L. Lumbar microdiscectomy: subperiosteal versus transmuscular approach and influence on the early postoperative analgesic consumption. *Eur Spine J* 2008; **17**(4): 518–22.

67. Wu HL, Tsou MY, Chao PW, *et al.* Evaluation of the relationships between intravenous patient-controlled analgesia settings and morphine requirements among patients after lumbar spine surgery. *Acta Anaesthesiol Taiwan* 2010; **48**(2): 75–9.

68. Mastronardi L, Pappagallo M, Tatta C, *et al.* Prevention of postoperative pain and of epidural fibrosis after lumbar microdiscectomy: pilot study in a series of forty cases treated with epidural vaseline-sterile-oil-morphine compound. *Spine (Phila Pa 1976)* 2008; **33**(14): 1562–6.

69. Noble M, Treadwell JR, Tregear SJ, *et al.* Long-term opioid management for chronic noncancer pain. *Cochrane Database Syst Rev* 2010; (1): CD006605.

70. Davis JJ, Swenson JD, Hall RH, *et al.* Preoperative "fentanyl challenge" as a tool to estimate postoperative

opioid dosing in chronic opioid-consuming patients. *Anesth Analg* 2005; **101**(2): 389–95.

71. Werner MU, Mjobo HN, Nielsen PR, Rudin A. Prediction of postoperative pain: a systematic review of predictive experimental pain studies. *Anesthesiology* 2010; **112**(6): 1494–502.

72. Knotkova H, Fine PG, Portenoy RK. Opioid rotation: the science and the limitations of the equianalgesic dose table. *J Pain Symptom Manage* 2009; **38**(3): 426–39.

73. Stamer UM, Zhang L, Stuber F. Personalized therapy in pain management: where do we stand? *Pharmacogenomics* 2010; **11**(6): 843–64.

74. Dai F, Belfer I, Schwartz CE, *et al.* Association of catechol-*O*-methyltransferase genetic variants with outcome in patients undergoing surgical treatment for lumbar degenerative disc disease. *Spine J* 2010; **10**(11): 949–57.

75. Finan PH, Zautra AJ, Davis MC, *et al.* COMT moderates the relation of daily maladaptive coping and pain in fibromyalgia. *Pain* 2011; **152**(2): 300–7.

76. Cassinelli EH, Dean CL, Garcia RM, Furey CG, Bohlman HH. Ketorolac use for postoperative pain management following lumbar decompression surgery: a prospective, randomized, double-blinded, placebo-controlled trial. *Spine (Phila Pa 1976)* 2008; **33**(12): 1313–17.

77. Jirarattanaphochai K, Thienthong S, Sriraj W, *et al.* Effect of parecoxib on postoperative pain after lumbar spine surgery: a bicenter, randomized, double-blinded, placebo-controlled trial. *Spine (Phila Pa 1976)* 2008; **33**(2): 132–9.

78. Dahmani S, Brasher C, Stany I, *et al.* Premedication with clonidine is superior to benzodiazepines. A meta analysis of published studies. *Acta Anaesthesiol Scand* 2010; **54**(4): 397–402.

79. Guo SL, Wu TJ, Liu CC, Ng CC, Chien CC, Sun HL. Meperidine-induced serotonin syndrome in a susceptible patient. *Br J Anaesth* 2009; **103**(3): 369–70.

80. Seidel S, Aigner M, Ossege M, Pernicka E, Wildner B, Sycha T. Antipsychotics for acute and chronic pain in adults. *J Pain Symptom Manage* 2010; **39**(4): 768–78.

81. Rajpal S, Gordon DB, Pellino TA, *et al.* Comparison of perioperative oral multimodal analgesia versus IV PCA for spine surgery. *J Spinal Disord Tech* 2010; **23**(2): 139–45.

82. Patorno E, Bohn RL, Wahl PM, *et al.* Anticonvulsant medications and the risk of suicide, attempted suicide, or violent death. *JAMA* 2010; **303**(14): 1401–9.

83. Emir E, Serin S, Erbay RH, Sungurtekin H, Tomatir E. Tramadol versus low dose tramadol-paracetamol for patient controlled analgesia during spinal vertebral surgery. *Kaohsiung J Med Sci* 2010; **26**(6): 308–15.

84. Sadhasivam S, Boat A, Mahmoud M. Comparison of patient-controlled analgesia with and without dexmedetomidine following spine surgery in children. *J Clin Anesth* 2009; **21**(7): 493–501.

85. Remerand F, Couvret C, Pourrat X, *et al.* Prevention of psychedelic side effects associated with low dose continuous intravenous ketamine infusion. *Therapie* 2007; **62**(6): 499–505.

86. Timm C, Linstedt U, Weiss T, Zenz M, Maier C. Sympathomimetic effects of low-dose *S*(+)-ketamine. Effect of propofol dosage. *Anaesthesist* 2008; **57**(4): 338–46.

87. Onaka M, Yamamoto H. Balanced anesthesia with continuous ketamine reduces adverse effects of remifentanil. *Masui* 2008; **57**(10): 1218–22.

88. Souzdalnitski D, Lerman I, Chung KS. Nicotine transdermal. In: Sinatra R, Jahr J, Watkins-Pitchford J, eds. *The Essence of Analgesia and Analgesics*. Cambridge: Cambridge University Press; 2010: 512–14.

89. Shiri R, Karppinen J, Leino-Arjas P, Solovieva S, Viikari-Juntura E. The association between smoking and low back pain: a meta-analysis. *Am J Med* 2010; **123**(1): 87.e7–35.

90. Sipko T, Chantsoulis M, Kuczynski M. Postural control in patients with lumbar disc herniation in the early postoperative period. *Eur Spine J* 2010; **19**(3): 409–14.

91. Thomas AN, Suresh M. Opiate withdrawal after tramadol and patient-controlled analgesia. *Anaesthesia* 2000; **55**(8): 826–7.

92. Fernandes P, Dolan L, Weinstein SL. Intrathecal baclofen withdrawal syndrome following posterior spinal fusion for neuromuscular scoliosis: a case report. *Iowa Orthop J* 2008; **28**: 77–80.

93. Bellinger A, Siriwetchadarak R, Rosenquist R, Greenlee JD. Prevention of intrathecal baclofen withdrawal syndrome: successful use of a temporary intrathecal catheter. *Reg Anesth Pain Med* 2009; **34**(6): 600–2.

Chapter

20

Pathophysiology of the pediatric patient

Stephen J. Kimatian and Kenneth J. Saliba

Key points

- Embryologic failure of normal development leads to predictable patterns of malformation in the pediatric spine. Intuitively, co-developing organ systems may be adversely affected as well. These most commonly are the genitourinary and cardiovascular systems.

- Failure of neural tube closure early in embryogenesis results in a variety of central nervous system defects requiring surgical correction. This leads to lifelong disability affecting not only the nervous system but musculoskeletal and genitourinary systems as well.

- The most prevalent type of scoliosis is acquired idiopathic, which affects mostly otherwise healthy adolescents. These patients present with a cosmetic defect requiring correction to prevent progressive compromise of underlying lung function and the potential for worsening restrictive lung disease from associated thoracic cage derangement.

- Recent evidence suggests that certain unidentified systemic mediators may produce a generalized skeletal muscle dysfunction in adolescents with thoracolumbar scoliosis.

- Several unique aspects of the immature, pediatric spine affect its reaction to trauma differently than in the adult spine.

Zach's back was out of whack
It swerved and curved like a railroad track
Where most backs lie in a line so straight
Zach's formed an S or a figure eight.
Zach discovered when he lay face down
That his back was used by the kids in town
Who played Parcheesi and their games
Or tattooed maps on his vertebrae.
There was nothing else
With quite the knack
As that
Singularly
Interesting
Back of Zach's

Rivian Bell

Introduction

Spine pathology in the pediatric patient has both social and physiologic manifestations that affect a patient's physical and emotional development. Whether surgery is undertaken to restore function, prevent progression, improve mobility, or for cosmesis, spine surgery contributes to both the immediate and long-term prognoses of the patient. These patients may have multiple hospital admissions, surgeries, and anesthetics with resultant absences from school, separation from family, and prolonged immobilization, which no doubt have significant impact on both physical as well as psychosocial development. Scoliosis can be classified as congenital, idiopathic, neuromuscular, traumatic, neoplastic, or syndromically associated. When considering the anesthetic management of the pediatric patient for spinal surgery, special consideration must be given to the fact that, unlike in adults, spine disease in the pediatric patient is often only one component

Table 20.1 Classification of scoliosis

I. Congenital scoliosis
a. Vertebral malformations
1. Failure of formation
2. Failure of segmentation
3. Mixed
b. Costal malformations
c. Spinal dysraphism
II. Acquired (idiopathic)
a. Infantile
b. Juvenile
c. Adolescent
III. Neuromuscular scoliosis
a. Neuropathic
1. Cerebral palsy
2. Syringomyelia
3. Spinal muscular atrophy (SMA)
b. Myopathic
1. Duchenne muscular dystrophy
2. Friedrich's ataxia
3. Arthrogryposis
IV. Traumatic
a. Fracture
b. Surgical
V. Neoplastic scoliosis
a. Secondary to tumor
b. Secondary to treatment for neoplasm
VI. Associated with syndrome
a. Neurofibromatosis
b. Marfan's syndrome
c. Osteogenesis imperfecta
d. Mucopolysaccharidoses
e. Rheumatoid arthritis
f. Ehlers–Danlos syndrome
VII. Functional
a. Leg-length discrepancy
b. Pelvic asymmetry

of a broader genetic or developmental pathology. The most frequent type of scoliosis is idiopathic scoliosis. Its onset often corresponds with growth spurts and subsequently is characterized as infantile, juvenile, or adolescent. Progression and prognosis is associated with age of onset and this requires that the anesthesiologist caring for the pediatric patient understand early growth and development, including embryologic

development, associated with spinal pathology. Table 20.1 lists the most common types of scoliosis.

Embryologic development

The embryologic development of the spine begins in the 4th week of gestation and is intimately related to the development of other midline structures including the spinal cord, the heart, and the genitourinary system. Primitive mesoderm located on either side of the midline of the developing embryo gives rise to organized, discrete segments known as somitomeres. Arranged along the long axis, these cell clusters further organize into somites. By the beginning of the 4th week, ventral and medial cell layers of the somite differentiate and are known as the sclerotome. At the end of the 4th week, these cells experience a positional shift, and migrate to the neural tube and notochord, eventually encompassing them, and forming the vertebral column (see Fig. 20.1).

Normal formation of a segmented vertebral column involves sclerotome segments condensing with each other in a cranial–caudal fashion, whereby one representative vertebral segment is created from a cranial half and caudal half of two adjacent sclerotomes that fuse together. Intersegmental mesenchyme makes up the annulus fibrosus portion of the disc whereas the notochord persists solely as the nucleus pulposus, thereby completing the comprehensive anatomic structure of the intervertebral disc.

Cell density varies within each sclerotome, so that only the cranial portion permits passage of developing axonal extensions emanating from the neural tube (see Fig. 20.2). Therefore, the cellular expression within the sclerotome is influential in the development of the peripheral nervous system.[1] The dorsolateral cells of the somite become myotomes, and will eventually provide musculature to their respective segment of the developing spine. Their arrangement after spinal segmentation bridges the intervertebral disc, thus granting movement to the vertebral column.[2]

Congenital scoliosis represents abnormal spinal curvature as a result of either a defect in formation of an intact vertebral segment, which is referred to as a hemivertebra, or fusion of multiple, immobile segments, resulting in what is known as a bar. Either of these may lead to an abnormal curvature during growth that, if progressive, may require surgical correction.[3] Associated costal abnormalities may exist as well. There is also an increased incidence of genitourinary malformations and congenital heart disease, typically

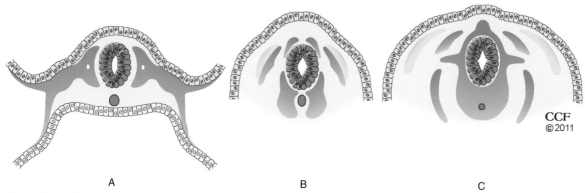

Figure 20.1 Differentiation of the somite, and formation of the axial skeleton and surrounding structures.
(A) During the 4th week of development, mesodermal cells comprising the paired somites migrate towards the neural tube and notochord. (B) The ventral and medial components of the somite differentiate into cells of the sclerotome, which encompass the neural tube and notochord, whereas the remaining dorsal somite cells develop into the dermomyotome. (C) The sclerotome now forms the bony elements surrounding the spinal cord, and the vertebral body encompassing the remnant of the notochord, which persists as the nucleus pulposus of the intervertebral disc. The dermomyotome differentiates into the dermis, and paraspinal musculature of the spinal column.

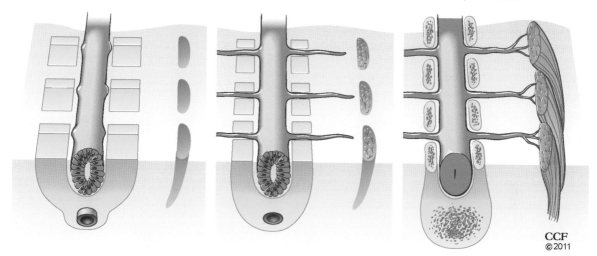

Figure 20.2 Formation of the vertebrae. An intersegmental boundary permits passage of growing axonal extensions of the spinal cord which will innervate the myotome. This resegmentation of the sclerotome is characterized by fusion of the cranial portion of one sclerotome with the caudal portion of the next segment, thus creating a vertebra.

a ventricular septal defect, patent ductus arteriosus, atrial septal defect, or stenosis of the pulmonary valve. Lateral hemivertebra represents embryologic failure of one of the paired lateral sclerotomes to properly develop.[1] However, if there is an anterior/posterior hemivertebra, the defect occurs further in development, during the ossification stage.[4]

The sacrum and coccyx develop solely out of the primitive tail bud, or caudal eminence, which gives rise to its own somites, in addition to providing its own neural tube (which will eventually fuse with the primary neural tube), neural crest, notochord, and mesenchyme. Therefore, it is very common to see malformations in the hindgut or urogenital system in sacral agenesis or

sacral dysplasia. Indeed, the association of anal atresia in infants afflicted with sacral agenesis is well known. These abnormalities typically spare the S1 vertebra, as its progenitor, somite #29 or 30, is derived from the primitive streak.[5] Over 50% of sacral agenesis patients have coexisting congenital scoliosis elsewhere in the spine.[6] Yet it is their life-threatening bowel obstruction, urinary collecting system malformation, or myelomeningocele that will require intervention earliest. Eventually, pelvic stabilization or vertebral fusion may be required.

Identification of congenital vertebral anomalies mandates the search for other organ system abnormalities that commonly occur together in a nonsyndromic manner, such as in the VATER association. Since embryologic evolving organ systems develop simultaneously, a nonrandom association of specific anomalies may exist. The VATER association, in addition to vertebral defects, includes **a**nal atresia, **t**rachea–**e**sophageal fistula, **e**sophageal atresia, and **r**adial limb anomalies. The addition of intra**c**ardiac defects or nonradial **l**imb anomalies extends the acronym to VACTERL. Lastly, bilateral renal malformations are not typical of the VATER complex, yet they are frequently present in afflicted infants.[7]

Spina bifida

Spina bifida (spinal dysraphism) encompasses a spectrum of congenital defects related to a failure of midline fusion of the developing neural tube. Spina bifida may occur along any portion of the spinal cord, but most commonly occurs in the lumbosacral region. The embryologic basis of neural tube defects begins with failure of the neural plate to normally fold over itself (typically by the 25th day after conception) to create a complete tube. This defect in neurulation, therefore, results in an open section, typically in the caudal end of the tube, which prevents migrating and differentiating sclerotome from forming a protective layer of bone over it.[8] When the neural elements and meninges remain intact inside the spinal canal despite an open vertebral defect dorsally (spina bifida occulta), there is typically no physical disability, and the defect is covered by skin, often with a patch of hair, or by a nevus, hemangioma, or lipoma.[9] Routine neurologic examination to assess for any spinal cord dysfunction that may manifest as difficulty in ambulation or sphincter control would seem to be prudent.[10] Physical disability may eventually manifest if multiple segments are involved in spina bifida occulta. Often associated with spondylolysis or spondylolisthesis, the prevalence of occult spinal dysraphism in the general population has been estimated at 12.4% following examination of over 3000 specimens.[11]

Protrusion of neural elements or spinal meninges outside the defect of the bony vertebral canal is known as myelodysplasia. Meningoceles contain cerebrospinal fluid and spinal meninges but the spinal cord remains intact, yet is frequently tethered caudally. There is far less risk of neurologic deficits with a meningocele. However, if the protruding sac contains the spinal cord, it is termed myelomeningocele, and patients experience significant neurologic dysfunction below the level of the lesion, consisting of bowel and bladder incontinence, and loss of strength and sensation of the lower extremities, in addition to tendon and joint abnormalities.[12]

Meningoceles and myelomeningoceles are surgical emergencies because of the high risk of infection associated with only partial, if any, epithelial coverage of the protruding defects, and the enhanced susceptibility to the rapid development of sepsis in newborns with this disease entity.

As mentioned earlier, following the repair of a myelomeningocele, children may develop a tethering of the spinal cord which is characterized clinically by weakness, gait abnormality, orthopedic deformity, urologic dysfunction, pain, or scoliosis. Cessation of symptom progression and relief of pain necessitate surgical release at the site where the spinal cord is attached to the thecal sac.[13]

Patients with myelodysplasia consistently have an Arnold–Chiari type II malformation of the hindbrain and upper cervical spinal canal. Although the entire brain is affected, the malformation is characterized by a crowded posterior fossa, herniation of the cerebellum and hindbrain into the foramen magnum, stretching of the medulla oblongata, and noncommunicating hydrocephalus.[14] Characteristic symptoms in infants include high-pitched, weak cries, frequent choking, swallowing dysfunction, gastroesophageal reflux, and poor feeding. Brainstem compression or cranial nerve traction may produce upper airway obstruction due to vocal cord paradoxical motion or paralysis evidenced by stridor, which may often be followed by oxyhemoglobin desaturation, cyanosis, and bradycardia.[15] Apnea may manifest even in surgically decompressed infants, culminating in respiratory failure and cardiac arrest.[16]

Scoliosis is frequently seen in patients with syringomyelia. Often, there may be an atypical left thoracic curve, which prompts MRI investigation, since the most common presentation is a right thoracic curve. Neurologic symptoms may be minor, or there may be sensory deficits, or cephalgia attributable to a coexisting Chiari I malformation, or the syrinx may be completely asymptomatic. Curve progression tends to be rapid, and neurosurgical decompression of the syrinx may halt scoliosis curve progression if intervention occurs at a younger age, ideally less than 10 years.[17]

Pulmonary function

Scoliosis, derived from the Greek word for "crooked," is a deformity of angulation, rotation, and translation of the vertebral spine. Its distortion of the rib cage may have pronounced influence on the maturation of the lungs, and may therefore adversely affect pulmonary function. A normal 9-fold increase in alveoli takes place from birth throughout the first 10 years of life.[18] However, early onset of scoliosis severely limits the multiplication of alveoli, leading to loss of gas exchange interface and to hypoplastic pulmonary arteries that become excessively muscularized, thus leading to subsequent hypoxemia.[19] Left unchecked, progressive impairment of cardiorespiratory function can result in pulmonary hypertension, right-sided heart failure, and death.

The most common pulmonary defect in children with thoracolumbar scoliosis is restrictive lung disease, defined as a decrease in FVC, FEV_1, and a normal FEV_1/FVC ratio. As scoliotic curvature progresses, spinous processes rotate toward the concave side of the curve. Ribs on the convex side are pushed posteriorly, while ribs on the concave side become prominent anteriorly. Idiopathic scoliosis patients with mild to moderate curves (20–45°) show no significant basal ventilatory abnormalities compared with healthy peers; however, at maximal exercise, they exhibit lower ventilatory efficiency.[20] Deleterious signs of worsening restrictive lung disease are hypoxemia, hypercapnia, and pulmonary hypertension, potentially resulting in cor pulmonale.[21]

Analysis of all three planes of the thoracic cage deformity in scoliosis reveals that all lung volumes are reduced significantly.[22] As the vertebral deformity progresses, thoracic cage mobility is reduced and normal lung compliance diminishes, leading to symptoms of exertional dyspnea, frequent pulmonary infections, and elevated resting respiratory rate. Three-dimensional imaging to study the kinematics of the chest and spine during breathing in scoliosis patients revealed a rigid, bony framework and a stiff thoracic spine, compared with healthy controls, which introduces mechanical inefficiency as a contribution to pulmonary impairment.[23] While a Cobb angle of less than 10° is considered normal, echocardiographic evidence of increased pulmonary artery pressures can be seen with angles of curvature as low as 25° and evidence of restrictive lung disease can be seen with angles above 60°. Evidence of pulmonary hypertension can be seen with Cobb angles in excess of 70°, progressing to pulmonary hypertension at rest as angles exceed 100°. Symptomatic lung disease manifesting as dyspnea on exertion and alveolar hypoventilation can often be found in Cobb angles in excess of 100°.[24,25]

In idiopathic scoliosis, despite the obvious cosmetic derangement, the primary purpose of corrective surgery is the reversal of the thoracic cage deformity and prevention of further curve progression while promoting recovery of lung function. However, in patients with neuromuscular disease, the underlying lung disease persists even after surgical correction.[26] This is attributable to the disease etiology (cerebral palsy, muscular dystrophy, or spinal muscular atrophy), which results in respiratory muscle weakness. Both inspiratory and expiratory muscle strength are reduced in patients with neuromuscular disease independent of the presence of scoliosis. However, the added impact of scoliosis significantly reduces FVC, FEV1, and FEF 25–75% further.[27]

The presence of respiratory symptoms may not correlate with abnormal pulmonary function tests, as up to 67.7% of adolescent idiopathic scoliosis patients with abnormal PFTs may be completely asymptomatic.[28] However, patients with earlier onset of scoliosis, and those with congenital or neuromuscular etiology, may present with more severe hypoventilation, possibly requiring noninvasive ventilation or mechanical ventilation preoperatively. Interestingly, Bowen et al. reported that adolescents with congenital scoliosis (including a cohort with prior thoracic fusion) have a 13.6 times higher chance of having a body mass index (BMI) more than 2 standard deviations below normal.[29] A decreased BMI may reflect a catabolic state secondary to a higher resting respiratory rate and therefore higher caloric expenditure, or possibly a preexisting poor nutritional state as well. This may place the young patient at risk for respiratory muscle fatigue in the perioperative period, as well as coagulation abnormalities intraoperatively and postoperatively secondary solely to malnutrition.

Infantile scoliosis

Infantile scoliosis is defined as spinal curvature presenting from birth to 3 years. Affecting males more frequently than females, there are often other associated abnormalities. In the absence of congenital vertebral anomalies, neuromuscular conditions, or syndromes, the etiology is termed idiopathic. Less commonly, a structural intraspinal abnormality is present, such as a syrinx, tethered cord, or an Arnold–Chiari malformation.[30] Plagiocephaly, which is an oblique, lateral deformity of the infant skull due to premature closure of unilateral coronal and lambdoidal sutures, is also a typical finding in a majority of infants diagnosed with scoliosis.[31] There is a suggestion, perhaps, that continuous placement of infants in the oblique supine position molds the postnatal cranium and spine in idiopathic infantile scoliosis.[32,33] Absent at birth, infantile scoliosis may progress during a growth phase, in which case it will undoubtedly have an adverse affect on normal growth of the ribs, thorax, lung parenchyma, and pulmonary vasculature, leading to severe cardiopulmonary compromise if left untreated.[34] Fortunately, over 80% of cases of infantile scoliosis resolve spontaneously.

Adolescent idiopathic scolosis

In contrast to infantile scoliosis, which is diagnosed at birth or shortly afterwards, adolescent idiopathic scoliosis (AIS) has its onset during late childhood usually after the age of 10 years but before the occurrence of skeletal maturity. If a Cobb angle of at least 10° is used as the basis for diagnosis, idiopathic scoliosis has a prevalence estimated at 1–3% of adolescents.[35] Its inheritance is complex, neither autosomal dominant nor recessive, but polygenic, with incomplete penetrance, variable expressivity, and familial clustering.[36] Adolescent scoliosis is the most common form of scoliosis in the United States, and affects predominately girls with a ratio of at least 4:1.

The etiology is complex and unquestionably multifactorial. Several theories acting alone or in combination have been submitted over the last few decades. The concept of asymmetric loading of the vertebral body during the pubertal growth surge results in a wedged deformity has been investigated and replicated in a rat model.[37] Imbalanced paravertebral muscle fiber composition has also been implicated as a potential causative factor. AIS biopsy specimens revealed atrophy of type I fibers (used to sustain posture) of paraspinal musculature and deltoid muscles on the concave side of the curve.[38] AIS acceleration during the adolescent growth surge would seem to implicate growth hormone as a potential etiologic factor. However, investigation of growth hormone secretion in 15 adolescents diagnosed with idiopathic scoliosis found levels within normal limits compared with healthy controls.[39]

Kearon *et al.* reported cardiovascular deconditioning and decreased peripheral muscularity in AIS patients after assessing their work capacity and exercise tolerance, suggesting an overall decrease in lean muscle mass and possible nutritional deficiencies that may be present in adolescents with idiopathic scoliosis. It also suggests that there may be a systemic response to the development of a thoracic scoliosis deformity.[40] Interestingly, a recent study examined the potential role for unknown systemic mediators that may account for a generalized skeletal muscle dysfunction in patients with AIS, which by definition is a diagnosis of exclusion. Building on Kearon's findings, Martinez-Llorens *et al.* assessed lung function, exercise capacity, and limb muscle endurance

in adolescents with significant spinal deformity and in healthy patients. As expected, AIS patients exhibited a mild to moderate impairment of pulmonary function of a restrictive pattern and a reduced exercise capacity. This was attributed to decreased endurance and marked dysfunction of both inspiratory and expiratory muscles of respiration and limb muscle deconditioning, mainly of the quadriceps. However, what was revelatory in their findings was that the degree of muscle dysfunction assessed was completely unrelated to the severity of the spinal deformity. This hints at a potential role for currently unknown systemic mediators that produce generalized skeletal muscle dysfunction in adolescents with idiopathic scoliosis, thereby limiting exercise capacity to a greater degree than what is attributable to ventilatory defects alone.[41]

Associated neurologic pathology

Abnormal spinal curvature is common in several neurologic conditions. Cerebral palsy (CP) is the leading cause of spastic neuromuscular scoliosis, which is seen in up to 64% of CP patients.[42] A nonprogressive neuromuscular disability arising from various anatomic lesions affecting the brain in its early development, cerebral palsy is associated with visual and auditory impairment, seizures, learning disability, and gastroesophageal reflux. In addition to scoliosis, which has been attributed to unbalanced musculature and asymmetric innervation, cerebral palsy patients may also demonstrate degenerative arthritis, foot deformities, and joint and soft tissue contractures, which may significantly complicate acquisition of intravenous access.[43] The frequency and degree of severity of the scoliosis typically parallels the neurologic impairment of the patient. Nonambulatory patients with spastic quadriplegia, thus, tend to have rapidly progressing, marked curves resistant to conservative management strategies.[44,45] The curve's severity may adversely align the pelvis, thereby preventing proper chair sitting posture and encouraging skin breakdown and decubitus formation.[46] The characteristic neuromuscular scoliosis curve is shaped as a long C extending from the upper thoracic region to the pelvis. Finally, in contrast to idiopathic scoliosis, patients with cerebral palsy may have their scoliosis progress after skeletal maturity.[47]

The most common flaccid neuromuscular disorders are Duchenne muscular dystrophy and spinal muscular atrophy. They are of different etiologies, affecting multiple organ systems, and yielding similar results on the developing spine when patients are nonambulatory.

Duchenne muscular dystrophy (DMD) is a flaccid neuromuscular disease of muscular origin characterized by a lack of the protein dystrophin in skeletal muscles. Dystrophin normally aids in attaching actin and myosin to the cell membrane, and maintaining sarcolemmal integrity. The deletion of dystrophin in this X-linked recessive disease results in profound muscle weakness. Typical progression of the disease leads to nonambulation and wheelchair confinement during the second decade; at which time it is common that spinal deformity appears.[48] Scoliosis in the nonambulatory child with DMD progresses at an accelerated rate, and will require surgical intervention.[49] Intervention is aimed at halting curve progression and improving seated posture, which may maximize function, reduce pain, and inhibit skin breakdown, thereby improving quality of life.[50]

The development of a spinal deformity in the early teen years in patients with DMD, although it does distort the thoracic cage, is not the sole contribution to the deterioration of lung function. The presence of both contractures and worsening muscle weakness are the implicating factors in the development of restrictive pulmonary disease, as FVC has often already decreased precipitously before the onset of scoliosis.[51] Scoliosis progression, therefore, contributes very little to worsening lung function in DMD patients, and spinal corrective surgery is aimed at improving nonambulatory posture and quality of life rather than reversing the decline in pulmonary function. In addition to underlying respiratory muscle weakness, the presence of cardiomyopathy, cardiac conduction defects, dysphagia with potential aspiration of gastric contents, and rhabdomyolysis and hyperkalemia in response to succinylcholine also complicate the care for these patients in the perioperative period. Although there is no clear link between DMD and malignant hyperthermia (MH), the literature is replete with case reports of rhabdomyolysis and hyperkalemia in DMD patients exposed to volatile anesthetics, although without the hypermetabolism inherent in MH. Therefore, DMD patients are not at risk for developing an MH crisis more so than the general population, yet it remains prudent to avoid volatile anesthetics when administering general anesthesia to these patients because of the possibility of rhabdomyolysis and the development of cardiac complications.[52]

Another type of flaccid neuromuscular disorder that is also implicated in the development of scoliosis when the child becomes nonambulatory is spinal muscular atrophy (SMA), which is a neurogenic neuromuscular disorder. It is autosomal recessive in inheritance and results in profound, debilitating weakness due to loss of the anterior spinal horn neurons. There are four types of SMA, based on age at presentation and level of weakness. Both in DMD and SMA type 2 (onset of weakness between 6 and 18 months, and nonambulatory very early in life), spinal deformity is consistently present, usually as a progressive thoracolumbar C-curve, and generates an oblique pelvis.[53] The spinal deformity reduces rib mobility, thereby compressing the thorax, thus restricting pulmonary function and compromising ventilation. In contrast to DMD (in which a small percentage do not develop scoliosis), all children with SMA type 2 develop scoliosis by 3 years of age, and it is recommended that they undergo surgical correction.[54]

Tumors and neoplasms

Pediatric spinal cord tumors are exceedingly rare, representing 0.5–1% of all CNS tumors. The overwhelming majority of pediatric spinal tumors are glial in origin. These rare tumors often manifest in children and adolescents as intermittent back pain, which can often be overlooked, misdiagnosed, or attributed to adolescent growth spurt or as a sports related injury. Less commonly, in addition to intermittent back pain, spinal tumors may present in children as mild motor weakness, progressive kyphoscoliosis, torticollis, or a disturbance in gait. Astrocytomas are far more common in pediatrics than in adults, whereas ependymomas occur with the highest frequency in the adult population. The diagnosis often takes place after more common causes of back pain in this patient population are systematically excluded and conservative therapy has failed. Once the diagnosis is made, a combination of neurosurgical resection, radiation treatment, and chemotherapy constitute treatment.[55,56]

Trauma

Traumatic injury to the pediatric spine is most frequently associated with blunt trauma suffered during motor vehicle accidents in children under 8 years of age, in which the cervical level is affected most often.[57] Children over eight years of age with C-spine injuries have sports-related trauma as their most common mechanism of injury.[58] Immature bone and joints, and ligamentous laxity afford a protective degree of hypermobility in pediatric patients under the age of 8 years, as most often traumatic forces result in ligamentous injuries rather than fractures of the cervical spine. However, there is a consistent association of closed

353

head injury (CHI) with pediatric cervical spine injuries related to motor vehicle trauma, in which the CHI is the predictor of patient outcome.[59] Children under 8 years also have a proportionally larger head and underdeveloped neck musculature, thereby placing the pivot point from traumatic forces much higher in the spine, at the level of the craniocervical junction, compared with adults, in whom the fulcrum occurs around C5–C7. In children over 8 years, the pivot point is displaced caudally, approaching the lower C-spine, and injuries tend to result more often in fractures.[60] Although rare in adults, the phenomenon known as SCIWORA (spinal cord injury without radiographic abnormality) exists in pediatric spinal cord injury patients in up to 67% of cases, and represents neurologic injury without evidence of vertebral fraction or dislocation.[61] Prognosis is predicated on neurologic symptoms at presentation. This clinical entity results when the malleable pediatric bony spine is subjected to flexion/extension or distraction forces, then reduces spontaneously, and thereby subjects the underlying cord, which is anchored caudally and cranially and thus not nearly as pliable, to injury. SCIWORA tends to disappear as the cervical spine matures beyond the age of 8 years, and the pediatric spine is then subjected to a more adult pattern of injury following trauma.[62] Anatomic changes incurred during the normal maturation process include the wedge-shaped vertebral bodies now becoming rectangular in shape, facets assuming a more vertical orientation, and ligaments increasing in tensile strength.

Lumbar disc herniation occurs in up to 40% of adults, but is relatively uncommon in the pediatric population, with a reported incidence of 0.8–3%. A traumatic injury related to sporting activities is typically the precipitating event in pediatric patients presenting with neurologic symptoms. This is in contrast to adults, who usually elicit sciatica after lifting or twisting motions and who also generally suffer from degenerative changes of the disc itself in advance of eliciting any irritating movements.[63] However, in adolescents, trauma may be an inciting event that aggravates a preexisting anatomic abnormality such as scoliosis, transitional vertebrae (lumbarization or sacralization), or spina bifida occulta, which was discovered in up to 18.5% of adolescents presenting with low back pain and signs of lumbar nerve root compression.[64] Children and adolescents of first-degree relatives who suffer from low back pain due to lumbar disc herniation are more likely to develop this disorder during adolescence, suggesting a genetic influence.[65]

Associated syndromes

Congenital vertebral fusion in the upper cervical region characterizes Klippel–Feil syndrome. The classic Klippel–Feil triad consists of low posterior hairline, decreased cervical mobility, and a short, "webbed" neck with reduced number of cervical vertebrae. In addition to congenital scoliosis, common associated findings may include renal anomalies and a ventricular septal defect.[66] Hypermobile segments may promote neurologic injury, and upon presentation for surgical stabilization these patients may present a challenge in airway management.

Children with Down's syndrome are at risk for occipitocervical and atlantoaxial instability. Congenitally abnormal bone formation in the cervical spine may produce ligamentous laxity; therefore, trisomy 21 children may be susceptible to progressive subluxation and consequent neurologic impairment. Thankfully, the majority of Down's syndrome patients are neurologically asymptomatic.[67] Coexisting endocardial cushion defects of the heart and developmental delay are common in children with Down's syndrome. Lastly, these patients may have considerable macroglossia that could complicate effective mask airway ventilation.

Atlantoaxial instability is also seen in Morquio's syndrome, which is an inherited defect of metabolism of keratan sulfate (mucopolysaccharidosis type IV). This results in its deposition in connective tissues throughout the body, namely the airway, skeletal system, blood vessels, and skin. In addition to a prominent maxilla, short neck, and receding mandible, the congenital abnormality at the craniocervical junction, secondary to a hypoplastic odontoid, may progress over several years leading to cervical cord damage.[68]

Another mucopolysaccharidosis (type II), Hunter's syndrome, exhibits kyphosis and hypoplasia in the lumbar spine, but results in the accumulation of dermatan sulfate and heparan sulfate throughout various tissues of the body. Hunter's syndrome is primarily associated with progressive, disabling arthropathies, especially of the hips. This is in addition to atlantoaxial instability due to a hypoplastic odontoid, and the potential for cervical myelopathy secondary to spinal canal narrowing, which is also common in Morquio's syndrome. The lower thoracic and upper lumber vertebrae may be abnormally developed in this syndrome and, compounded by hypotonic abdominal musculature, may exaggerate kyphosis and scoliosis, limiting chest excursion and leading to respiratory compromise.[69,70]

Goldenhar's syndrome is the most common craniofacial malformation syndrome, and is worth mentioning due to the high incidence (40%) of coexisting congenital vertebral anomalies. High thoracic hemivertebrae are quite common, which are typically unbalanced, producing congenital scoliosis.[71] Unilateral mandibular hypoplasia is the hallmark of Goldenhar's syndrome, necessitating great attention to maintaining airway patency when administering sedation or general anesthesia to these children.

References

1. Schoenwolf GC, Bleyl SB, Brauer PR, Francis-West PH. Chapter 8, Development of the musculoskeletal system. In: *Larsen's Human Embryology*. 4th ed. Philadelphia: Churchill Livingstone/Elsevier; 2009: 217–45.

2. Sadler TW, ed. *Langman's Medical Embryology*. 7th ed. Baltimore: Williams & Wilkins; 1995: 161–2.

3. Wright JG, Hedden DM. Bone and joint surgery: surgical considerations. In: Bissonette B, Dalens B, eds. *Pediatric Anesthesia: Principles & Practice*. Chicago: McGraw-Hill; 2002: 1078–80.

4. Ozonoff MB. Spinal anomalies and curvatures. In: Resnick D, ed. *Diagnosis of Bone and Joint Disorders*. 3rd ed. Philadelphia: WB Saunders; 1995: 4245–6.

5. Pang D. Sacral agenesis and caudal spinal cord malformations. *Neurosurgery* 1993; **32**(5): 755–79.

6. Renshaw TS. Sacral agenesis. *J Bone Joint Surg Am*. 1978; **60**(3): 373–83.

7. Kallen K, Mastroiacovo P, Castilla EE, Robert E, Kallen B. VATER non-random association of congenital malformations: study based on data from four malformation registers. *Am J Med Genet* 2001; **101**(1): 26–32.

8. Schoenwolf GC, Bleyl SB, Brauer PR, Francis-West PH. Chapter 4, Forming the embryo. In: *Larsen's Human Embryology*. 4th ed. Philadelphia: Churchill Livingstone/Elsevier: 2009: 103–30.

9. Northrup H, Volcik KA. Spina bifida and other neural tube defects. *Curr Prob Pediatr* 2000; **30**(10): 313–32.

10. Guggisberg D, Hadj-Rabia S, Viney C, *et al.* Skin markers of occult spinal dysraphism in children: a review of 54 cases. *Arch Dermatol* 2004; **140**(9): 1109–15.

11. Eubanks JD, Cheruvu VK. Prevalence of sacral spina bifida occulta and its relationship to age, sex, race, and the sacral table angle: an anatomic, osteologic study of three thousand one hundred specimens. *Spine* 2009; **34**(15): 1539–43.

12. Hamid RK, Newfield P. Pediatric neuroanesthesia. Neural tube defects. *Anesthesiol Clin North Am* 2001; **19**(2): 219–28.

13. Morioka T, Hashiguchi K, Mukae N, Sayama T, Sasaki T. Neurosurgical management of patients with lumbosacral myeloschisis. *Neurol Med Chir (Tokyo)* 2010; **50**(9): 870–6.

14. McLone DG, Naidich TP. Developmental morphology of the subarachnoid space, brain vasculature, contiguous structures, and the cause of the Chiari II malformation. *AJNR Am J Neuroradiol* 1992; **13**(2): 463–82.

15. Charney EB, Rorke LB, Sutton LN, Schut L. Management of Chiari II complications in infants with myelomeningocele. *J Pediatr* 1987; **111**(3): 364–71.

16. Bell WO, Charney EB, Bruce DA, Sutton LN, Schut L. Symptomatic Arnold–Chiari malformation: review of experience with 22 cases. *J Neurosurg* 1987; **66**(6): 812–16.

17. Ozerdemoglu RA, Transfeldt EE, Denis F. Value of treating primary causes of syrinx in scoliosis associated with syringomyelia. *Spine* 2003; **28**(8): 806–14.

18. Emery JL, Mithal A. The number of alveoli in the terminal respiratory unit of man during late intrauterine life and childhood. *Arch Dis Child* 1960; **35**: 544–7.

19. Davies G, Reid L. Effect of scoliosis on growth of alveoli and pulmonary arteries and on right ventricle. *Arch Dis Child* 1971; **46**(249): 623–32.

20. Barrios C, Perez-Encinas C, Maruenda JI, Laguia M. Significant ventilatory functional restriction in adolescents with mild or moderate scoliosis during maximal exercise tolerance test. *Spine* 2005; **30**(14): 1610–15.

21. Wazeka AN, DiMaio MF, Boachie-Adjei O. Outcome of pediatric patients with severe restrictive lung disease following reconstructive spine surgery. *Spine* 2004; **29**(5): 528–34.

22. Aaro S, Ohlund C. Scoliosis and pulmonary function. *Spine* 1984; **9**(2): 220–2.

23. Leong JC, Lu WW, Luk KD, Karlberg EM. Kinematics of the chest cage and spine during breathing in healthy individuals and in patients with adolescent idiopathic scoliosis. *Spine* 1999; **24**(13): 1310–15.

24. Primiano FP, Nussbaum E, Hirschfeld SS, *et al.* Early echocardiographic and pulmonary function findings in idiopathic scoliosis. *J Pediatr Orthop* 1983; **3**(4): 475–81.

25. Bergofsky EH. Respiratory failure in disorders of the thoracic cage. *Am Rev Respir Dis* 1979; **119**(4): 643–69.

26. Payo J, Perez-Grueso FS, Fernandez-Baillo N, Garcia A. Severe restrictive lung disease and vertebral surgery in a pediatric population. *Eur Spine J* 2009: **18**(12): 1905–10.

27. Inal-Ince D, Savci S, Arikan H, *et al.* Effects of scoliosis on respiratory muscle strength in patients with neuromuscular disorders. *Spine J* 2009; **9**(12): 981–6.

28. Vedantam R, Crawford AH. The role of preoperative pulmonary function tests in patients with adolescent idiopathic scoliosis undergoing posterior spinal fusion. *Spine* 1997; **22**(23): 2731–4.

29. Bowen RE, Scaduto AA, Banuelos S. Decreased body mass index and restrictive lung disease in congenital thoracic scoliosis. *J Pediatr Orthop* 2008; **28**(6): 665–8.

30. Pahys JM, Samdani AF, Betz RR. Intraspinal anomalies in infantile idiopathic scoliosis: prevalence and role of magnetic resonance imaging. *Spine* 2009; **34**(12): E434–8.

31. Hopper WC Jr, Lovell WW. Progressive infantile idiopathic scoliosis. *Clin Orthop Relat Res* 1977; (**126**): 26–32.

32. Mau H. The changing concept of infantile scoliosis. *Int Orthop* 1981; **5**(2): 131–7.

33. McMaster MJ. Infantile idiopathic scoliosis: can it be prevented? *J Bone Joint Surg Br* 1983; **65**(5): 612–17.

34. Branthwaite MA. Cardiorespiratory consequences of unfused idiopathic scoliosis. *Br J Dis Chest* 1986; **80**(4): 360–9.

35. Weinstein SL, Dolan LA, Cheng JC, Danielsson A, Morcuende JA. Adolescent idiopathic scoliosis. *Lancet* 2008; **371**(9623): 1527–37.

36. Ward K, Ogilvie J, Argyle V, *et al.* Polygenic inheritance of adolescent idiopathic scoliosis: a study of extended families in Utah. *Am J Med Genet A* 2010; **152A**(5): 1178–88.

37. Mente PL, Stokes IA, Spence H, Aronsson DD. Progression of vertebral wedging in an asymmetrically loaded rat tail model. *Spine* 1997; **22**(12): 1292–6.

38. Yarom R, Robin GC. Muscle pathology in idiopathic scoliosis. *Isr J Med Sci* 1979; **15**(11): 917–24.

39. Misol S, Ponseti IV, Samaan N, Bradbury JT. Growth hormone blood levels in patients with idiopathic scoliosis. *Clin Orthop Relat Res* 1971; **81**: 122–5.

40. Kearon C, Viviani GR, Killian KJ. Factors influencing work capacity in adolescent idiopathic thoracic scoliosis. *Am Rev Respir Dis* 1993; **148**(2): 295–303.

41. Martinez-Llorens J, Ramirez M, Colomina MJ, *et al.* Muscle dysfunction and exercise limitation in adolescent idiopathic scoliosis. *Eur Respir J* 2010; **36**(2): 393–400.

42. Madigan RR, Wallace SL. Scoliosis in the institutionalized cerebral palsy population. *Spine* 1981; **6**(6): 583–90.

43. Murphy KP. The adult with cerebral palsy. *Orthop Clin North Am* 2010; **41**(4): 595–605.

44. McCarthy JJ, D'Andrea LP, Betz RR, Clements DH. Scoliosis in the child with cerebral palsy. *J Am Acad Orthop Surg* 2006; **14**(6): 367–75.

45. Thomson JD, Banta JV. Scoliosis in cerebral palsy: an overview and recent results. *J Pediatr Orthop B* 2001; **10**(1): 6–9.

46. Comstock CP, Leach J, Wenger DR. Scoliosis in total-body-involvement cerebral palsy. Analysis of surgical treatment and patient and caregiver satisfaction. *Spine* 1998; **23**(12): 1412–24.

47. Thometz JG, Simon SR. Progression of scoliosis after skeletal maturity in institutionalized adults who have cerebral palsy. *J Bone Joint Surg Am* 1988; **70**(9): 1290–6.

48. Oda T, Shimizu N, Yonenobu K, *et al.* Longitudinal study of spinal deformity in Duchenne muscular dystrophy. *J Pediatr Orthop* 1993; **13**(4): 478–88.

49. Gozal D. Pulmonary manifestations of neuromuscular disease with special reference to Duchenne muscular dystrophy and spinal muscular atrophy. *Pediatr Pulmonol* 2000; **29**(2): 141–50.

50. Arun R, Srinivas S, Mehdian SM. Scoliosis in Duchenne's muscular dystrophy: a changing trend in surgical management. *Eur Spine J* 2010; **19**(3): 376–83.

51. Miller F, Moseley CF, Koreska J, Levison H. Pulmonary function and scoliosis in Duchenne dystrophy. *J Pediatr Orthop* 1988; **8**(2): 133–7.

52. Gurnaney H, Brown A, Litman RS. Malignant hyperthermia and muscular dystrophies. *Anesth Analg* 2009; **109**(4): 1043–8.

53. Mullender M, Blom N, De Kleuver M, *et al.* A Dutch guideline for the treatment of scoliosis in neuromuscular disorders. *Scoliosis* 2008; **3**: 14.

54. Evans GA, Drennan JC, Russman BS. Functional classification and orthopaedic management of spinal muscular atrophy. *J Bone Joint Surg Br* 1981; **63B**(4): 516–22.

55. Baleriaux DL. Spinal cord tumors. *Eur Radiol* 1999; **9**(7): 1252–8.

56. Huisman TA. Pediatric tumors of the spine. *Cancer Imaging* 2009; **9** Spec No A: S45–8.

57. Parent S, Dimar J, Dekutoski M, Roy-Beaudry M. Unique features of pediatric spinal cord injury. *Spine* 2010; **35**(21 Suppl): S202–8.

58. Platzer P, Jaindl M, Thalhammer G, *et al.* Cervical spine injuries in pediatric patients. *J Trauma* 2007; **62**(2): 389–96.

59. Brown RL, Brunn MA, Garcia VF. Cervical spine injuries in children: a review of 103 patients treated consecutively at a level 1 pediatric trauma center. *J Pediatr Surg* 2001; **36**(8): 1107–14.

60. Reynolds R. Pediatric spinal injury. *Curr Opin Pediatr* 2000; **12**(1): 67–71.

61. Pang D, Pollack IF. Spinal cord injury without radiographic abnormality in children – the SCIWORA syndrome. *J Trauma* 1989; **29**(5): 654–64.

62. Kriss VM, Kriss TC. SCIWORA (spinal cord injury without radiographic abnormality) in infants and children. *Clin Pediatr (Phila)* 1996; **35**(3): 119–24.

63. Grobler LJ, Simmons EH, Barrington TW. Intervertebral disc herniation in the adolescent. *Spine* 1979; **4**(3): 267–78.

64. Parisini P, DiSilvestre M, Greggi T, Miglietta A, Paderni S. Lumbar disc excision in children and adolescents. *Spine* 2001; **26**(18): 1997–2000.

65. Clarke NM, Cleak DK. Intervertebral lumbar disc prolapse in children and adolescents. *J Pediatr Orthop* 1983; **3**(2): 202–6.

66. Thomsen MN, Schneider U, Weber M, Johannisson R, Niethard FU. Scoliosis and congenital anomalies associated with Klippel–Fiel syndrome types I–III. *Spine* 1997; **22**(4): 396–401.

67. Hankinson TC, Anderson RC. Craniovertebral junction abnormalities in Down syndrome. *Neurosurgery* 2010; **66** (3 Suppl): A32–8.

68. Morgan KA, Rehman MA, Schwartz RE. Morquio's syndrome and its anaesthetic considerations. *Paediatr Anaesth* 2002; **12**(7): 641–4.

69. Benson PF, Button LR, Fensom AH, Dean MF. Lumbar kyphosis in Hunter's disease (MPS II). *Clin Genet* 1979; **16**: 317–22.

70. Morini SR, Steiner CE, Gerson LB. Mucopolysaccharidosis type II: skeletal-muscle system involvement. *J Pediatr Orthop B* 2010; **19**(4): 313–17.

71. Gibson JN, Sillence DO, Taylor TK. Abnormalities of the spine in Goldenhar's syndrome. *J Pediatr Orthop* 1996; **16**(3): 344–9.

Chapter

21

Preoperative evaluation of the pediatric patient

Sara P. Lozano and Julie Niezgoda

Key points

- Preoperative planning for scoliosis surgery includes assessment of the Cobb angle, the number of vertebrae to be fused, the surgical approach, and the type of instrumentation to be used.
- Patients with a curvature exceeding 60° have altered pulmonary function and those with >100° are at risk for respiratory failure and prolonged mechanical ventilation postoperatively and therefore baseline pulmonary function tests should be obtained.
- Patients with early-onset scoliosis or curvature >100° are at risk for progressive pulmonary hypertension and cor pulmonale. Echocardiography and ECG should be done to evaluate bi-ventricular function in patients with decreased exercise tolerance or respiratory function. Nonambulatory patients should have a preoperative cardiac work-up.
- Children with neuromuscular or congenital scoliosis are at much greater risk for surgical repair and require an extensive evaluation due to congenital anomalies, difficult IV access, cardiopulmonary compromise, hematopoietic and coagulation problems, and nutritional issues requiring preoperative optimization. A preoperative consultation with the parents or caregiver should be made to outline the perioperative expectations, including potential blood loss, administration of blood products, and possible prolonged mechanical ventilation.

Introduction

Children presenting for spine surgery most commonly have scoliosis, a complex deformity involving both the

Table 21.1 Classification of scoliosis

Idiopathic (70%)	▪ Infantile <3 years or ▪ Early onset <5 years ▪ Juvenile 3–10 years or ▪ Late onset >5 years ▪ Adolescent >10 years

Neuromuscular (15%)	▪ Neuropathic
	  • Upper motor neuron: cerebral palsy
	  • Lower motor neuron: poliomyelitis
	  • Spinal muscle atrophy
	▪ Myopathic
	  • Duchenne muscular dystrophy
	  • Friedreich's ataxia

Congenital	▪ Vertebral abnormalities
	▪ Rib abnormalities
	▪ Neural tube defects
	  • Spina bifida
	  • Myelomeningocele

Neurofibromatosis	
Mesenchymal	▪ Marfan's syndrome ▪ Arthrogryposis ▪ Osteogenesis imperfecta ▪ Mucopolysaccharidoses ▪ Rheumatoid arthritis
Neoplastic	▪ Primary tumors ▪ Secondary tumors
Traumatic	▪ Vertebral fractures ▪ Radiation

lateral curvature of the spine and rotation of the vertebrae resulting in an associated deformity of the rib cage. The spectrum of presentation for children with scoliosis can include the otherwise normal adolescent with idiopathic scoliosis (IS), the chronically ill child with neuromuscular disease, or the patient with congenital scoliosis and a myriad of associated congenital abnormalities. The most commons types of scoliosis are idiopathic, neuromuscular, and congenital (Table 21.1).

Scoliosis can potentially cause cardiopulmonary impairment, resulting in an increased risk of respiratory

Anesthesia for Spine Surgery, ed. Ehab Farag. Published by Cambridge University Press. © Cambridge University Press 2012.

complications after surgical correction. Therefore, the goal of the preoperative evaluation is to identify patients at high risk for postoperative complications, including prolonged mechanical ventilation (MV) in the intensive care unit. This chapter highlights specific issues related to the patient presenting for repair of scoliosis and discusses general aspects of the surgery.

General evaluation

The preoperative evaluation of any patient presenting for scoliosis surgery should include an assessment of the severity of problems relating to the scoliosis as well as the surgical plan, including the type of instrumentation, the surgical approach, and the number of vertebrae to be fused.

Cobb's angle is a measurement used for evaluation of the severity of the curves in scoliosis on an AP radiographic projection of the spine (Fig. 21.1). When assessing a curve the apical vertebra is first identified, which is the most affected vertebra in the curve. The apical vertebra is the spinal bone that has the most rotation and displacement from its ideal alignment. It also has the least amount of tilt, as measured by the angle of the end plates (top and bottom edges of vertebral body). The

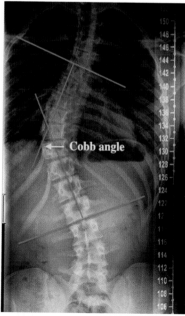

Figure 21.1 Anterior–posterior standing spinal radiograph showing the Cobb angle. The superior and inferior vertebrae involved in the curve are identified. Parallel lines are drawn along the top end plate of the superior vertebra and the bottom end plate of the inferior vertebra. Perpendiculars are drawn to these lines until they intersect; the resulting angle is the Cobb angle.

end/transitional vertebrae are then identified through the curve above and below. The end vertebrae are the most superior and inferior vertebrae that are the least displaced and rotated and have the maximally tilted end plate. A line is drawn along the superior end plate of the superior end vertebra and a second line is drawn along the inferior end plate of the inferior end vertebra. If the end plates are indistinct, the line may be drawn through the pedicles. The angle between these two lines (or lines drawn perpendicular to them) is measured as the Cobb angle. As a general rule a Cobb angle of 10° is regarded as a minimum angulation to define scoliosis.

Determination of the severity of the deformity is important, since different studies have found a direct correlation between respiratory dysfunction and the magnitude of the thoracic curve.[1–4] Furthermore, it has been suggested that the severity of the curvature is the most accurate predictor of lung impairment[4] in children with IS. However, Newton et al.[5] found an increased risk for moderate to severe pulmonary dysfunction in IS patients with a structurally cephalad curve, eight or more vertebral levels in the thoracic curve, or thoracic hypokyphosis. The most significant predictor of pulmonary function in this study was the number of vertebrae in the thoracic curve.

Scoliosis surgery, even in healthy patients, is associated with blood loss and large fluid shifts. The magnitude of blood loss is directly related to the number of vertebral levels to be fused, making it essential to know how many segments are involved for careful preoperative planning.

Basic tests that aid in the general assessment and preparedness of any patient presenting for spine surgery include a complete blood count (CBC) with platelets, basic metabolic panel (BMP), thrombin (PT), partial thromboplastin (PTT) time, and international normalized ratio (INR).

The following sections are divided into the different etiologies of scoliosis and will discuss the important aspects of the preoperative evaluation according to the specific underlying cause of the scoliosis.

Idiopathic scoliosis

Idiopathic scoliosis (IS) is the most common type of spinal deformity (70%). In IS, the curve progresses during periods of peak growth and is classified as infantile (<3 years old), juvenile (3–10 years old), or adolescent (>10 years old to skeletal maturity) depending on the period of onset. Since onset time bears a relationship to long-term prognosis, some clinicians refer to IS as early-

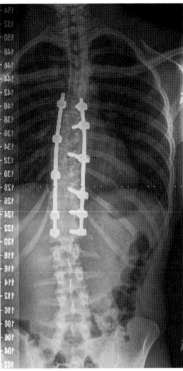

Figure 21.2 Posterior spinal fusion from T6 to L1 in a patient with adolescent idiopathic scoliosis.

onset (younger than 5 years) and late-onset (older than 5 years). Eighty percent of idiopathic scoliosis is of the adolescent variety and these patients are usually healthy apart from their spine deformity. Children with infantile IS present less frequently but they may have a more complicated perioperative course due to associated congenital heart defects, hip dysplasia, and mental disabilities.

The indication for surgery in IS is a progression of curve to greater than 40–50°.[6] The goal of the surgery is to prevent future worsening of the deformity and its effect on cardiopulmonary function while improving cosmetic appearance. A posterior approach is most commonly utilized during surgery (Fig. 21.2). Combined anterior and posterior approaches are used in more severe and rigid curves or where there is a need to prevent anterior growth.

The preoperative evaluation starts with a thorough history and physical examination with the primary focus on cardiopulmonary function and any hematopoietic or coagulopathy issues.

Assessment of respiratory function

Early-onset scoliosis produces progressive skeletal deformity, which interferes with lung growth. Patients whose scoliosis becomes prominent before 5 years of age show hypoplasia of the lung[7] and are at increased risk of severe morbidity and cardiorespiratory failure.[8] In contrast, there is little risk of long-term cardiopulmonary compromise in adolescent idiopathic scoliosis (AIS).[8] In a follow-up of 115 patients with untreated scoliosis, the mortality was significantly increased in infantile and juvenile scoliosis but not in adolescent scoliosis.[9]

As the degree of curvature progresses, all children with scoliosis develop narrowing of the chest cavity, resulting in changes in wall compliance and a restrictive lung defect. The three most common defects seen in pulmonary function testing (PFT) are decrease in vital capacity (VC), forced vital capacity (FVC), and forced expiratory volume in 1 second (FEV_1). In patients with curves greater than 35°, arterial blood gases (ABG) show a slight decrease in arterial oxygen tension (P_aO_2) with a normal arterial carbon dioxide tension (P_aCO_2). With curves >100°, the work of breathing increases, alveolar hypoventilation predominates, ventilation–perfusion mismatch occurs, and hypercapnia ensues. Respiratory failure is then the culmination of a spectrum of functional respiratory abnormalities caused by the deformity. Long-term cardiopulmonary complications such as pulmonary hypertension and cor pulmonale are more common in early-onset IS and rarely seen in AIS. A follow-up study of untreated AIS found that only patients with thoracic curves >100° were at risk of respiratory failure, cor pulmonale, and death.[10]

It is widely accepted that alterations in pulmonary function are seen when the curvature exceeds 60°[11] and that pulmonary function is not significantly impaired until the thoracic curve reaches 100–120°. This assumption is based on a follow-up of 219 patients with untreated AIS.[1] However, a recent prospective study of 631 patients with AIS found that a proportion of patients with thoracic curves <50° had moderate to severe pulmonary impairment measured with PFT.[5]

Further decreases in lung volumes up to 60% occur after scoliosis surgery; the FVC and FEV_1 reach a nadir at the third postoperative day and can remain significantly decreased at 1 week. Baseline values are reached 1–2 months after surgery. These postoperative changes in lung function are seen both in idiopathic and neuromuscular scoliosis, as well as in anterior and posterior spine fusions.[12]

In the preoperative evaluation, special attention must be given to respiratory symptoms and exercise tolerance. The most common initial complaint is dyspnea on exertion. An increased risk of shortness of breath is associated with the combination of a Cobb angle greater than 80° and a deformity with a thoracic apex.[10] Zhang et al.[13] found a significant correlation between abnormal preoperative PFT and preoperative pulmonary symptoms. While pulmonary function tests might be useful in evaluating patients with AIS, they are often not performed because these patients present with fewer respiratory symptoms or specific concerns. However, Newton et al.[5] suggested that PFT should be considered in patients with AIS, particularly in patients with radiographic findings such as a structural cephalad curve, more than eight vertebral levels in the thoracic curve, or thoracic hypokyphosis.

According to the American Thoracic Society guidelines, pulmonary function is considered normal when TLC, FVC, and FEV_1 are >80% of predicted values; mildly impaired when the parameters are between 65% and 80%; moderately impaired when they are between 50% and 65%; and severely impaired when they are less than 50% of predicted values.

In summary, abnormal cardiopulmonary function is more common in early-onset IS patients, or any patient with a thoracic curve >100°, but Newton et al.[5] reported significant pulmonary impairment in some adolescents with thoracic curves <50°. Decreased lung volumes reach a maximum 3 days postoperatively and may take several months to reach baseline values. Patients with an FVC of less than 50% of predicted values have severely impaired pulmonary function and FVC <30% denotes a patient at risk of postoperative respiratory insufficiency requiring chronic ventilatory support. Preoperative results in this range necessitate a consultation with the family prior to surgery.

Assessment of cardiac function

Untreated patients with IS can develop chronic hypoxemia, hypercapnia, and ultimately increased pulmonary vascular resistance, pulmonary hypertension (PHT), and cardiac dysfunction. Children with early-onset scoliosis and those with significant curvatures are at greatest risk for progression to pulmonary hypertension and cor pulmonale. However, some patients have evidence of increased pulmonary vascular resistance in the absence of abnormal pulmonary function in the early stages of scoliosis development. This pathology is believed to result from impairment in the development of the pulmonary vasculature rather than a consequence of physiologic changes caused by the thoracic deformity.[14]

A good exercise tolerance indicates an adequate cardiopulmonary status. Signs of right heart failure in the physical examination are jugular venous distension, hepatomegaly, and peripheral edema. Any child with a borderline respiratory status or with decreased exercise tolerance should have an electrocardiogram (ECG) and an echocardiogram to evaluate left and right ventricular function. Late ECG signs of right ventricular hypertrophy and PHT include right axis deviation, a tall P wave >2.5 mm, and R >S in leads V1 and V2.[15] Echocardiography is a useful noninvasive tool to evaluate right and left ventricular structure and to estimate the degree of PHT as indicated by tricuspid regurgitation and increased right ventricular pressure. In addition, echocardiographic evidence of mitral valve prolapse (MVP) is found in 25% of patients with AIS, and in 53% of patients with AIS plus a family history of skeletal abnormality. This suggests that the cardiac and skeletal systems may be affected by a generalized soft tissue defect.[16] Nevertheless, MVP is rarely of hemodynamic significance.

Other considerations

Surgery for correction of scoliosis in children and adolescents is associated with intraoperative and postoperative blood loss that often results in the administration of allogenic blood products. Blood loss is related to the length of procedure and number of segments fused. In a review of the literature concerning intraoperative blood loss in pediatric spine fusion surgery, Shapiro and Sethna[17] found that AIS patients treated with anterior spine fusions (ASF) had the lowest mean blood loss, with values ranging between 350 and 650 ml or 60–135 ml per vertebral level, while the same group of patients treated with posterior spine fusions (PSF) had a mean estimated blood loss (EBL) ranging between 600 and 1000 ml or 65–150 ml per vertebral level. A correlation between number of vertebrae fused and blood loss has also been recognized in other studies.[18,19] Therefore, blood type and crossmatching are necessary prior to surgery with sufficient time to obtain compatible blood products in case the patient has unexpected positive antibodies. PT, PTT, INR, and platelet count are also recommended.

In AIS, preoperative autologous blood donation reduces allogenic blood exposure and seems to be cost effective.[20] Another method used to avoid or reduce allogenic blood transfusion during AIS surgery is acute normovolemic hemodilution. A baseline hematocrit value is needed to evaluate the feasibility of autologous blood predonation and to estimate the amount of blood that can be removed during hemodilution. In addition, patients with low hematocrit levels may also benefit from a consultation with a hematologist for iron supplementation or recombinant erythropoietin to raise preoperative hematocrit levels and facilitate predonation.

A baseline neurologic evaluation is also needed in order to establish whether neurologic deficits are present before surgery. This is especially important if a wake-up test is going to be used.

The wake-up or Stagnara test is sometimes performed during surgery to evaluate the integrity of motor pathways. It requires that the patient be awake in order to undergo a quick neurologic evaluation in the middle of the procedure. Due to the critical need for cooperation during this test, only patients of appropriate developmental age who can follow commands are suitable for this evaluation. Patients need to be assessed during the preoperative examination. The wake-up test and the questions that will be asked should be explained to the patient and parents and the child should be reassured that no pain will be felt during the test.

Finally, since scoliosis surgery is associated with blood loss and extensive fluid shifts, the placement of intravenous lines and invasive monitors is required, and such anesthesia procedures should be explained to the patient and family in a reassuring way.

Neuromuscular scoliosis

Neuromuscular disorders include a wide variety of diseases causing, in many cases, severe progressive scoliosis (Fig. 21.3). Common etiologies include cerebral palsy (CP), Duchenne muscular dystrophy (DMD), and spinal muscular atrophy (SMA).

Patients with CP represent the vast majority of patients with neuromuscular disorders presenting for spine surgery. The clinical presentation ranges from the cognitively intact patient with mild monoplegia to the severely compromised patient with spastic quadriplegia and mental retardation. The severity of the deformity correlates with the degree of neurologic involvement and decline in functional activities. The incidence of scoliosis is approximately 66% in nonambulatory CP patients.[21] Indications for surgery in CP patients include curves greater than 40° in a skeletally immature person and curves greater than 50° in a skeletally mature person.[22]

Duchenne muscular dystrophy is the most common cause of myopathic neuromuscular scoliosis (NMS).

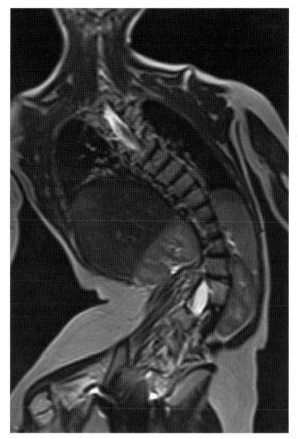

Figure 21.3 Spine MRI of a patient with spastic quadriplegia, showing severe scoliosis involving the thoracic and lumbar spine and pelvic obliquity.

Patients with DMD suffer from progressive muscular weakness resulting in increasing disability that leads to wheelchair dependence at about 10 years of age. The scoliosis then progresses with an acute deterioration seen during the adolescent growth spurt. Death commonly occurs in the second decade of life, usually from respiratory failure. Many centers operate on these children at an early stage of their scoliosis to improve quality and duration of life. Surgery is indicated once the curve reaches 20° since further progression at this point is inevitable.

Posterior instrumentation and fusion is the mainstay of surgical correction in NMS. Anterior release is reserved for severe deformities where a satisfactory correction cannot be obtained by posterior surgery alone. The aim of surgery for patients with NMS is to maximize the patient's function, prevent curve progression, and maintain a straight spine to allow comfortable sitting and aid nursing care. Correction of scoliosis does not affect decline in pulmonary function.

Patients with NMS have multiple comorbidities that may complicate the scoliosis repair. Furthermore, compared with patients with IS, surgery in these patients is usually extensive, involving more vertebral levels and is associated with blood losses sometimes exceeding the patient's estimated blood volume (EBV).

The preoperative evaluation of patients with NMS involves a multidisciplinary approach to carefully assess and understand the primary disease as well as to identify and optimize all the underlying medical conditions. Specific risks need to be evaluated prior to the surgical intervention to minimize postoperative complications. Key elements are the assessment of the patient's pulmonary, cardiovascular, hematologic, nutritional, gastrointestinal, and neurologic systems.

Assessment of pulmonary function

The cause of respiratory dysfunction in children with NMS is multifactorial. In addition to the mechanical distortion of the chest caused by the spine deformity, these patients have progressive muscle weakness due to lesions of the motor neurons or myopathy. Respiratory function may be further compromised by abnormalities in central respiratory drive, upper airway obstruction, nocturnal hypoventilation, poor cough reflexes, inability to clear secretions, pulmonary aspiration, and frequent respiratory infections. Chronic pulmonary aspiration can lead to fibrosis of pulmonary tissue and hypoxia. Also, reactive airway disease is common in patients with cerebral palsy. As a result, children with NMS have a more rapid deterioration in respiratory function with less severe curves than patients with AIS and are at risk of postoperative respiratory complications including atelectasis, bronchospasm, exacerbation of underlying chronic lung disease, and pneumonia and respiratory failure requiring prolonged mechanical ventilation and increased length of hospital stay.

In children with DMD, respiratory function steadily deteriorates throughout life, with an average reduction in vital capacity of 4% each year. A further 4% reduction is noted for every 10° progression of the Cobb angle.[23] A curve over 35° is usually associated with a VC ≤40% of the predicted normal.[24] Therefore, early surgical intervention is recommended prior to the development of large deformities and before forced vital capacity reaches <50% of the predicted values.

The surgical treatment of NMS has been associated with complication rates as high as 75%. In 1985, Anderson et al. reported an incidence of postoperative respiratory complications in children with NMS that was 5 times that of idiopathic scoliosis.[25] Similarly, Murphy et al. found that patients with NMS have higher rates of surgical wound infections and postoperative pneumonia, and are more likely to develop respiratory failure requiring mechanical ventilation.[26] Importantly, some studies have shown that patients with CP have the greatest complication rates.[25,27] A retrospective review of 107 patients with CP showed that postoperative complications after posterior spine fusion correlated with the severity of neurologic impairment, significant medical problems, and a spinal curvature >70°.[28]

Additional factors such as the duration of surgery, blood loss, and anterior or staged procedures influence the rate of respiratory complications and need for postoperative ventilation.[13,27,29] Recently, some surgeons have adopted a thoracoscopic approach to anterior release in an attempt to reduce pulmonary morbidity.

Although improvements in surgical and anesthetic techniques have reduced the complication rates in NMS, they remain higher than in other spinal deformities. Preoperative pulmonary function tests are an important parameter to predict the development of postoperative pulmonary complications and the need for postoperative ventilatory support.

Several studies have reported a strong association between decreased VC and increased postoperative pulmonary complications,[12,30,31] but others have shown that although pulmonary complications occur, surgery in patients with severe respiratory dysfunction can be undertaken successfully with a positive postoperative outcome.

In a retrospective review of 38 patients with NMS who underwent PSF, low preoperative VC correlated with pulmonary complications and the need for prolonged mechanical ventilation.[31] Similarly, Jenkins et al.[30] found that VC provided the best indicator for outcome and a VC <30% was associated with major respiratory complications in 48 children with DMD. Additionally, in a study of 125 patients who had scoliosis surgery, NMS patients with preoperative FEV_1 <40% were the most likely to require mechanical ventilation for more than 3 days while patients with IS were the least likely.[32] Likewise, VC and FEV_1 were significantly decreased in patients who required prolonged mechanical ventilation in a study of 46 NMS patients.[33]

Patients with progressive scoliosis and respiratory failure represent an anesthetic challenge. Frequently these patients are not considered surgical candidates on the basis of their respiratory status. Early reports even recommended preoperative tracheostomy in patients with severe restrictive lung disease.[15,34] AVC >35% was suggested by Weimann et al. for consideration of spinal surgery in DMD.[35]

In contrast to the previous studies mentioned, Rawlins et al.[36] looked at complications in 32 patients, 31 with congenital scoliosis and 1 with DMD with FVC <40%. The rate of major pulmonary complications was 19% and, although 3 patients required tracheostomy, there were no perioperative deaths. The authors concluded that spine surgery could be offered to patients with reduced FVC, but emphasized the importance of careful monitoring and a multidisciplinary approach in the perioperative care of these patients. Similarly, in a study of 21 patients with congenital and NMS with VC <45%, Wazeka et al. reported a complication rate of 33% with no perioperative deaths. Again, the authors emphasized the importance of a thorough preoperative evaluation including multiple subspecialties to optimize the patient before surgery.[37] Furthermore, Marsh et al. found similar complication rates and length of hospital stays when comparing DMD patients with a FVC >30% and patients with a FVC <30% after spinal surgery.[38] Finally, in a prospective study of 42 patients with nonidiopathic scoliosis, 76.2% of patients were safely extubated at the end of surgery without any further complications or need for re-intubation. An increased tendency for postoperative ventilation was observed in children with DMD and in those with a preoperative forced vital capacity <30%. The authors concluded that early extubation can be safely performed in this group of patients, but highlighted the importance of a comprehensive preoperative assessment and availability of intensive care support, as well as a standardized anesthetic technique including the use of short-acting anesthetics, drugs to reduce blood loss, and postoperative pain relief.[39]

The use of noninvasive positive-pressure ventilation (NIPPV) has improved significantly in the past 10 years, leading to improved perioperative care and improved survival, and has led to an increased number of high-risk surgeries being performed. Recent studies suggest that this therapy may decrease the need for prolonged mechanical ventilation or tracheostomy in patients with NMS and respiratory failure.

A prospective study of 45 DMD patients undergoing spinal surgery showed similar overall duration of respiratory support and hospital stay between patients with preoperative FVC >30% and <30%. In this study, all patients were transitioned to noninvasive

bilevel positive airway pressure (BiPAP) to facilitate early tracheal extubation, often with no more than 24 hours of mechanical ventilation.[40] Gill et al.[41] looked at 8 patients with underlying myopathy and progressive scoliosis with VC <30% who were on nocturnal noninvasive ventilation prior to spinal surgery. All patients were gradually weaned to BiPAP over 48 hours with no postoperative cardiac or pulmonary complications and a significant improvement in quality of life was observed in a follow-up. In addition, a study by Bach and Sabharwal followed 5 patients with DMD and SMA with VC <40% who were trained in the use of NIPPV and mechanically assisted coughing prior to spinal fusion. Patients were extubated by the third postoperative day to NIPPV despite ventilatory dependence and no patients developed pulmonary complications or required a tracheostomy.[42]

In summary, to minimize risk, a preoperative consultation with a pulmonologist, as well as close attention to postoperative ICU respiratory care should be anticipated. In our institution, all patients with NMS have a formal anesthesia consultation.

The importance of preoperative PFT in patients with NMS has been emphasized in many reviews.[43,44] PFT is recommended in patients who are able to cooperate. Most children with DMD are cognitively able to perform PFT. In patients with severe respiratory impairment, plans for postoperative ventilation and even tracheostomy should be discussed with the family or caregiver. However, PFT cannot be easily performed in patients with severe mental retardation or young age, but respiratory history, clinical examination, chest radiographs, and arterial blood gases can be valuable in the assessment of pulmonary status.

The history should include information about exercise tolerance in ambulatory patients, history of reflux and aspiration, and frequency and severity of respiratory infections, as well as symptoms of airway obstruction, nocturnal hypoventilation, and sleep apnea. Signs and symptoms that indicate restrictive lung disease include hypoxemia and dyspnea. The presence of rhonchi in the physical examination may indicate the inability to clear secretions. Upper airway obstruction can also be evident in the physical examination. The presence of an adequate cough is a good clinical indicator of a satisfactory forced expiratory volume. Patients with symptoms such as morning headache and daytime somnolence may need a polysomnographic evaluation and overnight continuous pulse oximetry to diagnose nocturnal hypoventilation or sleep apnea. The institution of nocturnal noninvasive ventilation probably helps to optimize these patients for surgery and should be continued postoperatively. The early use of nocturnal home ventilation has proved valuable for the survival of these children.[45] In addition, a chest radiograph is recommended to evaluate for signs of chronic aspiration and pneumonia and can also reveal cardiomegaly. Acute lower or upper respiratory infections should be treated aggressively before surgery.

Furthermore, arterial blood gases are indicated if the patient has resting hypoxemia or exertional dyspnea, or requires ventilatory support.

No evidence is available about the benefit of preoperative practice with noninvasive ventilation in patients with NMS. However, recently a multidisciplinary workgroup of experts recommended preoperative practice with noninvasive ventilation in patients with DMD and SMA with FVC <40% prior to spine surgery.[46]

In conclusion, the goal of the preoperative pulmonary evaluation in patients with NMS is to identify those children at increased risk of postoperative pulmonary complications or respiratory failure. Determining when it is no longer safe to anesthetize these children remains controversial and should be based on individual patient factors and not solely on results of PFT.

Assessment of cardiovascular function

Muscle disorders such as DMD affect not only skeletal muscle, but also cardiac and smooth muscle.[47] Although clinically significant cardiomyopathy rarely develops before 10 years of age, eventually all children with DMD will have cardiac dysfunction. Evidence of decreased cardiac function increases in frequency and severity from early adolescence and it has been found that over 90% of adolescents with DMD have subclinical or clinical cardiac involvement.[48] Severe cardiomyopathy that results in early death is seen in 10% of the patients.[45]

Assessment of cardiac function is necessary in all patients with DMD presenting for spinal surgery; however, exercise tolerance might be difficult to evaluate if the child is wheelchair bound.

Tests that aid in the cardiac evaluation include electrocardiography (ECG), echocardiography, chest radiography, and venous or arterial blood gases.

The cardiomyopathy of DMD is characterized by fibrosis of the posterobasal and lateral wall of the left ventricle and is associated with arrhythmias, ventricular dilatation and cardiac failure.

Classical ECG findings are sinus tachycardia, tall R waves in the right precordial leads, and deep Q waves in the left precordial leads and biventricular hypertrophy.[49] Other signs of cardiac dysfunction include prolongation of the PR interval, bundle branch block, and ST segment elevation or depression. In cases of arrhythmia, a 24-hour Holter monitor is required.

Echocardiography is recommended in patients with DMD. However, its value has been questioned due to some reports of acute intraoperative cardiac failure in patients with normal resting echocardiography undergoing spine fusion.[50,51] A normal echocardiogram might not indicate a normal cardiac reserve in this group of patients and does not evaluate the response of the myocardium to stress, such as that during major surgery. It has been proposed that more sensitive methods, such as stress echocardiography, be used to evaluate cardiac risk in these patients.[50] Additionally, intraoperative transesophageal echo may be necessary. An ejection fraction (EF) below 50% is associated with perioperative mortality. It is difficult to determine the point at which the risks of surgical complications outweigh the benefits of scoliosis surgery. Morris, in a recent editorial, considered a left ventricular ejection fraction (EF) of less than 50% and a forced vital capacity (FVC) of less than 25% a contraindication for elective surgery.[52] Similarly, in some centers an EF <30% is a contraindication for surgery in patients with DMD.[43]

In patients with CP, right ventricular dysfunction can develop as a result of increased pulmonary vascular resistance and PHT due to chronic hypoxia. A chest radiograph, an echocardiogram, and venous or arterial blood gases can assist in the screening for cardiac compromise in patients with CP and severe respiratory dysfunction in whom chronic hypoxia is suspected.

Hematologic considerations

Blood loss is a major issue in patients with NMS. A literature review of intraoperative blood loss in pediatric spine fusion surgery concluded that patients with NMS had the highest mean blood loss.[17] Similarly, other studies have shown that NMS patients have 6.9 times higher risk of bleeding more than 50% of their estimated blood volume (EBV)[53] and are 7.8 times more likely to receive an allogenic red blood cell transfusion than patients with other causes of scoliosis during spinal fusion surgery.[19] Meert et al.[19] found that NMS is the most important predictor of allogenic red cell transfusion.

365

The cause of increased blood loss in neuromuscular patients is not well understood and seems to be multifactorial. Often, these patients have multiple comorbidities and lower body weight, and undergo extensive fusions and longer surgeries than patients with IS. Patients with CP are often taking antiepileptic medications such as valproic acid, a known hepatotoxin and a cause of platelet dysfunction, as well as acquired von Willebrand factor type I deficiency. Although the potential association between valproic acid use and increased blood loss is controversial,[54,55] some centers check valproic acid levels preoperatively and surgery is delayed if the level is not in the low therapeutic range.[22]

Additionally, patients with neuromuscular disorders tend to be malnourished and underweight. Poor nutritional status can lead to impaired production of vitamin K-dependent clotting factors, increasing the risk of bleeding. Alterations in baseline coagulation factor levels and abnormal coagulation parameters early in the course of PSF have been documented in patients with spastic quadriplegia.[56] Furthermore, vascular smooth muscle dysfunction, increased fibrinolytic activity, and platelet function deficiency have all been reported in patients with DMD.[57–59] The platelet dysfunction in DMD patients may be the result of a reduction of expression of glycoprotein IV, also present in these patients.[57] Increased fibrinolytic activity seems to be induced by leakage of muscle components as a result of muscle degeneration and muscle destruction.[59]

Predonation of blood and acute normovolemic hemodilution are of less value in patients with NMS. Therefore, a CBC with platelet count, cross-matching of blood, and a coagulation profile are essential for these patients.

Awareness of the potential blood loss during scoliosis surgery, especially in children with NMS, warrants proper patient selection, careful preoperative planning, and implementation of strategies to minimize blood loss and transfusions.

Nutritional considerations

An adequate nutritional status is essential to meet the demands for the increased metabolic rate seen in the postoperative period. As previously stated, nutritional problems are common in patients with NMS. Patients with CP are often malnourished as a result of poor oropharyngeal control and gastroesophageal reflux that limits oral intake.

Poor nutritional status has been associated with higher complication rates after spine surgery[60,61] and can potentially lead to impaired production of vitamin K-dependent clotting factors, increasing the risk of bleeding. As a result, nutritional status needs to be carefully assessed during the preoperative evaluation of NMS patients.

A useful and simple tool for nutritional assessment is the growth chart. A weight for age below the 5th percentile is correlated with postoperative complications after scoliosis repair in CP patients.[28] Biochemical markers such as albumin, prealbumin, transferrin, and lymphocyte count are commonly used for the assessment of nutrition. Jevsevar and Karlin[61] evaluated 44 patients with CP and spastic quadriplegia who had spinal surgery for scoliosis. Patients with a preoperative albumin ≥ 3.5 g/dl and a total blood lymphocyte count $\geq 1.5 \times 10^3/\mu l$ had significantly lower rate of infection and a shorter period of tracheal intubation and hospitalization. The authors recommended that aggressive measures be used to improve the nutritional status when plasma albumin is <3.5 g/dl or the total lymphocyte count is $<1.5 \times 10^3/\mu l$.

Nutritional abnormalities should be addressed and corrected before spinal surgery. In some patients, a gastrostomy tube may be necessary to optimize the nutritional status before surgery. A gastrostomy tube also allows the administration of clear liquids up to 2 hours before the surgery, decreasing the risk of hypovolemia.

Gastrointestinal evaluation

Disorders of the swallowing mechanism, gastroesophageal reflux disease (GERD), and hiatal hernia are common in patients with CP. The most common signs and symptoms of these disorders are vomiting, tracheal aspiration, esophagitis, failure to thrive, malnutrition, and recurrent pneumonias. GERD can worsen after surgery. The Nissen fundoplication, a surgical treatment for GERD unresponsive to medical management, has had satisfactory results with control of the vast majority of the symptoms.

Preoperative assessment and treatment of gastroesophageal reflux is important in the prevention of aspiration pneumonia. Drvaric et al.[60] demonstrated a marked reduction in postoperative morbidity in patients with CP in whom surgical correction of esophageal abnormalities was done before spinal surgery, and recommended gastroesophageal and nutritional evaluation of all patients with CP before spinal surgery. If swallowing status has not been determined preoperatively, a barium swallow study is recommended to assess the risk of aspiration. For those patients with severe gastroesophageal reflux, a Nissen fundoplication should be done prior to surgery.

Neurologic evaluation

The neurologic evaluation in patients with NMS should include examination of motor function and tendon reflexes and should document any preexisting neurologic deficits and baseline neurologic status.

Seizures are present in approximately 30% of patients with CP. Optimum seizure control is required before surgery and antiepileptic medications should be continued until the morning of surgery and resumed as soon as possible in the postoperative period. Similarly, medications for the treatment of spasticity such as baclofen and diazepam should be continued in the perioperative period.

In patients who have vagal nerve stimulation (VNS) as part of their seizure treatment, the VNS device should be interrogated before the surgery to ensure that is working properly. As for a pacemaker, the use of electrocautery and external defibrillation can potentially damage the generator or electrodes. Although the VNS apparatus does not have to be deactivated before surgery, confirmation of correct functioning after surgery is recommended.[62]

Other considerations

Although it is now thought that DMD and other dystropinopathies are not associated with malignant hyperthermia (MH),[63] patients with Duchenne and Becker muscular dystrophy can develop a syndrome often confused with MH when exposed to potent inhalational anesthetics and succinylcholine. This MH-like syndrome consists of rhabdomyolysis, hyperkalemia, and cardiac arrest but often lacks the signs of hypermetabolism seen in MH. Some authors recommend that volatile agents and succinylcholine be avoided in these patients, especially now that intravenous anesthetics are readily available.[64,65] The history of hyperkalemia or cardiac arrest in previous anesthetics should alert the anesthesiologist about this possible complication.

Children with CP are exposed to multiple surgical procedures and latex allergens from an early age, increasing the risk of developing latex allergy. Therefore, the preoperative assessment of patients with NMS should also include screening questions for latex allergy. If latex allergy is present, the anesthesiologist and operating room staff should be notified with sufficient time to prepare a latex-free environment on the day of the surgery.

Many children with NMS have deformities and contractures of limb joints and have had prolonged neonatal intensive care units stays with multiple surgeries resulting in poor vascular access. These factors in addition to the presence of dehydration during the preoperative period can make vascular access extremely difficult. The preoperative evaluation should assess the patient for venous and central access difficulty. Planning may include consultation with the general surgeon to obtain adequate IV access before the surgery.

Ethical considerations

The decision-making process for spinal surgery in patients with NMS is often challenging. Evaluation of perioperative risks in patients with severe disability is difficult and social issues often complicate the preoperative assessment of these children. The likelihood of improving quality of life at the expense of increased morbidity and mortality needs to be considered.

Despite a high risk of postoperative complications and even death, Tsirikos et al.[66] found a mean predicted survival of 11 years for children with severe spastic CP after spinal scoliosis surgery. Furthermore, although there is little evidence that spine surgery improves respiratory function in this group of children, the overall satisfaction rate is high.[67-71] Parents and caregivers have reported improvement in overall health status, better sitting balance, and improved comfort and pain relief, as well as in activities of daily living and time required to provide care.

The preoperative evaluation should then assess individual patient's risks and the family's goals and expectations. A detailed and realistic explanation of risks of the anesthesia-related morbidity and the benefits of surgery is necessary before a decision can be made.

Children with normal intellect should be involved in the decision to accept the choice of surgery. The risk of death and resuscitation decision-making also needs consideration before surgery.

Congenital scoliosis

Congenital scoliosis is usually part of a generalized condition presenting at any age resulting from failure of vertebral segmentation and formation or a combination of both processes. The number of abnormal vertebrae and their location determines the severity

Table 21.2 Congenital syndromes and disorders associated with scoliosis[80–82]

Disorder/brief description	Clinical issues	Preoperative evaluation
Marfan's syndrome Autosomal dominant Tall stature Arachnodactyly with hyperextensibility	Cardiac abnormalities: 80%. Mitral and aortic valve insufficiency, ascending and descending aortic dilatation, dissecting aneurysm	Family history Cardiology consultation ECG, echocardiogram, cardiac MRI Pulmonary consultation PFT
Rett's syndrome Neurodevelopmental disorder Mutation of X chromosome MECP2 gene abnormality	Severe intellectual disability Seizures, nutritional problems, decreased bone density Progressive scoliosis	Preoperative evaluation in line with other neuromuscular disorders
Arthrogryposis Spectrum of different syndromes characterized by multiple joint contractures	Multiple joint contractures, decreased temporomandibular joint mobility, atlantoaxial instability, cardiac and renal abnormalities. Thoracic insufficiency syndrome.	Difficult peripheral and central venous access Careful assessment of the airway PFT, echocardiogram
Jarcho–Levin syndrome Autosomal recessive Short neck and trunk	Vertebral and rib congenital malformations Severe restrictive lung disease from chest hypoplasia, upper airway abnormalities, congenital diaphragmatic hernia, congenital heart disease	PFT or CT scan lung volumes ECG, echocardiography Cervical spine series Difficult intubation possible Noninvasive ventilation
Jeune's syndrome Autosomal recessive Rhizomelic dwarfism	Severe respiratory insufficiency, hepatic fibrosis, renal tubular dysplasia, cervical spine abnormalities	Cervical spine films Pulmonary consultation, PFT Liver function tests
Osteogenesis imperfecta Genetic disorder Autosomal dominant Short stature	Multiple fractures of long bones, growth deficiency Extremity deformities Restrictive pulmonary disease	High risk of bone fractures Careful intraoperative positioning Cardiac and pulmonary evaluation Calcium and phosphorus levels
Mucoplysaccharidosis Autosomal recessive Coarse features, protruding tongue Mental retardation	Metabolic storage disease with multiorgan involvement, coronary artery narrowing, cardiac valvular involvement, airway obstruction, excessive oral secretions	Pulmonary and cardiac evaluation Renal, liver evaluation Possible difficult ventilation/intubation
VACTER syndrome Autosomal recessive and X-linked forms	Vertebral anomalies, anal atresia, cardiac defects, tracheoesophageal fistula, renal and radial abnormalities	Pulmonary and cardiac assessment Evaluate neurologic and renal function
Neurofibromatosis Autosomal dominant Café-au-lait spots	Multiple neurofibromas of nerves and skin, seizures, skeletal anomalies, progressive thoracic scoliosis, renal artery stenosis, pheochromocytoma, laryngeal stenosis due to tumors	Evaluate for upper airway obstruction Cardiac evaluation, blood pressure measurement C-spine evaluation to rule out compression
Spinal muscle atrophy Autosomal recessive	Degeneration and loss of anterior horn cells, severe amyotrophic muscle weakness, with respiratory insufficiency	Evaluate extent of muscle weakness, pulmonary assessment, evaluate for pulmonary hypertension.

of the congenital curvature. The greatest progression usually occurs during periods of rapid growth such as the first three years of life and adolescence. Vertebral malformations with involvement of the thoracic cage may lead to the development of thoracic insufficiency and restrictive lung disease. Patients with congenital scoliosis may develop respiratory insufficiency with curves of less than 65°. Also, congenital scoliosis may be associated with other congenital defects in the cardiac, renal, or neurologic systems. In some cases, congenital scoliosis is a part of a syndrome.

The indications for surgery in congenital scoliosis depend on the underlying anomaly and the prediction for progression. Intraspinal abnormalities are found in 18–38% of patients with congenital spinal deformities[72–74] and their presence greatly increases the risk of neurologic injury during spine surgery. Hensinger et al. found a 14% incidence of congenital heart disease in patients with Klippel–Feil syndrome[75] and Basu et al.,[74] in a review of 126 patients with congenital scoliosis, found a 26% incidence of congenital heart disease. The most common anomalies were ventricular septal defects, patent ductus arteriosus, and tetralogy of Fallot. Additionally, the incidence of urologic abnormalities in patients with congenital spinal deformity ranges from 21% to 34%.[74-78] These patients should be carefully examined before spine surgery. Recently, Chan and Dormans reviewed and outlined the preoperative evaluation of patients with congenital vertebral malformations.[79]

Tests performed preoperatively include magnetic resonance imaging (MRI), echocardiography, and renal ultrasound. MRI is the more sensitive method for detecting intraspinal abnormalities. All patients with congenital scoliosis should have echocardiography as part of a preoperative work-up for spinal deformity surgery. Furthermore, a pulmonary function test should be obtained before surgery, but in the very young child who cannot tolerate pulmonary function testing a reasonable alternative is obtaining computed tomography lung volumes or a dynamic MRI. A cervical spine series with lateral flexion and extension to rule out instability should be obtained in children with cervical spine anomalies. Finally, airway evaluation is of particular importance, as many congenital syndromes are associated with difficult intubation.

Rare causes of scoliosis

There are many disorders and syndromes that are associated with scoliosis and other spine deformities. The preoperative evaluation in these patients requires an in-depth knowledge of the underlying pathology. The clinical issues of spine deformities in rare congenital syndromes have been recently reviewed.[80] Anesthetic considerations and recommendations for preoperative evaluation are outlined in Table 21.2.

References

1. Weinstein S, Zavala DC, Ponseti I. Idiopathic scoliosis: long-term follow-up and prognosis in untreated patients. *J Bone Joint Surg Am* 1981; **63**: 702.

2. Upadhyay S, Mullaji A, Luk K, *et al.* Relation of spinal and thoracic cage deformities and their flexibilities with altered pulmonary functions in adolescent idiopathic scoliosis. *Spine* 1995; **20**: 2415.

3. Jackson R, Simons E, Stripinis D. Coronal and sagittal plane spinal deformities correlating with back pain and pulmonary function in adult idiopathic scoliosis. *Spine* 1989; **14**: 1391.

4. Aaro S, Ohlund C. Scoliosis and pulmonary function. *Spine* 1984; **9**: 220.

5. Newton P, Faro F, Gollogly S, *et al.* Results of preoperative pulmonary function testing of adolescents with idiopathic scoliosis. a study of six hundred and thirty-one patients. *J Bone Joint Surg Am* 2005; **87**: 1937.

6. Gibson P. Anaesthesia for correction of scoliosis in children. *Anaesth Intensive Care* 2004; **32**: 548–59.

7. Barois A. Respiratory problems in severe scoliosis. *Bull Acad Nationale Méd* 1999; **183**: 721.

8. Branthwaite M. Cardiorespiratory consequences of unfused idiopathic scoliosis. *Br J Dis Chest* 1986; **80**: 360–9.

9. Pehrsson K, Larsson S, Oden A, *et al.* Long-term follow-up of patients with untreated scoliosis a study of mortality, causes of death, and symptoms. *Spine* 1992; **17**: 1091.

10. Weinstein S, Dolan L, Spratt K, *et al.* Health and function of patients with untreated idiopathic scoliosis: a 50-year natural history study. *JAMA* 2003; **289**: 559.

11. Muirhead A, Conner A. The assessment of lung function in children with scoliosis. *J Bone Joint Surg Br* 1985; **67**: 699.

12. Yuan N, Fraire J, Margetis M, *et al.* The effect of scoliosis surgery on lung function in the immediate postoperative period. *Spine* 2005; **30**: 2182.

13. Zhang J, Wang W, Qiu G, *et al.* The role of preoperative pulmonary function tests in the surgical treatment of scoliosis. *Spine* 2005; **30**: 218.

14. Primiano FP Jr, Nussbaum E, Hirschfeld S, *et al.* Early echocardiographic and pulmonary function findings in idiopathic scoliosis. *J Pediatr Orthop* 1983; **3**: 475.

15. Kafer E. Respiratory and cardiovascular functions in scoliosis and the principles of anesthetic management. *Anesthesiology* 1980; **52**: 339.

16. Hirschfeld S, Rudner C, Nash CL Jr. *et al.* Incidence of mitral valve prolapse in adolescent scoliosis and thoracic hypokyphosis. *Pediatrics* 1982; **70**: 451.

17. Shapiro F, Sethna N. Blood loss in pediatric spine surgery. *Eur Spine J* 2004; **13**: 6–17.

18. Guay J, Haig M, Lortie L, *et al.* Predicting blood loss in surgery for idiopathic scoliosis. *Can J Anesth* 1994; **41**: 775–81.

19. Meert K, Kannan S, Mooney JF. Predictors of red cell transfusion in children and adolescents undergoing spinal fusion surgery. *Spine* 2002; **27**: 2137.

20. Murray D, Forbes R, Titone M, *et al.* Transfusion management in pediatric and adolescent scoliosis surgery. efficacy of autologous blood. *Spine* 1997; **22**: 2735–40.

21. Hodgkinson I, Berard C, Chotel F, *et al.* Pelvic obliquity and scoliosis in non-ambulatory patients with cerebral palsy: a descriptive study of 234 patients over 15 years of age. *Rev Chir Orthop Réparatrice Appareil Moteur* 2002; **88**: 337.

22. Thomson J, Banta J. Scoliosis in cerebral palsy: an overview and recent results. *J Pediatr Orthop B* 2001; **10**: 6.

23. Kurz L, Mubarak S, Schultz P, *et al.* Correlation of scoliosis and pulmonary function in Duchenne muscular dystrophy. *J Pediatr Orthop* 1983; **3**: 347.

24. Smith AD, Koreska J, Moseley C. Progression of scoliosis in Duchenne muscular dystrophy. *J Bone Joint Surg* 1989; **71**: 1066.

25. Anderson P, Puno M, Lovell S, *et al.* Postoperative respiratory complications in non-idiopathic scoliosis. *Acta Anaesthesiol Scand* 1985; **29**: 186–92.

26. Murphy N, Firth S, Jorgensen T, *et al.* Spinal surgery in children with idiopathic and neuromuscular scoliosis. What's the difference? *J Pediatr Orthop* 2006; **26**: 216.

27. Sarwahi V, Sarwark J, Schafer M, *et al.* Standards in anterior spine surgery in pediatric patients with neuromuscular scoliosis. *J Pediatr Orthop* 2001; **21**: 756.

28. Lipton G, Miller F, Dabney K, *et al.* Factors predicting postoperative complications following spinal fusions in children with cerebral palsy. *J Spinal Disord Tech* 1999; **12**: 197.

29. Mohamad F, Parent S, Pawelek J, *et al.* Perioperative complications after surgical correction in neuromuscular scoliosis. *J Pediatr Orthop* 2007; **27**: 392.

30. Jenkins J, Bohn D, Edmonds J, *et al.* Evaluation of pulmonary function in muscular dystrophy patients requiring spinal surgery. *Crit Care Med* 1982; **10**: 645.

31. Padman R, Mcnamara R. Postoperative pulmonary complications in children with neuromuscular scoliosis who underwent posterior spinal fusion. *Delaware Med J* 1990; **62**: 999.

32. Yuan N, Skaggs D, Dorey F, *et al.* Preoperative predictors of prolonged postoperative mechanical ventilation in children following scoliosis repair. *Pediatr Pulmonol* 2005; **40**: 414–19.

33. Udink Ten Cate F, Van Royen B, Van Heerde *et al.* Incidence and risk factors of prolonged mechanical ventilation in neuromuscular scoliosis surgery. *J Pediatr Orthop B* 2008; **17**: 203.

34. Sakai DN, Hsu J, Bonnett C, *et al.* Stabilization of the collapsing spine in Duchenne muscular dystrophy. *Clin Orthop Relat Res* 1977; **128**: 256.

35. Weimann R, Gibson D, Moseley C, *et al.* Surgical stabilization of the spine in Duchenne muscular dystrophy. *Spine* 1983; **8**: 776.

36. Rawlins B, Winter R, Lonstein J, *et al.* Reconstructive spine surgery in pediatric patients with major loss in vital capacity. *J Pediatr Orthop* 1996; **16**: 284.

37. Wazeka A, Dimaio M, Boachie-Adjei O. Outcome of pediatric patients with severe restrictive lung disease following reconstructive spine surgery. *Spine* 2004; **29**: 528.

38. Marsh A, Edge G, Lehovsky J. Spinal fusion in patients with Duchenne's muscular dystrophy and a low forced vital capacity. *Eur Spine J* 2003; **12**: 507–12.

39. Almenrader N, Patel D. Spinal fusion surgery in children with non-idiopathic scoliosis: is there a need for routine postoperative ventilation? *Br J Anaesth* 2006; **97**: 851–7.

40. Harper C, Ambler G, Edge G. The prognostic value of pre-operative predicted forced vital capacity in corrective spinal surgery for Duchenne's muscular dystrophy. *Anaesthesia* 2004; **59**: 1160–2.

41. Gill I, Eagle M, Mehta J, *et al.* Correction of neuromuscular scoliosis in patients with preexisting respiratory failure. *Spine* 2006; **31**: 2478.

42. Bach J, Sabharwal S. High pulmonary risk scoliosis surgery: role of noninvasive ventilation and related techniques. *J Spinal Disord Tech* 2005; **18**: 527.

43. Soudon P, Hody JL, Bellen P. Preoperative cardiopulmonary assessment in the child with neuromuscular scoliosis. *J Pediatr Orthop B* 2000; **9**: 229–33.

44. Pruijs JE, Van Tol MJ, Van Kesteren RG, *et al.* Neuromuscular scoliosis: clinical evaluation pre- and postoperative. *J Pediatr Orthop B* 2000; **9**: 217–20.

45. Eagle M, Baudouin S, Chandler C, *et al.* Survival in Duchenne muscular dystrophy: improvements in life expectancy since 1967 and the impact of home nocturnal ventilation. *Neuromusc Disord* 2002; **12**: 926–9.

46. Mullender M, Blom N, De Kleuver M, *et al.* A Dutch guideline for the treatment of scoliosis in neuromuscular disorders. *Scoliosis* 2008; **3**: 14.

47. Boland BJ, Silbert P, Groover R, *et al.* Skeletal, cardiac, and smooth muscle failure in Duchenne muscular dystrophy. *Pediat Neurol* 1996; **14**: 7–12.

48. Finister J, Stollberger C. The heart in human dystrophinopathies. *Cardiology* 2003; **99**: 1–19.

49. Perloff J, Roberts W. The distinctive electrocardiogram of Duchenne's progressive muscular dystrophy: an electrocardiographic–pathologic correlative study. *Am J Med* 1967; **42**: 179–88.

50. Schmidt G, Burmeister M, Lilje C, *et al.* Acute heart failure during spinal surgery in a boy with Duchenne muscular dystrophy. *Br J Anaesth* 2003; **90**: 800.

51. Sethna N, Rockoff M, Worthen H, *et al.* anesthesia-related complications in children with Duchenne muscular dystrophy. *Anesthesiology* 1988; **68**: 462.

52. Morris P. Duchenne muscular dystrophy: a challenge for the anaesthetist. *Pediat Anesth* 1997; **7**: 1–4.

53. Edler A, Murray D, Forbes R. Blood loss during posterior spinal fusion surgery in patients with neuromuscular disease: is there an increased risk? *Pediatr Anesth* 2003; **13**: 818–22.

54. Winter S, Kriel R, Novacheck T, *et al.* Perioperative blood loss: the effect of valproate. *Pediat Neurol* 1996; **15**: 19–22.

55. Chambers H, Weinstein C, Mubarak S, *et al.* The effect of valproic acid on blood loss in patients with cerebral palsy. *J Pediatr Orthop* 1999; **19**: 792.

56. Brenn B, Theroux M, Dabney K, *et al.* Clotting parameters and thromboelastography in children with neuromuscular and idiopathic scoliosis undergoing posterior spinal fusion. *Spine* 2004; **29**: E310.

57. Forst J, Forst R, Leithe H, *et al.* Platelet function deficiency in Duchenne muscular dystrophy. *Neuromuscul Disord* 1998; **8**: 46–9.

58. Noordeen M, Haddad F, Muntoni F, *et al.* Blood loss in Duchenne muscular dystrophy: vascular smooth muscle dysfunction? *J Pediatr Orthop B* 1999; **8**: 212.

59. Saito T, Takenaka M, Miyai I, *et al.* Coagulation and fibrinolysis disorder in muscular dystrophy. *Muscle Nerve* 2001; **24**: 399–402.

60. Drvaric D, Roberts J, Burke S, *et al.* Gastroesophageal evaluation in totally involved cerebral palsy patients. *J Pediatr Orthop* 1987; **7**: 187.

61. Jevsevar D, Karlin L. The relationship between preoperative nutritional status and complications after an operation for scoliosis in patients who have cerebral palsy. *J Bone Joint Surg* 1993; **75**: 880.

62. Hatton K, Mclarney J, Pittman T, *et al.* Vagal nerve stimulation: overview and implications for anesthesiologists. *Anesth Analg* 2006; **103**: 1241.

63. Finsterer J. Current concepts in malignant hyperthermia. *J Clin Neuromuscul Dis* 2002; **4**: 64.

64. Yemen T, Mcclain C. Muscular dystrophy, anesthesia and the safety of inhalational agents revisited; Again. *Pediatr Anesth* 2006; **16**: 105–8.

65. Hayes J, Veyckemans F, Bissonnette B. Duchenne muscular Dystrophy: an old anesthesia problem revisited. *Pediatr Anesth* 2008; **18**: 100–6.

66. Tsirikos A, Miller F, Glutting J. Life expectancy in pediatric patients with cerebral palsy and neuromuscular scoliosis who underwent spinal fusion. *Dev Med Child Neurol* 2003; **45**: 677–82.

67. Bridwell K, Baldus C, Iffrig T, *et al.* Process measures and patient/parent evaluation of surgical management of spinal deformities in patients with progressive flaccid neuromuscular scoliosis (Duchenne's muscular dystrophy and spinal muscular atrophy). *Spine* 1999; **24**: 1300.

68. Comstock C, Leach J, Wenger D. Scoliosis in total-body-involvement cerebral palsy: analysis of surgical treatment and patient and caregiver satisfaction. *Spine* 1998; **23**: 1412.

69. Jones K, Sponseller P, Shindle M, *et al.* Longitudinal parental perceptions of spinal fusion for neuromuscular spine deformity in patients with totally involved cerebral palsy. *J Pediatr Orthop* 2003; **23**: 143.

70. Larsson E, Aaro S, Normelli H, *et al.* Long-term follow-up of functioning after spinal surgery in patients with neuromuscular scoliosis. *Spine* 2005; **30**: 2145.

71. Watanabe K, Lenke LG, Daubs MD, *et al.* Is spine deformity surgery in patients with spastic cerebral palsy truly beneficial? A patient/parent evaluation. *Spine (Phila Pa 1976)* 2009 Sep 15; **34**(20): 2222–32.

72. Bradford D, Heithoff K, Cohen M. Intraspinal abnormalities and congenital spine deformities: a radiographic and MRI study. *J Pediatr Orthop* 1991; **11**: 36.

73. Mcmaster M. Occult intraspinal anomalies and congenital scoliosis. *J Bone Joint Surg* 1984; **66**: 588.

74. Basu P, Elsebaie H, Noordeen M. Congenital spinal deformity: a comprehensive assessment at presentation. *Spine* 2002; **27**: 2255–9.

75. Hensinger R, Lang J, Macewen G. Klippel–Feil syndrome: a constellation of associated anomalies. *J Bone Joint Surg* 1974; **56**: 1246.

76. Bernard TN Jr, Burke S, Johnston CE 3rd, *et al.* Congenital spine deformities. a review of 47 cases. *Orthopedics* 1985; **8**: 777.

77. Guerrero G, Saieh C, Dockendorf I, *et al.* Genitourinary anomalies in children with congenital scoliosis. *Rev Chil Pediatr* 1989; **60**: 281–3.

78. Macewen G, Winter R, Hardy J. Evaluation of kidney anomalies in congenital scoliosis. *J Bone Joint Surg* 1972; **54**: 1451.

79. Chan G, Dormans J. Update on congenital spinal deformities: preoperative evaluation. *Spine* 2009; **34**: 1766.

80. Campbell R Jr. Spine deformities in rare congenital syndromes: clinical issues. *Spine* 2009; **34**: 1815.

81. Butler M, Hayes B, Hathaway M, *et al.* Specific genetic diseases at risk for sedation/anesthesia complications. *Anesth Analg* 2000; **91**: 837.

82. Downs J, Bergman A, Carter P, *et al.* Guidelines for management of scoliosis in Rett's syndrome patients based on expert consensus and clinical evidence. *Spine* 2009; **34**: E607.

22

Fluid management and monitoring of the pediatric patient

Tunga Suresh, Patrick M. Callahan, and Peter J. Davis

Key points

- A comprehensive knowledge of renal physiology in pediatrics is important in the management of fluid and electrolytes.
- Colloids have a defined but limited role in the pediatric patient undergoing spinal surgery.
- Glucose should be used cautiously in the perioperative period.
- The indications for blood and blood components vary even within this subgroup.
- Monitoring techniques in pediatrics are unique and the parameters specific for different age groups.

Introduction

This chapter will focus on fluid management of children undergoing spinal surgery and on the monitoring of such patients. Fluid management issues to be addressed will include the use of crystalloid versus colloid, transfusion triggers, and blood component administration. Monitoring issues will focus on the value of various monitoring modalities and their application in children.

Fluid management

Knowledge of the fluid compartments and a thorough understanding of renal physiology and the fundamental differences in the various age groups form the cornerstone in the management of fluid and electrolytes in the perioperative period in the pediatric patient. There are several peculiarities to contend with in the pediatric population undergoing spinal surgery, including but not limited to: the need for strict control of perioperative glucose levels; avoiding fluids that could cause a hypocoagulable state; maintaining perfusion to the vital organs; avoiding major changes

in the electrolytes; and maintaining a steady hemodynamic state to allow for a meaningful intraoperative neurophysiological monitoring. Though several controversies have erupted in the recent past regarding the type of fluid to be used and the aggressiveness with which to treat the child, basic concepts have amazingly remained the same for over half a century. Some of the concepts expounded by Holliday and Segar in their original description of the "maintenance need for water in parental fluid therapy in pediatrics" have survived the test of time, albeit with minor modifications.[1]

Body fluid compartments and their differences in the pediatric patient

The total body water and total blood volume vary considerably from the premature infant to the older child. *Total body water* is about 80% in the premature child,[2] decreasing to around 75% at term and eventually reaching the adult values of about 57% at the age of 18 years. Approximate *blood volumes* are around 90–105 ml/kg in the premature infant to about 65–70 ml/kg in the adult population (Table 22.1). The one-third rule holds true for the body fluid compartments. The total body fluid is distributed between the extracellular and intracellular spaces. One-third of the total body fluid is in the extracellular space and is known as extracellular fluid (ECF); the remaining two-thirds is in the intracellular space, and is known as intracellular fluid (ICF). One-third of the ECF is plasma; the rest is in the interstitial space. Fluid in bone and dense connective tissue is significant but is mobilized slowly; the rest of the interstitial fluid and plasma constitutes a functional space that is sometimes referred to as functional extracellular fluid. It should be recognized that all fluid compartments are in continuity and the differences between the various fluid compartments are purely a function and a result of the cell membranes separating them. The implications of this are quite profound. In a diseased state such as

Anesthesia for Spine Surgery, ed. Ehab Farag. Published by Cambridge University Press. © Cambridge University Press 2012.

sepsis the cell membranes are more porous and unable to function adequately, leading to equalization across the different fluid compartments.

The maintenance of plasma volume is essential for adequate tissue perfusion. The major ion in the intracellular compartment is potassium, whereas the major ion in the extracellular fluid is sodium. The difference in the sodium and potassium levels in the various compartments is maintained by the Na^+/K^+ ATPase pump in the cell membrane.

The renal system

The primary function of the kidney is as an excretory organ; however, it also has other vital functions including regulation of salt and water, acid–base balance, and secretion of hormones (Fig. 22.1). The kidneys of a newborn are still immature and have not developed fully. Glomerular filtration rate, which is used as a measure of renal function, is as low as $21\ ml/min/1.73\ m^2$ in the newborn. It increases to $60\ ml/min/1.73\ m^2$ by the age of 2 weeks and reaches adult values of $90\ ml/min/1.73\ m^2$ by about 2 years. This relative immaturity of the renal system in the newborn may lead to difficulties in handling salt and water loads.[3]

Osmotic regulation

The regulation of tonicity is primarily a function of vasopressin, which is synthesized by the hypothalamus and released by the posterior lobe of the pituitary gland (Fig. 22.2). The total body osmolality is the sum of the major ions in the body divided by the total body water ([sodium + potassium]/total body water). However the osmolality of the extracellular fluid is due in the main to the concentration of sodium in this compartment. A decrease in pure water is sensed through the osmotic receptors in the hypothalamus, leading to an increase in the production of arginine vasopressin (AVP), which is also known as the antidiuretic hormone (ADH) or argipressin or simply vasopressin. ADH in turn modulates the secretion of water via the kidney. It also has an effect on the intake of water. A neonate can concentrate urine to a maximum of 600 mOsm/l in response to water deprivation, compared to about 1200 mOsm/l in

Table 22.1 Blood volumes in different age groups

Age group	Approximate blood volume (ml/kg)
Premature infant <1.5 kg	90–110
Neonate (0–28 days)	80–90
Infant (1–12 months)	75–80
Preschoolers	75–85
4–6 years	80–85
7–18 years	85–90
Adult	65–75

Adapted from *Smith's Anesthesia for Infants and Children*. 7th edition, 2006 Table 11.2: Chapter 11, p. 367.

Figure 22.1 Functions of the kidney.

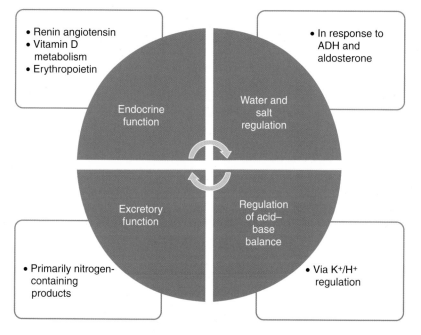

- Renin angiotensin
- Vitamin D metabolism
- Erythropoietin

Endocrine function

- In response to ADH and aldosterone

Water and salt regulation

Excretory function

- Primarily nitrogen-containing products

Regulation of acid–base balance

- Via K^+/H^+ regulation

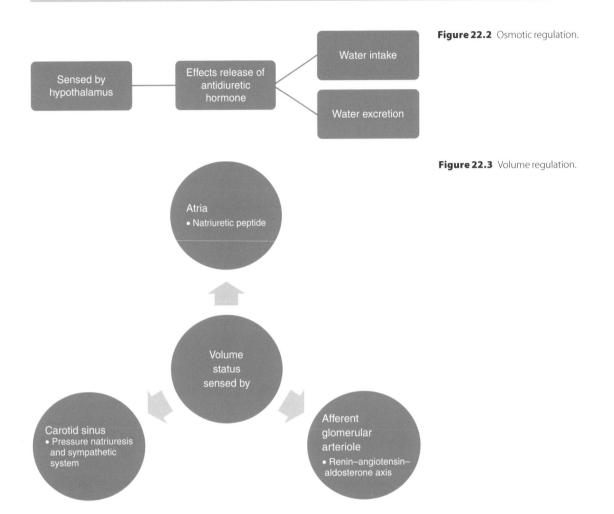

Figure 22.2 Osmotic regulation.

Figure 22.3 Volume regulation.

an adult. This ability improves rapidly over the first few weeks of life to almost adult levels by the first month. Although a full-term infant can conserve sodium, a preterm infant is unable to do so. This is the one of the main reasons that a neonate needs a fluid management plan that is quite distinct from the older child. On the other hand, the newborn is able to excrete very dilute urine in the range of 30–50 mOsmol/l.

Volume regulation

The body recognizes changes in the volume status in several ways (Fig. 22.3). Volume changes may be iso-osmotic as in situations where there is a loss of water and electrolytes such as in acute blood loss. These changes are sensed via baroreceptors that are present in the afferent arteriole of the glomerulus. This initiates a cascade of events leading to the activation of angiotensin II. Angiotensin II acts on the adrenal cortex to release aldosterone, which leads to conservation of sodium and water. Through its action on the hypothalamus, angiotensin II also releases antidiuretic hormone. Angiotensin II also has direct effects on the peripheral vasculature. The atria and the carotid sinus are equally important in sensing changes in the volume status. They effect their changes via the natriuretic peptides and the autonomic nervous system, respectively. From the carotid sinus afferent impulses travel via the nerve of Herring, through the glossopharyngeal nerve to synapse at the nucleus tractus solitarius. The nucleus tractus solitarius modulates the autonomic nervous system to effect changes in the vascular and cardiac responses.

Tenets governing perioperative fluid therapy in pediatrics

Osmolality

There appears to be a gradual shift in trends in the fluid management of patients undergoing neurosurgery, reflecting the better understanding of the pathophysiology of neuronal injury. It has been a strictly enforced rule to restrict fluids in neuroanesthesia. Conceptual awareness of the risks of hypotension-related ischemic injury has lead to the recognition of the need to maintain hemodynamic parameters such as mean arterial pressure and perfusion pressure to prevent this. In turn this has led to a measured but pragmatic use of intravenous fluids among neuroanesthesiologists.

It is worth reviewing the reasons behind the original dictum of restricting fluids and the potential implications of the changing trends. It is important to stress that the fluid strategies being discussed pertain mainly to patients with brain injury. However, an understanding of this will help with a formulation of a fluid plan based on scientific principles and available evidence.

There is a fundamental difference between the peripheral vasculature and the vessels in the brain. The desmosomes in the peripheral vessels along with the endothelial cells form a barrier membrane which maintains the integrity of the vessel. The membrane is relatively porous when compared with the intracranial vasculature, with pores as wide as 6–7 nm (60–70 Å) in the peripheral vasculature. The brain is kept immune from small changes in the extracellular fluid by the blood–brain barrier (BBB). The tight junctions in the intracranial vessels restrict the pore size to around 0.5–0.7 nm (5–7 Å), resulting in a more robust barrier. The implication of this is fairly simple. The peripheral vessel allows free exchange of small solutes such as the electrolytes, but larger molecules such as plasma proteins cross with greater difficulty. In the brain, particles cross the BBB depending on their fat solubility, rather than on size alone. The premise that this BBB is breached in injury is what has prompted anesthesiologists to be cautious in the use of fluids in general. In this situation, changes in the composition of the extracellular fluid will have a greater impact on solutes crossing this barrier along with the resultant movement of the solvent, leading to brain edema and potential increase in the intracranial pressure. There is evidence to suggest that excessive use of crystalloids, which leads to a decrease in colloid osmotic pressure, can result in brain edema even in the normal brain.[4] The colloid osmotic pressure – also known as the oncotic pressure – is the osmotic pressure exerted by the plasma proteins, which are larger molecules contained within the plasma. The capillary and interstitial oncotic pressures, the capillary and interstitial hydrostatic pressures, along with the filtration coefficient are the major variables in the

Starling equation. Hypertonic fluids can cause thromboses of the peripheral vein and can lead to fluid shift from inside the cell into the extracellular fluid.

The role of the endothelial glycocalyx is of considerable significance. The endothelial cells, along with this layer, which is composed of proteoglycans and glycoproteins, form a dual barrier that is fundamental to the integrity of the vascular endothelium. The endothelial glycocalyx also protects against platelet and leukocyte adhesion. Among mediators that affect the endothelial glycocalyx are proteases, tumor necrosis factor α, oxidized low-density lipoproteins, and atrial natriuretic peptide. Maintaining normovolemia (avoiding hypervolemia) in the perioperative period could be decisive in preserving this protective layer. This can help prevent pathological edema as a result of fluid shifts.

The administration of isotonic fluids is preferable to the administration of hypotonic or hypertonic fluids. Administration of nonisotonic fluids leads to increased changes in the presence of a decreased ability of the kidneys to concentrate, particularly in neonates. The lowest concentration of glucose in commercially available intravenous fluids for clinical use is currently 5% in the USA. This essentially means that fluids containing sodium *and* glucose that are isotonic (Dextrose 2.5% in 0.45 NaCl) can only have a maximum sodium concentration of about 70 mEq/l. The glucose in the intravenous fluid contributes to the rest of the osmolality. Once administered, the glucose in the solution is transported into the cell and is then metabolized. This leaves the remaining administered fluid hypotonic relative to plasma. In the context of tissue at risk during spine surgery, i.e., potential ischemia of the spinal cord, this becomes critical, predisposing and contributing to tissue edema of the injured tissue. Table 22.2 outlines the osmolality and electrolyte composition of different intravenous crystalloid solutions commonly used in pediatrics.

Water requirements

The basis for the common use of the 4–2–1 rule is the proposals put forth by Holliday and Segar in their paper "The maintenance need for water in parenteral fluid therapy" in 1957.[1] They recognized the close relationship of the calories utilized to the amount of water required from studies done by their peers and suggested a simplified formula for intravenous fluid management. These guidelines have stood the test of time, albeit with a few modifications. The fact that these guidelines have come in for criticism is rather a result of misinterpretation of their suggestions than due to a strict adherence

375

Table 22.2 Commonly used crystalloids and their electrolyte content

Fluid	Osmolarity (mOsmol/l)	Na (mEq/l)	Cl (mEq/l)	K (mEq/l)	Ca (mEq/l)	Calories (cal/l)
0.9% NaCl	308	154	154	–	–	–
0.45% NaCl	154	77	77	–	–	–
Lactated Ringer	272	130	109	4	3	9
Ringer solution	310	147.5	156	4	4.5	–
Dextrose 2.5% 0.45% NaCl	280	77	77	–	–	85
Dextrose 5% 0.45% NaCl	406	77	77	–	–	170
Dextrose 10% 0.2% NaCl	575	34	34	–	–	340
D10W	505	–	–	–	–	340
D10 0.45%NaCl	660	77	77	–	–	340
Plasmalyte-R	312	140	103	10	5	Acetate 47 lactate 8

Adapted from *Smith's Anesthesia for Infants and Children*. 7th edition, 2006, Table 4.8: Chapter 4, p. 122.

to their guidelines. It was estimated that the urinary losses along with insensible losses through the skin and lungs amount to 100 ml for every 100 kcal (418 kilojoues) metabolized. They then calculated that the calorific requirements for a child weighing 0–10 kg were about 100 kcal per kg per day. Since metabolism of 100 kcal requires 100 ml of water, they proposed that the maintenance water required for these children was 100 ml/kg/day or 4 ml/kg/h. Children who were a little older required less caloric intake. In summary, caloric requirements approximated to 100 kcal/kg/day for the first 10 kg and 50 kcal/kg/day for each of the next 10 kg. For every kilogram beyond 20, the child required a further 25 kcal per day. This amounts to 4 ml/kg/h for the first 10 kg, 2 ml/kg/h for the next 10 kg, and 1 ml/kg/h of water for every kilogram thereafter. This calculation of the water requirement has been relatively unchallenged to date and forms a perfectly acceptable basis for calculation of the maintenance needs.

The criticism leveled at Holliday and Segar's original proposal is aimed at the calculation of the amount of sodium required. They suggested that a child needs about 3 mEq of sodium, 2 mEq of potassium, and 2 mEq of chloride per 100 kcal per day. This was based on the amount of electrolytes in breast milk and cow's milk and the amount of milk consumed by a child; they then doubled it to ensure that the maintenance was adequate. They suggested that the maintenance fluid that was most appropriate was D5 in 0.2% normal saline. They also added, "as with any method, an understanding of the limitations and exceptions to the

system is required. Even more essential is the clinical judgment to modify the system as circumstances dictate." In addition they acknowledged that "with respect to maintenance need for electrolytes, less precise data are available and figures considerably in excess of minimum requirements are readily handled."

The most commonly used guidelines in the perioperative period are modifications and adaptations of the formula proposed by Holliday and Segar. Berry's modification is the most widely quoted in textbooks of pediatric anesthesia. Berry suggested that children younger than 3 years should receive a bolus of 25 ml/kg of basic salt solution over the first hour of surgery. For children older than 3 years Berry suggested that they should receive 15 ml/kg in the first hour. This was based on Furman's calculation of the fluid deficit of the child coming in for surgery. The assumption was that the child would be fasted for between 6 and 8 hours before surgery. Since the revised guidelines for preoperative fasting in children, where the child is allowed clear fluids up to 2 hours prior to surgery, the above formulae lead to an overestimation and overtreatment of the fluid deficit.[5]

Another method of calculating the maintenance requirement is to use the body surface as the index. It has been proposed that a child requires 1500 ml/m² per day; proponents of this formula also suggest that the sodium requirements are roughly 30–50 mEq/m² per day, and the potassium requirement is 20–40 mEq/m² per day. This formula does not appear to have gained favor amongst most anesthesiologists.

Assessment of water requirement should take into account the deficit, the maintenance needs and ongoing losses. Ongoing losses include loss into the third space, which can be difficult to assess. The excessive movement of fluid from the intravascular compartment into the interstitium is known as *third space loss*. The sequestration of fluid into the interstitium is pronounced in ischemic areas. The goal of therapy is to ensure an adequate plasma volume and this should guide fluid management. Replacement of third-space loss in the first instance should probably be with isotonic crystalloids.

Colloids versus crystalloids

The arguments for and against the use of colloids have been ongoing for a very long time. The pertinence of this argument with respect to fluid management of the patient undergoing spine surgery will be apparent when you consider the reasons put forth by the two groups. The "colloid group" argues that unless a colloid is used in the fluid administered, the fluid rapidly redistributes within the whole of the extracellular fluid compartment. It therefore takes a larger volume of infused fluid to achieve an effective plasma volume if a crystalloid is used. The corresponding increase in the interstitial fluid could be detrimental in tight spaces such as around the spinal cord. The use of a colloid in this situation allows for better containment of the administered fluid within the plasma along with preservation of the colloid osmotic pressure. They also argue that saline-based intravenous fluids, due to their higher chloride content have an effect on the bicarbonate regulation by the kidney, which can lead to hyperchloremic metabolic acidosis. Chloride also has an effect on the renal blood flow and appears to delay the recovery of renal function. However, it should be pointed out that colloids are in suspension in a crystalloid-based intravenous fluid and therefore the latter argument is a weak one. The typical content of sodium in colloids range from 130 to 160 mEq/l and the accompanying chloride is roughly in the same range.

The "crystalloid group" argues that while the above is true and holds good in a nondiseased state, it has a very different implication in the diseased state. In a critically ill patient or one in whom the vascular permeability is increased as in sepsis, the colloid will actually leak into the interstitial space, increasing the oncotic pressure within the interstitium. This can theoretically lead to a more intractable type of edema as mobilization of this fluid will require metabolism of the colloid that has left the plasma. It becomes apparent that in areas where there is a localized breach in the capillary/interstitial barrier (such as ischemic areas in the spine), the leakage of the given colloid could be counterproductive.

Colloids

The colloids can be grouped into natural colloids derived from plasma, such as albumin, and all the others, which are classified as synthetic colloids. The synthetic colloids include those that contain hydroxyethyl starch (HES), gelatins, or dextrans.

HES comprises modified polymers of amylopectin. Hydroxyethyl starches are a heterogeneous group of fluids. HES contains glycogen-like modified polysaccharides derived from either waxy maize starch or potato starch. The following factors define their characteristics.

(a) The molecular weight (MW). The various hetastarches in use have MWs ranging from 70 to 670 kDa. HES with higher MWs are associated with a higher side effect profile. HES with a lower MW are metabolized faster and have a shorter half-life in the body.

(b) The molar substitution (MS) ratio or degree of substitution (DS). Although the degree of substitution and the molar substitution reflect the same property, the way they are calculated is different.

The degree of substitution is calculated by dividing the number of substituted anhydrous glucose residues (G_s) by the total number of anhydrous glucose residues (G_t);

$$DS = \frac{G_s}{G_t}$$

The molar substitution is derived by calculating the average number of hydroxyethyl groups reacted to every anhydrous glucose residue:

$$MS = \frac{W_H \times 162}{1 - W_H \times 44}$$

where W_H is the weight fraction of the hydroxyl ethyl polymer and the numbers represent the mass of the hydroxyethyl group (44) and the anhydrous glucose residue (162).

MS is represented as a ratio and ranges from 0.4 to 0.7 in the commercially available HES. HES with a higher MS are metabolized slowly and as a result have a longer half-life in the body, but are also associated with greater side effects.

377

Table 22.3 Properties of commonly used HES

	6% HES 450/0.7	6% HES 670/0.7	6% HES 130/0.4	6% HES 70/0.5
Generation	1st	1st	3rd	2nd
Side effects	High	High	Low	Intermediate
MW	High 450	High 670	Medium 130	Low 70
MS	High 0.7	High 0.7	Low 0.4	Intermediate 0.5
C2:C6 substitution	4:1	4:1	9:1	4:1
Suspended in	Saline	Balanced solution	Saline	Balanced solution

Adapted from: Bailey AG *et al.*, Perioperative crystalloid and colloid fluid management in children: where are we and how did we get here? *Anesth Analg* 2010; 110(2): 375–90.

(c) C_2:C_6 substitution ratio. Not only is the degree of substitution important, but the *point* of substitution dictates the metabolism of HES. HES that have greater substitution of the glucose molecule by the hydroxyethyl group at the C2 position are metabolized more slowly than those that are substituted at the C6 position, without a corresponding increase in the side effects.

(d) The medium in which the colloid is suspended appears to be important too: i.e., normal saline or a plasma-based balanced crystalloid solution similar to lactated ringers.

(e) The concentration of the HES gives the HES their final characteristic. They are available as 3%, 6%, or 10% solutions. 6% solution is iso-osmotic, whereas 10% solution is hypertonic.

(f) Other important properties of HES include the viscosity, degree of branching, free phosphate levels and total phosphate levels, particularly in the third-generation tetrastarches.

The newer HES are designed to have a low MW and a low MS with a higher substitution involving the C2 position. Table 22.3 gives the properties of some of the commonly used HES.

Gelatins are polypeptides that are modified from bovine collagen. The main advantage with gelatins is that there is no dose limitation as there is for HES and dextrans. They also have much smaller molecular weight.

Dextrans are derived from bacteria and are available as 40 kDa or 70 kDa solutions. Their effect on coagulation has led to a decline in their general use but they do appear to lower the viscosity of blood.

Risks associated with colloids

Albumin 5% and 25% are prepared from human plasma by cold alcohol fractionation followed by treating the plasma to 60°C for 10 hours to eliminate the infectious risks. The donor is also screened for active viral diseases to decrease the potential risk for transmitted diseases. Creutzfeldt–Jakob disease (CJD), the variant CJD (vCJD), and viral diseases in particular are the potential risks.[6] Although to date there have been no reported incidents of transmission of either CJD, the FDA warns that the use of human albumin should always be preceded by a full discussion about the potential risk of transmitted diseases.

Studies have shown changes in the thromboelastogram (TEG) and thrombin generation assays reflecting a hypocoagulable state even with the use of albumin, which remains the gold standard for colloids. Evidence does suggest that the effect of albumin on coagulation is negligible as long as the amount of albumin used is less than 25% of the circulating blood volume.[7] HES with a higher molecular weight and higher molar substitution are associated with worse side effects than those with lower molecular weights and molar substitutions, particularly with regard to coagulation.[8] HES appears to impair the function of von Willebrand factor, factor VIII, and also platelets. The suggested maximum dose of hetastarch 130/0.4 (Voluven®) is 50 ml/kg/day in adults. Clinical data in children (2–12 years old) are limited and safety and efficacy have not been well established.

Allergic reactions are associated more with the synthetic colloids than with albumin. Life-threatening hypersensitivity reactions are again more frequent with the synthetic colloids. Pruritus is a complication that occurs at a variable frequency (0–22%) and could be a significant issue with some of the colloids. Renal toxicity as a result of the high oncotic pressure can usually be prevented by using colloids along with crystalloids. Renal tubular swelling, renal tubular obstruction, and medullary ischemia have all been described as potential risks.[9] HES are relatively contraindicated in patients with a decreased renal function.

The largest randomized, double-blinded trial comparing crystalloids with albumin is the multicenter Saline vs. Albumin Fluid Evaluation study involving over 7000 patients.[10] The study concluded that there was no advantage in using colloids over crystalloids. The only difference identified was in patients with traumatic brain injury (TBI), who appeared to do worse when resuscitated with albumin. A post hoc study involving this group did indeed confirm a slightly worse outcome in the group that received albumin.[11]

Finally, issues of cost-effectiveness of the various solutions must be considered. Albumin, at $80/500 ml (up to $190 in Europe), is more expensive than the synthetic colloids such as Volvulen at $45/500 ml, and 6% Hespan in NS at $15/500 ml, which are significantly more expensive than crystalloids (NS 70 cents/500 ml).[12]

Considering the side effect profile and the cost vs. benefit it is then easy to come to the conclusion that crystalloids should remain the primary fluid of choice in a patient undergoing spine surgery. Colloids still have a place, but their use should be tailored to the specific needs of the patient.

Sodium requirements

It is difficult to look at sodium requirements in isolation as the discussion often returns to water intoxication or hyperchloremic acidosis. There is, however, merit in reviewing what is turning out to be the most contentious issue regarding perioperative fluid therapy. The argument stems from the fact that the most common electrolyte abnormality in the hospitalized child is hyponatremia. For the development of hyponatremia two criteria have to be met. The first is the presence of excess pure water and the second is the inability of the kidney to excrete this excess water. The use of hypotonic solutions can contribute to the first, and the nonosmotic secretion of ADH in the immediate postoperative period can satisfy the second requirement. Acquired hyponatremia and its related complications are a significant concern. Like the issue of crystalloid and colloid, isotonic versus hypotonic postoperative fluid administration has become an area of contention. Hoorn and colleagues reported over 50 cases of neurologic complications related to hyponatremia including 26 deaths in a review of reported cases.[13] An in-depth analysis did reveal that the children who developed hyponatremia-related

complications received volumes well in excess of the calculated requirements based on the commonly used formulae. Moritz and Ayus suggest isotonic saline as the fluid of choice in the perioperative period as a defense against hospital-acquired hyponatremia.[14,15] In their counter-argument, Holliday and Segar suggest that both isotonic saline and 0.2% NS in D5 would work just as effectively when used judiciously, and that both regimes could lead to complications when used inappropriately. They also point out that hypernatremia like its counterpart is a cause of neurologic injury and even death.

Inappropriate secretion of ADH in the immediate postoperative period leads to the secretion of hypertonic urine along with the retention of water. Natriuresis along with the retention of free water leads to hyponatremia. In a study involving patients undergoing gynecological surgery, Steele and colleagues realized that the use of isotonic saline does not guarantee against the development of hyponatremia.[16]

When the above is taken into consideration along with the unique requirements of the pediatric spine patient, it becomes important to avoid hyponatremia and the resulting excess free water. This could further contribute to edema formation, which is particularly undesirable in this specific subgroup.

Glucose requirements

Glucose has traditionally been a component of fluids used in the perioperative period in children for several reasons. The protein-sparing effect of glucose is well recognized as is the fat-sparing effect. This prevents muscle breakdown during the catabolic phase of recovery; ketosis is also prevented by the fat-sparing effect. Glucose has been added to support the energy requirements of the brain. The addition of glucose also theoretically decreases sodium loss in the urine and allows for a lower concentration of sodium in the intravenous fluid while keeping the fluid isotonic.

The fear that fasting may lead to hypoglycemia has been dispelled by several studies that have shown that most children have normal blood glucose in spite of fasting. These have also shown that the majority of children undergoing surgery will respond to the routine administration of glucose by exhibiting significant hyperglycemia. Administration of 5% glucose-containing solutions does prevent hypoglycemia at the expense of moderate to severe hyperglycemia.[17] The above reasons have encouraged clinicians to suggest that glucose is not an essential component in the fluids used in the perioperative period and if, used, a lower concentration may be appropriate.[18] This should, however, be tempered by the fact that some children do develop asymptomatic hypoglycemia as a consequence of fasting. Hypoglycemia under anesthesia is just as undesirable as hyperglycemia, if not more so.[19-21]

Hyperglycemia is defined as a sustained elevation of plasma glucose to at least 7.8 mmol/l. It is well recognized that hyperglycemia exacerbates ischemic neurologic injury and contributes to a poor outcome.[22] Welborn et al. suggest that a fluid containing a lower concentration of glucose may be the answer to avoiding hyperglycemia.[17,18] An alternative approach would be to avoid using glucose-containing solutions and to base their use on intraoperative blood glucose measurements. According to the guidelines issued by the Association of Paediatric Anaesthetists of Great Britain and Ireland, children at risk of hypoglycemia should be given dextrose-containing solutions or have their blood glucose monitored during surgery. Such children are those on parenteral nutrition or a dextrose-containing solution prior to surgery, children of low body weight (<3rd percentile) or having surgery of more than 3 hours' duration, and children having extensive regional anesthesia.

Tissue perfusion

The goal of fluid therapy is to ensure adequate tissue perfusion. In a child undergoing spine surgery, tissues at risk include the spinal cord, the eyes, and other vital organs. The balance of oxygen supply and demand needs to remain net positive to prevent ischemia. The use of various monitoring techniques helps to assess the adequacy of perfusion. A decrease in the transcutaneous oxygen level, a transcutaneous to arterial oxygen ratio of less than 0.75, near-infrared spectrometry levels of less than 75%, the presence of lactic acidosis, a decrease in end-tidal CO_2 to arterial CO_2 ratio, and the response of the above to an increase in the F_iO_2 are all clinically useful indicators of poor tissue perfusion. Continuous oximetric catheters provide a trend in the central venous oxygen levels (S_vO_2), which reflects tissue perfusion fairly accurately. Recognizing the need for crystalloids, colloids, or blood products remains an important part of the decision making.

Blood transfusion

Perioperative blood and component therapy must be approached by strategies to conserve blood and strategies on how and when to replace blood. Those used to conserve blood are particularly important in the pediatric patient, but they are merely an adaptation of the strategies used in the adult patient and are discussed elsewhere in this book.

There has been a paradigm shift in the practices involving transfusion of blood components in pediatrics. These changes reflect practices outside the operating room, but the basis of the changes helps guide us in our practices involving blood component therapy. The two most important developments that have brought about the change in our practices are: (1) greater awareness of the infective risks associated with blood transfusion,[23] and (2) strong criticism of the use of the single criterion for perioperative blood transfusion of a hemoglobin level of 10 g/dl.[24]

This has led to a futile search until now for other indicators for the need to transfuse. In addition to the risks associated with blood component therapy in adults, transfusion has unique challenges in the pediatric population. Although children have a larger blood volume for weight, small-sized children actually have small total blood volumes. The overall prevalence of blood transfusion in pediatrics is about 5%. A review of these children who received blood products reveals that over two-thirds of the transfusions were in the perioperative period. The paucity of data dictates that guidelines for transfusion in children are mostly adaptations of guidelines that are available for adults. The following are some of the differences in the need for, and in the practice of blood transfusion between adults and children.

Differences in hemoglobin and their P$_{50}$ characteristics

P$_{50}$ and hemoglobin

There are two distinct groups within the pediatric population who have different requirements. It is customary to divide them into children less than 4 months old and those over 4 months old. In the first 4 months of life there is a decreased production of erythropoietin and smaller total blood volumes (even though they have a relatively larger blood volume for weight). There is a transition from the fetal type of hemoglobin to the adult variant over this period. Fetal hemoglobin has a higher affinity for oxygen and hence the oxygen dissociation curve is shifted to the left. The implications of this are important insofar as an acceptable hemoglobin level in an adult may not equate to an acceptable level in children. P_{50} is the pO_2 at 50% SO_2. The P_{50} of adult hemoglobin at 37°C and a pH of 7.4 is 27 mmHg. The P_{50} of fetal hemoglobin at 37°C and a pH of 7.4 is 19 mmHg. The P_{50} of an infant beyond 3 months of age rises to about 30 mmHg. A hemoglobin level of 7 g/dl will be able to carry the same amount of oxygen whether it is fetal Hb (HbF) or adult Hb (HbA); the unloading characteristics of the fetal hemoglobin could, however, mean that this level of hemoglobin is inadequate for the neonate. To give an example, a hemoglobin level of 10 g/dl in an adult with a P_{50} of 27 mmHg equates to just 6.8 g/dl in a 2-month-old child with a P_{50} of 24 mmHg. Using the above calculation, a neonate less than 2 months of age will require a hemoglobin level of at least 12 g/dl to be considered the equivalent of 8 g/dl in an adult.

Oxygen flux

From the above argument it becomes apparent that a neonate requires a higher hemoglobin than an adult. This is even before considering the increased metabolic demands and oxygen requirements of the child. Oxygen demands in the adult are 2–4 ml/kg/min; in the neonate this figure is between 5 and 8 ml/kg/min. Oxygen supply to the tissues is directly proportional to the cardiac output and the oxygen content. Oxygen supply = Cardiac output × Oxygen content. Oxygen supply should be greater than the oxygen demand.

As the cardiac output is already at a near maximal level in the neonate, the only way the oxygen supply can be enhanced is by increasing the oxygen-carrying capacity. The most important determinant of this is the hemoglobin level. However, the laboratory hemoglobin level in itself remains nothing more than a surrogate in assessing the adequacy of oxygen supply. A better indicator would be mixed venous oxygen levels and, if available, oxygen extraction ratios. They may not be applicable or available for every patient. Lactic acidosis indicates a decreased perfusion state, and improving oxygen-carrying capacity and therefore the oxygen delivery by increasing the hemoglobin may be beneficial even in the presence of mild anemia.

Trigger for transfusion or threshold for tolerance?

Liberal policy versus restrictive policy

The liberal policy on blood transfusion is to use a cut-off of Hb 10 g/dl or a Hct of 30% to transfuse the child.

A more restrictive policy is to adopt a lower Hb value of 7 g/dl or a Hct of 20% as a threshold below which one would transfuse. A review of the literature[25,26] does support this restrictive policy, but it is important to understand that these studies were done in children with chronic anemia, outside of the operating room.

Clinicians have sought for an easy method to fall back on to determine when to transfuse a child. The 10/30 rule used to be inviolable for any child coming to the operating room, i.e., all children with hemoglobin less than 10 g/dl or a hematocrit less than 30% would have required transfusion according to this rule. This has been challenged over the last 10 to 15 years, not least because of the risk of transmission of hepatitis, HIV, and other infections with blood transfusion. Other risks include transfusion-associated graft versus host disease (TA-GVHD), transfusion-related acute lung injury (TRALI), transfusion-associated circulatory overload (TACO), allergic and nonallergic reactions, and risks associated with the anticoagulants and preservatives used. In spite of this, clinicians have been cautious about lowering their threshold for transfusion as most of the studies done have been outside the operating room. In fact the studies involving children tend to focus on the issue of chronic anemia. There is obviously a clear distinction between chronic anemia and acute anemia, with readjustment in the oxygen dissociation curve in chronic anemia to enable better delivery of oxygen. Lacroix et al. looked at transfusion policy within the pediatric intensive care unit (PICU) and concluded that even in critically ill children, if stable, a hemoglobin threshold of 7 g/dl for red cell transfusion can decrease transfusion requirements without increasing adverse outcomes.[26] Perioperative visual loss is a dreaded complication sometimes seen in patients undergoing spine surgery. The risk factors associated with this include anemia, glaucoma, diabetes, hypertension, smoking, obesity, prolonged surgery, prone position, and massive blood loss. A practice advisory by the American Society of Anesthesiologists seems to suggest, but falls short of making it an advisory, that a minimum hemoglobin of 9.4 g/dl or a hematocrit of 28 should be maintained. This advisory was for all patients at risk of perioperative visual loss and was not specific for pediatrics. It would stand to reason that this should be the very minimum in pediatric patients undergoing spine surgery. Based on the above discussion a reasonable recommendation for transfusion would be as shown in Box 22.1).

> **Box 22.1. Guidelines for perioperative blood transfusion in pediatrics**
>
> The following are guidelines for perioperative blood transfusion.
> - A hematocrit of 30 or less with
>   - Ongoing blood loss
>   - Evidence of decreased perfusion (lactic acidosis, decreased S_vO_2)
>   - Hemodynamic instability not as a result of cardiac function.
> - In the absence of the above, a lower Hct threshold may be appropriate (25–30), but should always take into account the potential for risks associated with a low hemoglobin including but not limited to ischemic optic neuropathy.
> - A blood loss of more than 20% of the blood volume usually requires blood transfusion.
> - Blood loss of 10–20% when associated with the criteria in the first indication may need transfusion.
> - Neonates and children less than 4 months old require a higher hematocrit due to the characteristics of fetal hemoglobin.
> - In children with cyanotic heart disease and those with severe lung disease the trigger should be set at a higher Hct (at least 38–40).
> - Children with sickle cell disease also need special consideration and a higher hematocrit.

Choosing the right product

Packed red blood cells

Packed red blood cells (PRBCs) are the products of choice when the aim is to improve oxygen delivery. The hematocrit in PRBC units ranges from 50–65 depending on the preservative used. The life of the unit is also dependent on the preservative used: 28 days when CPDA-1 (citrate, phosphate, dextrose, and adenine) is used to 42 days when (Adsol) AS-1 and AS-2 are used. As a general rule neonates and small children should receive blood that is relatively new. The longer the blood has been preserved the greater the degree of cell destruction and risks associated with it such as hyperkalemia. When the risk of hyperkalemia related to PRBCs is high, washed red blood cells should be used.

Washed PRBCs

Washed PRBCs are indicated in children with a history of severe transfusion reaction related to plasma proteins. Washing cells also reduces the potassium content in the transfused PRBCs.

Leukoreduced PRBCs

Knowledge about nonhemolytic transfusion reactions and the methodology of transmission of certain diseases such as Cytomegalovirus (CMV) have led to the use of leukoreduced PRBCs. Leukoreduction decreases the white blood cells in the preserved unit of PRBCs. TA-GVHD is another complication that has been attributed to the presence of white blood cells in PRBCs. Leukoreduction reduces the risk of transmission of CMV and that of TA-GVHD but does not eliminate it. Leukoreduced blood also prevents alloimmunization and delayed platelet refractoriness.

Irradiated PRBCS

Irradiated blood is aimed at eliminating the risk of TA-GVHD and should be used in those susceptible. The dose of radiation used is very small and does not protect against transmission of CMV. Neonates are the most susceptible as their immunological system is immature and therefore they should receive washed, leukoreduced, and irradiated PRBCs. This indication should probably be extended to children below 6 months of age. Others such as those immunosuppressed and those awaiting a transplant should be considered at risk.

Volume to be transfused

A transfusion of 15 ml/kg with PRBCs that have a hematocrit of 65% will raise the hemoglobin by about 3 g/dl. Another distinction that needs to be made is that the lowest tolerable hemoglobin is not necessarily the optimal hemoglobin. Having exposed the child to one donor, one should aim to achieve a hemoglobin level of at least 12 g/dl without overloading the child. The volume to be transfused can also be calculated using the following formula (Table 22.4).

$$\text{Volume to be transfused} = \text{Weight (kg)} \times \frac{\text{Desired Hct} - \text{Observed Hct}}{\text{Hct of PRBCs}}$$

Other products

The use of products such as fresh frozen plasma, platelets, and cryoprecipitate should always be done on the basis of tests such as thromboelastogram (TEG) and clotting studies. The role of the TEG in this situation cannot be overemphasized, even though it needs to be corroborated with laboratory studies.

Platelets. Leukocyte-reduced platelet pheresis units in 200–300 ml of plasma equate to 5–6 random units of platelet concentrate. The dose of platelets to be used

Table 22.4 Reference for transfusion of blood products

	PRBC	FFP	Cryoprecipitate	Platelets
Cross-match	Required	Not required	Not required	Not required
Dose	10–20 ml/kg	10–20 ml/kg	1 unit/10 kg	10–20 ml/kg
ABO	Compatible	Compatible	Compatible	Compatible[a]
Rh compatibility	Consider	(Consider)[b]	Not required	Consider

[a] If ABO-compatible platelets are not available consider volume-reduced platelets in children less than 12 years old.
[b] Consider Rh compatibility in women of child-bearing age.

in children less than 10 kg is 10–20 ml/kg. In children 10–15 kg, one-third of a pheresis unit should be used. In children 15–25 kg, one-half of a pheresis can be used. In children more than 25 kg, one pheresis unit should be used while awaiting laboratory confirmation. Platelets should be ABO and Rh compatible but do not require a cross-match. Platelets may need to be irradiated in the specific groups discussed above.

Fresh frozen plasma (FFP) may be needed if the prothrombin time (PT) and partial thromboplastin time (PTT) are greater than 1.5 times normal. If more than one blood volume has been transfused, FFP may be administered while waiting for laboratory confirmation. Warfarin overdose or reversal in a child who requires emergent surgery is another indication for FFP. FFP may be needed in children with plasma anticoagulant deficiency such as protein C, protein S, or antithrombin III when specific therapy is not available. FFP should also be considered in the clinical setting of disseminated intravascular coagulation. ABO-identical or -compatible FFP must be transfused. Matching tests are not necessary No consideration needs to be given to rhesus (D) compatibility when administering FFP; however, when large volumes are required in women with child-bearing potential this may be a consideration (FFP may contain some RBC stroma). The dose of 10–20 ml/kg when used for replacement of factors will raise the factors by 10–20%.

Cryoprecipitate should be used when there is a qualitative or quantitative deficiency of fibrinogen. Cryoprecipitate when used should be given at a dose of 1 unit for every 10 kg. This will raise the fibrinogen level by 60–100 mg/dl. The precipitate should be ABO compatible; Rh need not be considered.

Recombinant activated factor VII. The mechanism of action of recombinant activated factor VII appears to be complex and difficult to elucidate. The tissue factor-dependent mode of action appears to be the primary mechanism. The complex of tissue factor and rVIIa activates platelets and factors leading to a deposition of thrombin and fibrin. To a lesser extent rVIIa directly activates platelets and factor X to generate thrombin in a tissue factor-independent mode of action. The use of rVIIa is a rescue technique and should be used after consultation with the hematologist. Coagulation studies done at the earliest signs of coagulopathy and thromboelastography provide clues to the treatment of abnormal hemostasis.

Monitoring of the pediatric patient for spine surgery

The following discussion about monitoring of the pediatric patient is directed specifically toward one undergoing spine surgery. Exciting innovations in equipment used for monitoring show tremendous promise in this field. It is also important to understand that the basic parameters used as reference vary significantly with age. To emphasize the point, a systolic pressure of 60 mmHg could be considered life-threatening in the adult, but is perfectly acceptable in the neonate.

Pulse oximetry

Modern pulse oximeters provide much more information than just the peripheral oxygen saturation. Though the principles behind the measurement of S_pO_2 remain the same, advances in the technology allow us to assess fractional saturation as opposed to functional saturation:

Fractional Hb saturation

$$= \frac{HbO}{HbO + Hb + MetHb + COHb}$$

Functional Hb saturation

$$= \text{Percentage of} \left[\frac{HbO}{HbO + Hb} \right]$$

where HbO is oxyhemoglobin, Hb is reduced hemoglobin, MetHb is methemoglobin, and COHb is carboxyhemoglobin.

Table 22.5 Information that can be obtained from an arterial catheter

Direct arterial pressure measurement
Abnormal waveforms
Anacrotic – aortic stenosis
Collapsing – aortic regurgitation, hyperdynamic circulation such as fever, anemia, hyperthyroidism
Bisferiens – aortic stenosis with regurgitation
Alternans – heart failure
Damping – air bubble, compliant tubing
Resonant – catheter too long
Information that can be derived from an arterial catheter
Rate
Rhythm
Arterial blood pressure
Mean arterial pressure – can be derived from integrating the area under the pressure curve
Contractility – the rate of the upstroke
Peripheral vascular resistance – the downstroke indicates the PVR
Continuous blood gas monitoring with fiberoptic sensors
Volume status – by assessing the variation with positive-pressure ventilation

Adapted from: Yentis SM, Hirsch NP, Smith GB. *Anesthesia and Intensive Care A-Z: An Encyclopedia of Principles and Practice*, 3rd edition. Elsevier, 2009.

They also incorporate methods of indexing variations in the plethysmography curve to give us valuable information such as plethysmography variability index (PVI).

The variation reflects changes in the stroke volume, which in turn is a reflection of the volume status (with limitations). Other additions to the pulse oximeter are the ability of modern units to provide continuous and noninvasive monitoring of hemoglobin levels (SpHb) and, in addition, to filter motion artifacts (signal extraction technology – SET). Both SpHb and PVI have been validated in the adult population and need independent validation in the pediatric subgroup. The ability of modern machines to eliminate the motion artifact is useful in patients undergoing neurodiagnostic monitoring where muscle twitching could interfere with pulse oximetry.

Blood pressure measurement

Direct arterial pressure measurements are desirable in children undergoing lengthy procedures on the spine. A plethora of information can thus be obtained (Table 22.5). The radial artery remains the preferred site even in the neonate. Larger arteries such as the femoral and the axillary may be considered if attempts to cannulate the radial artery fail. Direct arterial pressure monitoring also allows for arterial sampling, which helps with the management of fluid and blood products in the child. A baseline thromboelastogram should be drawn soon after the placement of the catheter along with hemoglobin, glucose, and blood gas samples. There is a large variation in blood pressure with age. Table 22.5 is provided as a guide to the management of the pediatric patient under anesthesia.

Central venous catheter, pulmonary artery catheter, and continuous S_vO_2 monitoring

A child undergoing spine surgery is subject to large fluid shifts, with blood loss very often in excess of 20% of the blood volume. They may need vasoactive support and frequent blood draws. They may therefore be appropriate candidates for placement of a central venous catheter with the capability of monitoring mixed venous oxygen saturation continuously. S_vO_2 is a good measure of the adequacy of tissue perfusion and may help guide transfusion in children. The availability of continuous oximetric catheters in sizes appropriate even for neonates has led to the increased utilization of these catheters. A pulmonary artery (PA) catheter may be needed in the presence of cardiac disease such as valvular heart disease, heart failure, and left ventricular dysfunction; respiratory indications include acute respiratory failure and chronic obstructive pulmonary disease, and a PA catheter may also be placed when large fluid shifts are anticipated.

ECG

Maturational changes of the heart are reflected in electrocardiographic parameters[27] (Table 22.6). Quite simply, the distances needed to be traveled are much shorter and hence the various intervals are also shorter. They gradually lengthen with age to reach adult values by about 16 to 18 years. There is right ventricular dominance in the newborn which gradually reverts to a left ventricular dominance by the age of 1 year. The other important difference is the rapid resting heart rate in the smaller child. As a result, definitions of tachycardia, bradycardia, and a normal rate are all individualized to different age groups. The resting heart rate in a newborn is between 120 and 160 beats per minute. The high rate is necessary to maintain the cardiac output as the ability to increase the stroke volume is limited by the poor compliance of the ventricles.

The PR interval is 0.08–0.15 seconds in the newborn until about 2 years. It eventually reaches the adult value of 0.12–0.20 seconds by 16 years. The QRS interval is

Table 22.6 Age-related differences in vital signs

Age	HR (bpm)	BP (mmHg)	RR (per min)	PR interval (s)	QRS width (s)
Preemie	120–170	55–75/35–45	40–70	0.08–0.15	0.03–0.08
0–3 months	100–180	65–85/45–55	35–55	0.08–0.15	0.03–0.08
3–6 months	105–180	70–90/50–65	30–45	0.08–0.15	0.03–0.08
6–12 months	110–170	80–100/55–65	25–40	0.07–0.16	0.03–0.08
1–3 years	90–165	90–105/55–70	20–30	0.08–0.16	0.03–0.08
3–6 years	65–140	95–110/60–75	20–25	0.09–0.17	0.04–0.08
6–12 years	60–130	100–120/60/75	14/22	0.09–0.18	0.04–0.09
16+ years	55–85	110–135/65/85	12–18	0.12–0.20	0.05–0.10

Adapted from: Sharieff GQ, Rao SO, The pediatric ECG. *Emerg Med Clin North Am* 2006; 24: 196.

0.03–0.08 seconds in the newborn until about 2 years. It gradually increases to the adult values of 0.05–0.10 seconds by 16 years.

Another fact that is useful to remember is that the types of arrhythmia that are prevalent in the pediatric population are very different from those found in adults. In the absence of congenital heart disease, supraventricular tachycardias are the most common type of arrhythmia. Bradyarrhythmias are always assumed to be a result of hypoxia unless proven otherwise. In a child with congenital heart disease the nature of the disease and the intervention the child has had will influence the type of abnormality seen in an ECG.

Temperature monitoring

Accurate monitoring of the child when under anesthesia is very important as both hypothermia and hyperthermia are real risks and need to be recognized early. Maintaining the temperature of the child under anesthesia is difficult and early detection of hypothermia will help prevent complications related to it (Table 22.7). Temperature is regulated through the preoptic nucleus in the anterior hypothalamus. Esophageal, rectal, bladder, and tympanic temperatures are better indicators of core temperature.[28] Axillary temperature reflects surface or shell temperature and is not as reliable. A rise in temperature is a late sign of malignant hyperthermia and is usually preceded by tachycardia and hypercapnia.

End tidal CO_2

Capnography remains one of the most reliable ways of confirming the placement of the endotracheal tube. Both a rise in end-tidal carbon dioxide and a decrease can be significant. A rise in $ETCO_2$ may be indicative of inadequate ventilation or an increased metabolic rate as in malignant hyperthermia. A decrease in $ETCO_2$ similarly could be a result of hyperventilation

Table 22.7 Complications of hypothermia

Cardiovascular	Neurologic
Decreased cardiac output	Confusion
Ventricular arrythmias	Delayed awakening
Vasoconstriction	Decreased MAC
Increased afterload	Recurarization
Hematological	Other effects
Increased viscosity	Diuresis
Thrombocytopenia	Decreased drug metabolism
Increased hematocrit	Metabolic acidosis
Sickling	Hyperkalemia
Coagulopathy	Hyperglycemia
Respiratory	Wound
Apnea	Delayed healing
Reduced O_2 delivery	Infection
Shift of the O_2 dissociation curve to the left	
Pulmonary hypertension	
Respiratory acidosis	

Adapted from: Sharieff GQ, Rao SO, The pediatric ECG. *Emerg Med Clin North Am* 2006; 24: 196.

or decreased pulmonary blood flow. In children with congenital heart disease this could be due to pulmonary hypertension or dynamic right ventricular outflow tract obstruction, as in tetralogy of Fallot.

Bispectral index

There is increasing interest in the use of the bispectral index (BIS) in children undergoing spinal surgery. As these children usually receive a low dose of inhaled anesthetic along with other intravenous agents, amnesia cannot be reliably provided. The studies to date suggest that BIS appears to be reliable in children above the age of 1 year.[29] There is a large interpatient variability and BIS does not appear to correlate well when halothane and ketamine are used. There is, however, little evidence at present that BIS decreases the incidence of awareness or recall in children.

Other monitors

Children have sensitive skin, and frequent monitoring of the pressure points and the eyes is important. A precordial stethoscope provides invaluable information and is often underrated. Similarly, an esophageal temperature probe with the ability to connect to an esophageal stethoscope is a useful tool. Neurodiagnostic monitoring is discussed in Chapter 6.

Summary

Sanctorius in his book *De Statica Medicina* (1614) says

> If a Physician who has the Care of another's Health, is acquainted only with the sensible Supplies and Evacuations, and knows nothing of the Waste that is daily made by Insensible Perspiration, he will only deceive his Patient, and never cure him.

Today our understanding of the anatomy, the physiology, and the pathology of the pediatric patient allows us to tackle this difficult but exciting challenge of perioperative fluid therapy head on and to develop a unique plan to fit the needs of each child. The guidelines regarding fluid therapy and blood products are intended as a basis for the formulation of such a plan, but they cannot replace the judgment of the clinician (Box 22.2).

Box 22.2 Guidelines for perioperative fluid management.

1. Hypovolemia should be corrected rapidly to maintain cardiac output and organ perfusion. (Initially with crystalloids.)
2. In the child, a fall in blood pressure is a late sign of hypovolemia.
3. Maintenance fluid requirements should be calculated using the formula of Holliday and Segar.

Body weight daily fluid requirement

0–10 kg	4 ml/kg/h
10–20 kg	40 ml/h + 2 ml/kg/h above 10 kg
>20 kg	60 ml/h + 1 ml/kg/h above 20 kg

4. A fluid management plan for any child should address deficits, maintenance requirements, and ongoing losses

---

5. The assessment and treatment of deficit based on current formulae probably overestimates the requirements;[20] hence a more restrictive approach may be appropriate.
6. During surgery, all of these requirements should initially be managed by giving isotonic fluids such as normal saline or lactated Ringer's solution in all children over 1 month of age.
7. When cost and benefit are assessed, colloids have a very limited and defined role in the fluid management of the pediatric patient undergoing spine surgery.
8. The majority of children over 1 month of age will maintain a normal blood sugar if given non-dextrose-containing fluid during surgery.
9. Children at risk of hypoglycemia should have frequent blood sugar measurements and glucose supplemented as required.
10. Fluid therapy should be monitored by daily electrolyte estimation, use of a fluid input/output chart and daily weighing if feasible.
11. Transfusion of blood and products may be required depending on the clinical situation (Box 22.1).

Modified from the consensus guidelines for perioperative fluid management put forth by the Association of Pediatric Anesthetists of Great Britain and Ireland (APAGBI).

Perioperative use of blood and blood products requires decisiveness based on the fundamentals of transfusion medicine. Blood and products carry a significant risk, but can be very effective in avoiding complications. Although we have striven to move away from the use of a single trigger for transfusion, we appear to have set different thresholds for the use of blood and products. It is hoped the framework here will provide the essence of an appropriate plan for the use of blood and blood products in the pediatric patient undergoing spinal surgery.

The advent of newer monitoring techniques allows for a better understanding of the needs of each patient. Miniaturization, computerization, digitization, and the ability to access data in real time have all led to the proclamation of a new era in monitoring. Anesthesiologists have been in the forefront of innovations in monitoring over the last few decades and have been enthusiastic in embracing new technology. An understanding of the limitations of the technology and the techniques is just as important as adopting them into clinical practice.

References

1. Holliday MA, Segar WE. The maintenance need for water in parenteral fluid therapy. *Pediatrics* 1957; **19**(5): 823–32.

2. Friis-Hansen B. Body water compartments and fluid metabolism in children. *Acta Paediatr Suppl* 1955; **44** (Suppl 103): 31–4.

3. Aperia A, Broberger O, Herin P, Thodenius K, Zetterström R. Postnatal control of water and electrolyte homeostasis in pre-term and full-term infants. *Acta Paediatr Scand Suppl* 1983; **305**: 61–5.

4. Tommasino C, Moore S, Todd MM. Cerebral effects of isovolemic hemodilution with crystalloid or colloid solutions. *Crit Care Med* 1988; **16**(9): 862–8.

5. Jacob M, Chappell D, Conzen P, *et al.* Blood volume is normal after pre-operative overnight fasting. *Acta Anaesthesiol Scand* 2008; **52**(4): 522–9.

6. Foster PR. Assessment of the potential of plasma fractionation processes to remove causative agents of transmissible spongiform encephalopathy. *Transfus Med* 1999; **9**(1): 3–14.

7. Tobias MD, Wambold D, Pilla MA, Greer F. Differential effects of serial hemodilution with hydroxyethyl starch, albumin, and 0.9% saline on whole blood coagulation. *J Clin Anesth* 1998; **10**(5): 366–71.

8. Falk JL, Rackow EC, Astiz ME, Weil MH. Effects of hetastarch and albumin on coagulation in patients with septic shock. *J Clin Pharmacol* 1988; **28**(5): 412–15.

9. Legendre C, Thervet E, Page B, *et al.* Hydroxyethylstarch and osmotic-nephrosis-like lesions in kidney transplantation. *Lancet* 1993; **342**(8865): 248–9.

10. Finfer S, Norton R, Bellomo R, *et al.* The SAFE study: saline vs. albumin for fluid resuscitation in the critically ill. *Vox Sang* 2004; Suppl **2**: 123–31.

11. Myburgh J, Cooper DJ, Finfer S, *et al.* Saline or albumin for fluid resuscitation in patients with traumatic brain injury. *N Engl J Med* 2007; **357**(9): 874–84.

12. Bailey AG, McNaull PP, Jooste E, Tuchman JB. Perioperative crystalloid and colloid fluid management in children: where are we and how did we get here? *Anesth Analg* 2010; **110**(2): 375–90.

13. Hoorn EJ, Geary D, Robb M, *et al.* Acute hyponatremia related to intravenous fluid administration in hospitalized children: an observational study. *Pediatrics* 2004; **113**(5): 1279–84.

14. Moritz ML, Ayus JC. Prevention of hospital-acquired hyponatremia: a case for using isotonic saline. *Pediatrics* 2003; **111**(2): 227–30.

15. Moritz ML, Ayus JC. The pathophysiology and treatment of hyponatraemic encephalopathy: an update. *Nephrol Dial Transplant* 2003; **18**(12): 2486–91.

16. Steele A, Gowrishankar M, Abrahamson S, Mazer CD, Feldman RD, Halperin ML. Postoperatie hyponatremia despite near-isotonic saline infusion: A phenomenon of desalination. *Ann Intern Med* 1997; **126**(1): 20–5.

17. Welborn LG, McGill WA, Hannallah RS, *et al.* Perioperative blood glucose concentrations in pediatric outpatients. *Anesthesiology* 1986; **65**(5): 543–7.

18. Welborn LG, Hannallah RS, McGill WA, *et al.* Glucose concentrations for routine intravenous infusion in pediatric outpatient surgery. *Anesthesiology* 1987; **67**(3): 427–30.

19. Kinnala A, Rikalainen H, Lapinleimu H, *et al.* Cerebral magnetic resonance imaging and ultrasonography findings after neonatal hypoglycemia. *Pediatrics* 1999; **103**(4 Pt 1): 724–9.

20. Anderson JM, Milner RD, Strich SJ. Effects of neonatal hypoglycaemia on the nervous system: a pathological study. *J Neurol Neurosurg Psychiatry* 1967; **30**(4): 295–310.

21. Burns CM, Rutherford MA, Boardman JP, Cowan FM. Patterns of cerebral injury and neurodevelopmental outcomes after symptomatic neonatal hypoglycemia. *Pediatrics* 2008; **122**(1): 65–74.

22. Sieber FE, Traystman RJ. Special issues: glucose and the brain. *Crit Care Med* 1992; **20**(1): 104–14.

23. Strong DM, Katz L. Blood-bank testing for infectious diseases: how safe is blood transfusion? *Trends Mol Med* 2002; **8**(7): 355–8.

24. Consensus conference. Perioperative red blood cell transfusion. *JAMA* 1988; **260**(18): 2700–3.

25. Kirpalani H, Whyte RK, Andersen C, *et al.* The premature infants in need of transfusion (PINT) study: a randomized, controlled trial of a restrictive (low) versus liberal (high) transfusion threshold for extremely low birth weight infants. *J Pediatr* 2006; **149**(3): 301–7.

26. Lacroix J, Hebert PC, Hutchison JS, *et al.* Transfusion strategies for patients in pediatric intensive care units. *N Engl J Med* 2007; **356**(16): 1609–19.

27. Rautaharju PM, Davignon A, Soumis F, *et al.* Evolution of QRS-T relationship from birth to adolescence in Frank-lead orthogonal electrocardiograms of 1492 normal children. *Circulation* 1979; **60**(1): 196–204.

28. Bissonnette B, Sessler DI, LaFlamme P. Intraoperative temperature monitoring sites in infants and children and the effect of inspired gas warming on esophageal temperature. *Anesth Analg* 1989; **69**(2): 192–6.

29. Degoute CS, Macabeo C, Dubreuil C, *et al.* EEG bispectral index and hypnotic component of anaesthesia induced by sevoflurane: comparison between children and adults. *Br J Anaesth* 2001; **86**(2): 209–12.

Chapter

23

Surgical techniques in the pediatric patient

23.1 Scoliosis

David P. Gurd

Key points

- Scoliosis surgery is indicated for curves greater than 45–50° or curves with continued deformity progression.
- Most scoliosis cases are performed through a posterior approach.
- Maintaining a mean arterial pressure of 70 mmHg during spine exposure can help to minimize intraoperative blood loss.
- Pedicle screws are the best modality for spine fixation and curve correction.
- The insertion of pedicle screws can be performed safely.

Spine deformity correction is a common procedure performed in the pediatric operating room. Scoliosis (lateral curvature of the spine) affects approximately 2–3% of the population with 0.1–0.3% progressing to significant curvature.[1-3] A measurement of 45–50° is the accepted minimum curvature to begin operative discussion as the deformity is likely to continue to progress[4-6] (Fig. 23.1). The younger the patient and the larger the curve, the more likely it is for progression to occur.[7] Curve progression has also been identified during the adolescent growth spurt.[8] Indications for operative intervention include curvature greater than 45–50°, progression of deformity, loss of spine balance, and thoracic lordosis. The main goal of surgery is to prevent further progression of the deformity and to achieve spinal balance. With improved instrumentation and the ability to monitor nerve function

intraoperatively, significant curve correction can be achieved while ensuring patient safety. Definitive fusion of the spine is typically delayed until the majority of spine growth is established (triradiate cartilage closed) to prevent pulmonary dysfunction and avoid the crankshaft phenomenon.[9,10] Triradiate cartilage closure closely correlates with a downswing in the adolescent growth spurt; therefore, surgery at this point will have limited growth concerns. There is no specific degree of deformity at which intervention offers the best results, although as a deformity progresses the curve becomes more stiff, which can make deformity correction more difficult and pulmonary function can be detrimentally affected.[11-19]

Surgery for scoliosis is a significant undertaking. The entire surgical team must be competent in the operative planning and procedure to limit possible complications. This team includes the surgeon, anesthesiologist, nursing, and neurology. The two most important factors for nonneurologic complications are increased anesthetic time and surgical time,[20] so efficiency from each team member is of great importance. It is paramount to ensure that each team member understands their role and performs it with professionalism and efficiency is paramount. This begins with room preparation. Thorough room cleansing and limiting unnecessary "traffic" within the room can help to minimize infection. Preparation of all surgical instruments, neurologic monitoring, and Cell Saver (Haemonetics intraoperative blood salvage) should be done prior to anesthetic administration to help diminish anesthetic time. General endotracheal anesthesia is required with appropriate intravascular access.

Anesthesia for Spine Surgery, ed. Ehab Farag. Published by Cambridge University Press. © Cambridge University Press 2012.

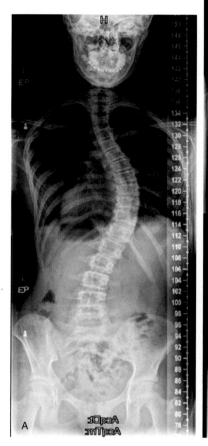
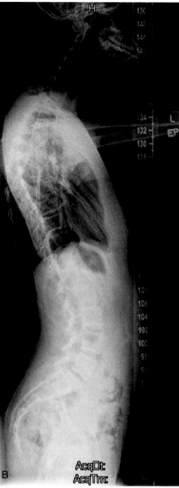

Figure 23.1 (A) PA radiograph demonstrating scoliosis (mainly right thoracic) with Cobb angle greater than 50°. (B) Lateral radiograph of the same patient with hypokyphosis and rib hump deformity.

Spinal cord monitoring equipment for somatosensory evoked potentials (SSEPs) and motor evoked potentials (MEPs) is placed once the patient is anesthetized.[21-23] Hemodilution can also be performed at this time.

Scoliosis surgery can be performed using different approaches. The anterior approach is done with the patient in a lateral decubitus position with rib removal and exposure through the pleura or diaphragm to gain access to the vertebral bodies. While this is still a very useful approach for some curve types, it is used less frequently due to concerns for harmful effects on the pulmonary function[24,25] and concerns for scar irritation and flank pain.[26] Thoracoscopic techniques have been used, which are less invasive than open anterior approaches and may have fewer problems with pain and pulmonary function while allowing for a shorter hospital stay.[27-29] The posterior approach has become the most common form of treatment for scoliosis

surgery. When comparing anterior and posterior fusion for a thoracolumbar curve, posterior spinal fusion demonstrated better curve correction, better maintenance of correction, and shorter hospital stay.[30] The posterior approach combined with pedicle screws offers excellent correction while avoiding pulmonary injury. Studies have shown improved pulmonary function after posterior spinal fusion.[31-35] Even for very large curves (greater than 90°), posterior-only surgery can be very effective.[36,37] This chapter, therefore, will focus on posterior spinal fusion.

Once anesthetized and ready for surgery, the patient is placed in a prone position on a Jackson table or its equivalent (Fig. 23.2). The abdomen should be free of pressure to help prevent blood loss. Distributing stress over the thighs with sufficient padding helps to decrease the incidence of lateral femoral nerve irritation.[38] Positioning is very important as the patient

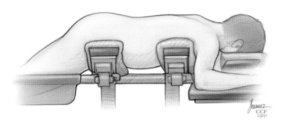

Figure 23.2 Example of patient positioning in a prone position when looking from the side. Notice the free abdomen with padding to the pelvis and chest. Arms should be in a comfortable position with less than 90° of abduction.

can be immobilized in this position for some time and minimizing skin pressure and nerve stretch is important. Padding to all pressure points is imperative. For females, areolar irritation can occur from pressure on the chest pad and should be appropriately protected. The arms are abducted and extended less than 90° for brachial plexus protection and padding should be applied under the axilla. Supination of the arm tends to diminish ulnar nerve irritation.[39] The knees should be flexed and the feet supported with the toes dangling freely. The skin of the back is then cleansed and prepped. Antibiotics are administered within an hour of incision. The surgeon must have a good preoperative plan as far as understanding levels of the spine requiring fusion and any special equipment that may be required during the case. Fusion should be limited to those levels of structural curvature. Lenke's classification[40] is useful to determine structural curves by using bend radiographs to determine the flexibility of the curves and lateral radiographs to help determine junctional kyphosis. Minimizing levels fused helps to limit surgical intervention and surgical time while allowing for more flexible levels of the spine postoperatively.

Posterior spinal surgery for scoliosis can be broken down into three steps, each of equal importance: first is exposure of the spine; second is anchor placement within the spine; third is deformity correction, bone grafting, and closure. To gain exposure, an incision is made over the midline of the spine from the most cranial level to the most caudal level of instrumentation. Fluoroscopy or intraoperative radiographs are useful to confirm correct levels. Electrocautery and collagen shrinkers such as Aquamantis (Salient Surgical Technologies, Portsmouth, NH, USA) are very helpful to minimize intraoperative blood loss. Maintaining mean arterial pressure (MAP) near 70 mmHg can be helpful for minimizing bleeding while allowing for safe blood flow to the spinal cord. A MAP of less than

55–60 mmHg may be associated with an increased risk of spinal cord ischemia.[41] Ophthalmologic injuries may also occur due to relative hypotension.[42] Inhalation agents should be limited to allow for good function of the neurological testing. Dissection is taken through the dermis and subdermal adipose to the supraspinous ligament and the spinous processes. Maintaining a midline dissection avoids vasculature, which minimizes blood loss as dissection in this area occurs through a relatively avascular plane. Once the spinous processes are identified, it is important again to verify correct spine levels as dissection and disruption of normal anatomy too proximally or distally may increase the risk for junctional kyphosis. Sharp dissection is undertaken midline through the cartilaginous caps of the spinous process. At each level, subperiosteal dissection is performed along the spinous process, over the lamina, and laterally to the tip of the transverse process. Extraperiosteal dissection (into the paraspinal musculature) may also increase blood loss and, therefore, should be avoided. At each level, packing is placed which helps with further dissection and limits blood loss. With this performed bilaterally at each level, retractors are placed to allow for ease of visualization. Multiple assessments should be performed throughout the case to ensure that there is no active bleeding.

The next step is to gain anchor fixation to the spine. This can be done by many methods including hooks, cables, wires, and screws. As pedicle screws have shown improved fixation and ability for curve correction[43-48], this chapter will focus on pedicle screw placement (Figs. 23.3–23.5). To limit the risks involved with pedicle screw placement, one must understand spine anatomy and the typical three-dimensional changes that can occur with the specific deformity present at that level (Fig. 23.6). For lumbar pedicle screws, the facet joint is removed, which allows for the cancellous entry point to the pedicle (Fig. 23.7). At the mid aspect of the transverse process and just lateral to the lateral aspect of the lamina (Fig. 23.8), a "gear shift" is inserted and passed through the pedicle into the cancellous bone of the vertebral body (Fig. 23.9). A probe is then passed into this tract to ensure an intact medial, lateral, superior, inferior, and anterior wall (Fig. 23.10). This probe can be measured to determine appropriate length of screw (Fig. 23.11). The path is then tapped with an appropriately sized tap and the pedicle screw can be inserted (Fig. 23.12). Screw placement can be done with CT or fluoroscopic guidance, but can also be done safely through the "free-hand" technique.[49,50] If done by the

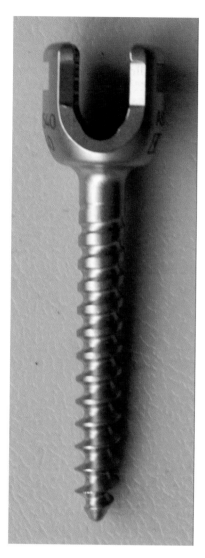

Figure 23.3 A pedicle screw as seen from the front. The U-shaped head allows for rod attachment and threads are located at the top of this area for a locking bolt to secure the rod to the screw.

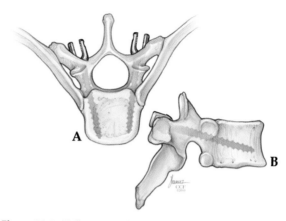

Figure 23.5 (A) Illustration of pedicle screws within the pedicle of a thoracic vertebral body. Just medial to the pedicle is the neural canal. (B) The same screw from the lateral view.

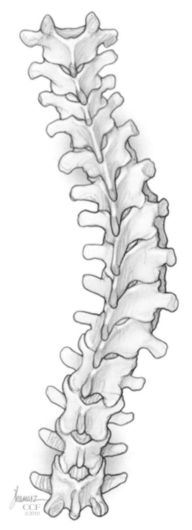

Figure 23.6 Example of rotational deformity that occurs with scoliosis. Notice how the vertebral body rotates out toward the apex and convexity of the curve. The majority of the rotation is located nearest to the apex, less away from the apex.

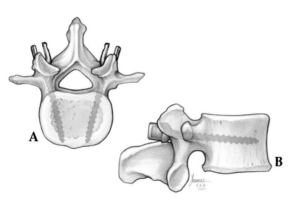

Figure 23.4 (A) Illustration of pedicle screw within the pedicle of a lumbar vertebral body. Just medial to the pedicle is the neural canal. (B) The same screw from the lateral view.

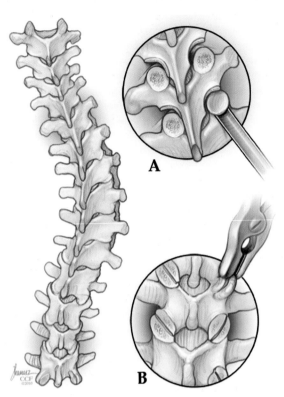

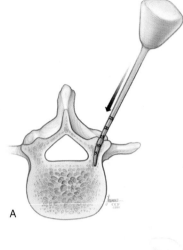

Figure 23.9 (A) Gearshift insertion through the cancellous bone of the pedicle toward the vertebral body. Initially the gear shift is pointed laterally to avoid medial breech. (B) Once past the neural canal, the tip of the gearshift can be directed medically.

Figure 23.7 (A) Demonstrating facetectomy in the thoracic spine with removal of the inferior facet. (B) Facetectomy of the lumbar spine. Note: this bone is saved and used later for bone grafting.

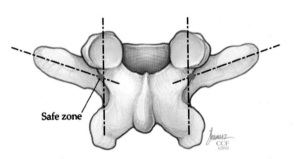

Figure 23.8 Illustration of the lumbar spine delineating the safe area for pedicle screw insertion. The dot represents the starting point, which is typically just lateral to the axilla of the lamina and transverse process and near the midpoint of the transverse process.

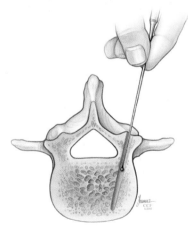

Figure 23.10 A probe is used to feel the walls of the pedicle to ensure that no breech has occurred.

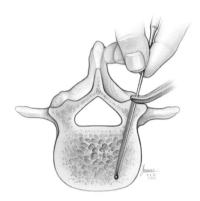

Figure 23.11 This probe can be used to measure the depth of the tract to help determine the correct length of the pedicle screw. Screw length should be slightly shorter than what is measured to avoid anterior penetration.

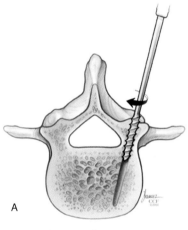

A

Figure 23.12 (A) A tap is used to prepare the pedicle for screw placement. (B) The screw has been inserted into this path.

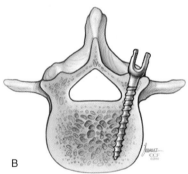

B

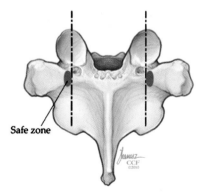

Safe zone

Figure 23.13 Illustration of the portion of the thoracic spine delineating the safe area for pedicle screw insertion.

"free-hand" technique, fluoroscopic check can be performed to ensure that each screw is in good position. MEPs should also be checked frequently to ensure that there is no neurologic change. In the thoracic spine, the inferior facet of the above vertebrae can be removed (Fig. 23.7A). The starting point can vary with regard to the superior and inferior starting point for each level, but should always be just lateral to the middle aspect of the superior facet (Fig. 23.13). Typically, a burr can be used to gain access to the medullary canal and then similar entry can be performed as described in the lumbar spine. Similar probing, tapping, and screw placement can be performed. Facet osteotomies, such as the Ponte osteotomy, can be useful for allowing mobility of the spine. Further osteotomies such as pedicle subtraction osteotomy or vertebral column resection can be performed for severe deformities but are beyond the scope of this chapter. Once all screws are placed, it is important to recheck for bleeding, assess alignment of screws fluoroscopically, and recheck MEPs. If there is bleeding difficulty with screw placement, a thrombin gel, such as Floseal (Baxter International Inc., Deerfield, IL, USA), can be used safely. If a screw can be placed efficiently and safely, then this may be the best way to tamponade any cancellous bone bleeding. There are multiple types of screws that can be used; I prefer uniaxial screws as they may help to improve sagittal alignment while allowing for coronal stability.

With the anchors placed, a rod is measured for the concavity of the curve. This rod is cut, prebent, and loosely locked in to the concavity of the curve. Rotation of this rod in a 90° derotation maneuver helps to straighten the coronal alignment while improving the sagittal alignment. It is important prior to this maneuver to elevate the MAP to greater than 90° as stretch during correction may cause arterial spasm and lead to neurologic compromise. Increasing MAP may improve arterial flow and lessen neurologic risk. As correction occurs, close attention should be given to the SSEP and MEP monitoring. If there is change, less correction should be accepted. Elevating the patient's blood pressure, hematocrit, and oxygenation is also helpful.[51] If spinal cord monitoring is unchanged, further deformity correction can be performed with spine derotation. Special connectors are attached to the screws and axial alignment correction is performed (Fig. 23.14). It is important to avoid pushing down on the spine as this can create hypokyphosis.[52] Further distraction to the concavity and compression of the convexity or in-situ bending can be done to maximize the correction.

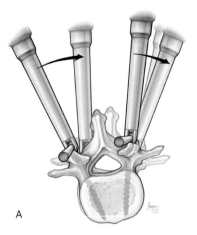

Figure 23.14 (A) Illustration of the spine derotation technique with screw connectors attached. Arrows depict the rotation maneuver. (B) With derotation performed, axial alignment of the spine is much improved.

A

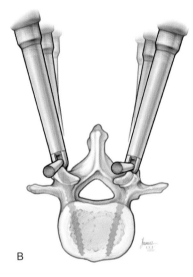

B

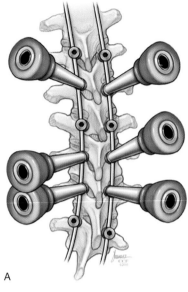

Figure 23.15 (A) Derotation connectors visualized from the posterior view. Typically connectors would be at each screw. (B) Posterior view illustration after correction maneuvers have been performed.

A

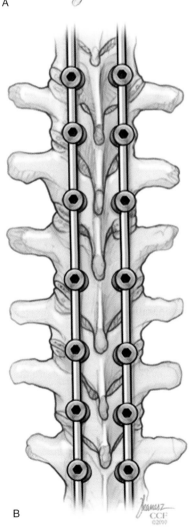

B

The convex rod is often placed with mild decrease in sagittal alignment rod bending to help with axial derotation. Final tightening of the locking bolts can be performed once acceptable alignment has been achieved (Fig. 23.15). Fluoroscopy or plain radiography can be used to check fixation and spine balance, and to view the pulmonary fields for pneumothorax (Fig. 23.16). An adequate field for bone healing must be created. Decortication of the spinous process, lamina, and transverse process can be performed with a burr or an osteotome. Bone taken during the case can be used as autograft and other forms of bone graft material may be used for supplementation. Deep fascia and skin are closed in layers after thorough irrigation.

Postoperatively, close monitoring of the patient is required. Oxygenation, blood pressure, and hematocrit should be followed closely. Late-onset neurologic changes within the immediate postoperative

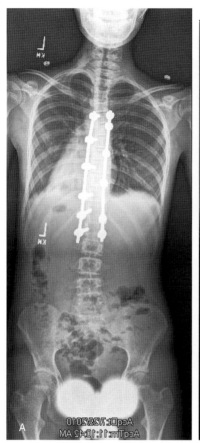
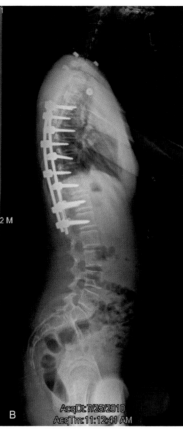

Figure 23.16 Example of postoperative imaging with PA (A) and lateral (B) radiographs from the same patient in Fig. 23.1.

period may be the result of spinal cord ischemia in patients due to relative hypotension.[53] Postoperative pain control can be treated with epidural anesthesia, intrathecal morphine injection, or patient-controlled analgesia.[54,55] Ketorolac can be used postoperatively as it has not been shown to increase risk of pseudoarthrosis.[56] Early mobilization is important for pulmonary and bowel function. Most patients will tolerate sitting and standing on postoperative day 1 and progressive ambulation can be expected over the next few days. Typical hospital stay is between 4 and 7 days. Over the next 6 months, the patient is allowed to do low-impact activities and activities of daily living, but should limit forward bending, twisting, and lifting greater then 5 kg (ca. 10 lbs). Return to school should be expected by 6 weeks. After 6 months, the patient can return to most activities including noncollision sports.

References

1. Bruszewski J, Kamza Z. [Incidence of scoliosis based on an analysis of serial radiography.] *Chir Narzadow Ruchu Ortop Pol* 1957; **22**: 115–16.

2. Kane WJ, Moe JH. A scoliosis prevalence survey in Minnesota. *Clin Orthop Relat Res* 1970; **69**: 216–18.

3. Willner S, Uden A. A prospective prevalence study of scoliosis in Southern Sweden. *Acta Orthop Scand* 1982; **53**: 233–7.

4. LaGrone MO, King HA. Idiopathic adolescent scoliosis: indications and expectations. Chapter 33. In: Bridwell KH, DeWald RL, eds. *The Textbook of Spinal Surgery*. 2nd ed. Philadelphia: Lippincott–Raven; 1997: 425–50.

5. Edgar M, Mehta M. Long-term follow-up of fused and unfused idiopathic scoliosis. *J Bone Joint Surg* 1988; **70B**: 712–16.

6. Weinstein SL. Idiopathic scoliosis. Natural history. *Spine* 1986; **11**: 780–3.

7. Lonstein JE. Carlson JM. The prediction of curve progression in untreated idiopathic scoliosis during growth. *J Bone Joint Surg*. 1984; **66**: 1061–71.

8. Duval-Beaupere G. Pathogenic relationship between scoliosis and growth. In: Zorab PA, ed. *Scoliosis and Growth*. Edinburgh: Churchill Livingstone; 1971: 58–64.

9. Sanders JO, Herring JA, Browne RH. Posterior arthrodesis and instrumentation in the immature

(Risser-grade-0) spine in idiopathic scoliosis. *J Bone Joint Surg* 1995; **77A**: 39–45.

10. Sponseller PD, Betz R, Newton PO, *et al.* Differences in curve behavior after fusion in adolescent idiopathic scoliosis with open triradiate cartilages. *Spine* 2009; **34**: 827–31.

11. Vedantam R, Crawford AH. The role of preoperative pulmonary function tests in patients with adolescent idiopathic scoliosis undergoing posterior spinal fusion. *Spine* 1997; **22**: 2731–4.

12. Vedantam R, Lenke LG, Bridwell KH, *et al.* A prospective evaluation of pulmonary function in patients with adolescent idiopathic scoliosis relative to the surgical approach used for spinal arthrodesis. *Spine* 2000; **25**: 82–90.

13. Aaro S, Ohlund C. Scoliosis and pulmonary function. *Spine* 1984; **9**: 220–2.

14. Leong JC, Lu WW, Luk KD, *et al.* Kinematics of the chest cage and spine during breathing in healthy individuals and in patients with adolescent idiopathic scoliosis. *Spine* 1999; **24**: 1310–15.

15. Wood KB, Schendel MJ, Dekutoski MB, *et al.* Thoracic volume changes in scoliosis surgery. *Spine* 1996; **21**: 718–23.

16. Weinstein SL, Zavala DC, Ponseti IV. Idiopathic scoliosis: long-term follow-up and prognosis in untreated patients. *J Bone Joint Surg Am* 1981; **63**: 702–12.

17. Upadhyay SS, Mullaji AB, Luk KD, *et al.* Relation of spinal and thoracic cage deformities and their flexibilities with altered pulmonary functions in adolescent idiopathic scoliosis. *Spine* 1995; **20**: 2415–20.

18. Kearon C, Viviani GR, Kirkley A, *et al.* Factors determining pulmonary function in adolescent idiopathic thoracic scoliosis. *Am Rev Respir Dis* 1993; **148**: 288–94.

19. Newton PO, Faro FD, Gollogly S, *et al.* Results of preoperative pulmonary function testing of adolescents with idiopathic scoliosis. A study of six hundred and thirty-one patients. *J Bone Joint Surg Am* 2005; **87**: 1937–46.

20. Puno R, Lenke L, Richards S, Sucato D, Emans J, Erickson M. Non-neurologic complications following surgery for adolescent idiopathic scoliosis. *Spine J* 2006; **6**(5): 80S.

21. Padberg AM, Wilson-Holden TJ, Lenke LG, Bridwell KH. Somatosensory motor-evoked potential monitoring without a wakeup test during idiopathic scoliosis surgery. An accepted standard of care. *Spine* 1998; **23**: 1392–400.

22. Padberg AM, Komanetsky RE, Bridwell KH, *et al.* Neurogenic motor evoked potentials: A prospective comparison of stimulation methods. *J Spinal Dis* 1997; **11**: 21–4.

23. Papin P, Arlet V, Marchesi D, *et al.* Unusual presentation of spinal cord compression related to misplaced pedicle screws in thoracic scoliosis. *Eur Spine J* 1999; **8**: 156–9.

24. Kim, YJ, Lenke, LG. Prospective pulmonary function comparison of anterior spinal fusion in adolescent idiopathic scoliosis: thoracotomy versus thoracoabdominal approach. *Spine* 2008; **33**: 1055–60.

25. Kim YJ, Lenke LG, Bridwell KH, *et al.* Prospective pulmonary function in adolescent idiopathic scoliosis relative to the surgical procedure. *J Bone Joint Surg Am* 2005: **87**; 1534–41.

26. Kim, YB Lenke, LG. The morbidity of an anterior thoracolumbar approach: adult spinal deformity patients with greater than five-year follow-up. *Spine* 2009; **34**: 822–6.

27. Sucato DJ, Erken YH, Davis S, *et al.* Prone thoracoscopic release does not adversely affect pulmonary function when added to a posterior spinal fusion for severe spine deformity. *Spine* 2009; **34**: 771–8.

28. Picetti GD, Pang D. Thoracoscopic techniques for the treatment of scoliosis. *Childs Nerv Syst* 2004; **20**: 802–10.

29. Sucato DJ, Newton PO, Betz RR, *et al.* Defining the learning curve for performing a thoracoscopic anterior spinal fusion and instrumentation for AIS: a multi-center study. Presented at the annual meeting of the Pediatric Orthopaedic Society of North America, Ottawa, Ontario, Canada, 2005.

30. Geck MJ, Rinella A, Hawthorne D, *et al.* Comparison of surgical treatment in Lenke 5C adolescent idiopathic scoliosis: anterior dual rod versus posterior pedicle fixation surgery: a comparison of two practices. *Spine* 2009; **34**: 1942–51.

31. Cheng I, Kim Y, Gupta MC, *et al.* Apical sublaminar wires versus pedicle screws-which provides better results for surgical correction of adolescent idiopathic scoliosis? *Spine* 2005; **30**: 2104–12.

32. Liljenqvist U, Lepsien U, Hackenberg L, *et al.* Comparative analysis of pedicle screw and hook instrumentation in posterior correction and fusion of idiopathic thoracic scoliosis. *Eur Spine J* 2002; **11**: 336–43.

33. Kim YJ, Lenke LG, Kim J, *et al.* Comparative analysis of pedicle screw versus hybrid instrumentation in posterior spinal fusion of adolescent idiopathic scoliosis. *Spine* 2006; **31**: 291–8.

34. Karatoprak O, Unay K, Tezer M, *et al.* Comparative analysis of pedicle screw versus hybrid instrumentation in adolescent idiopathic scoliosis surgery. *Int Orthop* 2008; **32**: 523–8; discussion 529.

35. Lehman, RA. Operative treatment of adolescent idiopathic scoliosis with posterior pedicle screw-only

constructs: minimum three-year follow-up of one hundred fourteen cases. *Spine* 2008; **33**: 1598–604.

36. Luhmann SJ, Lenke LG, Kim YJ, *et al.* Thoracic adolescent idiopathic scoliosis curves between 70° and 100°. Is anterior release necessary? *Spine* 2005; **30**: 2061–7.

37. Kuklo TR, Lenke LG O'Brien MF, *et al.* Accuracy and efficacy of thoracic pedicle screws in curves more than 90°. *Spine* 2005; **30**: 222–6.

38. Mirovsky Y, Neuwirth M. Injuries to the lateral femoral cutaneous nerve during spine surgery. *Spine* 2000; **25**: 1266–9.

39. Prielipp RC, Morell RC, Walker FO, *et al.* Ulnar nerve pressure: influence of arm position and relationship to somatosensory evoked potentials. *Anesthesiology* 1999; **91**: 345–54.

40. Lenke LG, Betz RR, Harms J, *et al.* Adolescent idiopathic scoliosis: anew classification to determine extent of spinal arthrodesis. *J Bone Joint Surg* 2001; **83**: 1169–81.

41. Owen JA. The application of intraoperative monitoring during surgery for spinal deformity. *Spine* 1999; **24**: 2649–62.

42. Myers MA, Hamilton SR, Bogosian AJ, *et al.* Visual loss as a complication of spine surgery: A review of 37 cases. *Spine* 1997; **22**: 1325–9.

43. Liljenqvist U, Hackenberg L, Link T, *et al.* Pullout strength of pedicle screws versus pedicle and laminar hooks in the thoracic spine. *Acta Orthop Belg* 2001; **67**: 157–63.

44. Hackenberg L, Link T, Liljenqvist U. Axial and tangential fixation strength of pedicle screws versus hooks in the thoracic spine in relation to bone mineral density. *Spine* 2002; **27**: 937–42.

45. Kostuik JP, Munting E, Valdevit A. Biomechanical analysis of screw load sharing in pedicle fixation of the lumbar spine. *J Spinal Disord* 1994; **7**: 394–401.

46. Kwok AW, Findelstein JA, Woodside T. Insertional torque and pull-out strengths of conical and cylindrical pedicle screws in cadaveric bone. *Spine* 1996; **21**: 2429–34.

47. Mahar AT, Bagheri R, Oka R, Akbarnia BA. Biomechanical comparison of different anchors for the pediatric dual growing rod technique. *Spine* 2008; **6**: 933–9.

48. Jones GA, Kayanja M, Lieberman I. Biomechanical characteristics of hybrid hoof-screw constructs in short-segment thoracic fixation. *Spine* 2008; **33**: 173–7.

49. Kim YW, Lenke LG. Free-hand pedicle screw placement during revision spinal surgery: analysis of 552 screws. *Spine* 2008; **33**(10): 1141–8.

50. Kuklo TR, Lenke LG, Bridwell KH, Cho YS, Riew KD. Free hand pedicle screw placement in the thoracic spine, is it safe? *Spine* 2004; **29**: 333–42.

51. Bridwell KH, Lenke LG, Baldus C, Blanke K. Major intraoperative neurologic deficits in pediatric and adult spinal deformity patients. Incidence and etiology at one institution. *Spine* 1998; **23**: 324–31.

52. Vora V, Crawford A, Babekhir N, *et al.* A pedicle screw construct gives an enhanced posterior correction of adolescent idiopathic scoliosis when compared with other constructs: myth or reality. *Spine* 2007; **32**: 1869–74.

53. Paonessa KJ, Hutchings F. Delayed postoperative neurologic deficits following spinal deformity surgery. Paper presented at the Scoliosis Research Society Annual Meeting, New York, NY, Sept. 16–20, 1998.

54. Sucato DJ, Duey-Holtz A, Elerson E, *et al.* Postoperative analgesia following surgical correction for adolescent idiopathic scoliosis: a comparison of continuous epidural analgesia and patient-controlled analgesia. *Spine* 2005; **30**: 211–17.

55. Milbrandt TA, Singhal M, Minter C, *et al.* A comparison of three methods of pain control for posterior spinal fusions in adolescent idiopathic scoliosis. *Spine* 2009; **34**: 1499–503.

56. Sucato DJ, Lovejoy JF, Agrawal S, *et al.* Postoperative ketorolac does not predispose to pseudoarthrosis following posterior spinal fusion and instrumentation for adolescent idiopathic scoliosis. *Spine* 2008; **33**: 1119–24.

23.2 Tethered cord: surgical release

Mark Luciano

Key points

- A tethered cord results from a variety of anatomical anomalies and clinical settings. The surgical indication, goal, method, and outcome vary depending on the specific disorder.

- The clinical decision to surgically release may result from the anticipation of progressive spinal cord stretch and injury in the growing asymptomatic infant or in a patient of any age with progressive neurologic deficits.

- The common surgical goal is release of the tether via a dorsal approach. Complete resection of the pathology is not always required.
- Surgical preparation varies with the age and nature of tether but may involve special consideration for limb deformity, latex allergy, and electrophysiological monitoring.
- The surgical procedure varies from a simple, one-level laminectomy to a multiple-level laminectomy with lesion resection, use of the operative microscope, laser, and plastics closure.

Introduction

Surgical release of a tethered spinal cord is a procedure seen in both adult and pediatric neurosurgical practices. The common pathological feature in all cases is a form of adhesion between the caudal spinal cord and the caudal spinal canal. The primary goal of a tether release is to separate the caudal spinal cord or conus from canal elements that, as a result of skeletal growth or movement, pull the spinal cord, stretching its neural and vascular elements. The anatomical reasons for tether are multiple and thus the "tethered cord syndrome" may be treated in varied clinical settings of spinal anomaly and presents from infancy to adulthood. The difficulty and outcome of this surgical release depend greatly on the cause of tethering. For example, in the case of a thickened filum terminali, release is a relatively straightforward procedure requiring a single or partial laminectomy and 1–2 hours of operative time. On the other hand, a lipomeningocele represents a complex tether with intermingled nerves that may require electrophysiological monitoring, hours of microsurgery, laser reduction, and more elaborate closure techniques. Because of this variability, appropriate planning for a "tether release" procedure requires a broader understanding of its context.

Tethered cord pathology: clinical setting and work-up

While a spinal cord can be tethered anywhere along its course in the spinal canal, the most common type is seen as tethering of the spinal cord terminus or "conus" secondary to developmental abnormality. Cord tethering is a significant part of the pathology in the open spinal defect of myelomeningocele where the caudal cord is open, exposed, and contiguous with lumbar skin.[1,2] Tethered cord also accompanies closed skin defects such as lipoma, dermal sinus tract, split cord malformation, or thickened filum terminali[7]. These forms of tethered cord are commonly suspected in the neonate when a dimple, angioma, or abnormal hair tuft is seen in the lumbar or sacral region. In this case the next step in diagnosis is usually a lumbar spine ultrasound that can identify a low-lying conus below the L1/2 level and possibly identify the structures causing the tether. If suspected clinically or by ultrasound, MRI is important to verify the exact anatomy of the tethering lesion or anomaly before a surgical procedure is performed. This MRI may be done separately before the day of operation or, because of the requirement for general anesthesia for MRI in the infant, may be performed just preoperatively on the day of surgery.

As noted above, a fundamental finding in the diagnosis of tethered cord is the low-lying spinal cord conus. In the period of rapid skeletal growth just before and in the months after delivery the length of the skeletal spinal canal rapidly outstrips that of the spinal cord itself, resulting in an apparent "ascent" of the conus in the canal.[8] During this period any anatomical anomaly tethering the conus to the "descending" skeletal elements stretches the spinal cord. Although spinal cord pathology and symptoms may arise directly from elongated neural elements, research has indicated a role for stretched spinal vessels resulting in spinal cord ischemia that may not be reversible.[5] The severity of the tethered cord and potential for progressive spinal cord injury are not well predicted by the degree of conus descent, which may vary from high lumbar to sacral. In fact, though controversial, a mild form of tether called "tether 0" has been treated where the conus is in normal position but progressive symptoms consistent with tethered cord exist along with some other spinal abnormality.[9]

The likelihood of progressive spinal cord stretch with the dramatic skeletal growth of childhood and adolescence combined with the concern for irreversible spinal cord injury has been the main argument for prophylactic release of an asymptomatic tethered cord when diagnosed in infancy. This is especially the case where the morbidity of release is considered low as a result of simple pathology and experienced microsurgery. Asymptomatic tethered cord incidentally found in adulthood may not require release, though symptoms may develop in adulthood perhaps secondary to the effect of persistent stretch and movement. Progressive neurologic deterioration consistent with tethered cord is an indication for release at any age. Patients with tethered cord, before and after release, are followed closely for any progressive neurologic deficit usually proceeding in a caudal to rostral direction. Common presenting symptoms may be back and leg pain and urological symptoms. Urodynamics are often useful in detecting progression.[6] Re-tether is possible secondary to adhesive scarring at the surgical site and repeated release may be attempted several times, though with diminishing returns.

Types of spinal cord tethering

1. *Myelomeningocele*: Seen in the perinatal period and released with myelomeningocele cyst closure usually within the first 72 hours of birth. The result of closure is most commonly a secondary tether, which has to be monitored for symptoms throughout development and may require later re-release.[2]
2. *Lipomeningocele, spinal lipoma*: A closed skin defect most often identified in the infant with a subcutaneous fatty mass that extends through the dura into the spinal canal. Lipomas may also be entirely intradural with adhesion to the cord or spinal roots. The complexity of resection depends largely on the lipoma's position dorsal or caudal to the spinal cord and nerve roots (Fig. 23.17).
3. *Meningocele*: A meningocele is usually diagnosed in infancy as a midline cystic mass in the lumbar, thoracic, or cervical region. It is the skin-covered meningeal sac which usually has no or minimal neuronal content, yet the cord may be tethered to the dorsal canal at the cyst origin and nerve roots may be pulled into the sac.
4. *Dermal sinus tract*: The dermal sinus tract is often suspected in the neonatal period on the basis of a dimple or lump in the lumbar region, occasionally with active fluid drainage. Resection may be done in infancy for tether release as well as for avoidance of meningitis[3] (Fig. 23.18).
5. *Split cord malformation*: A split cord malformation is often diagnosed in infancy on the basis of lumbar stigmata and/or extremity deformity. It may be associated with other spinal cord anomalies such as a spinal cord syrinx. The tethering is based on a bony spicule dividing the dural sac and cord (type 1) or a cartilaginous divide within a singe dural sleeve (type 2).[4] Resection may be performed in infancy or at any age as symptoms develop (Fig. 23.19).
6. *Thickened filum terminale*: A thickened filum may be suspected at birth with lumbar skin stigmata or after becoming symptomatic in childhood, young adulthood, or later adulthood. Tethering is based

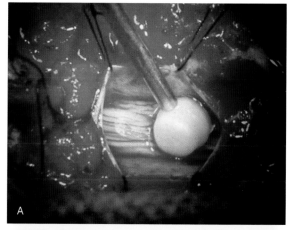

A

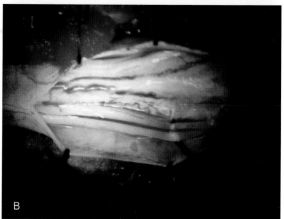

B

Figure 23.17 (A) Dorsal spinal lipoma. (B) Caudal spinal cord lipoma.

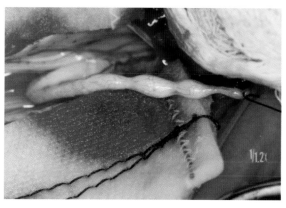

Figure 23.18 Dermal sinus tract.

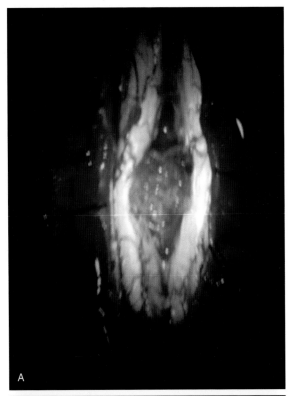

on the less elastic filum, which is greater than 2 mm and may be fibrous and fatty[3] (Fig. 23.20).

7. *Postsurgical tethering*: Any etiology of tethered cord or intradural spinal surgery of any kind, including tether release, may result in a tethered cord from scarring and adhesion of the spinal cord to the surgical site. Re-tether from a myelomeningocele or lipomeningocele is more likely than from sectioning of a thickened filum.

Preoperative considerations

The variety of clinical settings creating a tether results in specific considerations and expectations for each kind of tether. Nevertheless, common elements of positioning, approach, monitoring, and goals exist for most tethered cord release procedures.

Positioning

In most cases of tethered cord release a dorsal approach to the sacral, lumbar, thoracic, or cervical spinal cord

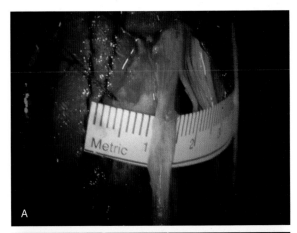

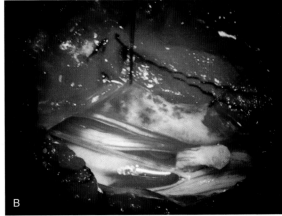

Figure 23.19 (A) Split cord malformation type I. (B) Bony spur resection.

Figure 23.20. (A) Intact fatty and fibrous filum. (B) Thickened filum after resection.

is required, utilizing a prone position. Positioning may be made more difficult by limb deformity, contractures, or kyphosis. Access to a broad area of the dorsal trunk or limbs may be required should a skin or muscle flap be required. Positioning is usually performed after placement of monitoring electrodes and a Foley catheter.

Monitoring

Sensory and/or motor potentials and EMG with intraoperative stimulation are useful for following spinal cord status and differentiating nerves from adhesion during dissection. Sensory evoked potentials are not obtained in infancy. The usual application includes placement of electrodes on lower extremities and sphincter. While such monitoring is uncommon in the myelomeningocele closure of neonatal surgery, it may be very helpful during resection of a lipoma with adhered or included nerve roots. It is of some use in identifying nerve roots surrounding a thickened filum or dermal sinus tract. In this situation EMG recording during monopolar or bipolar electrostimulation without muscle relaxation is utilized.

Allergy

Children with myelomeningocele require a latex-free environment for potential latex allergy.

Surgical technique

General surgical approach

The surgical approach is usually via a midline dorsal incision over the area of suspected tether in the lumbosacral sacral region. In the case of skin-covered lesions this incision may be single or elliptical lines surrounding an area of a subcutaneous lipoma or exiting dermal sinus tract. If the tether involves a lesion coming to the surface it may be resected subcutaneously and then followed deeply to approach the spinal dorsal elements and dura. Normal dura above and, if possible, below this lesion is identified and may be opened with a midline incision or elliptically around the entering structures. In case of thickened fatty filum, the skin and subcutaneous tissue posterior elements and dura may be entirely normal in the midline and a simple midline incision approach and laminectomy is used. The goal of the surgery in each case is to obtain a spinal cord and conus without attachments to the spinal canal and with as much free space as possible to reduce the possibility of recurring tether. The entire adhering structure,

such as filum or lipoma, need not be entirely resected when benign, though lipomas are often reduced where entangled nerve roots and the conus are not threatened by dissection. Closure may be simple and primary or involve a duraplasty or muscle and skin flaps. The lateral monitoring EMG and nerve stimulation are used to help with the dissection of the tethering mass.

Special considerations in specific disorders

Myelomeningocele

In the newborn with myelomeningocele the nervous elements are exposed at the surface cystic mass, which may be closed and dry or leaking CSF at the time of birth. Myelomeningoceles are usually closed within 1–3 days post-delivery. With the high incidence of hydrocephalus in these infants, CSF shunting may be performed at the same time or at a later date. During patient positioning care is taken not to add injury to the exposed spinal cord plaque by keeping it moist and as clean as possible, and by avoiding compression. Skin preparation involves a saline-diluted povidone-iodine solution over the exposed plaque with a more rigorous scrub over a wide area of the back to allow for skin mobilization or flap placement. The operation proceeds with an elliptical incision isolating the spinal cord plaque. The dura is identified under normal lamina just rostral to the emergence of the myelomeningocele. A layered closure proceeds with new formation of a neural tube using a 7-0 sutured closure of the spinal cord terminus under microscopy or loupe magnification. The dura is closed through an inward folding of the lateral sac's fascia in layers. Subsequently, the lumbar fascial sleeve and subcutaneous and skin closures are performed in separate layers if possible. In the case of a shallow canal or severely kyphotic spine, a corrective vertebral body resection may be performed with suture fixation of the spinal elements. With most defects, lateral skin undermining and mobilization is sufficient for closure. On occasion, plastic surgery assists in skin or muscle mobilization over the larger defects.

Lipomeningocele

Lipomeningocele often presents as a soft, fatty subcutaneous mass under completely closed skin. It may be resected in the neonatal period in childhood or adulthood. Repeated resection and release is not uncommon. The level of difficulty and duration of the

401

release vary greatly depending on the anatomy of the lipomeningocele. Lipomas that enter through the dorsal dura and remain dorsal to the spinal cord, adhering to the dorsal aspect of the spinal cord conus, may be resected at the level of the conus without injury to the spinal cord or the cauda equina. The lipoma may not be entirely removed as it fuses with the spinal cord, but it may be reduced effectively at the conus with the use of a CO_2 laser. It should be emphasized that the goal of the surgery is to release a tethered spinal cord and not necessarily removal of the entire lipoma. This is especially true with a lipoma that extends caudally from the conus and intermingles with roots of the cauda equina. Lipomas are commonly fibrous and tough, and dissection from nerve roots that may run through is impossible without severe injury. This dissection is most often done under loupe or operative scope magnification or electrophysiological monitoring and may proceed on a millimeter-by-millimeter basis. Large areas of lipoma may be unresected depending on nerve root involvement. Release of a lipomeningocele often results in a significant dural opening defect that may require a dural patch for closure. The risk of CSF leakage may be reduced by horizontal position in the postoperative period.

Thickened filum

Sectioning of a thickened filum terminale is the simplest, shortest, and most straightforward of the tether release procedures. It is also the least likely to re-tether, though even in this case the rate may be as high as 8–9%.[8] The approach is a simple midline incision and laminectomy in the lumbar or sacral region below the level of the conus. The overlying skin and lamina may be entirely normal, though spina bifida occulta may be present. After a dural opening through a one- or two-level laminectomy, the cauda equina can be visualized and often the final terminale itself appears as a larger dorsal and neurovascular band. It may be further identified by areas of yellow fat and ultimately by a lack of response to electric stimulation. Nerve roots are often adherent to the surface of the filum and must be carefully dissected after inspection of the full circumference. After isolation of the filum bipolar cautery may be used gently over a 1–2 mm segment before sectioning with microscissors or scalpel. The chances of recurrent tether via a filum reconnection are almost zero, though adhesion of the cord or filum to the scar at the laminectomy site itself is possible. The dura may be closed primarily in a watertight fashion. Patients may be up and often discharged the next day.

Dermal sinus tract

Dermal sinus tract is most often diagnosed in infancy as a lumbar dimple that may actively conduct fluid from the spinal canal to the skin surface. Nodular dermoids may also be found that produce sebaceous dermal elements. The tract tethers through its rostral extension, attaching to the caudal spinal cord. The indications for surgery include tether and risk of infection and meningitis. Similarly to other tether release procedures, the release proceeds from a midline lumbar incision that in this case includes an ellipse around the tract's terminus at the skin. Though not all sinuses extend into the spinal canal, it may be followed inward toward the posterior spine elements and dura, where it may enter the canal. The dura is exposed at, and rostral to, the entering tract. It is opened elliptically around the tract, which is then followed rostral to its tether at the spinal cord. Again, intraoperative stimulation and monitoring may be helpful for identifying and protecting adherent nerve roots. The tract is resected to avoid possible irritation, mass effect, or re-tethering. The dura may be closed primarily or with a small patch.

Meningocele

Meningoceles are skin-covered, fluid-filled meningeal out-pouchings that are largely devoid of neural elements. It is not uncommon, however, for a tethered cord to be associated with its exit from the spinal canal or for nerves to be pulled up into it. Although often resected in the neonatal period, they may be resected in children or even in older adults. After midline or elliptical incision the membrane is identified and separated from the overlying skin. A transillumination or previous imaging helps identify areas of suspected infolded neural elements. With opening of the sac, nerve elements and spinal cord can be identified and released. After resection of the redundant membranes the incision is closed in layered fashion.

Postsurgical tether

Essentially all children with surgically closed myelomeningocele have tethered cords that may require release in later life if symptomatic. Other forms of tethered cord release surgery or any other lumbar sacral procedure may cause scarring and tethering that subsequently becomes symptomatic with growth, movement, or aging. These procedures vary in their spinal level and extent of required dissection and requirement for surgical adjuvants such as magnification, laser, or neural monitoring.

Special equipment and procedures

Electrophysiological monitoring

Sensory evoked potentials have limited utility but may be used with dissection of tethering lesions off the dorsum of the spinal cord. EMG recording and intraoperative stimulation is rarely used in neonatal surgery such as myelomeningocele closure, but it may be used in many tethered pathologies in identifying neural elements in the dissection. This is most important in lipomeningocele where nerve roots are admitted and run through the fibrous and fatty mass. However, it can also be important in identifying nerve roots adherent to thickened filum terminale or dorsal spinous tract. Electrical stimulation with a monopolar electrode provides greatest sensitivity, and bipolar probes may be used when more specific localization is needed. Muscle paralysis is avoided during this procedure.

Laser

The CO_2 laser is a useful adjunct in dissection of scar and the reduction of the lipoma's mass. The laser can be used in conjunction with operative microscopy or as a free handheld tool. The advantage of this procedure is its minimal spread of thermal energy, allowing a safer and less traumatic reduction or lysis.

Skin and muscle flaps

In most cases the closure of even open defects such as myelomeningocele can be performed without the use of skin and muscle flaps secondary to the loose skin and inability to mobilize large areas laterally to the skin and muscle defect. Closure of larger defects sometimes requires mobilization of skin and muscle flaps. With repeated surgery, plastic closures are occasionally required.

Endoscopic

There have been reports of minimally invasive spinal procedures including release of tethered cord using endoscopic techniques. This method is not generally performed but may be feasible with simpler procedures such as filum sectioning. In this case the endoscope may be considered in the same way as the operative microscope in its purpose and use.[9]

Postoperative considerations

Lower extremity sensory motor function must be assessed immediately postoperatively. Postoperative pain may derive not only from the lumbar incision but also from irritation of nerve roots or dorsal spinal cord in the dissection. A PCA pump for maximal control of what may be severe acute pain is helpful whenever age-appropriate. These patients often have had or will have chronic pain and medication coverage must reflect previous use. The patient is most often kept horizontal for the night of surgery and may need to be horizontal for several days depending of the risk of CSF leakage.

Summary/conclusions

Spinal cord tethering results in stretched neural elements and vessels that lead to reversible and then irreversible spinal cord injury and symptoms. The goal of release is the separation of the cord from any tethering element that binds it to the caudal canal. This release may be performed in the asymptomatic infant and in patients with progressive symptoms. It is performed in neonates and in adults and in a variety of clinical settings. Knowledge of the specific pathology is needed to understand the extent of the planned procedure and any special procedures or equipment being considered such as monitoring, laser, dural substitutes, or flaps. With this variability in procedure, communication about the specific goals and surgical course becomes especially important.

References

1. Cochrane DD. Occult spinal dysraphism. In: Albright AL, Pollack IF, Adelson PD, eds. *Principles and Practice of Pediatric Neurosurgery*. 2nd ed. New York: Thieme; 2008: 367–89.

2. Regel DH. Tethered myelomeningocele. In: McLone DG, ed. *Pediatric Neurosurgery: Surgery of the Developing Nervous System*. 4th ed. Philadelphia, PA. WB Saunders; 2001: 279–86.

3. Roth M. Cranio-cervical growth collision: another explanation of the Arnold–Chiari malformation and of basilar impression. *Neuroradiology* 1986; **28**: 87–194.

4. Yamada S, Iacono RP, Andrade T, Mandybur G. Yamada BS. Pathophysiology of tethered cord syndrome. *Neurosurg Clin N Am* 1995; **6**(2): 311–23.

5. Tubbs RS, Elton S, Grabb P, Dockery SE, Bartolucci AA, Oakes WJ. Analysis of the posterior fossa in children with the Chiari malformation. *Neurosurgery* 2001; **48**(5): 1050–5.

6. Zomorodi A, George TM. Tethered cord syndrome. In: Kim DH, Betz RR, Huhn SL, Newton PO, eds. *Surgery of the Pediatric Spine*. New York: Thieme; 2008: 207–16.

7. Tye GW, Ward JD, Myseros JS. Occult spinal dysraphism and the tethered spinal cord. In: Benzel EC,

ed. *Spine Surgery: Techniques, Complication Avoidance, and Management*. 2nd ed. Philadelphia, PA: Elsevier Churchill Livingstone; 2005: 1131–43.

8. Young RL, Harbrook-Bach T, Vaughn M, *et al.* Symptomatic retethering of the spinal cord after section of a tight filum terminale. *Neurosurgery* 2011; **68**(6): 1594–602.

9. Xiao D. Endoscopic spinal tethered cord release: operative technique. *Childs Nerv Syst* 2009; **25**: 577–81.

24

Spinal surgery for patients with congenital heart disease and other associated conditions

Patrick M. Callahan, Tunga Suresh, and Peter J. Davis

Key points

- Knowledge of the anatomy of the specific heart defect and the surgical interventions is essential.
- Congenital heart disease is often associated with other congenital anomalies.
- Ventilatory strategies have a significant effect on the cardiovascular stability of the patient with congenital heart disease.
- Have additional invasive monitoring available, i.e., arterial and central catheters and echocardiography.
- Emergency drugs and a defibrillator need to be readily available.

Introduction

This chapter will focus on the anesthetic concerns of children with congenital or acquired pediatric cardiac disease undergoing scoliosis surgery. In addition to the myriad of cardiovascular physiological perturbations, these children frequently have other associated congenital abnormalities that affect anesthetic management. An understanding of the physiology of the underlying defect as well as the physiology of the corrective repair is essential for ensuring a good patient outcome.

Although most pediatric patients presenting for scoliosis surgery have the idiopathic form of the disease, a significant number of patients with spinal pathology have other associated congenital or acquired anomalies. While scoliosis affects roughly 1% of the general population, as many as 4–12% of patients with cardiac disease have scoliosis.[1] With advances in both surgical and medical management of patients with pediatric heart disease, more of these patients are surviving, and as a consequence, more

patients with congenital heart disease are presenting for non-cardiac surgery.

Thus, the anesthesiologist must have an understanding of the pathophysiology of the underlying heart lesion as well as have an understanding of the physiological consequences that occur with either correction or palliation of the defect. In addition, patients with cardiac defects also have an increased incidence of associated syndromes and other congenital abnormalities. Recognition of these associated syndromes and their anesthetic implications is essential for the anesthetic management of these patients.

This chapter will focus on the most common forms of pediatric heart disease, the medical and surgical management of these common defects, the pathophysiology involved, and their anesthetic implications. In addition, syndromes associated with congenital heart defects will be reviewed.

Atrial septal defects

Overview

Atrial septal defects (ASDs) are very common congenital heart lesions discovered in syndromic or otherwise healthy patients. ASDs occur in 1 in 1500 live births. They are defined as a communication between the left and the right atrium through the interatrial septum. Their classification is based upon their location within the septum. Defects may be present in or near the ostium secundum, ostium primum, sinus venosus, or coronary sinus. Secundum atrial septal defects are some of the more common heart defects found in children, accounting for almost 10% of congenital heart disease.

Blood flow is influenced by pressure and compliance differentials as well as the size of the defect. The physiological effects are determined by the degree of shunting.

Anesthesia for Spine Surgery, ed. Ehab Farag. Published by Cambridge University Press. © Cambridge University Press 2012.

There are a number of factors that limit the free flow of left-to-right shunt across an atrial septal defect. Infants are born with elevated pulmonary vascular tone, which gradually decreases over the first few months of life to normal adult levels. In addition, the right ventricle is stiff and much less compliant than its adult counterpart. These variables result in right-sided pressures that may minimize the amount of left-to-right shunting that occurs early in life, particularly in the setting of small defects. As the patient grows and pulmonary vascular resistance decreases, an increase in left-to-right shunting occurs.

Most patients with isolated atrial septal defects will be asymptomatic and may remain healthy and active well into adulthood. However, too much pulmonary blood flow will, over time, lead to right atrial and ventricular dilatation and hypertrophy. In addition, the pulmonary vascular bed remodels in the setting of volume overload, and pulmonary hypertension may ensue. Pulmonary vascular occlusive disease develops in 5–10% of unrepaired ASD patients, and shunt flow changes to right to left (Eisenmenger's syndrome).

Management

Patients with small defects that are detected early in life are typically followed for some time prior to intervention. In most patients, small defects have been shown to shrink or even close. If the defects are larger than 8 mm, the chance of spontaneous closure is low.[2] These patients, along with patients symptomatic from smaller defects, are candidates for closure. Closure can be performed either percutaneously or surgically.

Operative closure is done with the patient on cardiopulmonary bypass. Small defects can be closed with a few stitches, and larger defects can be closed with a piece of pericardium or prosthetic material. Percutaneous closure is performed in the catheterization laboratory.

Anesthetic considerations

Patients presenting for spinal procedures may have atrial septal defects that are open and being followed or already closed either spontaneously or via intervention. Preoperative evaluation of these patients should include inquiry for evidence of heart failure. It is important to review the ECG for evidence of right heart enlargement which is signaled by large p waves and right axis deviation. ECG may also provide information about arrhythmias that may have developed secondary to distorted electrical pathways in the setting of an enlarged heart.

Patients who have had atrial septal defects closed may still have residual shunts that were not closed or perhaps have reopened. Any path across the atrial septum is an opportunity for a paradoxical embolus; therefore, strict precautions against air embolism should be followed while administering fluids and medications.

Atrioventricular canal defects

Overview

Atrioventricular (AV) canal defects, also known as atrioventricular septal defects, span a variety of pathology. Typically there is a low atrial level defect, in the ostium primum, a ventricular septal defect and varying degrees of atrioventricular valve abnormalities. AV canal defects account for approximately 5% of congenital heart disease and are frequently associated with Down's syndrome.

Shunting depends on the size and location of the defects but typically occurs at both the atrial and ventricular levels. Due to the abnormal attachments, atrioventricular valve dysfunction is also common.

Most patients suffer from left-to-right shunting, which often leads to right-sided enlargement, failure, and/or arrhythmias. Clues to excessive pulmonary blood flow and an overworked heart include patients presenting with recurrent respiratory infections and failure to thrive. If patients are not diagnosed early, pulmonary vascular resistance increases and surgical intervention may no longer be an option. Repairing the defect in the setting of pulmonary hypertension can place the right ventricle under excessive strain and predispose it to failure.

Management

Early operative intervention is key for patients with complete AV canal defects. The goals of the surgical repair are to close both the atrial and ventricular level defects and reconstruction of both atrioventricular valves in a competent fashion. Surgeons may use a variety of techniques to repair these defects. Some use two separate patches, one for the atrial and one for the ventricular defect, while others may use a single patch closing both defects.

Anesthetic considerations

There are several factors that need to be considered while formulating an anesthetic plan for a child who is to have a repair of an AV canal defect. The conduction system is in close proximity to the area of surgical repair. As a result, rhythm disturbances are not uncommon. Also, the reconstruction of the atrioventricular valves is a daunting process that does not always achieve an ideal result. Preoperative echocardiography will frequently reveal some degree of mitral and or tricuspid insufficiency.

Ventricular septal defects

Overview

Ventricular septal defects are the most common form of congenital heart disease with more than 5 infants affected per 1000 live births. The defects are typically classified by their location within the ventricle. They may be subarterial, perimembranous, inlet, or muscular. Perimembranous lesions are the most common. The physiological effects are determined by the degree of shunting. The degree of shunting is a function of the size of the defect and the relative pulmonary and systemic resistances. A critical factor when evaluating a defect in the ventricular septum is its size. Smaller defects limit the degree of shunting, while larger defects offer little resistance to flow. Increased left-to-right shunting with increased pulmonary blood flow leads to pulmonary vascular changes, increased pulmonary vascular resistance, and pulmonary hypertension. Unrepaired, large defects dramatically increase the workload of the heart. Increased return to the left atrium leads to left atrial dilation and left ventricular hypertrophy. Congestive heart failure can occur very early in life if the defect is not detected and addressed.

Management

The clinical course of a patient with a known ventricular sepal defect may vary dramatically. Smaller defects are typically asymptomatic and may not benefit from medical or surgical management. Moderate to large defects are initially treated with diuretics to improve the symptoms of congestive heart failure. A majority of ventricular septal defects will close spontaneously. Patients undergo surgical repair if the symptoms of heart failure do not respond to medical management or if left ventricular dilatation progresses. Stunted growth and recurrent respiratory infections are often a hallmark of congestive heart failure. Ventricular septal defects associated with elevated pulmonary artery pressures are also closed regardless of whether the patient is symptomatic.

Anesthetic considerations

Spinal surgery patients may have small ventricular septal defects that are being followed or one that has been closed. Medically managed patients should be examined for evidence of worsening failure as well as electrolyte abnormalities in the setting of chronic diuretic use. Some patients who have had their ventricular septal defects repaired and those who have had repairs but have residual defects will be candidates. Patients with unrepaired defects are at risk for paradoxical embolus.

Myocardial and pulmonary function are likely to be normal if complete repair is done within the first year of life. Patients with repaired ventricular septal defects may have evidence of residual defects, myocardial dysfunction, tricuspid insufficiency, right bundle branch block, subaortic obstruction, and aortic insufficiency.

Tetralogy of Fallot

Overview

Tetralogy of Fallot (TOF) is one of the most common forms of cyanotic congenital heart defects. The classic findings seen in patients with TOF include obstruction to blood flow from the right ventricular outflow tract, right ventricular hypertrophy, a ventricular septal defect, and an aorta that overrides the ventricular septum. Variants of TOF include patients with complete pulmonary atresia where pulmonary blood flow depends on a patent ductus arteriosus and in many cases multiple aortopulmonary collateral arteries (MAPCAs).

Patients' symptoms range from no cyanosis in situations where obstruction to pulmonary blood flow is mild, to dramatic cyanosis, secondary severe obstruction of the right ventricular outflow tract, and subsequent right-to-left shunting. In most patients the degree of obstruction is dynamic and minor changes in physiology can lead to significant alterations in pulmonary blood flow. "Tet" spells, or episodes of desaturation, are triggered by increases in the subpulmonic obstruction. This obstruction is thought to be mediated by alterations in contractility, systemic vascular resistance, and intravascular volume. Innocent events such as crying and defecation may trigger profound cyanosis. Such spells, while alarming, are rarely fatal. Children experiencing a spell may instinctively squat. Squatting increases systemic vascular resistance by kinking the femoral arteries, thereby reducing right-to-left shunting.

Unrepaired patients are unlikely to live beyond the age of 10 years.[3] The effects of chronic hypoxia and the persistent systemic pressure delivered to the right side make heart failure inevitable. Associated cardiac abnormalities include a right-sided aortic arch, a second VSD, and coronary artery abnormalities. TOF is also associated with chromosomal abnormalities, 22q11 deletion, and DiGeorge and velocardiofacial syndromes.

Management

Small patients or patients at increased risk of complications from a repair are palliated using a modified Blalock–Taussig (BT) shunt. The BT shunt is a prosthetic tube that connects the subclavian artery to the pulmonary artery, guaranteeing pulmonary blood flow. This allows the patient to grow until definitive surgical intervention can take place.

Current surgical strategies are aimed at performing the complete repair early in life, thereby avoiding the complications associated with palliative procedures. Surgical goals during a complete TOF repair are to obtain unobstructed blood flow to the lungs and to minimize shunting of blood. Surgeons typically use a patch to close the ventricular septal defect and then carefully inspect the right ventricular outflow tract. In some, the obstruction is entirely below the level of the pulmonary valve. In these instances resection of muscle below the valve may be sufficient. Obstruction that traverses across the pulmonary valve may require a transannular patch to relieve the obstruction.

Closing the VSD and relieving the right ventricular outflow tract obstruction early in life prevents myocardial fibrosis. Despite early intervention, a stiff, thickened right ventricle may be difficult to fill in the early postoperative period following repair. With time the ventricle is able to remodel and obtain more normal anatomy and function.

TOF patients frequently require further interventions later in life. The pulmonary valve often becomes regurgitant and requires either replacement or repair.

Anesthetic considerations

While having an unrepaired TOF patient present for elective spinal surgery is highly unlikely, anesthetic concerns for unrepaired TOF patients are focused on preventing further desaturation and maintaining cardiac output. Treatment strategies for cyanotic spells include the following: (1) Prior to induction keeping the child calm and limiting fasting to a minimum; if a spell occurs prior to obtaining IV access,

administering oxygen to reduce pulmonary resistance and bending the child's legs to their chest to increase afterload. (2) If intravenous access has been established, fluid administration will distend the right ventricle and reduce the degree of obstruction. Vasoconstrictors such as phenylephrine will help increase afterload, and beta blockers will decrease the heart rate to allow for more diastolic filling of the ventricle and reduce contractility and infundibular spasm. Volatile agents decrease contractility and decrease subpulmonic obstruction.

A more probable scenario is a patient with corrected TOF presenting for a spinal procedure. Although corrected, these patients frequently have residual sequelae from their repair. The major issue following TOF repair is abnormal right ventricular (RV) pressure loading from residual shunts and obstruction as well as RV volume loading from pulmonary regurgitation. Long-term progressive RV dysfunction is associated with arrhythmias and the risk of sudden death. Many patients following repair may be asymptomatic and ventricular dysfunction may be evident on exercise testing. Patient's records should be inspected for evidence of residual shunts and/or obstruction. As mentioned, pulmonary insufficiency is common and should be evaluated preoperatively. Rhythm disturbances are also seen with regularity following tetralogy repairs, and thus the ECG should be inspected for evidence of heart block and other abnormalities. Tricuspid regurgitation may be a surrogate marker for RV dysfunction.

Hypoplastic left heart syndrome and single ventricle physiology

Overview

Hypoplastic left heart syndrome (HLHS) is a rare congenital heart defect that results in an underdeveloped left side of the heart. While only 2 infants in 10 000 may be born with the disease, it accounts for almost a one-quarter of cardiac deaths early in life.[4]

Typically the mitral valve is stenotic or atretic along with the left ventricle, aortic root, and ascending aorta. Survival of these infants is dependent on a patent ductus arteriosus to allow pulmonary blood flow to maintain systemic circulation and perfusion to vital structures. A defect in the atrial septum allows oxygenated blood returning to the left atrium to mix with right-sided systemic venous return, which empties into the right atrium. The right ventricle provides both pulmonary circulation and systemic circulation (via the patent ductus arteriosus). Coronary perfusion is usually dependent on retrograde filling of the proximal aorta by flow across the ductus arteriosus.

Ideally, there is a balance between the systemic perfusion and pulmonary perfusion with the amount of blood flowing to the lungs equal to that to the rest of the body. Following the ratio of cardiac output to the lungs (Qp) to cardiac output to the body (Qs) allows one to determine the efficiency of work that the heart is performing and the degree of shunting that is present. In the balanced HLHS patient with the Qp/Qs equal to 1, the expected arterial saturation will be 75%. Manipulations in inspired oxygen content and ventilation radically alter the resistance in the pulmonary vasculature and can consequently affect systemic blood flow and perfusion. As pulmonary vascular resistance decreases, blood preferentially flows to the lungs. This increase in arterial saturation occurs at the expense of systemic perfusion. Conversely, if pulmonary vascular resistance increases, blood flow through the lungs is reduced and the blood is poorly oxygenated, but the systemic output is increased.

In the first week of life, most hypoplastic left heart patients will undergo a Norwood procedure that transitions the right ventricle into the systemic pump for the patient. This is achieved by fabricating a new aorta by joining the pulmonary trunk with the diminutive existing aorta and supplementing the new arch with a homograft (Fig. 24.1). As the main pulmonary artery is sacrificed, pulmonary blood flow is reestablished with a shunt from the subclavian artery (BT) or right ventricle (Sano) to the remaining branch pulmonary arteries. Following this procedure, the patient's arterial saturation is expected to be in the high 70s to mid 80s.

Once the child reaches 2–4 months of age, they return to the operating room for a Glenn procedure. The Glenn procedure involves ligation of the connection of the superior vena cava (SVC) to the right atrium and the anastomosis of the SVC to the branch pulmonary arteries. At this point the shunt created during the previous operation is taken down. The Glenn procedure relieves the right ventricle of unnecessary work. However, patients remain desaturated as the inferior vena cava still empties into the right atrium and mixes with saturated pulmonary venous blood across the atrial septum.

The final stage of the procedure, the Fontan, is undertaken at approximately 2 years of age. This procedure routes blood returning from the IVC through or around the heart to the branch pulmonary arteries

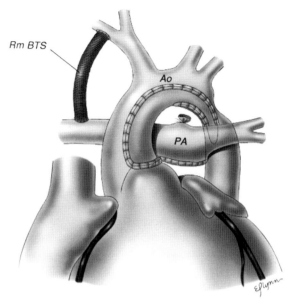

Figure 24.1 Norwood operation. (Reprinted from reference [24], O'Brien P, Boisvert JT. Current management of infants and children with single ventricle anatomy. *J Pediatr Nurs* 2001;16(5):338–50 with permission from Elsevier.)

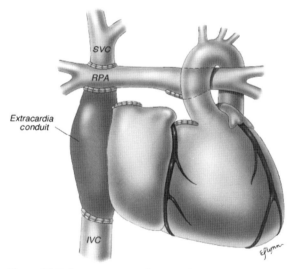

Figure 24.2 Fontan operation. (Reprinted from reference [24], O'Brien P, Boisvert JT. Current management of infants and children with single ventricle anatomy. *J Pediatr Nurs* 2001;16(5):338–50 with permission from Elsevier.)

such that a vast majority of venous return now bypasses the heart completely and flows passively to the lungs (Fig. 24.2). Occasionally, the surgeon will create a small hole or fenestration in the Fontan circuit that allows blood to empty into the right atrium if pressures in the circuit increase. This, in essence, increases systemic

409

blood flow but with desaturated blood. Following the Fontan, the HLHS patient should have an arterial saturation in the mid to high 90s.

At the conclusion of these procedures the patient has a single systemic pump in the right ventricle and passive venous return to the pulmonary vascular bed via the IVC and SVC. Ideal Fontan physiology will include a mean systemic venous pressure of 10–15 mmHg and a common atrial pressure of 7–10 mmHg. Optimum physiology necessitates adequate volume, normal sinus rhythm, low pulmonary vascular resistance, unrestricted ASD, and AV valve competency. Over time, RV dysfunction occurs and arrhythmias develop. Diastolic dysfunction is common. In addition, recurrent pleural effusions, peripheral edema, ascites, and protein-losing enteropathy frequently occur. Because of elevated venous pressures, cerebral blood flow may require higher systemic blood pressures. Because the right ventricle is not designed to handle systemic pressures, by the early 4th decade of life the right ventricle begins to show signs of failure.

Anesthetic considerations

The outcome of these procedures, while providing a decent quality of life for patients, leaves an anatomic and physiologic scenario that may be unfamiliar and intimidating to the anesthesiologist charged with their care. While the Fontan, or single ventricle, physiology is much more stable than the tenuous circulation that the patients were born with, there are many things to take into careful consideration.

Physiologic changes that increase pulmonary vascular resistance dangerously reduce forward flow to the lungs and subsequently comprise cardiac output. Avoiding hypercarbia, hypoxia, and acidosis helps ensure that pulmonary vascular resistance is minimal and that pulmonary blood flow is maintained.

Patients do not tolerate hypovolemia, since the systemic venous pressure is the driving force for blood flow to the lung. Vasodilation during induction of a dehydrated Fontan patient can dramatically impair blood flow to the lung and compromise cardiac output. Dehydration should be aggressively corrected once IV access is obtained.

In addition, positive intrathoracic pressures with mechanical ventilation further reduce the return of blood to the lungs. Peak inspiratory pressures should be closely monitored and patients extubated as soon as possible. During mechanical ventilation, large tidal volumes with low respiratory rates provide low mean airway pressures and long expiratory times enhancing pulmonary blood flow. PEEP to maintain FRC is also instrumental in minimizing pulmonary vascular resistance.

Because the patient is dependent on a single right ventricle, the anesthetic should be tailored to minimize the degree of myocardial depression and increases in pulmonary vascular resistance. Careful titration of volatile and intravenous anesthetics is essential.

Heart transplantation

Overview

Heart transplantation is performed on an increasing number of pediatric patients for reasons including congenital heart disease and cardiomyopathy. While improvements in immunosuppression have dramatically improved recipient outcomes, there simply are not enough organs available. Thirty percent of patients on the list will die waiting for their new heart.

Management

After a heart has been successfully transplanted, the greatest risk to the transplanted organ is rejection. Acute rejection is the leading cause of death for several years following transplantation. As a result, patients are managed with a variety of immunosuppressant drugs and routinely brought to the heart catheterization laboratory for surveillance endomyocardial biopsies. Biopsies are performed monthly over the first 6 months when risk of rejection is highest. After this period, the biopsies are spaced out and performed on an annual basis.

Anesthetic considerations

Performing an anesthetic on a heart transplant recipient requires attention to certain details. Recognition of the signs of rejection, such as tachycardia, malaise, fever, weight loss, and rhythm disturbances, is vital. Any elective surgery should be postponed if rejection is suspected such that appropriate medical intervention can occur.

In addition to rejection, transplanted hearts also have an increased incidence of coronary artery disease. Inflammation within the walls of the coronary vessels eventually compromises blood flow. Since these hearts are denervated, myocardial ischemia may not present with chest pain.

Transplant patients are immunocompromised secondarily to their immunosuppressant regimens.

Consequently, they are prone to life-threatening infections. Posttransplant lymphoproliferative disorder (PTLD) is another unfortunate complication that is seen in this population. PTLD is characterized by B-cell proliferation typically induced by Epstein–Barr virus (EBV) in a context of immunosuppression. Untreated, patients who acquire PTLD suffer from a very high rate of mortality.

Immunosuppressive drugs may lead to hypertension, diabetes, renal insufficiency, and growth retardation.

A transplanted heart does not have the innervation of a native heart. Transplanted hearts have abnormal responses to drugs and stress. Typical increases in heart rate from hypotension and increased need for oxygen supply are not present. Instead, peripheral vasoconstriction increases preload and augments cardiac output. Also, circulating catecholamines directly stimulate the heart to increase the heart rate. Beta blockade markedly reduces the heart's response to circulating catecholamines. Indirect-acting agents such as atropine have no effect on the denervated heart, while direct-acting agents like epinephrine work well.

Cardiomyopathy

Overview

Cardiomyopathy is a disease of the myocardium that affects a significant number of infants and children. The two main forms are dilated and hypertrophic.

Dilated cardiomyopathy results in diminished systolic function and cardiac dilatation. Causes are numerous but include infectious, genetic, and toxic agents. Symptoms usually present gradually unless related to an acute viral myocarditis. In infants and children, typical presenting signs are nonspecific and include tachypnea, irritability, and poor feeding. Heart dilatation frequently leads to incompetence of the right and left atrioventricular valves.

Hypertrophic cardiomyopathy is a genetically inherited cardiac disease that is the most common cause of sudden cardiac death in children over 10 years of age, with as many as 1 in 500 births affected globally. It is characterized by a thickened but not dilated ventricle. This thickening leads to left ventricular outflow tract obstruction in a majority of patients. In addition to obstructive symptoms, patients may have coronary ischemia and diastolic dysfunction secondary to an increase in left ventricular mass.

Management

Treatment of dilated cardiomyopathy aims at improving cardiac output, resolving fluid overload, and dilating the peripheral vascular bed (afterload reduction). Phosphodiesterase inhibitors are frequently used as they tend to diminish pulmonary and systemic vascular resistance while providing much-needed inotropy to the heart. Longer-term improvement in function of symptomatic patients may be achieved using digoxin. Meanwhile, diuretics such as furosemide are frequently utilized in this population. Those patients with larger ventricular and atrial chambers may require anticoagulation to minimize risk of clot formation. If the patients are unresponsive to medical management, transplantation is offered.

Diuretics may be added in patients with evidence of pulmonary congestion. Patients thought to be at high risk of sudden cardiac death may have an implantable cardioverter-defibrillator. Patients who do not respond to medical management may be referred to a surgeon for a septal myectomy, in which obstructive muscle bundles in the left ventricular outflow tract are removed.

Anesthetic considerations

The successful anesthetic management of dilated cardiomyopathy requires careful attention to fluid management, afterload reduction, and inotropic support. While excessive fluid may push a patient into pulmonary edema, these patients should not be allowed to become dehydrated because the ventricles of these patients function on the higher end of the Frank–Starling curve. Cardiac output is very sensitive to an adequate preload. Milrinone should be considered intraoperatively as it helps to improve inotropy as well as reduce vascular resistance. Volatile agents should be used judiciously as their myocardial depressant effects may be poorly tolerated.

Hypertrophic cardiomyopathy requires slightly different intraoperative strategies. Afterload needs to be maintained as reductions in coronary perfusion pressure place a thickened ventricle at significant risk of ischemia. Also, the preload should be maintained at normal to high. A full ventricle reduces the dynamic outflow track obstruction.

Valvular lesions

While an in-depth discussion of the various valvular lesions is beyond the scope of this chapter, stenotic and

Table 24.1 Hemodynamic goals for valvular lesions

Lesion	HR and rhythm	Preload	Afterload	Contractility
AS	Slow, sinus	Full	Maintain	–
AI	Normal	Maintain	Lower	May need support
MS	Slow	Full	–	–
MR	Normal, sinus	Maintain	Lower	May need support

HR, heart rate; AI, aortic insufficiency; AS, aortic stenosis; MR, mitral regurgitation; MS, mitral stenosis
Adapted from reference [5]: Yao F-SF, Artusio JF. *Yao & Artusio's Anesthesiology: Problem-oriented Patient Management*. 5th ed. Philadelphia: Lippincott Williams & Wilkins, 2003.

regurgitant valves effect the management of many cardiac patients presenting for noncardiac surgery. Table 24.1 provides a brief review of the hemodynamic goals associated with the most common valvular pathologies.[5]

Approach to the cardiac patient for spinal surgery

The anesthetic approach to any patient with congenital heart disease should be systematic. There are several questions that must be answered prior to surgery. First, what is the defect? Second, was it repaired and if so, how? Third, how is their cardiac condition currently impacting the patient's physiology? Finally, what do you need to do to safely guide a patient with this condition through their spinal surgery?

While a majority of elective procedures will wait until the cardiac disease has been optimally managed or corrected, appropriate assessment of patients with heart disease is essential. Minor defects such as repaired atrial septal defects may not need much additional preparation, while children with single ventricle physiology require a meticulous evaluation and understanding of the underlying physiology.

Preoperative assessment

History and physical examination

Preparing an anesthetic for a pediatric patient with heart disease requires a careful history and physical examination. Details picked up during this process can alter the anesthetic plan considerably and in some cases help identify patients not medically optimized for elective surgery.

A complete surgical history is essential. Often, the complexity of the surgeries may limit the family's utility in obtaining a proper history. In these cases, hospital records and operative reports are more reliable for

Table 24.2 New York Heart Association Heart Failure Classification

Class I	No limitation to their activity by their disease
Class II	Mild symptoms including fatigue and shortness of breath in the setting of moderate activities
Class III	Pronounced symptoms with activities that would not typically elicit strain
Class IV	Unable to perform any activity without discomfort

understanding the patient's current anatomy and physiology. For example, if a child has had a previous BT shunt, blood pressures on the effected upper extremity limb will be low or nonexistent.

Once the current configuration of the heart is visualized, the child's functional status must be determined. Recognizing evidence of heart failure can be particularly challenging in the pediatric population. Heart failure in adult patients is graded by The New York Heart Association (NYHA) classification (Table 24.2). The scale is readily carried over to the older adolescent; however, younger children require more directed questions to determine their cardiac function. Classic signs of decompensation are nonspecific but include failure to gain weight, tachypnea, tachycardia, hepatomegaly, and difficulty with feeding.

Heart failure in patients with congenital heart disease may be caused by pressure or volume overload. Failure secondary to pressure overload is related to increased resistance or obstruction. Volume overload is found in those patients with significant shunts and regurgitant valves. If any element of heart failure or decompensation is present, it warrants careful consideration and delay of any elective procedure until sufficient medical management can be achieved.

Many pediatric patients with heart disease suffer from chronic desaturation, a state that may impact every organ system. On examination, patients may have a high heart rate, clubbing of their nail beds, and cyanosis. The polycythemia that results from chronic desaturation may lead to headaches, visual loss, and paresthesias.

This population will often have greatly elevated cardiac workloads, forcing their bodies to conserve energy by stunting growth. Hence, pediatric cardiac patients are routinely small for their age.

Many pediatric cardiac patients suffer from high pulmonary artery pressures. Pulmonary hypertension is a significant risk factor for intraoperative cardiac arrest and increased mortality. Enlarged pulmonary arteries may result in small-airway compression, predisposing patients to respiratory infections, atelectasis, and an increase in the work of breathing.

Airway compression is common in patients with congenital heart defects. Airway compression can occur in both cyanotic and acyanotic forms of congenital heart disease. Cardiac defects with large left-to-right shunts, tetralogy of Fallot with absent pulmonic valve, or tetralogy of Fallot with pulmonary atresia or truncus arteriosus are the more common associated lesions. Compression of the airway can occur at different levels of the tracheal bronchial tree. Airway obstruction can result from compression by vascular structures, i.e., rings and slings, or by compression of dilated pulmonary arteries, left atrial enlargement or cardiomegaly, or intraluminal bronchial obstruction. (Fig. 24.3)

The preoperative work-up should also look for evidence of significant nerve injuries. The location of the phrenic and recurrent laryngeal nerves within the chest puts them at significant risk of damage during open heart operations. Procedures on or near the aortic arch may damage the recurrent laryngeal nerve, causing vocal cord paresis and increasing the risk of perioperative aspiration. Damage to the phrenic nerve is less common, but can markedly reduce the efficiency of respiratory efforts and lead to unanticipated respiratory complications.

Laboratory values

Any number of abnormalities can be picked up in the pediatric cardiac population by examining their routine preoperative laboratory investigations. Hypoxic patients often have polycythemia, as low oxygen levels stimulate the kidney to release erythropoietin, driving an increase in red cell production. Higher than normal red cell mass compensates for the desaturated blood and increases oxygen delivery. Patients with abnormally high hematocrit are prone to hyperviscosity and are more susceptible to sludging and strokes, particularly in the setting of dehydration. Preoperative phlebotomy should be considered when hematocrits rise to levels greater than 65%.

Pediatric cardiac patients often have substantial clotting abnormalities that need to be evaluated. Patients may have low platelets, dysfunctional platelets, low levels of key clotting factors, and low levels of fibrinogen. One study looking at congenital heart patients found that 19% had significant coagulation anomalies, with elevations in PT and PTT being the most frequent finding.[6] Cyanotic patients are particularly affected by thrombocytopenia, as platelet count has been shown to be directly related to their oxygen saturation and inversely related to hemoglobin concentration. While the cause of this decrease is unknown, it is related to a reduced circulating lifespan of the platelets.

In addition, some patients in this population may be taking anticoagulants to minimize thrombus formation around prosthetic materials or in enlarged cardiac chambers where stasis of blood can occur. Discussion with the surgeons and cardiologists should help determine an appropriate management strategy for their perioperative anticoagulation.

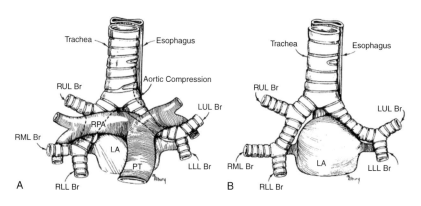

Figure 24.3 Relationship of the pulmonary arteries to the tracheobronchial tree. (From reference [25], Berlinger NT, Long C, Foker J, Lucas RV Jr. Tracheobronchial compression in acyanotic congenital heart disease. *Ann Otol Rhinol Laryngol* 1983;92(4 Pt 1):387–90.)

Electrolyte evaluation of patients on diuretics may reveal alterations that require correction preoperatively, although this may not be as frequent as once thought.[7]

ECG

All pediatric cardiac patients should have a recent ECG for review. Familiarity with the patient's baseline ECG will help decipher important perioperative changes and guide intervention. Arrhythmias may be evidence of worsening heart failure or physical trauma to the heart's electrical pathways from previous procedures. Procedures close to the sinoatrial node such as atrial switch procedures and repairs of high atrial septal defects lead to supraventricular rhythm disturbances in 20–45% of patients.[8] Disruption of the atrioventricular node is more common during repairs of atrioventricular canals, membranous ventricular septal defects, and tetralogy of Fallot. Procedures that manipulate or distort the ventricular septum may lead to right and/or left bundle branch blocks.

Subtle alterations in axis and wave size can point to ventricular hypertrophy. Likewise, large P waves may be indicative of atrial enlargement.

In addition, there are some syndromes that exhibit prolongation of the QT interval. Baseline QT prolongation warrants avoidance of drugs that could further increase the QT interval.

Pacemakers

Some patients with cardiac disease and associated arrhythmias may have already had the rhythm disturbances addressed with a pacemaker or an implantable cardiac defibrillator (ICD). Prior to entering the operating room, it is important to know where the device is located, what mode the device is in, whether the device is functioning appropriately, the patient's inherent rhythm, and whether the device needs to be turned off before heading to the operating room. Often the patient has already seen a cardiologist and this information is readily available. In situations where the device has not recently been interrogated, this should be done prior to entering the operating room.

Echocardiography

Transthoracic echocardiography is an easy noninvasive means of following a pediatric patient's cardiac status. Assessment of a patient's most recent study prior to surgery provides information regarding anatomy, existing or residual shunts, valves, pressure gradients, and function.

Perioperative management

Induction

There is no universal technique to anesthetize a pediatric cardiac patient for a spinal procedure. The variations of physiology in these patients demand tailored anesthetic plans. The drugs and techniques used to induce these patients must aim to maintain the patient's baseline performance and when possible improve it. Success hinges on appropriate airway management, avoidance of hypotension, elevated pulmonary vascular resistance, increases in oxygen demand, and dehydration.

Premedication with oral midazolam 0.5–1 mg per kilogram is reasonable in most patients, often facilitating smoother inductions. Inhalational inductions are rarely contraindicated, although careful attention to cardiac rhythm and function is essential. Preoperative measures to obtain intravenous access on an alert child often have greater physiologic consequences than bringing the child into a controlled environment and administering volatile anesthetic. This is particularly true considering that intravenous access in this population may be challenging secondary to prolonged hospital stays.

Patient positioning is always an important consideration in patients presenting for spinal surgery. Pediatric patients with cardiac disease deserve careful attention as the patient's physiology may be negatively affected by certain positions. Prone positioning has been shown to decrease cardiac index by up to 24%.[9] Other studies have shown that prone position leads to a measurable increase in heart rate and peripheral vascular resistance.[10] Careful inspection to ensure that the abdomen is free from compression helps prevent obstruction to blood flow within the inferior vena cava, a particularly important consideration in those with Fontan physiology.[11]

Emergency drugs

In addition to the standard emergency drugs that are available for routine procedures, these patients may require additional preparation. Hemodynamic lability during induction is not uncommon. Having appropriate concentrations of drugs such as atropine, epinephrine, phenylephrine, and calcium ready for administration can quickly recover a patient's ideal physiologic state while changes in the anesthetic can be made.

Defibrillators

Patients with previous heart surgery are subject to a number of arrhythmias. Stress of surgery may

Table 24.3 Candidates for antibiotic prophylaxis for endocarditis (2007 AHA Guidelines)

Patients with prosthetic valves
History of previous endocarditis
Congenital cyanotic lesions that are unrepaired
Congenital lesions repaired with a prosthetic device or material up to 6 months following the procedure
Repaired defects with residual shunts
Heart transplant recipients with a valvulopathy

Table 24.4 Effects of anesthetic agents on somatosensory evoked potentials

Agent	Amplitude	Latency
Desflurane	↓	↑
Isoflurane	↓	↑
Sevoflurane	↓	↑
Nitrous oxide	↓	↔
Barbiturates	↓	↑
Etomidate	↑	↔
Ketamine	↑	↔
Midazolam	↓	↔
Opioids	↔	↔
Propofol	↔	↔
Dexmedetomidine	↔	↔

↓Decreases; ↑, increases; ↔, remains the same.

predispose patients to enter into a rhythm that is poorly tolerated by their condition. The ability to quickly recognize and treat rhythm disturbances is crucial. Consider the placement of defibrillator pads in patients prone to or sensitive to intraoperative arrhythmias.

Antibiotics

Guidelines for antibiotic prophylaxis to prevent infective endocarditis in patients undergoing procedures were last updated by the American Heart association in 2007. These guidelines are listed in Table 24.3. If the patient meets one of these criteria and is having a procedure that disrupts the gingival tissue or respiratory tract mucosa, or involves operating on infected skin or musculoskeletal tissues, prophylaxis is recommended.[12]

Monitoring

Standard ASA monitors are used in all cases. Additional monitors should be determined by the nature of the surgical procedure and the patient's clinical condition. This varies on a patient-to-patient basis. A low threshold for the placement of an arterial catheter is reasonable in many of these patients. Arterial catheters may be important to follow the patient's blood pressure closely and to draw intraoperative laboratory samples. If patients have shunts that use or have sacrificed a subclavian artery, avoidance of the involved side will prevent inaccurate arterial pressure measurements.[11]

Central venous catheters are useful for the measurement of central venous pressures and the administration of drugs perioperatively. Providers must be aware of the abnormal venous connections present in Fontan and Glenn circulations. The catheters may still provide useful information regarding venous pressure and pulmonary artery pressures; however, they may not be reliable monitors of ventricular filling pressures.[13]

In light of the abnormal physiology of the Fontan patient, some authors have argued for the intraoperative monitoring of ventricular filling and function using transesophageal echocardiography. Constant visualization of the cardiac chambers throughout surgery provides real-time evaluation of preload, contractility, and cardiac output.[14]

Management

Intraoperative management of pediatric cardiac patients for spinal procedures should focus on keeping up with necessary fluid and blood requirements as well as preventing large fluctuations in pulmonary and systemic pressures.

Intraoperative inotropic and vasoactive drips should be available for patients with more complex cardiac lesions. A lower threshold in starting these medications may be necessary to maintain delicately balanced hemodynamics and prevent depression of an already weakened heart.

Spinal surgery often employs intraoperative electrophysiological monitoring to detect insults to sensitive neurologic structures. It is important to maintain a physiologically stable condition, including blood pressure, oxygen saturation, hematocrit, glucose, and temperature, as changes may disrupt the amplitude and latency of monitored waveforms. In addition the drugs given may strongly affect neurophysiological monitoring. Table 24.4. Total intravenous anesthetic techniques may be used in the cardiac population without a significant increase in risk to the patient; although avoiding volatile agents altogether is rarely necessary.

415

As discussed earlier, many of these patients will have abnormal coagulation profiles. Studies have also shown that pediatric cardiac patients with normal coagulation tests demonstrate an increased susceptibility to intraoperative blood loss.[6] Intraoperative cell salvage and the availability of blood and blood products should be investigated prior to incision.

Just as important as the concern over blood loss is the awareness that these patients may also be at risk of abnormal clot formation. Fontan patients have been shown to have an increased susceptibility to thrombus formation secondary to increased levels of factor VIII.[15] Careful attention to perioperative anticoagulation strategies is imperative in these patients.

During the emergence phase, it is important to reverse any residual neuromuscular blockade. Weakness in this patient population leads to hypoventilation and hypoxia and hypercardia may ensue. Fluctuations in pulmonary vascular resistance are poorly tolerated in many cardiac patients.

Syndromes associated with spinal and cardiac pathology

There are a myriad of pediatric syndromes associated with spinal deformities, and a large proportion of these syndromes are associated with congenital cardiac defects. Textbooks on these syndromes have been published, which describe the disease as well as the associated anesthetic implications.[16] This section will review eight of the more common syndromes that might impact anesthetic management.

Marfan's syndrome

Overview

Marfan's patients suffer from a multisystem autosomal dominant connective tissue problem, manifested by long bone overgrowth, dislocation of the ocular lens, pneumothorax, hyperextensible joints, mitral valve prolapse, and dilatation of the aortic root. Roughly 1 in 5000 patients suffer from Marfan's syndrome where a loss of strength of collagen leads to weakness in the walls of vessels, predisposing the formation of aneurysms. Cardiac problems typically do not arise until the twenties or thirties; however, infant forms of the disease have been described.[17]

Anesthetic considerations

Most Marfan's syndrome patients will be managed with (beta-blocking agents to reduce the stress on the aortic wall and reduce the incidence of dissection. Intraoperative management should avoid wide fluctuations in arterial pressure to achieve this same goal. Ventilatory strategies should be monitored carefully to avoid high airway pressures in a population prone to pneumothoraces. Also, positioning of these patients requires attention to avoid trauma and dislocation to joints.

Down's syndrome

Overview

Down's syndrome or trisomy 21 is the most common chromosomal syndrome, with approximately 1 in 800 live births affected. In addition to the characteristic facial appearance, these patients also have varying degrees of cervical spine instability, subglottic stenosis, heart defects, duodenal atresia, imperforate anus, xerodermia, hypothyroidism, and other related problems.[18]

Anesthetic considerations

Airway assessment is particularly important in Down's syndrome patients. Macroglossia, midface hypoplasia, and cervical spine instability can be a challenge to the management of the airway. In selecting an endotracheal tube, using a tube one-half to one full size smaller than what would normally be indicated for the patients' age avoids complications associated with their subglottic stenosis.

Cervical instability is reported to occur in up to 30% of Down's syndrome patients. Most guidelines recommend cervical neck films to evaluate for this when the child starts ambulating. While neck films examining atlantooccipital instability are not mandatory prior to proceeding to the operating room, they should be reviewed if available. Typically, direct laryngoscopy maintaining a neutral head position is safe in these patients, although fiberoptic intubation may be warranted in patients with suspicious neurologic findings or documented cervical spine instability. Neutral head position should be maintained in these patients throughout the course of their procedure.

Cardiac defects occur in up to 50% of Down's syndrome patients. Most frequently encountered defects include atrioventricular canal defects, atrial septal defects, and ventricular septal defects.[19] Sensitivity to anesthetic agents with respect to bradycardia has been reported in patients with Down's syndrome. Thickened skin may hinder attempts at intravenous access as well as invasive intraoperative monitoring.

Friedreich's ataxia

Overview

This autosomal recessive disorder, affecting 1 in 50 000 people, involves the progressive deterioration of the posterior spinal cord, cerebellum, and peripheral nervous system leading to loss of ambulatory ability.[20]

Onset occurs between the ages of 5 and 15 years when patients develop difficulty walking. Over time a majority of patients will become wheelchair-bound. No definitive treatment is currently available; however, aggressive screening for cardiomyopathy, arrhythmias, scoliosis, and diabetes mellitus improves life expectancy and quality of life.

Anesthetic considerations

Many anesthesiologists avoid regional techniques in these patients citing the baseline neurologic problems; however, there are reports of successful neuraxial blockade without adverse events.

Patients with Friedreich's ataxia are routinely found to have some degree of hypertrophic cardiomyopathy. Perioperative management must focus on maintaining a normal to high venous pressure while avoiding increases in heart rate, decreases in systemic vascular resistance, and increases in contractility.

These patients have altered responses to neuromuscular blocking drugs. Depolarizing agents have caused hyperkalemia-associated cardiac arrhythmias in these patients and therefore should be avoided. Nondepolarizing drugs may demonstrate exaggerated effects. Thus, appropriate monitoring of neuromuscular function is important.

Klippel–Feil syndrome

Overview

This syndrome typically involves fusion of cervical vertebrae limiting neck movement. These patients may have associated ventricular septal defects and hearing loss. Approximately 1 in 40 000 births will have the disorder, with females affected more than males. Several types of the syndrome are described, depending on the location and severity of the orthopedic abnormalities. Fifteen percent of patients will present with congenital heart disease. Scoliosis occurs in up to 60% of cases. Genitourinary abnormalities are also common.[10]

Anesthetic considerations

A difficult intubation should be anticipated and appropriately planned for. Preoperatively these patients should have neck films with proper interpretation to rule out instability. Airway management involves maintaining the head in a neutral position both during laryngoscopy and during surgical positioning. Patients may develop significant neurologic deficits in the setting of minor injuries or manipulations of the neck.

Noonan's syndrome

Overview

Noonan's syndrome affects 1 in 2000 live births in an autosomal dominant fashion with variable penetration. Features of these patients include abnormal facies, short stature, scoliosis, and heart defects. Other important features include a propensity for clotting abnormalities and mental retardation. Fifty percent of patients have congenital heart defects. Pulmonary stenosis, hypertrophic cardiomyopathy, ASD, and tetralogy of Fallot[21] are the more common cardiac defects.

Anesthetic considerations

Face and airway anomalies in these patients can cause difficulty with intubation. Also preoperative laboratory examination may reveal significant coagulopathy and guide intraoperative management.

Duchenne muscular dystrophy

Overview

Duchenne muscular dystrophy is a progressive disease of muscle fibers affecting 1 in 3500 males. The mutation, spontaneous in some patients but inherited in a majority, causes the protein dystrophin to be produced in an abnormal fashion. Absence of dystrophin leads to a destabilization of muscle fibers. Muscle then has a tendency to break down and be replaced with scar and fatty tissue. Some areas, commonly the calves, experience pseudohypertrophy whereby a majority of muscle is filled with scar and is nonfunctional.[22]

Patients may not show signs of the disease early in life. Most of the sequelae are identified as the child starts to walk. Muscle weakness is recognized between the ages of 2 and 5 years. Children with Duchenne muscular dystrophy may have difficultly standing and adopt a characteristic technique to do so, known as Gower's sign. Eventually, patients become wheelchair-dependent. Cardiac muscle involvement of the disease is universal. The heart muscle gradually thickens then dilates.

Anesthetic considerations

Patients with muscular dystrophy are at risk from a number of complications during an anesthetic. Dilated cardiomyopathy must be suspected and investigated prior to entering the operating room. As the patient is frequently immobile, assessing the patient for signs and symptoms of heart failure may be difficult. Availability of appropriate emergency drugs and careful titration of anesthetic agents are essential to preserve myocardial function. Careful attention to fluid management is also important in these patients.

The depolarizing muscular blocker succinylcholine is absolutely contraindicated in these patients as the abnormal muscle tissue releases large amounts of potassium and can lead to cardiac arrest.

Duchenne patients are not prone to malignant hyperthermia. However, volatile agents are avoided because their use may lead to rhabdomyolysis, myoglobinuria, renal failure, and hyperkalemia. While depolarizing neuromuscular blockers are contraindicated, even nondepolarizing neuromuscular blockers should be used with caution secondary to prolonged affects in these patients.

Rett's syndrome

Overview
Rett's syndrome is a disorder that primarily affects the central nervous system. Patients progressively develop symptoms of autism, dementia, difficulty walking, and difficulty using their hands. It is an X-linked dominant syndrome that only affects females. While the child may develop normally to the age of 1 year, problems start to surface with language and gait. Hand tremors may also be seen in the ages of 2–3 years. Cardiac involvement of this syndrome is a prolonged QT interval.

Anesthetic considerations
Several anesthetic agents should be avoided or minimized in this setting to avoid dangerous arrhythmias (Table 24.5).[23]

Arthrogryposis multiplex congenita

Overview
Arthrogryposis patients have multiple limb contractures and can be classified as either type 1 or type 2. Approximately 1 in 1000 live births will demonstrate evidence of the syndrome. Some cases are known to be sporadic while most type 1 cases demonstrate an autosomal dominant pattern of inheritance. Children with type 1 arthrogryposis typically have involvement of their hands and feet, but do not have issues with neurologic development. Children with type 2 arthrogryposis

Table 24.5 Drugs that prolong the QT interval (anesthetic highlights)

Well documented	Moderate association
Amiodarone	Nicardipine
Procainamide	Gatifloxacin
Sotalol	Levofloxacin
Clarithromycin	Lithium
Erythromycin	Risperidone
Chlorpromazine	Chloral hydrate
Haloperidol	Fosphenytoin
Droperidol	Octreotide
Methadone	Ondansetron
Organophosphates	Tacrolimus
	Voriconazole

often have more significant joint contractures and present with additional anomalies involving the heart, lung, kidney, skin, and neurologic systems.

Anesthetic considerations
Preparation for patients with arthrogryposis having spinal surgery should include anticipation of potentially difficult airways. Patients have also been reported to have a higher incidence of fevers intraoperatively, although it does not appear that these patients are more susceptible to malignant hyperthermia.

References

1. Coran DL, Rodgers WB, Keane JF, et al. Spinal fusion in patients with congenital heart disease – predictors of outcome. *Clin Orthop Relat Res* 1999; (**364**): 99–107.

2. Radzik D, Davignon A, van Doesburg N, et al. Predictive factors for spontaneous closure of atrial septal defects diagnosed in the first 3 months of life. *J Am Coll Cardiol* 1993; **22**(3): 851–3.

3. Bertranou EG, Blackstone EH, Hazelrig JB, et al. Life expectancy without surgery in tetralogy of Fallot. *Am J Cardiol* 1978; **42**(3): 458–66.

4. Fyler D. Report of the New England Regional Infant Cardiac Program. *Pediatrics* 1980; **65**(2 Pt 2): 375–461.

5. Yao F-SF, Artusio JF. *Yao & Artusio's Anesthesiology: Problem-oriented Patient Management.* 5th ed. Philadelphia: Lippincott Williams & Wilkins; 2003.

6. Colon-Otero G, Gilchrist GS, Holcomb GR, et al. Preoperative evaluation of hemostasis in patients with congenital heart disease. *Mayo Clin Proc* 1987; **62**(5): 379–85.

7. Hastings LA, Wood JC, Harris B, et al. Cardiac medications are not associated with clinically

important preoperative electrolyte disturbances in children presenting for cardiac surgery. *Anesth Analg* 2008; **107**(6): 1840–7.

8. Gatzoulis MA, Freeman MA, Siu SC, *et al.* Atrial arrhythmia after surgical closure of atrial septal defects in adults. *N Engl J Med* 1999; **340**(11): 839–46.

9. Pump B, Talleruphuus U, Christensen NJ, *et al.* Effects of supine, prone, and lateral positions on cardiovascular and renal variables in humans. *Am J Physiol Regul Integr Comp Physiol* 2002; **283**(1): R174–80.

10. Farid IS, Omar OA, Insler SR. Multiple anesthetic challenges in a patient with Klippel–Feil Syndrome undergoing cardiac surgery. *J Cardiothorac Vasc Anesth* 2003; **17**(4): 502–5.

11. Bailey PD Jr., Jobes DR. The Fontan patient. *Anesthesiol Clin* 2009; **27**(2): 285–300.

12. Wilson W, Taubert KA, Gewitz M, *et al.* Prevention of infective endocarditis: guidelines from the American Heart Association: a guideline from the American Heart Association Rheumatic Fever, Endocarditis, and Kawasaki Disease Committee, Council on Cardiovascular Disease in the Young, and the Council on Clinical Cardiology, Council on Cardiovascular Surgery and Anesthesia, and the Quality of Care and Outcomes Research Interdisciplinary Working Group. *Circulation* 2007; **116**(15): 1736–54.

13. Leichtle CI, Kumpf M, Gass M, *et al.* Surgical correction of scoliosis in children with congenital heart failure (Fontan circulation): case report and literature review. *Eur Spine J* 2008; **17**(Suppl 2): S312–17.

14. Vischoff D, Fortier LP, Villeneuve E, *et al.* Anaesthetic management of an adolescent for scoliosis surgery with a Fontan circulation. *Paediatr Anaesth* 2001; **11**(5): 607–10.

15. Odegard KC, Zurakowski D, DiNardo JA, *et al.* Prospective longitudinal study of coagulation profiles in children with hypoplastic left heart syndrome from stage I through Fontan completion. *J Thorac Cardiovasc Surg* 2009; **137**(4): 934–41.

16. Bissonnette B. *Syndromes: Rapid Recognition and Perioperative Management.* New York: McGraw-Hill; 2005.

17. Keane MG, Pyeritz RE. Medical management of Marfan syndrome. *Circulation* 2008; **117**(21): 2802–13.

18. Meitzner MC, Skurnowicz JA. Anesthetic considerations for patients with Down syndrome. *AANA J* 2005; **73**(2): 103–7.

19. Borland LM, Colligan J, Brandom BW. Frequency of anesthesia-related complications in children with Down syndrome under general anesthesia for noncardiac procedures. *Pediatr Anesth* 2004; **14**(9): 733–8.

20. Lynch DR, Farmer JM, Balcer LJ, Wilson RB. Friedreich ataxia – effects of genetic understanding on clinical evaluation and therapy. *Arch Neurol Chicago* 2002; **59**(5): 743–7.

21. Campbell AM, Bousfield JD. Anaesthesia in a patient with Noonan's syndrome and cardiomyopathy. *Anaesthesia* 1992; **47**(2): 131–3.

22. Morris P. Duchenne muscular dystrophy: a challenge for the anaesthetist. *Paediatr Anaesth* 1997; **7**(1): 1–4.

23. Kies SJ, Pabelick CM, Hurley HA, *et al.* Anesthesia for patients with congenital long QT syndrome. *Anesthesiology* 2005; **102**(1): 204–10.

24. O'Brien P, Boisvert JT. Current management of infants and children with single ventricle anatomy. *J Pediatr Nurs* 2001; **16**(5): 338–50.

25. Berlinger NT, Long C, Foker J, Lucas RV Jr. Tracheobronchial compression in acyanotic congenital heart disease. *Ann Otol Rhinol Laryngol* 1983; **92**(4 Pt 1): 387–90.

Chapter

25

Postoperative pain control in pediatric patients

Rami Karroum, Loran Mounir Soliman, and John Seif

Key points

- Children and adolescents undergoing correction of scoliosis deformation are known to suffer from increased pain sensation compared with adults. Postoperative pain control can be challenging and often a multimodal approach to pain management is necessary.
- Dual epidural catheters have demonstrated superiority over intravenous patient-controlled analgesia in postoperative pain control. Their major disadvantage lies in a high initial failure rate.
- Intrathecal administration of narcotics is an effective technique with an acceptable adverse effect profile. The major disadvantage lies in the limited duration of action: 18–24 hours at best.
- The addition of NSAIDs such as ketorolac, and central antispasmodics such as diazepam, to a narcotic analgesic regimen in lumbar spine surgery provides better pain control than opioid analgesics alone.
- Tramadol may offer a distinct advantage over typical opioid analgesics for the relief of postoperative pain in children. Its effect on respiration is apparently negligible.

Introduction

Major spine surgery for correction of scoliosis deformation causes severe acute postoperative pain that lasts for at least 3 days.[1] Patients undergoing this operation are most often children or adolescents and are known to suffer from increased pain compared with adults.[2,3] They are usually receiving potent opioid pain relief postoperatively for 10–15 days.[4] Patients undergoing spinal surgery also represent a very diverse group having various diseases including idiopathic scoliosis, neuromuscular conditions, and cerebral palsy. Moreover, the efficacy of regional anesthetic in these patients is difficult to determine because of variations in the type, volume, and dosage of medications infused, the route and modes of delivery, and the number of catheters used in different studies.[5]

Postoperative pain management for these patients can be challenging and often a multimodal approach to pain management is necessary.[6] The goal is to provide safe and efficacious analgesia in the postoperative period in order to minimize postoperative respiratory complications by allowing deep breathing, early ambulation, chest physiotherapy, and rehabilitation.

Mechanism of postoperative pain

Postoperative pain following major scoliosis surgery is multifactorial. It results from multilevel surgical injury to bony tissues, decortication, and the corrective forces applied to the spine with instrumentation. Tissue injury and inflammatory changes initiate activation of both the peripheral and central pain pathways. However, the relative importance of these nociceptive mechanisms in the intensity of postoperative pain is not well established. Release of chemical mediators such as bradykinin, prostaglandins, and cytokines as a result of tissue damage and inflammation alters the response of high-threshold nociceptors (A-δ and C fibers), causing them to fire at a much lower threshold.[7] Sensitization of the spinal cord dorsal horn neurons causes allodynia and hyperalgesia. Although increased excitability of the dorsal horn neurons is a known mechanism of chronic pain, it has also been demonstrated in acute pain models.[8,9]

Methods of pain control after posterior spinal fusion

Various methods have been explored for postoperative pain control following posterior spinal fusion (PSF).

Anesthesia for Spine Surgery, ed. Ehab Farag. Published by Cambridge University Press. © Cambridge University Press 2012.

The most commonly used methods comprise placement of single or double epidural catheters, intrathecal opioids, and intravenous patient-controlled analgesia (IV PCA).

Epidural analgesia

Introduction

The use of epidural anesthesia for orthopedic surgery has been well established; however, the use of this technique for spinal fusions is more limited. Although several studies using various combinations of local anesthetics and opioids demonstrate the efficacy of the technique, fewer studies have demonstrated its superiority over conventional patient-controlled analgesia (PCA).

A single or double epidural catheter can be placed to provide postoperative analgesia following PSF.

Single epidural catheter

In general, clinical experience with the single epidural catheter emphasizes the frequent occurrence of pain localized in the upper or lower parts of the surgical field as a result of incomplete analgesia administration. Of three randomized controlled trials, only one concluded that epidural catheters provide modestly improved analgesia compared with IV PCA.[10–12] This study randomized patients to receive either patient-controlled epidural analgesia (PCEA) with 0.1% bupivacaine + hydromorphone 10 µg/ml at 8 ml/h and PCEA bolus dose of 2 ml allowed every 30 minutes; IV PCA with hydromorphone 2 µg/kg/h continuous infusion; or 2 µg/kg bolus dose. A high failure rate of the epidural catheter (37%) was noted in this study.[12] Two additional controlled randomized trials failed to show superiority of the single epidural catheter over IV PCA. One study used a mixture of bupivacaine 0.125% with fentanyl 2.5 µg/ml and administered it at a rate of 0.3 ml/kg per hour. They concluded that the lack of analgesic benefit may have resulted from the use of the low concentrated bupivacaine with the addition of a low dose of the lipophilic opioid fentanyl to cover 10–12 dermatomes.[10] In another randomized controlled study, two epidural failures occurred because the catheter could not be inserted; and no differences were observed between groups in mean visual analog scores or total morphine usage. The authors attributed the results to a failure to deliver an adequate amount and volume of local anesthetic and opioid.[11]

A large retrospective study comparing epidural catheter injection (EPI) with PCA in patients who had undergone either anterior or posterior spinal fusion established that the epidural technique was safe and that it effectively controlled postoperative pain for a longer period of time than did PCA. Thirteen percent of patients had their epidural catheters discontinued within 24 hours of spinal fusion surgery due to excessive pain, which was attributed to incorrect catheter positioning. The rate of respiratory depression and transient neurologic change, defined as "asymmetric differences in light touch sensation," was 10%.[13]

A prospective study collected data regarding epidural analgesia in 12 pediatric patients after PSF. The surgeon inserted the epidural catheter before wound closure. One patient received an intraoperative bolus and the other 11 were dosed postoperatively in the pediatric intensive care unit (PICU). The bolus included 30–50 µg/kg of morphine with 5–10 ml of 0.1–0.25% bupivacaine. The bolus was followed by a continuous infusion of bupivacaine with morphine supplemented by nurse-controlled analgesia or PCA. The total hourly doses of epidural medications varied from 4 to 10 ml/h of 0.0625–0.125% bupivacaine and 5–10 µg/kg/h of morphine. Postoperative analgesia was satisfactory in all patients. One patient with Duchenne muscular dystrophy developed atelectasis and respiratory failure requiring re-intubation. However, the emergence of these conditions was thought to be unrelated to the epidural infusion.[14]

A large study described the use of epidural analgesia after spinal surgery in 71 pediatric patients. Prospective data were reported for 41 patients and retrospective data were reported for 30 patients. The surgical procedure was PSF in 50 patients, anterior spine fusion (ASF) in 5 patients, and ASF/PSF in 16 patients. For the five anterior approaches, the epidural catheter was placed percutaneously by the anesthesiologist, whereas all other catheters were placed intraoperatively by the surgeon at the T9 level. Postoperative infusions consisted of hydromorphone (10–50 µg/ml) in 61 patients. The remaining 10 patients received either epidural fentanyl or morphine. In all cases, the infusion also included 0.0625–0.125% bupivacaine with a final infusion rate of 2–10 ml/h. Twenty-three patients also received intermittent IV doses of ketorolac; however, this was later determined to be unnecessary. Analgesia was successful in 64 patients. Of the remaining 7 patients, 5 were considered failures and 2 could not be assessed.[15]

In addition to the above studies, which used continuous epidural infusion, other studies used intermittent boluses of narcotics, with or without local anesthetics.

In a retrospective review, one group of patients had a single epidural catheter placed at L1–2. The catheter was intermittently bolused with 30–50 µg/kg of morphine every 12 to 24 hours. The other group of patients received intermittent IV/IM morphine. Opioid consumption was significantly less in the epidural morphine group on postoperative days 1 and 2.[16]

In an open-label trial with no control group, the epidural catheter was dosed with 2 mg of morphine and 4 ml of 0.25% bupivacaine when patients complained of pain. Eighteen of 22 patients had complete pain relief with dosing by catheter. The catheters were left in place for an average of 4.1 ± 0.7 days (range 3–5 days). The catheters were dosed an average of 5.5 ± 1.9 times a day (range 3–9 days).[17]

Double epidural catheters

Several studies have demonstrated the superiority of the double catheter technique.[18–20] In an uncontrolled study, the efficacy of the double epidural catheter in providing analgesia after PSF was investigated in 14 children who had mixed underlying conditions. Before wound closure, two epidural catheters were placed by the surgeon. A portion of the ligamentum flavum was removed to insert the epidural catheters. Under fluoroscopy, the tip of the upper catheter was positioned at T1–4 and the tip of the lower catheter was positioned at L1–4. The catheters were first dosed with a solution containing 1 µg/kg of fentanyl and 5 µg/kg of hydromorphone diluted in 0.3 ml/kg of preservative-free saline. The solution was divided and 0.2 ml/kg was injected into the lower catheter and 0.1 ml/kg was injected into the upper catheter. After the patients recovered from anesthesia and showed normal results of a neurologic examination, the catheters were dosed with local anesthetic solution. This included 0.2% ropivacaine (0.1 ml/kg into the upper catheter and 0.2 ml/kg into the lower catheter). A continuous infusion was started, which consisted of 0.1% ropivacaine plus hydromorphone 10 µg/ml, infused at 0.1 ml/kg/h into the upper catheter and 0.2 ml/kg/h into the lower catheter. Intravenous diazepam was used as needed to control muscle spasms. Intravenous ketorolac was used for mild to moderate pain. Effective analgesia was provided for the 14 patients without adverse effects. However, 9 patients (62%) had episodes of significant pain. It is possible that the opening of the epidural space allowed some drug to escape from the epidural space, which explained the decreased level of successful analgesia.[21]

In another uncontrolled study, a double epidural catheter was used for postoperative analgesia after spine deformity surgery in 23 adolescents who had mixed underlying conditions. Before wound closure, the cephalad catheter was positioned at T4–6 and the lower catheter was positioned at T10–L1. Once a normal postoperative neurologic examination was documented, an initial bolus was administered of 0.0625% bupivacaine (8 ml for patients weighing more than 50 kg and 5 ml for those weighing ≤50 kg). This was followed by continuous infusion of a mixture of bupivacaine 0.0625%, fentanyl 2 µg/ml, and clonidine 3 µg/ml at 10 ml/h for 48 hours. Complete analgesia was obtained at rest in all patients. Acceptable analgesia was provided during mobilization in 83% of patients.[22]

In another study,[19] the upper catheter was inserted at the cranial end of the wound, with the tip directed 4–5 cm cephalad to T1–4. The lower catheter was inserted at the caudal end of the wound, with the tip directed 4–5 cm to a position L1–4. Correct placement was confirmed radiographically at the end of the operation, with 3 ml contrast medium through each catheter to obtain anteroposterior and lateral chest radiographs. Postoperative analgesia was maintained with the ongoing remifentanil target-controlled infusion (TCI) device until the first postoperative morning, but without activating the epidural catheters, so that neurologic assessment could be performed. The catheters were flushed every 8 hours with 2 ml saline before activation.

On the first postoperative morning at 08:00 (T0), study medication was initiated as follows: continuous intravenous morphine with 0.05 mg/kg/h in the morphine group or, in the epidural group, epidural ropivacaine 0.3% with 4–8 ml boluses according to the height of the patients through each catheter. This was followed by a continuous epidural infusion of ropivacaine 0.3% using two separate infusion pumps. The epidural infusion rate was maintained at 4–10 ml/h in each catheter to obtain a sensory blockade from T2 to T12. This study demonstrated that after major scoliosis correction, continuous epidural infusion with plain ropivacaine 0.3% through two epidural catheters provides greater pain control than intravenous morphine, at rest and during coughing; less pruritus; less nausea and vomiting; and earlier return of bowel function.

The use of ropivacaine 0.3% in this study was based on other studies that demonstrated a more comprehensive analgesia with increasing concentrations of ropivacaine: 0.1%, 0.2%, and 0.3%.[23,24] The investigators did

Table 25.1 Commonly used epidural solutions for postoperative pain control in pediatric spinal fusion patients

Solution	Rate	Side effects	Comments
Ropivacaine 0.1% + hydromorphone 10 μg/ml[21]	0.1 ml/kg/h into the upper catheter and 0.2 ml/kg/h into the lower catheter	Local anesthetics: sympathectomy and local anesthetic toxicity Hydromorphone: sedation, nausea and vomiting, pruritus, delayed respiratory depression, urinary retention, and postoperative ileus (incidence of side effects lower than morphine	Double epidural catheters
Bupivacaine 0.0625%, fentanyl 2 μg/ml, and clonidine 3 μg/ml for 48 h[22]	10 ml/h in each catheter	Fentanyl: sedation, nausea and vomiting, pruritus, respiratory depression, urinary retention, and postoperative ileus Clonidine: sedation	Double epidural catheters
Ropivacaine 0.3%[19]	4–10 ml/h in each catheter		Double epidural catheters Delay initiating epidural infusion until first postoperative morning at 08:00
0.1% bupivacaine + hydromorphone 10 μg/ml[12]	8 ml/h and PCEA bolus dose of 2 ml allowed every 30 min		Single catheter
Bupivacaine 0.125% + fentanyl 2.5 μg/ml[10]	0.3 ml/kg/h		Single catheter

not use epidural opioids, because previous studies had shown that epidural opioids did not improve the quality of analgesia on dynamically evoked pain, such as is induced by coughing or mobilization.[25]

Other studies also demonstrated less frequent incidences of nausea, vomiting, and pruritus in children who received epidural ropivacaine than in those who received an epidural bupivacaine–hydromorphone mixture (Table 25.1).[26]

Placement of the epidural catheter

The surgeon usually places the catheter under direct visualization before closing the wound. A single catheter is usually placed at the midpoint of the incision and advanced 3–5 cm cephalad as described by Shaw *et al.*[27] The position of the double epidural catheter varies according to the literature. The epidural catheter is usually tunneled under the skin to decrease the risk of infection and to maintain the catheter's position.

The necessity for radiologic confirmation of the catheter's position is supported by some observational studies. In a study of 12 pediatric patients, the epidural catheter was inserted by the surgeon before wound closure. Variability was demonstrated in the location of the distal tip of the catheter. It was located at T5–6 in 1 patient, T6–7 in 5 patients, T7–8 in 4 patients, T8–9 in 1 patient, and T11–12 in 1 patient.[14] A prospective observational study of 14 patients after spinal fusion surgery reported epidural catheter placement

by Omnipaque (iohexol) injection and confirmation by chest radiography. In 5 patients no dye was noted in the epidural space and consequently, no analgesia was obtained. In 7 patients dye was seen in the epidural space; and in 2 patients dye was seen in the paravertebral gutters. These 9 patients were given adequate analgesia. The authors concluded that correctly placed catheters provided effective analgesia.[28]

In another study, the surgeons placed the epidural catheters under direct visualization without radiographic confirmation of placement. The incidence of epidural failure to provide adequate analgesia during the early postoperative recovery period was 37%. This study concluded that due to the high early failure of epidural catheters, intraoperative verification of catheter placement and patency might improve the epidural success rate.[29]

Initiating local anesthetic infusion through the epidural catheter

The most critical period for the development of early secondary neurologic complications occurs during the first 14–18 hours.[30–32] The recognition of motor blockade during this period is therefore extremely important, because early detection may prevent the occurrence of irreversible deficits. However, the probability of motor blockade resulting from local anesthetic can delay the diagnosis. Therefore, some studies recommend delaying the start of postoperative

423

epidural infusion to the morning following surgery, in order to allow for continuous neurologic assessment. Alternative methods of pain control, such as continuous infusion of IV narcotics, IV PCA, epidural narcotics, or intrathecal narcotics, can be used until epidural infusion is started.

On the other hand, epidural infusion can be started in the immediate postoperative period once the results of neurologic examination have proved normal. The use of dilute solutions of local anesthetics should eliminate the potential for sensory or motor changes induced by the local anesthetic. If postoperative weakness or other neurologic changes do develop, epidural infusion should be postponed, and the patient immediately evaluated. However, neurologic changes should not be attributed to the epidural catheter because doing so may delay diagnosis of potentially reversible surgical conditions.

The two most common methods used to administer drugs through an epidural catheter are intermittent dosing or continuous infusion. Patient-controlled epidural analgesia (PCEA) has been successfully used in children older than age 5 for orthopedic surgery and thoracotomies but experience after scoliosis surgery is limited.[33]

Adverse effects of epidural catheters

Adverse effects of local anesthetics

1. **Systemic toxicity.** Current recommendations to decrease the potential for systemic toxicity include limiting the initial bolus dose to 2.5 mg/kg of bupivacaine and limiting the infusion to 0.3–0.4 mg/kg/h.
2. **Sympathectomy.** Sympathectomy can result in hypotension. A highly placed thoracic catheter can potentially result in bradycardia. These effects may be potentiated by perioperative hypovolemia, a common occurrence in pediatric patients.

Adverse effects of neuraxial opioids

Adverse effects of neuraxial opioids include sedation, nausea and vomiting, pruritus, delayed respiratory depression, urinary retention, and postoperative ileus.[26–34.] These problems may be more common with neuraxial morphine,[35] which has an incidence as high as 30–60% according to some studies. Some investigators prefer to use hydromorphone and fentanyl with a dual epidural catheter technique, in order to limit the need for hydrophilic opioids, and thereby achieve greater dermatomal spread.

Hydromorphone, with intermediate hydrophilic and lipophilic properties, has fewer reported side effects than morphine.[36,37] Other studies show that a combination of epidural morphine and butorphanol may effectively prevent pruritus, nausea, and vomiting and improve the analgesic efficacy of the epidural technique.[38] Other investigators use only plain local anesthetics to avoid the side effects of neuraxial opioids

Adverse effects of the catheter

1. **Risk of infection.** Although infection is a potential risk, to our knowledge there are no reports of infectious complications related to the neuraxial anesthetic technique for spine surgery. Also, clinical experience has demonstrated the efficacy of prolonged use of tunneled catheters.[39]
2. **Potential for neurologic damage.** Transient neurologic changes and respiratory depression have been reported.[13] These led to either a temporary or permanent interruption of the epidural infusion. Although these complications did not require re-intubation to maintain oxygenation or transfer to an intensive care unit, such complications are nevertheless disconcerting and require heightened vigilance by all caregivers to assure respiratory and/or neurologic recovery.
3. **Paresthesia** is also known to occur, and is one of the reasons that patients stop using the epidural catheter. However, no formal study of this adverse effect has been undertaken.[40]
4. **Isolated reports of neurologic deficits.** A case report on a 12-year-old girl indicated that she developed a persistent Horner's syndrome after PSF.[41] Another case report described lower extremity paralysis in the immediate postoperative period after PSF in an 11-year-old patient.[42] The child was returned to the operating room, and the spinal instrumentation was removed. Motor and sensory function gradually returned and was back to baseline 9.5 hours after dosing of the epidural catheter. Although no definitive cause of the problem was identified, the authors offered as possible explanations spinal cord compression, ischemia, or problems related to the epidural anesthesia.
5. **Epidural hematoma.** To our knowledge, the risk of epidural hematoma does not increase when epidural catheters are placed for postoperative pain control following PSF. The lack of increase

may stem from the fact that most patients undergoing this type of surgery are otherwise healthy adolescents with no coagulation abnormalities.

Intrathecal narcotics

Introduction

Studies on the use of intrathecal (IT) morphine for postoperative pain control following PSF are reproducible. The use of intrathecal morphine to provide analgesia was first reported in 1979.[43] Since then, intrathecal morphine has been used to provide postoperative analgesia for numerous types of surgery, including spinal fusion.[44–47] This approach seems to be an effective technique with an acceptable adverse effect profile.

Advantages and disadvantages of using intrathecal narcotics

Intrathecal morphine, when given before the start of surgery, can decrease the amount of remifentanil required intraoperatively and therefore may minimize the development of acute opioid tolerance that may be seen after the use of high-dose remifentanil infusions.[48,49]

Intrathecal morphine has not been found to interfere with the monitoring of intraoperative somatosensory evoked potentials in children undergoing spinal fusion.[50] Some studies have shown that intrathecal morphine, when given before the beginning of surgery, may decrease intraoperative blood loss.[46] The major disadvantage of intrathecal morphine is its limited duration of action: 18–24 hours at best.

Mechanism of action

Analgesia is produced by morphine action on opioid receptors within the dorsal horn.[51]

Since morphine is hydrophilic, it remains in the CSF for an extended period of time, allowing it to migrate in a cephalad direction after injection at the lumbar level. Migration results in measurable levels of morphine at the level of the brainstem within 1–5 hours.[52]

As the terminal elimination half-life of morphine from the CSF is approximately 3 hours, desired and adverse effects of morphine may continue for up to 24 hours.[53]

Dosage of intrathecal morphine

Review of the literature shows wide variation in the dosing of intrathecal morphine. Ranges between 2 and 25 µg/kg have been reported.[44–46] One study evaluated

the efficacy of two doses of IT morphine (2 or 5 µg/kg) versus saline in 30 children ranging in age from 9 to 19 years who underwent PSF. Both doses were effective in pain control at rest during the first 24 hours.[46] Another study evaluated 20 pediatric patients undergoing either anterior spinal fusion (5 patients) or PSF (15 patients).[44] IT morphine (25 µg/kg) was administered at the lumbar level before the start of the surgical procedure. The tracheas of all of the patients were extubated within 30 min of completion of the procedure. Excellent analgesia was obtained and no patient required postoperative analgesics until the 36th postoperative hour.

Yet another study reported administration of IT morphine in 33 pediatric patients undergoing PSF.[45] IT morphine (mean dose 10 µg/kg; range 7–19 µg/kg) was administered in a volume of 10 ml at the lumbar level approximately 1 hour before the end of surgery. This large volume (10 ml) was used to minimize the consequences of extrathecal leakage of morphine from the injection site. The average duration of pain relief was 18.8 hours (range 0–40 h), but 2 patients did not experience any pain relief. Early respiratory depression was noted in 3 patients. Late respiratory depression, occurring 6 hours postoperatively, was noted in 5 patients and was successfully treated with naloxone. The higher incidence of respiratory depression may have been caused by the larger volume used for the IT injection.

A retrospective analysis of postoperative pain scores in 407 consecutive patients with idiopathic scoliosis who underwent PSF divided them into three groups: no dose ($n = 68$); moderate dose of 9–19 µg/kg, mean 14 µg/kg ($n = 293$); and high dose of 20 µg/kg or greater, mean 24 µg/kg ($n = 46$). Effective decrease in pain scores was noticed for up to 23.9 hours in the two groups that received intrathecal morphine. The major difference between the low-dose group and the high-dose group was found in the rate of respiratory depression. The study showed close to 8 times as many respiratory depressions with the high-dose group as with the low-dose group (15.2% vs. 2.6%).[54] This study concluded that intrathecal morphine in the moderate dose range of 9–19 µg/kg (mean 14 µg/kg) provides safe and effective postoperative analgesia. Higher doses did not result in significantly improved analgesia; moreover, the higher doses led to a higher frequency of respiratory depression, which required admission to the PICU.[54]

In a study of 80 pediatric patients, 40 patients received lumbar IT morphine (2 µg/kg) and sufentanil

(50 μg), before the start of the surgical procedure and the other 40 patients received IV sufentanil (1–3 μg/kg). The authors found prolonged pain relief with minimal respiratory depression in the intrathecal group. In addition, postoperative mobilization was better tolerated in the patients who had received IT morphine. Although the $PaCO_2$ levels were higher in the IT group, no respiratory depression was noted.[55]

A retrospective study reviewed 138 patients divided into three groups. The first group (41 patients) received PCA morphine (demand dose of 0.01–0.02 mg/kg, lockout interval from 6 to 10 min +/− basal rate of 0.02 mg/kg/h with a maximum dose of 0.5 mg/h. The second group (42 patients) received a single dose of preoperative intrathecal morphine (7 μg/kg) and PCA pump for breakthrough pain after recovery from anesthesia (IT/PCA). The third group (55 patients) had an epidural infusion without PCA (EPI). At the end of the surgery, the epidural catheter was placed by the operating surgeon under direct visualization. It was usually placed at the thoracolumbar junction. Upon completion of the surgery and after the patient demonstrated spontaneous movement of the lower extremities, a bolus dose of hydromorphone (10–20 μg/kg) was given through the epidural catheter. A continuous infusion of hydromorphone (20 μg/ml) and bupivacaine (0.1%) was then started at an initial rate of 0.1–0.2 ml/kg/h. If pain relief was inadequate, a bolus dose of 50–60% of the infusion rate was given, and the infusion rate was increased by 10%.

This study concluded that EPI controls postoperative pain for the longest period of time and allows for a quicker return to consumption of solid foods. A single preoperative intrathecal morphine injection controls the pain equally for the first 24 hours with less pruritus, fewer adverse events, and less need for nursing and physician intervention.[56]

Adverse effects of intrathecal narcotics

Neuraxial opioids, particularly morphine, can produce pruritus, nausea and vomiting, urinary retention, and respiratory depression.[57] Therefore, an optimal dosing range should be selected that provides adequate analgesia with minimal adverse effects. Pruritus is due to the superior migration of the drug and the drug's interaction with opioid receptors in the trigeminal nucleus of the medulla.[57] It usually occurs around the eyes and face of the patient and is self-resolving. Infusion of low-dose naloxone to minimize the pruritis has been explored.[58–61] As a hydrophilic agent, morphine can result in rostral spread, leading to delayed respiratory depression.

Intravenous patient-controlled analgesia

Whether intravenous patient-controlled analgesia (IV PCA) is superior to epidural analgesia for postoperative pain control in PSF patients remains controversial. Some studies show no difference between the two; others conclude that epidural analgesia is superior.[10–12,18–20]

The advantage of IV PCA resides in the fact that plasma concentrations of opioids are maintained in a narrower range, with lower peak levels and higher trough levels than levels of intermittent injection. As a result, respiratory and central nervous system depression is minimized, and the patient therefore experiences greater satisfaction. Opioids that can be used in PCA include morphine, hydromorphone, and fentanyl (Table 25.2). Anecdotal reports show that many patients seem to prefer hydromorphone and claim that they feel less dizzy and less nauseated.

The use of continuous basal infusion (CBI) of the opioid to supplement child-administered doses remains controversial. CBI tends to maintain near-therapeutic plasma opioid levels, particularly during periods of sleep. This can decrease nocturnal awakening due to pain, thereby improving sleep patterns and analgesic effectiveness. A retrospective study showed that continuous postoperative morphine infusion without a demand dose is a safe and effective method of pain management in patients with idiopathic scoliosis following PSF.[62] However, the use of CBI can cause respiratory depression.[63]

There is wide variation (from 0% to 25%) in the reported incidence of respiratory depression in children receiving PCA.[63–68] The Anesthesia Patient Safety Foundation (APSF) has recommended continuous respiratory monitoring, minimally invasive pulse oximetry, and a continuous measure of respiratory rate for children receiving PCA, neuraxial, or serial doses of parenteral opioids.[69] Other side effects related to opioids include nausea, vomiting, constipation, and pruritus.

Adjuvant medications

Gabapentin

In spinal surgery, peripheral tissue injury results in sensitization of peripheral and central pathways.[70] Anticonvulsants, such as gabapentin, suppress spontaneous neuronal firing and have been effective in treating chronic, centrally mediated neuropathic pain syndromes.[71–74] Several studies have used gabapentin

Table 25.2 Suggestions for initial settings of PCA opioids

Drug	Continuous basal infusion (μg/kg/h)	Demand dose (μg/kg)	Lockout interval (min)	4-hour limit (μg/kg)
Fentanyl	0–0.5	0.5	6–10	7–10
Morphine	0–20	10–20	6–15	250–400
Hydromorphone	0–4	2–4	6–15	50–80

in adult surgical patients in a single-dose design as well as in continued use 1 week after surgery. These studies have demonstrated that gabapentin has an opioid-sparing effect.[75,76]

In a prospective randomized controlled study, 59 patients were randomized to have preoperative gabapentin (15 mg/kg) or placebo (29 gabapentin and 30 placebos).[77] After surgery; all patients received IV PCA opioid and continued on either gabapentin (5 mg/kg) or placebo 3 times a day for 5 days. Total morphine consumption was significantly lower in the gabapentin group following surgery and through postoperative day 2. No difference was found for days 3 through 5. The gabapentin group also had significantly reduced first pain scores in the recovery room and the morning after surgery. Afterward, pain scores were not significantly different between the two groups. The study concluded that up to 2 days after surgery, an initial preoperative loading dose and continued use of oral gabapentin decreased early total morphine consumption and pain scores in pediatric patients undergoing spinal fusion. The study recommended further research on other dosing regimens of gabapentin in pediatric spinal fusion.

Acetaminophen

Acetaminophen acts mainly in the central nervous system. It is believed to act as a central COX inhibitor, producing prostaglandin inhibition and hence providing analgesia and antipyresis.[78] It is available orally (pill form and elixir) and rectally. Intravenous paracetamol was approved by the Federal Drug Administration (FDA) in 2010 for use in the United States. The IV form may play a more important role as adjuvant pain medication in the immediate postoperative period when oral intake is not usually well tolerated.

Acetaminophen is a relatively safe drug. However, one main concern regarding it is that overdosing can cause severe hepatotoxicity.[79] Another concern is that because of its antipyretic properties, acetaminophen can mask febrile states in the immediate postoperative period.[80]

It is used as a sole agent for mild postoperative acute pain. However, in the context of moderate to severe pain, it has to be used in conjunction with opioids or NSAIDs. Together with NSAIDs, it has emerged as a useful adjunct in multimodal analgesic regimes.[81] It can help reduce the need for opioids during the postoperative period. When combined with oral opioids such as oxycodone (Percocet), it facilitates transition to the enteral route for pain control. The patient can be discharged home on these prescription medications.

Acetaminophen can be administered orally at a dose of 10–15 mg/kg every 4 hours. The maximum daily dose is 90 mg/kg/day and should not exceed 4 g/day. For intravenous administration the recommended dose for children who weigh less than 50 kg is 15 mg/kg every 6 hours or 12.5 mg/kg every 4 hours with a maximum single dose of 750 mg/dose and a maximum total daily dosage of 75 mg/kg/day ($\leq$3750 mg/day). For children who weigh $\geq$50 kg the recommended dose is 650 mg every 4 hours or 1000 mg every 6 hours with a maximum single dose of 1000 mg and a maximum total daily dosage of 4000 mg/day.[82]

NSAIDs

Nonsteroidal anti-inflammatory drugs have proven efficacy as the sole analgesic agent for management of mild to moderate pain. They can also be used as adjuvants to other analgesics after major surgery.[83,84] They have a synergistic action with many other analgesic interventions, particularly with opioid analgesia. In addition, they enhance the effect of narcotics and decrease narcotic requirement.[85–91] The benefits of NSAIDs include reduced pain, improved postoperative ambulation, shorter hospitalization, and decreased nausea, emesis, and sedation.[85] They act via nonselective inhibition of cyclooxygenase enzymes (COX-1, COX-2). COX-2 is a source of prostaglandins during inflammatory processes. On the other hand, COX-1 has protective effects on the stomach, where it mediates the production of prostaglandins.[92] The availability of the injectable NSAID ketorolac has extended perioperative use to patients who cannot tolerate oral medications after surgery. The side effects of NSAIDS include bleeding, gastrointestinal ulcers, and renal failure.[93–103]

One main concern regarding the use of NSAIDs following PSF is that they can delay bone healing. NSAIDs inhibit bone metabolism in animal models through disrupting the synthesis of prostaglandins and inhibiting osteoblast cell production at endosteal bone surfaces.[104-107] However, evidence suggests that nonunion of the spine is associated with a large dose, not a low dose, of ketorolac.[108] A study of adult patients showed that the use of ketorolac after spinal fusion surgery in humans, limited to 48 hours after surgery, had no significant effect on ultimate fusion rates.[109] These results contrast with those of a study of adult patients who had instrumented fusion from L4 to the sacrum. This latter study showed a significant increase in the incidence of pseudoarthrosis in the ketorolac group.[110]

In a retrospective cohort study of 405 patients who had adolescent idiopathic scoliosis, ketorolac did not predispose to pseudoarthrosis following posterior spinal fusion and instrumentation with autologous bone grafting.[111]

Another concern with the use of ketorolac is its potential for postsurgical bleeding through reversible inhibition of platelet function.[112] However, the frequency of life-threatening bleeding due entirely to ketorolac remains low.[113-116] Nevertheless, it is preferable to administer this medication toward the end of surgery after hemostasis is achieved. In addition, the operating surgeon should be consulted before ketorolac is administered.

NSAIDs can lead to acute kidney injury particularly in patients with volume depletion.[117-121] This effect is believed to arise from the inhibition of prostaglandins, which act to preserve renal blood flow and glomerular filtration rate by relaxing preglomerular resistance.[122]

One study compared the relative risk of renal failure in two groups, one treated with opioids and the other with ketorolac. When treatment with ketorolac was for less than 5 days, the risk of renal failure was the same in the two groups. However, when patients were treated for more than 5 days, the relative risk for renal failure was higher in the ketorolac group; but the overall incidence of renal failure was only 1%. Therefore, to avoid kidney injury it is recommended that treatment with ketorolac is not to exceed 5 successive days.[123]

The recommended dose for IV ketorolac is 0.5 mg/kg every 6 hours, not to exceed 30 mg per dose and no more than 120 mg/day.

Another subclass of NSAIDs is the selective COX-2 inhibitors. The COX-2 inhibitors are less likely to cause bleeding (platelet effects), particularly GI bleeding (unprotected GI mucosa), but carry the same risk of the other adverse effects as standard NSAIDs, in addition to cardiovascular and thrombotic risks.[124] Because of these risks, the use of COX-2 inhibitors is limited for postoperative pain control.

Diazepam

Diazepam is a long-acting benzodiazepine. It binds to benzodiazepine receptors and enhances GABA effects. It appears to have a specific role as an adjuvant analgesic for pain arising from skeletal muscle spasm.[125] Its use as adjuvant medication following posterior spinal fusion can reduce opioid requirements, which in turn reduces opioid-induced side effects such as nausea and vomiting. The commonly used dose is 0.05–0.1 mg/kg IV; maximum 5 mg every 6 hours as needed for muscle spasms.[12]

Oxycodone

Oxycodone is a familiar opioid in the United States in the form of Percocet (oxycodone with acetaminophen). It is used for the treatment of moderate to severe acute pain. It is also used to gradually replace parenteral opioid in the postoperative period. It has 60% bioavailability after oral administration. Analgesia begins within 20–30 minutes and peaks at between 1 and 2 hours. Elimination half-time is 2.5–4 hours and duration of effect is 4–5 hours.

Oxycodone and its active metabolite oxymorphone may accumulate in patients with renal insufficiency, leading to respiratory depression if the dose and interval are not adjusted. It is 10 times more potent than codeine when given orally. The recommended dose is 0.05–0.15 mg/kg every 4 hours as needed.[126]

Nalbuphine

Nalbuphine possesses agonist properties at the κ receptors and antagonist effects at the μ receptors. It is metabolized mainly in the liver and has a plasma half-life of about 5 hours. The mean elimination half-life of nalbuphine in adults is 2.2–2.6 hours but is shorter in children, in which it is approximately 0.9 hour.[127-130] Nalbuphine appears to have a ceiling effect, as further increase in the dose does not result in greater analgesia.

Nalbuphine has been used to antagonize μ-mediated side effects such as nausea, vomiting, pruritus, urinary retention, and respiratory depression in patients receiving morphine, fentanyl, or hydromorphone. Nalbuphine has been known to antagonize pruritus at doses of 25–50 µg/kg q6h PRN, and some studies have found this to be effective.[131,132]

Naloxone

Naloxone is a potent µ, δ, and κ antagonist. It is rapidly metabolized in the liver and has a plasma elimination half-life of 60 minutes.

A syndrome of hypertension tachycardia, dyspnea, tachypnea, pulmonary edema, nausea, vomiting, and ventricular fibrillation has been reported in patients who receive high doses of opioids for severe pain and who receive excessive doses of naloxone rapidly for the treatment of respiratory depression.[133,134]

In patients with oversedation and diminished respiratory rate due to opioids; naloxone in small IV increments of 0.5–1 µg/kg is given every few minutes until side effects are reversed. This dosage can be followed by a continuous microinfusion of 0.25 µg/kg/h if needed to prevent recurrence of symptoms. More profound respiratory depression such as apnea must be treated more aggressively. Opioid infusion should be discontinued, positive-pressure ventilation with oxygen instituted, and 5–10 µg/kg of naloxone administered intravenously.

Pruritus is a common side effect associated with epidural or intrathecal opioid use, occurring in as many as 30–70% of children. Antihistaminics are usually ineffective in treating pruritus because the mechanism of pruritus is a central opioid effect not a histamine effect. Naloxone infusion at a rate of 0.25 µg/kg/min can be used to treat intractable pruritus. The same dose can reverse the incidence of nausea without affecting the analgesia or opioid consumption.[135]

In addition to naloxone for the treatment of postoperative nausea and vomiting, metoclopramide 0.10–0.15 mg/kg can be given intravenously. It is a dopamine receptor antagonist and an effective antiemetic but may cause sedation and dystonia. Serotonin receptor antagonists such as ondansetron and dolasetron comprise another class of effective antiemetics. They have the advantage of virtually eliminating the risk of dystonic or oculogyric reactions that occur with metoclopramide. However, headache is a common side effect.

Tramadol

Tramadol, a synthetic 4-phenyl-piperidine analogue of codeine, is a centrally acting atypical opioid.[136] Although tramadol's mode of action is not completely understood, at least two complementary mechanisms contribute to its effect. Tramadol opioid activity results from low affinity binding of the parent compound to µ-opioid receptors and higher binding of the M_1 receptor.[137] Tramadol is also a weak inhibitor of norepinephrine and serotonin reuptake.[138] The opioid and monoaminergic mechanisms of action are thought to extend the analgesic benefit to both opioid-sensitive and opioid-insensitive pain. Clinical experience indicates that tramadol does not have many of the side effects typically associated with opioid agonists.

Tramadol has an apparently negligible effect on respiration, as demonstrated in studies in adults and children. It may offer a distinct advantage over typical opioid analgesics for the relief of postoperative pain in children.[139–141] Its use for severe pain is limited by the fact that it has a ceiling effect. It may be useful particularly in patients who refuse opioids or tolerate them badly. Recommended is a dose of 1–2 mg/kg orally (maximum single dose 100 mg), every 4 to 6 hours, with a maximum daily dose of the lesser of either 8 mg/kg or 400 mg. (Table 25.3).

Summary

Epidural analgesia

1. If epidural analgesia is used for postoperative pain control, the dual catheter technique is preferred.
2. The surgeon should place the catheters before wound closure. Intraoperative radiologic verification of catheter placement and patency might improve the epidural success rate.
3. Usually the cephalad catheter is positioned at T4–6 and the lower catheter is positioned at T10–L1. The catheter should be advanced 3–5 cm into the epidural space.
4. Delay the start of epidural infusion postoperatively to the following morning, to allow for continuous neurologic assessment, because the most critical period for the development of early secondary neurologic complications is the first 14–18 hours. Motor blockade resulting from local anesthetic can delay the diagnosis.
5. Other methods of pain control such as continuous infusion of IV narcotics, IV PCA, epidural narcotics, or intrathecal narcotics can be used until the epidural infusion is started.
6. Subsequent use of dilute solutions of local anesthetics should eliminate the potential for sensory or motor changes caused by the local anesthetic.

Table 25.3 Adjuvant medications used in the postoperative period

Medication	Mechanism of action	Pharmacokinetics	Dose
Gabapentin	Antiepileptic Binds to an undefined neuroreceptor in the brain, suppresses spontaneous neuronal firing	Absorption: very rapid; facilitates transport Bioavailability: 60%	Not FDA-approved for management of acute postoperative pain Suggested use in pediatric spinal fusion patients: preoperative gabapentin (15 mg/kg), followed by postoperative gabapentin (5 mg/kg) for 2 days.[77]
Ketorolac	NSAID: inhibits cyclooxygenases, reducing prostaglandins and thromboxane synthesis	Protein binding: 99% Time to peak serum concentration: IV: 1–3 min	0.5 mg/kg IV; maximum 30 mg/dose, 120 mg/day up to 5 days Some studies limit use for 48 h to avoid pseudoarthrosis
Diazepam	Long-acting benzodiazepine; antispasmodic	Protein binding: 98% Metabolism: hepatic	0.05–0.1 mg/kg IV; maximum 5 mg every 6 h as needed for muscle spasms
Acetaminophen	Analgesic, antipyretic. Reduces production of prostaglandins centrally	Primarily absorbed from small intestine Time to peak serum concentration–oral: immediate release 10–60 min IV: 15 min	Oral tablets or elixirs 10–15 mg/kg q4–6h; maximum 90 mg/kg/day
Oxycodone	Binds to various opioid receptors	Metabolism: hepatic Half-life, elimination– Children 2–10 years: 1.8 h Adults: 3.7 h	0.05–0.15 mg/kg PO q4–6h
Nalbuphine	κ receptor agonist μ receptor antagonist	Half-life, elimination– Children: 0.9 h Adults: 2.2 2.6 h	25–50 µg/kg q6h PRN for pruritus
Naloxone	Potent µ, δ, and κ antagonist	Metabolism: hepatic Plasma elimination half-life 60 min	Infusion at 0.25 µg/kg/h for treatment of nausea, pruritus
Ondansetron	Selective 5-HT$_3$ receptor antagonist	Plasma protein binding: 70–76%	0.1 mg/kg with a recommended maximum dose of 4 mg for treatment of PONV
Tramadol	Weak µ receptor agonist Norepinephrine and serotonin reuptake inhibitor	Absorption: rapid and complete Metabolism: hepatic Half-life: 6–8 h	1–2 mg/kg orally every 4–6 h Max. single dose: 100 mg Max. daily dose: lesser of either 8 mg/kg or 400 mg

PONV, postoperative nausea and vomiting.

7. Alternatively, the epidural can be dosed once a normal postoperative neurologic examination is documented. An initial bolus of 0.0625% bupivacaine (8 ml for patients weighing more than 50 kg and 5 ml for those weighing ≤50 kg) can be given, followed by a continuous infusion of dilute solutions of local anesthetics.

8. If postoperative weakness or other neurologic changes develop, epidural infusion should be held, and the patient should be immediately evaluated.

9. Neurologic changes should not be attributed to the epidural catheter, as this assumption may delay the diagnosis of potentially reversible surgical conditions.

Intrathecal preservative-free morphine

1. The average duration of pain relief is 18 hours.

2. Preservative-free morphine at a dose range of 9–19 µg/kg, mean 14 µg/kg, can be administered. Smaller doses of 2–5 µg/kg have been used successfully in other studies. We use 5–10 µg/kg.

3. Higher doses are associated with a longer duration of pain control, but also with a higher incidence of respiratory depression.

4. The surgeon can administer it at the end of surgery before wound closure.

5. Other modalities of pain control, such as IV PCA should be started as soon as the patient experiences pain.

Intravenous patient-controlled analgesia (IV PCA)

In the absence of epidural or intrathecal opioids, start with hydromorphone with a CBI of 2 µg/kg/h and demand of 2–4 µg/kg with lockout interval every 10 minutes. The demand dose can be increased by 10% increments every hour until pain is controlled, or until the maximum 4-hour limit of 50–80 µg/kg is reached. CBI should be stopped once the patient starts oral intake, usually on postoperative day 1.

References

1. Weldon BC, Connor M, White PF. Pediatric PCA: the role of concurrent opioid infusions and nurse-controlled analgesia. *Clin J Pain* 1993; **9**: 26–33.

2. Johnston CC, Strada ME. Acute pain response in infants: A multidimensional description. *Pain* 1986; **24**: 373–82.

3. Gillies ML, Smith LN, Parry-Jones WL. Postoperative pain assessment and management in adolescents. *Pain* 1999; **79**: 207–17.

4. Czarnecki ML, Jandrisevits MD, Theiler SC, Huth MM, Weisman SJ. Controlled-release oxycodone for the management of pediatric postoperative pain. *J Pain Symptom Manage* 2004; **27**: 379–86.

5. Tobias JD. A review of intrathecal and epidural analgesia after spinal surgery in children. *Anesth Analg.* 2004; **98**: 956–65.

6. Raw DA, Beattie JK, Hunter JM. Anaesthesia for spine surgery. *Br J Anaesth* 2003; **91**: 886–904.

7. Dahl JB, Moiniche S. Pre-emptive analgesia. *Br Med Bull* 2004; **71**: 13–27.

8. Lascelles BDX, Waterman AE, Cripps PJ, Livingston A, Hendersen G. Central sensitization as a result of surgical pain: an investigation of the effect of the pre-emptive value of pethidine for ovarian hysterectomy in the rat. *Pain* 1995; **62**: 201–12.

9. Dirks J, Moiniche S, Hilsted KL, Dahl JB. Mechanisms of post-operative pain: clinical indications for a contribution of central sensitization. *Anesthesiology* 2002; **97**: 1591–6.

10. Cassady JF Jr, Lederhaas G, Cancel DD, *et al.* A randomized comparison of the effects of continuous thoracic epidural analgesia and intravenous patient-controlled analgesia after posterior spinal fusion in adolescents. *Reg Anesth Pain Med.* 2000; **25**: 246–53.

11. O'Hara JF Jr., Cywinski JB, Tetzlaff JE, *et al.* The effect of epidural versus intravenous analgesia for posterior spinal fusion surgery. *Paediatr Anaesth* 2004; **14**: 1009–15.

12. Gauger VT, Voepel-Lewis TD, Burke CN, *et al.* Epidural analgesia compared with intravenous analgesia after pediatric posterior spinal fusion. *J Pediatr Orthop* 2009; **29**: 588–93.

13. Sucato DJ, Duey-Holtz A, Elerson E, *et al.* Postoperative analgesia following surgical correction for adolescent idiopathic scoliosis: a comparison of continuous epidural analgesia and patient-controlled analgesia. *Spine* 2005; **30**: 211–17.

14. Arms DM, Smith JT, Osteyee J, Gartrell A. Postoperative epidural analgesia for pediatric spine surgery. *Orthopedics* 1998; **21**: 539–44.

15. Shaw BA, Watson TC, Merzel DI, *et al.* The safety of continuous epidural infusion for postoperative analgesia in pediatric spine surgery. *J Pediatr Orthop* 1996; **16**: 374–7.

16. Amaranth L, Andrish JT, Gurd AR, *et al.* Efficacy of intermittent epidural morphine following posterior spinal fusion in children and adolescents. *Clin Orthop Relat Res* 1989; **249**: 223–6.

17. Adu-Gyamfi Y. Epidural morphine plus bupivacaine for relief of postoperative pain following Harrington rod insertion for correction of idiopathic scoliosis. *J Int Med Res* 1995; **23**: 211–17.

18. Blumenthal S, Min K, Nadig M, *et al.* Double epidural catheter with ropivacaine versus intravenous morphine: a comparison for postoperative analgesia after scoliosis correction surgery. *Anesthesiology* 2005; **102**: 175–80.

19. Blumenthal S, Borgeat A, Nadig M, *et al.* Postoperative analgesia after anterior correction of thoracic scoliosis: a prospective X2 randomized study comparing continuous double epidural catheter technique with intravenous morphine. *Spine* 2006; **31**: 1646–51.

20. Saudan S, Habre W, Ceroni D, *et al.* Safety and efficacy of patient controlled epidural analgesia following pediatric spinal surgery. *Paediatr Anaesth* 2008; **18**: 132–9.

21. Tobias JD, Gaines RW, Lowry KJ, *et al.* A dual epidural catheter technique to provide analgesia following posterior spinal fusion for scoliosis in children and adolescents. *Paediatr Anaesth* 2001; **11**: 199–203.

22. Ekatodramis G, Min K, Cathrein P, Borgeat A. Use of a double epidural catheter provides effective postoperative analgesia after spine deformity surgery. *Can J Anaesth* 2002; **49**: 173–7.

23. Zaric D, Nydahl PA, Philipson L, *et al.* The effect of continuous lumbar epidural infusion of ropivacaine (0.1%, 0.2% and 0.3%) and 0.25% bupivacaine on sensory and motor block in volunteers: a double-blind study. *Reg Anesth* 1996; **21**: 14–25.

24. Scott DA, Chamley DM, Mooney PH, *et al.* Epidural ropivacaine infusion for postoperative analgesia after

major lower abdominal surgery: a dose finding study. *Anesth Analg* 1995; **81**: 982–6.

25. Gall O, Aubineau JV, Bernière J, Desjeux L, Murat I. Analgesic effect of low-dose intrathecal morphine after spinal fusion in children. *Anesthesiology* 2001; **94**: 447–52.

26. Moriarty A. Postoperative extradural infusions in children: preliminary data from a comparison of bupivacaine/diamorphine with plain ropivacaine. *Paediatr Anaesth* 1999; **9**: 423–7.

27. Shaw BA, Watson TC, Merzel DI, *et al.* The safety of continuous epidural infusion for postoperative analgesia in pediatric spine surgery. *J Pediatr Orthop* 1996; **16**: 374–7.

28. Turner A, Lee J, Mitchell R, *et al.* The efficacy of surgically placed epidural catheters for analgesia after posterior spinal surgery. *Anaesthesia* 2000; **55**: 370–3.

29. Gauger VT, Voepel-Lewis TD, Burke CN, *et al.* Epidural analgesia compared with intravenous analgesia after pediatric posterior spinal fusion. *J Pediatr Orthop* 2009; **29**: 588–93.

30. Bridwell KH, Lenke LG, Baldus C, Blanke K. Major intraoperative neurologic deficits in pediatric and adult spinal deformity patients. *Spine* 1998; **23**: 324–31.

31. Mineiro J, Weinstein SL. Delayed postoperative paraparesis in scoliosis surgery. *Spine* 1997; **22**: 1668–72.

32. Taylor BA, Webb PJ, Hetreed M, Mulukutla RD, Farrell J. Delayed postoperative paraplegia with hypotension in adult revision scoliosis surgery. *Spine* 1994; **19**: 470–4.

33. Birmingham PK, Wheeler M, Suresh S, *et al.* Patient-controlled epidural analgesia in children: can they do it? *Anesth Analg* 2003; **96**: 686–91.

34. Cucchiaro G, Dagher C, Baujard C, Dubousset AM, Benhamou D. Side effects of postoperative epidural analgesia in children: a randomized study comparing morphine and clonidine. *Paediatr Anaesth* 2003; **13**: 318–23.

35. Goodarzi M. Comparison of epidural morphine, hydromorphone and fentanyl for postoperative pain control in children undergoing orthopaedic surgery. *Paediatr Anaesth* 1999; **9**: 419–22.

36. Chaplan SR, Duncan SR, Brodsky JB, *et al.* Morphine and hydromorphone epidural analgesia. A prospective, randomized comparison. *Anesthesiology* 1992; **77**: 1090–4.

37. Goodarzi M. Comparison of epidural morphine, hydromorphone and fentanyl for postoperative pain control in children undergoing orthopaedic surgery. *Paediatr Anaesth* 1999; **9**: 419–22.

38. Lawhorn CD, Boop F, Brown R, Andelman P. Epidural pain management in the post-rhizotomy patient. *Pediatr Neurosurg* 1994; **20**: 198–202.

39. Aram L, Krane EJ, Kozloski LJ, Yaster M. Tunneled epidural catheters for prolonged analgesia in pediatric patients. *Anesth Analg* 2001; **92**: 1432–8.

40. Hered RW, Cummings J, Helffrich R. Persistent Horner's syndrome after spinal fusion and epidural analgesia. *Spine* 1998; **23**: 387–90.

41. Purnell RJ. Scoliosis correction and epidural analgesia: prolonged block following Harrington rod insertion. *Anaesthesia* 1982; **37**: 1115–17.

42. Taenzer AH, Clark C. Efficacy of postoperative epidural analgesia in adolescent scoliosis surgery: a meta-analysis. *Paediatr Anaesth* 2010; **20**: 135–43.

43. Wang JK, Nauss LE, Thomas JE. Pain relief by intrathecally applied morphine in man. *Anesthesiology* 1979; **50**: 149–51.

44. Dalens B, Tanguy A. Intrathecal morphine for spinal fusion in children. *Spine* 1998; **13**: 494–8.

45. Blackman RG, Reynolds J, Shively J. Intrathecal morphine: dosage and efficacy in younger patients for control of postoperative pain following spinal fusion. *Orthopedics* 1991; **14**: 555–7.

46. Gall O, Aubineau J, Bernière J, *et al.* Analgesic effect of low-dose intrathecal morphine after spinal fusion in children. *Anesthesiology* 2001; **94**: 447–52.

47. Urban MK, Jules-Elysee K, Urquhart B, *et al.* Reduction in postoperative pain after spinal fusion with instrumentation using intrathecal morphine. *Spine* 2002; **27**: 535–7.

48. Gibson PR. Anaesthesia for correction of scoliosis in children. *Anaesth Intensive Care* 2004; **32**: 548–59.

49. Crawford MW, Hickey C, Zaarour C, *et al.* Development of acute opioid tolerance during infusion of remifentanil for pediatric scoliosis surgery. *Anesth Analg* 2006; **102**: 1662–7.

50. Goodarzi M, Shier NH, Grogan DP. Effect of intrathecal opioids on somatosensory-evoked potentials during spinal fusion in children. *Spine* 1996; **21**: 1565–8.

51. Cousins MJ, Mather LE. Intrathecal and epidural administration of opioids. *Anesthesiology* 1984; **61**: 276–310.

52. Chaney MA. Side effects of intrathecal and epidural opioids. *Can J Anaesth* 1995; **42**: 891–903.

53. Nordberg G, Hedner T, Mellstrand T, *et al.* Pharmacokinetic aspects of intrathecal morphine analgesia. *Anesthesiology* 1984; **60**: 448–54.

54. Tripi PA, Poe-Kochert C, Potzman J, *et al.* Intrathecal morphine for postoperative analgesia in patients

with idiopathic scoliosis undergoing posterior spinal fusion. *Spine* 2008; **33**: 2248–51.

55. Goodarzi M. The advantages of intrathecal opioids for spinal fusion in children. *Paediatr Anaesth* 1998; **8**: 131–4.

56. Milbrandt TA, Singhal M, Minter C, *et al.* A comparison of three methods of pain control for posterior spinal fusions in adolescent idiopathic scoliosis. *Spine* 2009; **34**: 1499–503.

57. Chaney MA. Side effects of intrathecal and epidural opioids. *Can J Anaesth* 1995; **42**: 891–903.

58. Han DW, Hong SW, Kwon JY, *et al.* Epidural ondansetron is more effective to prevent postoperative pruritus and nausea than intravenous ondansetron in elective cesarean delivery. *Acta Obstet Gynecol Scand* 2007; **86**: 683–7.

59. Lockington PF, Fa'aea P. Subcutaneous naloxone for the prevention of intrathecal morphine induced pruritus in elective Caesarean delivery. *Anaesthesia* 2007; **62**: 672–6.

60. Gulhas N, Erdil FA, Sagir O, *et al.* Lornoxicam and ondansetron for the prevention of intrathecal fentanyl-induced pruritus. *J Anesth* 2007; **21**: 159–63.

61. Iatrou CA, Dragoumanis CK, Vogiatzaki TD, *et al.* Prophylactic intravenous ondansetron and dolasetron in intrathecal morphine-induced pruritus: a randomized, double-blinded, placebo-controlled study. *Anesth Analg* 2005; **101**: 1516–20.

62. Poe-Kochert C, Tripi PA, Potzman J, Son-Hing JP, Thompson GH. Continuous intravenous morphine infusion for postoperative analgesia following posterior spinal fusion for idiopathic scoliosis. *Spine* 2010; **35**: 754–7.

63. Berde CB, Solodiuk J. Multidisciplinary programs for management of acute and chronic pain in children. In: Schechter NI, Berde CB, Yaster M, eds. *Pain in Infants, Children and Adolescents.* Philadelphia: Lippincott Williams & Wilkins, 2003.

64. Voepel-Lewis T, Marinkovic A, Kostrzewa A, *et al.* The prevalence and risk factors for adverse events in children receiving patient-controlled analgesia by proxy or patient-controlled analgesia. *Anesth Analg* 2008; **107**: 70–5.

65. McDonald AJ, Cooper MG. Patient-controlled analgesia: an appropriate method of pain control in children. *Paediatr Drugs* 2001; **3**: 273–84.

66. Beaulieu P, Cyrenne L, Mathews S, *et al.* Patient-controlled analgesia after spinal fusion for idiopathic scoliosis. *Int Orthop* 1996; **20**: 295–9.

67. Rauen KK, Ho M. Children's use of patient-controlled analgesia after spine surgery. *Pediatr Nurs* 1989; **15**: 589–93, 637.

68. Goodarzi M, Shier NH, Ogden JA. Epidural versus patient-controlled analgesia with morphine for postoperative pain after orthopaedic procedures in children. *J Pediatr Orthop* 1993; **13**: 663–7.

69. Weinger MB. Dangers of postoperative opioids: APSF [Anesthesia Patient Safety Foundation] workshop and white paper addresses prevention of postoperative complications. *APSF Newsletter* 2006.

70. Woolf CJ, Chong MS. Preemptive analgesic – treating postoperative pain by preventing the establishment of central sensitization. *Anesth Analg* 1993; **77**: 362–79.

71. Rusy LM, Troshynski TJ, Weisman SJ. Gabapentin in phantom limb pain management in children and young adults: report of seven cases. *J Pain Symptom Manage* 2001; **21**: 78–82.

72. Bone M, Critchley P, Buggy D. Gabapentin in post amputation phantom limb pain: a randomized, double blind, placebo controlled, cross-over study. *Reg Anesth Pain Med* 2002; **27**: 481–6.

73. Backonja NM. Gabapentin monotherapy for the symptomatic treatment of painful neuropathy: a multicenter, double blind, placebo controlled trial in patients with diabetes mellitus. *Epilepsia* 1999; **40**: S57–9.

74. Pandey CK, Bose N, Garg G, *et al.* Gabapentin for the treatment of pain in Guillain–Barré syndrome: a double blind, placebo controlled, cross-over study. *Anesth Analg* 2002; **95**: 1719–23.

75. Menigaux C, Adam F, Guignard B, Sessler DI, Chauvin M. Preoperative gabapentin decreases anxiety and improves early recovery from knee surgery. *Anesth Analg* 2005; **100**: 1394–9.

76. Fassoulaki A, Patris K, Sarantopoulos C, Hogan Q. The analgesic effect of gabapentin and mexiletine after breast surgery for cancer. *Anesth Analg* 2002; **95**: 985–91.

77. Rusy LM, Hainsworth KR, Nelson TJ, *et al.* Gabapentin use in pediatric spinal fusion patients: a randomized, double-blind, controlled trial. *Anesth Analg* 2010; **110**: 1393–8.

78. Anderson BJ, Holford NH, Wollard GA, *et al.* Perioperative pharmacodynamics of acetaminophen analgesia in children. *Anesthesiology* 1999; **90**: 411–21.

79. American Academy of Pediatrics: Committee on Drugs. Acetaminophen toxicity in children. *Pediatrics* 2001; **108**: 1020–4.

80. Mayoral CE, Marino RV, Rosenfeld W, *et al.* Alternating antipyretics: Is this an alternative?" *Pediatrics* 2000; **105**: 1009–12.

81. Aleksandrovich IuS, Sukhanov IuV, Volykhin IV. [Evaluation of the efficacy of paracetamol as a component of postoperative combined analgesia in

433

children]. [Article in Russian]. *Anesteziol Reanimatol* 2009; **1**: 58–62.

82. Duggan ST, Scott LJ. Intravenous paracetamol (acetaminophen). *Drugs* 2009; **69**: 101–13.

83. Souter AJ, Fredman B, White PF. Controversies in the perioperative use of non-steroidal antiinflammatory drugs. *Anesth Analg* 1994; **79**: 1178–90.

84. Dahl JB, Kehlet H. Non-steroidal anti-inflammatory drugs: rationale for use in severe postoperative pain. *Br J Anaesth* 1991; **66**: 703–12.

85. Kinsella J, Moffat AC, Patrick JA, *et al.* Ketorolac trometamol for postoperative analgesia after orthopaedic surgery. *Br J Anaesth* 1992; **69**: 19–22.

86. Gillis JC, Brogden RN. Ketorolac. A reappraisal of its pharmacodynamic and pharmacokinetic properties and therapeutic use in pain management. *Drugs* 1997; **53**: 139–88.

87. Sevarino FB, Sinatra RS, Paige D, *et al.* Intravenous ketorolac as an adjunct to patient-controlled analgesia (PCA) for management of postgynecologic surgical pain. *J Clin Anesth* 1994; **6**: 23–7.

88. Sutters KA, Shaw BA, Gerardi JA, *et al.* Comparison of morphine patient-controlled analgesia with and without ketorolac for postoperative analgesia in pediatric orthopedic surgery. *Am J Orthop* 1999; **28**: 351–8.

89. Picard P, Bazin JE, Conio N, *et al.* Ketorolac potentiates morphine in postoperative patient-controlled analgesia. *Pain* 1997; **73**: 401–6.

90. Le Roux PD, Samudrala S. Postoperative pain after lumbar disc surgery: a comparison between parenteral ketorolac and narcotics. *Acta Neurochir (Wien)* 1999; **141**: 261–7.

91. Munro HM, Walton SR, Malviya S, *et al.* Low-dose ketorolac improves analgesia and reduces morphine requirements following posterior spinal fusion in adolescents. *Can J Anaesth* 2002; **49**: 461–6.

92. Gajraj NM. Cyclooxygenase-2 inhibitors. *Anesth Analg* 2003; **96**: 1720–38.

93. Gillis JC, Brogden RN. Ketorolac. A reappraisal of its pharmacodynamic and pharmacokinetic properties and therapeutic use in pain management. *Drugs* 1997; **53**: 139–88.

94. Saag KG, Cowdery JS. Nonsteroidal anti-inflammatory drugs. Balancing benefits and risks. *Spine* 1994; **19**: 1530–4.

95. Connelly CS, Panush RS. Should nonsteroidal anti-inflammatory drugs be stopped before elective surgery? *Arch Intern Med* 1991; **151**: 1936–46.

96. Feldman HI, Kinman JL, Berlin JA, *et al.* Parenteral ketorolac: the risk for acute renal failure. *Ann Intern Med* 1997; **126**: 193–9.

97. Nuutinen LS, Laitinen JO, Salomaki TE, *et al.* A risk-benefit appraisal of injectable NSAIDs in the management of postoperative pain. *Drug Saf* 1993; **9**: 380–93.

98. Toto RD, Anderson SA, Brown-Cartwright D, *et al.* Effects of acute and chronic dosing of NSAIDs in patients with renal insufficiency. *Kidney Int* 1986; **30**: 760–8.

99. Kenny GN. Potential renal, haematological and allergic adverse effects associated with nonsteroidal anti-inflammatory drugs. *Drugs* 1992; **44**: 31–6.

100. Strom BL, Berlin JA, Kinman JL, *et al.* Parenteral ketorolac and risk of gastro-intestinal and operative site bleeding: a postmarketing surveillance study. *JAMA* 1996; **275**: 376–82.

101. RuDusky BM. Severe postoperative hemorrhage attributed to single-dose parenteral ketorolac-induced coagulopathy. *Angiology* 2000; **51**: 999–1002.

102. Kallis P, Tooze JA, Talbot S, *et al.* Preoperative aspirin decreases platelet aggregation and increases post-operative blood loss – a randomized, placebo-controlled, double-blind clinical trial in 100 patients with chronic stable angina. *Eur J Cardiothorac Surg* 1994; **8**: 404–9.

103. Haws MJ, Kucan JO, Roth AC, *et al.* The effects of chronic ketorolac tromethamine (toradol) treatment on wound healing. *Ann Plast Surg* 1996; **37**: 147–51.

104. Dimar JR, Ante WA, Zhang YP, *et al.* The effects of nonsteroidal anti-inflammatory drugs on posterior spinal fusions in the rat. *Spine* 1996; **21**: 1870–6.

105. Keller J, Bunger C, Andreassen TT, *et al.* Bone repair inhibited by indomethacin. Effects on bone metabolism and strength of rabbit osteotomies. *Acta Orthop Scand* 1987; **58**: 379–83.

106. Martin GJ, Boden SD, Titus L. Recombinant human bone morphogenetic protein-2 overcomes the inhibitory effect of ketorolac, a nonsteroidal anti-inflammatory drug (NSAID), on posterolateral lumbar intertransverse process spine fusion. *Spine* 1999; **24**: 2188–93; discussion 2193–4.

107. Reikeraas O, Engebretsen L. Effects of ketoralac tromethamine and indomethacin on primary and secondary bone healing. An experimental study in rats. *Arch Orthop Trauma Surg* 1998; **118**: 50–2.

108. Ho ML, Chang JK, Wang GJ. Effects of ketorolac on bone repair: a radiographic study in modeled demineralized bone matrix grafted rabbits. *Pharmacology* 1998; **57**: 148–59.

109. Sucato DJ, Lovejoy JF, Agrawal S, *et al.* Postoperative ketorolac does not predispose to pseudoarthrosis following posterior spinal fusion and instrumentation for adolescent idiopathic scoliosis. *Spine* 2008; **33**: 1119–24.

110. Glassman SD, Rose SM, Dimar JR, *et al.* The effect of postoperative nonsteroidal anti-inflammatory drug administration on spinal fusion. *Spine* 1998; **23**: 834–8.

111. Pradhan BB, Tatsumi RL, Gallina J, *et al.* Ketorolac and spinal fusion: does the perioperative of ketorolac really inhibit spinal fusion? *Spine* 2008; **19**: 2079–82.

112. Camu F, Lauwers MH, Vanlersberghe C. Side effects of NSAIDs and dosing recommendations for ketorolac. *Acta Anaesthesiol Belg* 1996; **47**: 143–9.

113. Gupta A, Daggett C, Ludwick J, *et al.* Ketorolac after congenital heart surgery: does it increase the risk of significant bleeding complications? *Paediatr Anaesth* 2005; **15**: 139–42.

114. Gupta A, Daggett C, Drant S, *et al.* Prospective randomized trial of ketorolac after congenital heart surgery. *J Cardiothorac Vasc Anesth* 2004; **18**: 454–7.

115. Vitale MG, Choe JC, Hwang MW, *et al.* Use of ketorolac tromethamine in children undergoing scoliosis surgery: an analysis of complications. *Spine J* 2003; **3**: 55–62.

116. Chauhan RD, Idom CB, Noe HN. Safety of ketorolac in the pediatric population after ureteroneocystostomy. *J Urol* 2001; **166**: 1873–5.

117. Patrono C, Dunn MJ. The clinical significance of inhibition of renal prostaglandin synthesis. *Kidney Int* 1987; **32**: 1.

118. Oates JA, FitzGerald GA, Branch RA, *et al.* Clinical implications of prostaglandin and thromboxane A2 formation (2). *N Engl J Med* 1988; **319**: 761.

119. Huerta C, Castellsague J, Varas-Lorenzo C, García Rodríguez LA. Nonsteroidal anti-inflammatory drugs and risk of ARF in the general population. *Am J Kidney Dis* 2005; **45**: 531.

120. Rose BD, Post TW. *Clinical Physiology of Acid–Base and Electrolyte Disorders.* 5th ed. New York: McGraw-Hill; 2001: 192–6.

121. Murray MD, Brater DC. Renal toxicity of the nonsteroidal anti-inflammatory drugs. *Annu Rev Pharmacol Toxicol* 1993; **33**: 435.

122. Takahashi K, Schreiner GF, Yamashita K, *et al.* Predominant functional roles for thromboxane A2 and prostaglandin E2 during late nephrotoxic serum glomerulonephritis in the rat. *J Clin Invest* 1990; **85**: 1974.

123. Feldman HI, Kinman JL, Berlin JA, *et al.* Parenteral ketorolac: the risk for acute renal failure. *Ann Intern Med* 1997; **126**: 193.

124. Gajraj NM, Joshi GP. Role of cyclooxygenase-2 inhibitors in postoperative pain management. *Anesthesiology Clin N Am* 2005; **23**: 49–72.

125. Blumenkopf B. Combination analgesic-antispasmodic therapy in postoperative pain. *Spine (Phila Pa 1976)* 1987; **12**: 384–7.

126. Olkkola KT, Hamunen K, Maunuksela EL. Clinical pharmacokinetics and pharmacodynamics of opioid analgesics in infants and children. *Clin Pharmacokinet* 1995; **28**: 385–404.

127. Lo MW, Schary WL, Whitney CCJ. The disposition and bioavailability of intravenous and oral nalbuphine in healthy volunteers. *J Clin Pharmacol* 1987; **27**: 866–73.

128. Lo MW, Lee FH, Schary WL, Whitney CCJ. The pharmacokinetics of intravenous, intramuscular, and subcutaneous nalbuphine in healthy subjects. *Eur J Clin Pharmacol* 1987; **33**: 297–301.

129. Sear JW, Keegan M, Kay B. Disposition of nalbuphine in patients undergoing general anaesthesia. *Br J Anaesth* 1987; **59**: 572–5.

130. Jaillon P, Gardin ME, Lecocq B, *et al.* Pharmacokinetics of nalbuphine in infants, young healthy volunteers, and elderly patients. *Clin Pharmacol Ther* 1989; **46**: 226–33.

131. Kjellberg F, Tramer MR. Pharmacological control of opioid-induced pruritus: a quantitative systematic review of randomized trials. *Eur J Anaesthesiol* 2001; **18**: 346–57.

132. Cohen SE, Ratner EF, Kreitzman TR, *et al.* Nalbuphine is better than naloxone for treatment of side effects after epidural morphine. *Anesth Analg* 1992; **75**: 747–52.

133. Johnson C, Mayer P, Grosz D. Pulmonary edema following naloxone administration in a healthy orthopedic patient. *J Clin Anesth* 1995; **7**: 356–7.

134. O'Malley-Dafner L, Davies P. Naloxone-induced pulmonary edema. *Am J Nurs* 2000; **100**: 24AA–JJ.

135. Maxwell LG, Kaufmann SC, Bitzer S, *et al.* The effects of a small-dose naloxone infusion on opioid-induced side effects and analgesia in children and adolescents treated with intravenous patient-controlled analgesia: a double-blind, prospective, randomized, controlled study. *Anesth Analg* 2005; **100**: 953–8.

136. Dayer P, Desmeules J, Collart L. Pharmacology of tramadol. *Drugs* 1997; **53**: 18–24.

137. Raffa RB, Friderichs E, Reimann W, *et al.* Opioid and nonopioid components independently contribute to the mechanism of action of tramadol, an "atypical" opioid analgesic. *J Pharmacol Exp Ther* 1992; **260**: 275–85.

138. Bamigbade TA, Langford RM. The clinical use of tramadol hydrochloride. *Pain Reviews* 1998; **5**: 155–82.

139. Houmes RM, Voets MA, Verkaaik A, *et al.* Efficacy and safety of tramadol versus morphine for moderate and severe postoperative pain with special regard to respiratory depression. *Anesth Analg* 1992; **74**: 510–14.

140. Vickers MD, O'Flaherty D, Szekely SM, *et al.* Tramadol: pain relief by an opioid without depression of respiration. *Anaesthesia* 1992; **47**: 291–6.

141. Tarkkila P, Tuominen M, Lindgren L. Comparison of respiratory effects of tramadol and oxycodone. *J Clin Anesth* 1997; **19**: 582–5.

Index

437